Psychological Management of Stroke

Psychological Management
of Stroke

Nadina B. Lincoln, Ian I. Kneebone,
Jamie A.B. Macniven and Reg C. Morris

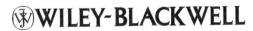

WILEY-BLACKWELL

A John Wiley & Sons, Ltd., Publication

Library of Congress Cataloging-in-Publication Data
Psychological management of stroke / Nadina B. Lincoln ... [et al.].
    p. cm.
  Includes bibliographical references and index.
   ISBN 978-0-470-68427-6 (cloth) – ISBN 978-0-470-68426-9 (pbk.)
  1. Cerebrovascular disease–Psychological aspects. 2. Cerebrovascular disease–Treatment. I. Lincoln, Nadina B.
  RC388.5.P79 2012
  616.8′106–dc23   2011024712

A catalogue record for this book is available from the British Library.

This book is published in the following electronic formats: ePDFs 9781119961314; Wiley Online Library 9781119961307; ePub 9781119954972; eMobi 9781119954989

Set in 10.5/13pt. Galliard by Thomson Digital, Noida, India

1   2012

Contents

About the Authors

Nadina Lincoln is Professor of Clinical Psychology at the University of Nottingham and honorary consultant clinical neuropsychologist at Nottingham University Hospitals NHS Trust. She has conducted an extensive programme of research to evaluate clinical stroke services.

Ian Kneebone is a Consultant Clinical Psychologist and a visiting reader at the University of Surrey. He has published on screening measures to detect psychological problems after stroke and on psychological interventions to manage them.

Jamie Macniven was until recently a Consultant Clinical Neuropsychologist for Nottingham University Hospitals NHS Trust and course director of the MSc programme in clinical neuropsychology at the University of Nottingham. He has now taken up the post of consultant clinical neuropsychologist at Waikato Hospital, Hamilton, New Zealand.

Reg Morris is Programme Director of the South Wales Doctorate Programme in Clinical Psychology, honorary professor at the Cardiff University and consultant clinical psychologist in Wiltshire NHS Trust and has published widely about facets of stroke care.

Ken Walters: The Cover Artist

Ken Walters was 30 years old, happily settled with a successful career in engineering. At that time he had no idea that he was about to enter a 19-year-period of unhappiness and bad luck. He broke his back while working briefly on a farm, and was so badly injured he didn't get up for a year and had severe persistent pain. Financial stresses triggered two heart attacks and when he was taken into hospital in 2005 and told he'd had a stroke, it was yet another disaster in his life. He was bedridden, paralysed down one side, with only a pad and pen to communicate. On his first day, after writing a note to the nurse, he found himself doodling. From then on he was drawing from dawn to dusk and couldn't stop. He had never had the slightest interest in art in his life. He was a practical person, an engineer by trade, and now, suddenly, memories and thoughts appeared as abstract images. In 2007, he heard about Second Life, and decided to show his work on-line for the first time. Now he is a professional artist, selling pictures worldwide. He cursed the stroke at the time, but it has changed his life in ways he could never have imagined. It has brought him interests and a new source of self-respect.

In Ken's words: 'In my art I try to bring together my experiences, skills and emotions. I draw on my experiences, filtered through my emotions and moods and use my skills to paint with light on my pc. I use my own software to translate what I see and feel into still frame images, I've replaced the brush and pencil with an electronic pen and tablet. Unlike with paint, I can vary the intensity of light in the images to reflect my thinking and emotions. I find it far more liberating and intensive than paint, and I control powerful computing ability to render my imagination into digital reality. This brings a unique aspect to my art, an aspect not known or understood by many. My chronic fatigue is a major driver of my emotions; it can also bring them to a halt.' Ken Walters kindly donated the cover image for this book. More of his images can be seen on http://kenwalters.deviantart.com/gallery

Foreword by The Stroke Association

The psychological consequences for people living with stroke are frequently neglected or inadequately addressed, yet may have a major impact on quality of life.

The Stroke Association is grateful to the authors for collating and presenting the evidence to facilitate improved stroke management in this important area. We urge healthcare professionals to read this book and take action to improve the quality of life for those affected by stroke.

Joanne Knight BSc DPhil MRSC
Director of Research & Development
The Stroke Association

The Stroke Association is the only charity solely concerned with helping everyone affected by stroke across the United Kingdom. Our vision is to have a world where there are fewer strokes and all those touched by stroke get the help they need.

www.stroke.org.uk
Stroke Helpline 0303 3033 100

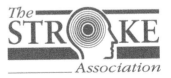

Preface

This book came about in response to several requests for information from professionals working in stroke services. In the United Kingdom and worldwide, there has been an increasing recognition that stroke has important psychological dimensions. The management of these presents a challenge to staff working in public health, voluntary organisations, primary care, emergency services as well as dedicated stroke services. Therefore, clinical psychologists have been increasingly recruited to work with survivors of stroke and to advise other professionals, particularly members of multidisciplinary stroke teams, on psychological assessment and interventions.

The aim of the book was to provide professionals working in stroke services with the evidence base to support their role. The aim was also to demonstrate the wide range of psychological skills which are relevant in helping people who have had strokes, or who are at risk of stroke. The inclusion of practical examples and case histories is intended to illustrate the application of psychological skills and knowledge in a real-world context. It is also hoped that it will give 'life' and relevance to the research literature.

The overall aim is to improve clinical services and outcomes for those who have suffered a stroke and for their families. Increasing recognition of the psychological aspects of stroke management and the development of psychological skills by all members of the multiprofessional team will help achieve these goals.

Acknowledgements

Many people have assisted us with the preparation of this book, and our thanks to them all for their help.

In particular, we would like to thank the following for commenting on draft chapters: Emmanuel Akinwuntan, Jane Barton, Audrey Bowen, Vanessa Dale, Avril Drummond, Vicki Hacker, Helena Harder, Samantha Hull, Valerie Morrison, Julie Wilcox, Paul Willner and Linda Worrall. Other people have contributed illustrations and unpublished information. These include Jane Barton, Audrey Bowen, Vanessa Dale, Robert Dineen and Luke Williams. In addition, we thank Caroline Watkins, who contributed some components of chapter 1.

The case studies in this book are based on real patients and carers. In some cases their details have been changed to preserve anonymity, but real names have been included for some, at their own request. In some instances, information has been slightly modified to illustrate particular points. We would like to thank all the patients and carers who provided information as well as the following professionals for contributing material for case studies: Mal Auton, Jane Barton, Vanessa Dale, Vicki Hacker, Gemma Wall, Roshan das Nair and Luke Williams.

The book was written as a collaboration between all four authors. However, each author was responsible for the majority of material provided in individual chapters. Ian Kneebone provided the major contribution to chapters on the management of mood and related problems (15, 16, 17 and 19), Jamie Macniven to chapters relating to neuropsychological aspects (3, 4, 6, 10 and 12), Reg Morris to chapters on lived experience, service delivery, decision making, social dimensions and prevention (1, 2, 9, 20, 21 and 22) and Nadina

Lincoln to chapters on both neuropsychological and emotional aspects (5, 7, 8, 11, 13, 14 and 18). Nadina Lincoln was responsible for devising the chapter plan, allocating and coordinating the work, editing drafts and attempting to ensure consistency across chapters.

   The Stroke Association provided initial funding for a meeting of the authors to get this book off the ground.

Section 1

Background to Stroke and Stroke Services

Chapter 1

Experiences and Effects of Stroke and Its Aftermath

Prosperity doth best discover vice, but adversity doth best discover virtue.
Francis Bacon (1625/2009)

Experiences and effects of stroke: the survivor's perspective

Stroke is a life-changing condition for survivors and those around them. In addition to the many and varied physical symptoms, such as reduced mobility, difficulty in controlling basic body functions and impaired speech, it also has a profound psychological impact. The effect of stroke on lives is clearly illustrated in the conclusions of a review of 39 studies of life after stroke (Bays, 2001a). Studies conducted in most nations found quality of life following stroke declined markedly, and it was consistently lower than that experienced by healthy adults. Stroke survivors were less able to engage in everyday activities and in social activities and were more depressed than healthy adults of similar age and background. These three things were also strongly associated with their self-reported quality of life. We are fortunate to be able to achieve a detailed insight into how life is affected by stroke through the accounts of stroke survivors who retain, or regain, the ability to communicate and are able to recount their experiences. The accounts of about 1000 survivors, from childhood to over 90 years of age, have been collected and analysed in research articles (Table 1.1), and several have produced in-depth autobiographies of their stroke experiences while many others have published their stories on stroke-related websites (Table 1.2). Such accounts are inevitably retrospective, and cannot hope to capture all the complexities and nuances of moment to moment streams of experiences. In some cases, moreover, they have been written despite impaired mental processes. However, they provide

Psychological Management of Stroke, First Edition. Nadina B. Lincoln, Ian I. Kneebone, Jamie A.B. Macniven and Reg C. Morris.
© 2012 John Wiley & Sons, Ltd. Published 2012 by John Wiley & Sons, Ltd.

Table 1.1 Qualitative Studies of Experiences of Stroke Survivors

Article	Number of survivors	Time since stroke (discharge)	Age	Method
Akinsanya, Diggory, Heitz and Jones (2009)	1	First 6 hours	47	Biographic article, with professional commentary
Alaszewski, Alaszewski and Potter (2004)	31	Unknown interval after discharge	40–89	Interviews
Backe, Larsson and Fridlund (1996)	6	3 weeks	50–66	Interviews
Banks and Pearson (2003)	50	Up to 15 months after discharge	18–49	Interviews, diaries
Bays (2001b)	9	After discharge, mean 30 months since stroke	Mean 68.2	Interviews
Bendz (2003)	15	3 to 12 months	Under 65	Interviews
Burton (2000a)	6	12 months	52–81	Interviews
Chest, Heart and Stroke Scotland, Scottish Association of Health Councils (2001)	114	Unknown interval after discharge	unknown	Interviews, focus groups
Cox, Dooley, Listo and Miller (1998)	39	Less than 4 years	63–93, mean 78.5	Interviews
Davidson and Young (1985)	29	1–7 and 12–18 months after discharge	40–82	Interviews
Doolittle (1992)	13	3 days to 6 months	Unknown	Interviews
Dowswell, Lawler, Dowswell, Young, Forster and Hearn (2000)	30	13–16 months	60–94	Interviews
Eaves (2002)	8	Up to 4 months	56–79	Interviews

(continued)

Study	N	Timing	Age	Method
Ellis–Hill, Payne and Ward (2000)	8	In hospital and 12 months after discharge	56–82	Interviews
Faircloth, Boylstein, Rittman, Young and Gubrium (2004)	57	1 to 12 months after discharge	46–88	Interviews
Faircloth, Boylstein, Rittman and Gubrium (2005)	111	1 to 24 months after discharge	Mean 67	Interviews
Folden (1994)	20	Within 2 weeks and 3–4 weeks after discharge	65–78	Interviews
Gillen (2005)	63	Soon after stroke, 5–7 days after admission to rehabilitation unit	Mean 61	Interviews
Haggstrom, Axelsson and Norberg (1994)	29	Unknown	60–91	Narratives
Jones, Mandy and Partridge (2008)	10	6 weeks to 13 months	Mean 61.8	Interviews
Kaufman (1988)	64	Unspecified	Over 45	Interviews
Kirkevold (2002)	9	1 week to 12 months	40–83	Interviews
McLean, Roper-Hall, Mayer and Main (1991)	20	Unknown interval after discharge	Mean age men 69, women 78	Interviews
Morris, Payne and Lambert (2007)	10	4–18 months	45–81	Focus group
Mumma (1986)	30	Over 3 months	Middle-aged	Interviews
Murray and Harrison (2004)	10	4–20 years	38–81	Interviews
Nilsson, Jansson and Norberg (1997)	10	1 and 3 months after discharge	53–81	Interviews
O'Connell, Hanna, Penney, Pearce, Owen and Warelow (2001)	Less than 40 survivors	2 to 180 months, mean 4.5 years	Mean 58.4, 20–89	Focus groups

Table 1.1 (*Continued*)

Article	Number of survivors	Time since stroke (discharge)	Age	Method
Olofsson, Andersson and Carlberg (2005)	9	4 months	64–83	Interviews
Pilkington (1999)	13	Unknown interval after discharge	40–91	Interviews
Pound, Gompertz and Ebrahim (1998)	40	10 months	Mean 71	Interview
Rittman, Faircloth, Boylstein, Gubrium, Williams, Van Puymbroeck and Ellis (2004)	51	1 month after discharge	46–84	Interviews
Rochette, Tribble, Desrosiers, Bravo and Bourget (2006)	10	3 weeks to 6 months	61–86	Interviews
Roding, Lindstrom, Malm and Ohman (2003)	5	Unknown interval after discharge	37–54	Interviews
Sabari, Meisler and Silver (2000)	6	8 months to 5 years	45–75	Group session
Sisson (1998)	11	1 week to 6 months	33–70	Interviews
Stone (2007)	83	Less than 2 years to over 10 years	Under 50	Internet narratives
Thomas and Parry (1996)	15	Unknown interval after discharge	45–77	Interviews

Table 1.2 Autobiographical Accounts of Stroke Survivors

Author/date or website	Title
McCrum (1998)	My year off: rediscovering life after stroke
Ripley (2006)	Surviving a stroke: recovering and adjusting to living with hypertension
Bauby (2002) (book)	The diving bell and the butterfly
Bauby and Schnable (2008) (film/DVD)	
Douglas (2002)	My stroke of luck
McCann (2006)	Stroke survivor: a personal guide to recovery
Bolte-Taylor (2008)	My stroke of insight
Stephens (2008)	Diary of a stroke
Kant (1997)	Rehabilitation following stroke: a participant perspective
Stroke Association: http://www. stroke.org.uk/information/ my_story/index.html	Information/my story
NHS Tayside: http://www. heartstroketayside.org.uk	Stroke patient stories. heart & stroke information point
http://www.pilgrim.myzen.co.uk/ patientvoices/naoconn.htm	Patient voices: reconnecting with life: stories of life after stroke
NHS Choices: http://www.nhs.uk/ Conditions/Stroke/Pages/ Jimstory.aspx?url=Pages/ Realstories.aspx	Real stories: stroke
Stroke Alliance for Europe (SAFE): http://www.safestroke.org/Facts/ StrokeStories/tabid/373/Default. aspx	Stories from stroke survivors, their carers and families
Different Strokes: http://www. differentstrokes.co.uk	Survivors' stories: adulthood, childhood and adolescence, achievements

an illuminating record of what survivors recall and believe to be their most salient perceptions and most significant feelings about stroke and its aftermath. McKevitt, Redfern, Mold and Wolfe (2004) reviewed 95 qualitative studies of stroke survivors and carers and concluded that such studies highlight the human experience of stroke and enable the identification of perceived needs, reveal differences in priorities between patients and professionals and may also signpost barriers to best-quality care. In addition, stroke survivors reported that they valued reading the personal accounts of other survivors (Wachters-Kaufmann, 2000); it increased their sense of understanding and reduced their sense of isolation. Almost one half of the respondents in this study reported that they found solutions to practical and emotional problems through reading, and one third felt motivated to make contact with other survivors.

Despite the variability in the type, location and severity of strokes, and the diversity of survivors themselves, there is a surprising degree of congruence between their stories, and the similarities often transcend gender differences (Stone, 2007) and appear consistently in different ethnic groups (Faircloth, Boylstein, Rittman & Gubrium, 2005). An exception to the uniformity of experience is the influence of the age of the survivor. While there is a measure of concordance across age groups (O'Kelly, 2002), differences in the age of survivors do determine perceptions of the significance of stroke, priorities and the types of goals that are pursued (O'Connell, Hanna, Penney, Pearce, Owen & Warelow, 2001; Banks & Pearson, 2003; Bendz, 2003; Roding, Lindstrom, Malm & Ohman, 2003). Another important source of difference is whether the stroke is located in the dominant hemisphere and affects communication and logical reasoning (Bolte-Taylor, 2008) or is in the nondominant hemisphere, in which case language abilities are largely unaffected.

For those who have not had the experience of stroke, including carers of stroke survivors, professionals, families and volunteers alike, the personal accounts of survivors may seems fragmentary and incomplete, like a light that casts the images of figures on a wall rather than illuminating the figures themselves. The observer must interpret and extrapolate from these accounts if they are to appreciate the reality that faces the stroke survivors in ways that will enable them to reach out and make meaningful connections. For the many survivors who do not regain the ability to recount their experiences, we must rely on the uncertain metric of our own experience, lived and vicarious, to guess what they are experiencing and guide our endeavours to meet their needs and expectations. In doing so, healthcare professionals should be mindful of evidence that staff and patients have different expectations and priorities (Becker & Kaufman, 1995; Bendz, 2003; Hafsteins-dóttir & Grypdonck 1997; Morris, Payne & Lambert, 2007) as well as differing perceptions of the care provided (Luther, Lincoln & Grant, 1998). In view of this, it is unsurprising that several personal accounts are critical of aspects of care and make uncomfortable reading for healthcare professionals.

Aspects of the experience of stroke survivors

Table 1.3 provides a schematic representation of psychologically significant aspects of the journey of a typical stroke survivor, derived from the qualitative studies and biographies listed in Tables 1.1 and 1.2, and categorised into symptoms, phases and features, psychological tasks and processes and important elements. To improve continuity and flow, the following account of experiences is provided without specific references in the text for each point. Interested readers will find instances in the literature cited in Tables 1.1 and 1.2.

The first stage is the onset of symptoms which usually develop rapidly and 'out of the blue'. Most accounts describe initial attempts to normalise symptoms, for example, as a migraine, numbness due to sleeping awkwardly on a limb, an infection or tiredness. There is frequently a sense of indifference and sometimes

Table 1.3 Psychologically Significant Aspects of Stroke Revealed by Biographies

Symptoms	Phases and features	Psychological tasks and processes	Elements
Onset and intensification	Stroke event / Seeking help	Normalisation, denial-acceptance	*(see Elements column listing below)*
	Diagnosis	Body, not self as focus	
	Emergency treatment	Consent to treatment	
	Health care staff (doctors)	Connection with staff as people / Accepting uncertain recovery prognosis	
Stabilize and (partially) resolve: Movement, perception, swallow, continence, pain, speech, cognition, balance, fatigue, appearance	Hospital care (nursing and environment)	Adjustment to personal care, expectations of behaviour, routines and new surroundings	
	Therapy: Arduous Effortful	Setting personal goals / Fatigue	
	Recovery: Leaving hospital	Small gains building hope / Fear of another stroke / Influence of other survivors	
Residual symptoms; disabilities and deficits	Community re-integration: Restriction, constriction and loss. Integration of former life and stroke within a new life. Employment and money. Changed identity and roles. New appreciation of life, greater reflection, new learning and new goals.	Acceptance and appreciation of changes versus need for restitution of former life	

Elements (columns shown at right of the table):
Resilience and adaptation versus depression and anxiety; Autonomy and control versus dependence and compliance; Developing health-beliefs about stroke; Family and friends; Other Survivors; Staff; Paramedical services; Hospital services; Community Services

frank denial of even severe symptoms. This may be a consequence of anosagnosia due to cognitive impairments. However, some survivors cite the lack of any pain and of any visible cause as reasons for their sense of unreality and failure to acknowledge symptoms. Many expect that symptoms will be transient and see them as an unwelcome interruption to their habitual routine which they often vigorously attempt to continue. If the stroke occurs in public, then the symptoms and the reactions of others may lead to feelings of embarrassment and attempts to conceal or explain away the effects.

> I'm typical of many patients who, when they have had a stroke, spend precious hours fighting the truth instead of fighting the illness. So I continue to deny what is happening because the truth is too stark and horrible to contemplate. (Stephens, 2008)

Eventually the survivor, or someone else, accepts the significance of the symptoms and obtains assistance. Where the person was alone at the time of the stroke there may be a delay of many hours, and efforts to obtain assistance when affected by hemiparalysis and aphasia may be protracted and traumatic. In cases where a survivor is alone and in real danger, some experience hearing helpful 'voices' commanding or urging them seek help. Hearing voices that give advice and encouragement (called auditory 'pseudo-hallucinations' because the person is aware the voices have no physical source) has also been reported by healthy, psychologically normal people in highly stressful or life-threatening situations (Spivak, Trottern, Mark, Bleich & Weizman, 1992; Brugger, Regard, Landis & Oelz, 1999), and is vividly described in Joe Simpson's book about surviving a mountaineering accident (Simpson, 1998).

> But resounding like thunder from deep within my being, a commanding voice spoke clearly to me: **'If you lie down now you will never get up'**. (Bolte-Taylor, 2008)

The next phase is usually the attendance of paramedics and transfer to an accident and emergency department. The initial diagnosis of stroke is now normally completed by the paramedics at the scene, and this stage is often enveloped in a fog of confusion for the survivor, and, in those with haemorrhagic strokes, also accompanied by excruciating headache. Some survivors find it hard to accept the diagnosis of stroke.

> What the hell are they talking about? A stroke! Strokes are for elderly people, with slurred speech, moving about in walkers or wheelchairs. I was only eighty; how can a stroke happen to me? (Douglas, 2002)

Survivors frequently report a sense of powerlessness and feeling extremely sleepy at this stage and resent being bombarded with questions and requests to perform neurological tests and undergo investigations; they experience diagnosis as impersonal and find it incongruous that their body, rather than their 'self', is the focus of others' attentions. Where communication is affected this early experience of healthcare staff may be extremely disturbing; it may appear that staff are speaking foreign languages or in code, and this may fuel fearful thoughts about something being hidden from the survivor. Survivors may not appreciate that their speech is affected and may become angry and frustrated when staff do not understand them. Frustration about providing staff with information, while not receiving any in return is common. Once diagnosis is complete, treatment decisions must often be made rapidly.

> Medical personnel swarmed about my gurney. The sharp lights and intense sounds beat upon my brain. ... 'Answer this, squeeze that, sign here!' I thought, 'How absurd! Can't you see I've got a problem here?' ... I wanted to scream 'leave me alone!' but my voice had fallen silent. They couldn't hear me because they couldn't read my mind. (Bolte-Taylor, 2008)

Survivors' accounts differ sharply about consent to treatment, with some reporting that they were not enabled to provide proper consent despite wishing to do so, and others feeling that being required to consent was burdensome and unrealistic and that they would have preferred staff to act in their best interests without requiring the survivor's consent.

> [T]here was one nurse I came to think of as my guardian angel, ... with ... a lovely smile and the most gentle manner of any nurse I'd experienced then or subsequently. ... For her sweetness towards me in those first few dreadful hours. ... I shall always be profoundly grateful. (McCrum, 1998)

Interactions with staff are crucial in this and subsequent stages, and the accounts are almost unanimous in identifying the personal qualities of staff as vital determinants of the survivor's trust and confidence as well as their general sense of safety and security. One account suggested that a lesion in the left hemisphere affecting language and sequential reasoning accentuated the prominence of personal characteristics and heightened sensitivity to body language and social cues (Bolte-Taylor, 2008). However, there may be other explanations, and heightened attention to the personal qualities that define kindness, compassion and a willingness to provide care may be a common psychological response to a sudden incapacity that spurs a person to make contact with those who are motivated to provide assistance. The actual personal qualities that engender trust and confidence are rather ineffable and writers of autobiographies of stroke struggle to elucidate them. However, being gentle and calm and genuinely interested in helping survivors, focussing on the person as well as their body, taking time and not rushing the survivor, making eye contact and using touch and other reassuring body language and creating a sense of being available for the survivor all seem to be manifestations of traits that engender an intuitive sense of trust. While the professionalism and apparent competence of staff are regarded as important, the centrality of impressions created by these personal attributes dominates almost all survivors' accounts.

> I'm full of an overwhelming desire to please the doctor. She is very cold, going through the routine of the examination with clinical precision, a screen behind her eyes rather like the cellophane on the display screen of a new mobile phone. . . . Why do none of the people who see me in this place treat me as if I have a brain? (Stephens, 2008)

In cases where diagnosis was initially incorrect or delayed, and treatment or investigations were perceived to be incomplete or inappropriate, survivors may experience anger at staff and continue to do so for many years. Many accounts of stroke indicate surprise at how few medical treatments were required and the infrequency of contact with medical doctors after the initial diagnosis phase. However, younger survivors in particular, may continue to have investigations to establish the cause of their early stroke for months or even years after the event.

Reports of the experiences of the direct symptoms of stroke are understandably very diverse due to variations in nature, size and location of the lesion. Hemiparesis is principally experienced through its effect on mobility and self-care capabilities. Not being able to use the toilet independently is a particular source of distress and embarrassment for most survivors. Another experience is that paralysis engenders a sense of mind–body separation highlighting the distinction between an intention to perform an act and the actual act itself. Many survivors find the lack of muscular response puzzling and difficult to accept and recount periods when they experiment with a kind of mind–body dialogue where they use concentration and the power of their mind to 'will' immobile parts of their body to respond. In some, this may evolve into a form of 'self-talk', in which the person issues mental instructions to limbs. For example, 'right arm reach out, move right, move up a bit. Now right hand grasp toothbrush. Now arm move back', and so on. Immobile limbs, particularly arms, take on special significance and may be described as 'appendages', 'flippers' and the like. Hemiparesis is also personally significant because it alters appearance, particularly through facial droop, and many survivors report being disturbed by looking at themselves in mirrors and may avoid doing so. Sensory loss and numbness are sometimes reported as imbuing a sense of unreality, and numbness of the tongue hampers eating and risks injury through biting. Impaired swallowing causes distress through the inability to eat a normal diet and appreciate the tastes and textures of foods. Eating is also a source of pleasure and a distraction from boredom. Pain of various kinds may be experienced: headache, joint pain, muscular cramps and also neuropathic pain. All pain engenders distress, and in some cases may provoke anxiety about being moved and hamper engagement in therapy. Incontinence and constipation are often experienced as deeply humiliating and embarrassing. Visual problems such as diplopia are distressing and disorienting and, while the partial loss of visual fields may not always be noticed, its effect on functions, such as driving, makes it significant. Vertigo, which often occurs in cases of posterior stroke, is incapacitating and acutely distressing. In addition, survivors are often puzzled and frustrated by ataxia. The effects of language and speech impairments are profoundly disturbing and frustrating and have been discussed above when considering admission and diagnosis. Many survivors are fearful of cognitive impairments, and may spend hours doing memory puzzles or engaging in private mental exercises to reassure themselves. In contrast, survivors with actual profound cognitive impairments are frequently unaware and unconcerned about them. Fatigue and the need for a lot of sleep are almost universal experiences. Sleep is regarded positively as a restorative, but many reports indicate that it may interfere with schedules, plans and activities. Fatigue is seen as a barrier to therapy and return to activities of daily life and employment. If a function which is seen as vital to a person's family role or employment is affected, then a person may experience very severe sense of loss and anxiety about the future. For example, several of the accounts of stroke were written by professional writers who were extremely concerned about losing the ability to type.

> The first part of my escape plan is to reclaim as much normalcy as possible: to do things I would normally do and not just sit around waiting for something to happen. . . . I must not play be the rules the stroke wants to impose on me. (Ripley, 2006)

After diagnosis and initial treatment, most survivors spend time in hospital with the expectation that the person will conform to unfamiliar routines, adopt the 'patient role' and accept personal care which is initially experienced as embarrassing and humiliating. An important psychological dimension at this stage is the person's perception of the balance between autonomy and control on the one hand and dependence and compliance on the other. Highly dependent survivors find it reassuring that they can influence the behaviour of staff even in small ways, for example by the way they greet them or make eye contact. Fear of not receiving enough care co-exists with the fear of restriction and over-protection. Imagination and fantasy are important, especially for the very disabled, and allow survivors to transcend the present and find solace and escape.

> My cocoon becomes less oppressive, and my mind takes flight like a butterfly. There is so much to do. You can wander off in space or time, set out for Tierra del Fuego or for King Midas's court. (Bauby, 2002)

Routine helps to structure days, and nights are often experienced as the worst part of each day with many survivors reporting anxiety, disturbing thoughts and problems with sleeping. Fear of recurrence of stroke and dying during sleep is often a source of distress. Weekends, when there is no therapy and few staff are available, are also regarded as bleak periods. Some survivors find rules and regulations applied in wards restrictive and oppressive, especially when there is no clear reason for them or staff flaunt them (e.g. smoking and bans on mobile phones), and survivors who inadvertently or deliberately contravene rules may come into conflict with staff. Relationships with nursing staff are crucial and, once again, personal qualities and gentleness are major determinants of survivors' reactions to staff. Being treated as an individual person with thoughts, feeling and a personality rather than as a 'body' is important, as is attention to wider human needs such helping with access to meaningful activities and personal contacts. Most survivors have 'favourite' nurses or therapists and miss them when they are away. Family members usually become indispensable at this stage, and young, previously independent, survivors may welcome their parents returning to their previous parenting role. Friends and other visitors are normally much appreciated for their company and as a link to the outside world, but survivors may sometimes feel like a captive audience, especially if visitors focus on their own concerns and not those of the survivor. Several accounts describe the automatic assumption that the survivor requires a visit from a minister of religion as inappropriate and unwelcome. However, religion is frequently a theme, and most survivors explore their orientation to spirituality or what happens after death at some stage during their recovery. Older survivors in particular may perceive religious faith as hope sustaining and their relationship to God as an important source of psychological 'connectedness' that has parallels their sense of connection with their family.

Fellow survivors emerge as important influences at this stage, visits from those who have recovered from stroke are particularly uplifting, and comparisons with other patients with greater impairments often make survivors feel fortunate and thankful. A camaraderie may develop with some fellow patients which provides mutual support and boosts morale through the realisation that the survivor is not alone. However, exposure to very ill or frail patients, and the medical and personal care procedures that they require in the ward, may be unpleasant and disturbing for less disabled survivors who see at firsthand how the human body can deteriorate and the undignified and sometimes painful measures that may be required to support life. Similarly, survivors may be upset by patients who exhibit confused or aggressive behaviour, and there are many reports of broken sleep caused by patients who repeatedly call out, and of intrusive behaviour by confused patients. Survivors may also feel compassionate towards other patients and can experience a strong urge to help them with self-care, such as with getting to the toilet or feeding, especially if staff are too busy to do these things and a helpless patient becomes distressed. At a later stage in their recovery, many survivors also make contact with the experiences of others through reading autobiographies of stroke survivors, and this is usually a very helpful and positive experience.

Therapy is perceived as vital and as the 'route back to normal life'. Participation in therapy satisfies an urge to become actively engaged in something that improves functioning and promotes recovery, and the achievement of therapy goals is a major source of hope. However, survivors generally find it arduous and demanding and fatigue is frequently a barrier to full engagement. Many survivors develop strong and usually very positive relationships with their therapists. However, relationships are not always harmonious and therapists are sometimes seen as overly demanding or inconsiderate of the survivor's needs. Some therapy tasks are perceived as childish, and their relevance to recovery is not appreciated. Survivors set themselves personal goals and targets for their recovery, such as walking or getting to the toilet unaided, and there may be frustration and anger with therapists if the therapist's and survivor's goals are not concordant. Survivors may become despairing if they do not achieve goals, and this can result in avoidance of therapy. Most reports of this stage emphasise how important it is that therapists maintain hope and are not overly pessimistic about achieving personally significant goals. Some survivors feel a need to take the initiative and fill the time between professional rehabilitation sessions by developing their own rehabilitation routines and exercises.

The perception of recovery begins as symptoms stabilise and begin to diminish. Even tiny gains, such as the movement of a finger, can have immense personal significance. Indeed, many severely affected survivors focus on areas in which tiny but progressive improvements occur and derive hope and encouragement from any change, however small. The written accounts of survivors clearly describe how important functions continue to recover for ten years or more, and several are keen to dispel the professional 'myth' that most of recovery takes place over the first six to eight weeks. Hope for recovery may be bolstered by recollections of recovery from previous illness or injuries, and by recalling and employing strategies and approaches that were helpful in the past. Survivors may start to re-engage in activities at this stage, including reading, watching television or keeping a diary. Some may begin to look forward to the future and start to make plans for their return to home, work and life after the stroke. This may provide a welcome respite from a bleak and restricting present. The accounts of survivors differ in the extent to which they regard restitution of their former life as the primary goal of recovery, or whether they seek a new and changed life that integrates their stroke experience into a new lifestyle. The opportunity provided by time in hospital to reflect and plan is usually viewed as a very beneficial experience, and many survivors regard it as one positive outcome of their stroke. New perspectives engendered by the stroke may enable them to see their previous lives in a new light. Some survivors start to make far-reaching plans for change and a profound separation of 'old life and old self' from 'new life and new self' begins to emerge.

As well as looking forwards, survivors have time to reflect on the causes of their stroke, and some come to view it as a kind of punishment for their past lives and become assailed with regret and remorse. Another common area for remembrance and reflection are the illnesses and deaths of parents and other loved ones. The survivor may draw parallels with their own current predicament, and feel that they achieve greater insight into how their relatives felt and behaved when they were ill. Although depression may occur at any stage after stroke, the period after the initial shock, when survivors have time to take stock and reflect, is often the occasion for clinical depression, in which both body and the mind are affected, or an existential crisis that affects mental equilibrium, adjustment and relationships but has few physical effects. Survivors report difficulty with the regulation of their emotions and many are labile and have angry outbursts which they subsequently regret, often targeted at those they love and depend upon. Surprisingly some see lability as a positive change and feel they have 'rediscovered' a lost ability to express feelings. Survivors' perceptions of their capacity to be resilient and adaptable in facing the challenges that confront them are important in determining the degree of depression, despair and anxiety that they experience.

> But I didn't want to see anybody. I didn't want anyone to see me. . . . I lay like that, in the darkness, almost comatose, my head stuffed in the pillow for a long time. Sometimes, my wife, sons, friends came in to see me, but I didn't see them. I didn't hear them. Sometimes, I didn't know whether it was day or night. It seemed as though I was in a black cave far down below the surface of the earth. (Douglas, 2002)

During recovery, survivors begin to consolidate what they have learned about stroke into an internal model of the condition. This often reflects the common-sense model of illness described by Leventhal, Diefenbach and Leventhal (1992) in which the dimensions of identity, timeline, consequences, cause and cure/control are central. This set of beliefs displaces older beliefs based upon vicarious experiences of the strokes of relatives and friends. Survivors often supplement information imparted by staff with reading leaflets or books about stroke. What they find is not always comforting, particularly statistics about recurrent stroke, its link with dementia and the side effects of treatments. Fear of recurrence of stroke often surfaces at this time, as does the effect of the trauma of the stroke itself, and many survivors report a sense of anxiety, especially about going home, if that is where they had the stroke and the event was traumatic or they struggled to summon help.

> Unfortunately it at this time I came across a newspaper headline, which stated that strokes double the risk of Alzheimer's disease. This was a difficult thought to deal with. ... The next thing I discovered was that recurrent strokes are frequent ... the fear of a second, and worse stroke, was very potent. (McCann, 2006)

The milestone of going home or to a placement is reached during this stage, and occurs increasingly sooner in the stroke care pathway due to early discharge policies. Leaving hospital frequently becomes an important goal, even an obsession that drives up motivation to engage in rehabilitation activities. Some survivors describe their discharge from hospital as a welcome 'escape' from what they perceived to be an alien and unsympathetic world. Unfortunately, reports of difficulties in the planning of the transition from hospital to home are frequent. Pringle, Hendry and McLafferty (2008) reviewed 28 studies of experiences soon after discharge and highlighted the importance of the profound personal and social changes that occur following stroke. Personal accounts often describe how returning home is initially experienced as liberating, but this is followed by a realisation of the impact of residual disabilities, and the extent to which former activities are inaccessible and must be curtailed: a person may 'discover' their disabilities through comparison with their former capabilities in the same home environment. Impaired movement, communication, memory and sensation may limit self-care, leisure and social activities. The impact of these disabilities may be accentuated by the reduction or termination of input from professional care staff and a home environment which is less adapted to support people with disabilities than the hospital setting. When they occur, restricted mobility and the inability to drive are serious losses and may provoke a sense of imprisonment. Walking may be limited by fear of falling, and, if and when walking recovers, it is perceived as a major marker of recovery, as is the resumption of driving. A proportion of survivors also endure episodes of confusion and disorientation.

Survivors often report being abruptly abandoned by services once they return home, and wish that therapy had continued over a longer period. Many note that care staffs' and therapists' visits to home are frequently delayed and curtailed, and they are liable to be distracted by phone calls. This is sometimes described as a feeling of being 'dumped' by support services following discharge. One gap in our knowledge of survivors' experiences after discharge is an autobiographical account by someone discharged to a care home. Bauby's (2002) book about being cared for in a naval hospital provides some insights, but he suffered from locked-in syndrome which is an unusual and extremely severe condition. One response to the reduction in professional input may be the development of exercise and mind training routines. These may involve basic tasks such as walking in a straight line and catching or squeezing a ball, or more sophisticated activities like playing computer games or doing crosswords. Survivors may make resolutions about exercising to stay fit and adopting healthier diets and lifestyles. Progress is often variable, with good days and setbacks. Survivors report being elated when they make new achievements, but experiencing episodes of depression and gloom when they seem to be making no progress. In younger people this recovery phase is often when the investigations into the causes of their stroke take place. This may require them to attend hospitals and to endure tiring or painful examinations and procedures. There may be fear of reoccurrence and frustration with professionals if a cause cannot be found and treated.

At first, it was a massive relief to be home again, a milestone in my slow return to the world I'd lost, but then depression began to set in. I became more and more obsessed with my disabilities, and more and more frustrated. (McCrum, 1998)

After some time at home most survivors begin to experience the effects of their stroke on their social world, valued roles and sense of identity. The social circle often contracts to close family and friends. Relationships with family members often change as a result of dependency and the need to accept assistance from them. Changed emotions and emotional expression and communication impairments also affect family relationships. Survivors normally seem to come to terms with accepting assistance and generally express appreciation towards caregivers. Many report that relationships become closer and more meaningful as a result of dependency, and in some cases a sense of reciprocity develops in which the survivor develops an appreciation of their own contribution to the well-being and fulfilment of their carers. However, a sense of being burdensome to relatives is also common, and a significant proportion of survivors experience marital breakdown which contributes to disruption and distress. Survivors may not be able to perform accustomed roles, such as that of breadwinner, or tasks, such as housework or cooking, that defined their former roles. They may be unable to attend meetings and events that were important sources of social contact and role identity. Younger survivors in particular may feel that their gender identity and capacity to form romantic attachments is diminished. Misinterpretation of disabilities as drunkenness or mental handicap and being reprimanded or 'talked down to' can cause distress and may induce avoidance of public places and social withdrawal that accentuates isolation. However, many survivors make contact with stroke groups and stroke clubs at this stage and derive major benefits in terms of emotional support and practical help. Survivors and their carers may continue to feel the sense of professional abandonment that began with the cessation of intensive rehabilitation therapy following discharge from hospital, and it is common to experience difficulty in locating and accessing needed services. Financial provision for the future emerges as a concern and returning to work is a theme for those employed at the time of their stroke. Some dread the first contact with former colleagues and feel shame about their disabilities. There may be concerns about how colleagues and managers will view the survivor, and about changes that have occurred at work since their absence. Attitudes towards returning to work differ markedly; some survivors view re-engagement as impossible and undesirable, and the stroke as an opportunity to invest energy in leisure activities or to make employment changes, while others long to return to their former job and find that not being able to work is a significant and enduring loss. When a person does return to work, or work-related activities, it is usually viewed as a major achievement and a milestone in their recovery. Many survivors find it deeply rewarding to substitute or supplement work by helping other survivors in various ways; by visiting them, writing letters, writing and disseminating their own stories or by joining support groups and stroke clubs.

> My stroke taught me so much, and for all that it stole, it gave me even more. In the process of healing, my life has changed for the better. Now I want to share what I have learned. (Douglas, 2002)

Survivors may find that the stroke prompts them to make provision for their families in the form of wills or gifts, and also to plan for possible future incapacity by making advance directives and donating powers of attorney. Some survivors adopt alternative medicine, such as acupuncture, reflexology or herbal remedies, and generally report that it is beneficial. There are also personal accounts of engaging in psychotherapy and of its role in achieving a better understanding the reasons for depression and anxiety. Therapy may also help to put the survivor's previous life and the effects of stroke into perspective. However, timing is crucial, and reports suggest that psychotherapy with a focus on general adjustment is most useful after returning home when the full implications of the stroke are clear. There are also many accounts of coping strategies that have been found to be helpful in dispelling depressive feelings and improving adjustment. These include looking on the bright side, drawing comparisons with more disabled individuals and feeling grateful, helping others, taking responsibility for self-care and making decisions, slowing down the pace of life, developing patience, developing routines, staying motivated, having faith in God, having a sense of humour, maintaining friendships and staying active.

As recovery progresses, some survivors feel that life has changed for the better. They may experience an accentuated appreciation of life and the world, new insights into the evaluation of what is meaningful and valuable, an intensification of feelings of love towards family members and friends and a greater sense of connectedness with other people in general. A person may feel that formerly submerged qualities have blossomed and that they have become more compassionate, tolerant and sympathetic. At a practical level a person may achieve a better work–life balance, a healthier lifestyle, new friends, new knowledge and insights and new outlets for their creativity and energy. These positive outcomes of stroke, 'the silver lining', have recently been recognised and studied (Gillen, 2005; Gangstad, Norman & Barton, 2009). An improved understanding of the factors that promote such positive outcomes could be a significant step in helping professionals to improve psychological recovery.

Implications

The powerfully moving personal accounts of stroke and its aftermath listed in Tables 1.1 and 1.2 graphically depict the life-changing nature of this condition and the events and forces that determine individual reactions to stroke and its consequences. For these insights, we should be thankful those who have shared their experiences of times of great personal adversity. (See also Table 1.4 for another personal account of stroke.) Many aspects of the experience of stroke survivors, such as the loss of muscle control and feelings of depression and desolation, have been extensively researched, and approaches to assessment and treatment have been, and are being, developed. Other experiences, such as the potential for positive, life-enhancing outcomes, have only more recently been recognised. Others, such as the way some people have the capacity to make contact and reassure people soon after their stroke when they are in mental turmoil and anguish, have yet to be fully explored.

This section will have succeeded in its purpose if it provides readers with a glimpse of the world of stroke survivors and the lived experiences that underlie some of the topics covered in the remainder of this text. It would be an immense bonus if it also helped some readers, including those who work with stroke survivors, to understand something of the fractured and tumultuous word of those who have recently experienced stroke in ways that inform and guide their endeavours to reach out, make connections and relieve psychological suffering and enhance well-being. More formally, some of the experiences revealed by survivors might be incorporated into staff training programmes and service elements. These might include training to foster an appreciation of the devastating effects of impaired communication ability during the early stages of stroke, training in approaches that reassure and develop the trust of newly admitted stroke survivors, training in approaches to goal setting that are sensitive to survivors' priorities and expectations, the development of service configurations that acknowledge and respect survivors' individuality and humanity, enhanced monitoring (and psychological support if necessary) in the crucial period following discharge and increased opportunities to make contact with, and receive support from, other stroke survivors.

Table 1.4 Linda's Story

One ordinary December day in 2005 when I was 37, I was sitting in my car preparing to leave work and go home. It was really cold so I had the heater on to warm the car up. I started to drive along the road, and got into second gear and then forgot how to drive the car! I was not in any pain, just simply bewildered. I managed to call my work colleague Lesley and told her I'd forgotten how to drive my car. Initially she thought I was mucking about (part of my pre- and post-haemorrhage character was that of a 'funster'). I actually had to convince her I was serious and asked her to come and collect me.

Lesley drove me home. By which time I was experiencing severe pains in the left hand side of my forehead. It felt like someone had stuck a knife into my head and was twisting it round. I really wanted Lesley to go so I could just lie down and sleep, but luckily she realised that something was very wrong. She called the out-of-hours doctor who told her to dial 999.

The next time I was fully conscious was four weeks later, and I was in the Neurology Unit of Frenchay Hospital, Bristol. During that time I was drifting in a dreamlike state without realising what had happened. I could see my son Stuart (who lived in Australia) and he looked like he'd been crying and I thought 'If I shut my eyes he might go away'. The nursing staff kept coming up and asking me puerile question; the name of the queen, the prime minister, which month we were in, etc.? I thought I answered them correctly, but actually I still don't know if I did.

All my family was present and the priest came and gave me the last rites. None of this panicked me as I thought I was in a dream. The knife twisting pain was ever present, then, and after recovering consciousness. I had it for months and even morphine didn't relieve it. Curiously, when I tried ibuprofen it did the trick. The whole experience was really weird, rather like the film 'Groundhog Day' reliving the same 'dream' – I thought – for months!

I was moved to Bath RUH and I still felt like I was dreaming. I thought all the nurses were foreign as none of them could understand me. When I needed a wash I tried to tell the nurse what I needed. To me my voice sounded completely normal, but I ended up having to sign it to make him understand. (All of which was difficult because I'd been left paralysed down the right side of my body – as luck wouldn't have it I am right handed). The nurse didn't understand, however, and subsequently went and got an air freshener to spray around the bed. He obviously thought I was complaining of the smell in the ward!

I was not at all horrified by my predicament because I still assumed I was dreaming. My prevailing emotion was irritation at not being able to communicate. Visitors were coming and going and smiling, but I simply thought I was in a big dream bubble! It wasn't until I actually realised what had happened to me, about eight weeks after the stroke, that I got upset. It was while still in Bath RUH that it slowly sank in that this was reality and I had actually suffered a huge subarachnoid haemorrhage.

A neurologist told me I would be transferred to Chippenham Hospital. This fact horrified me as I had worked there years ago when it was a geriatric hospital. In retrospect I think I was shielding myself from my 'real' problems by worrying about insignificant things.

(continued)

Table 1.4 (*Continued*)

When I was a patient I felt like I was transparent and that the staff weren't listening to me. My family and friends (many of whom lived in Kent) came to visit me regularly. My son came back, three times, from Australia to visit me in hospital. I was able to communicate with friends and family much more easily than the staff. I sounded as though I was drunk and incoherent.

I hated it in Chippenham hospital. I felt like I was in an old people's home. But fortunately I was in a room on my own.

I had a gradual realisation of how physically limited I had become; horrifically I was doubly incontinent and catheterised. I was very keen to get physiotherapy. However, with the added staffing pressures on the nurses I often missed my appointment slot with the physiotherapist. I became really frustrated that I could not push forward with my recovery and at being unable even to sit up in bed. I had learnt to eat with my left hand; I could even peel an orange one handed. I also learnt to write left handed. Radio 4 and talking books from the hospital library keep me sane!

At the hospital I religiously performed all the physical exercises given to me. I also had psychological counselling which I found a great help. I felt isolated in my predicament because all other patients were old enough to be my parents.

I was in Chippenham hospital for eight months. My home was adapted so I could return to it in my electric wheel chair. By the time I left hospital my speech was slow but understandable. I was on copious amounts of medication.

Coming home I was very scared having become more or less institutionalised in the hospital regime. Where I (still) live is quite isolated. I did not have a partner at the time. I had brought up my children on my own. In retrospect the fact that I had lived many years as an independent, career minded, person probably helped me cope better. I have never been scared of being on my own. I had three visits a day from a personal assistant (PA), and the Care in the Community Team came in three times a week. I was house-bound, but fortunately my incontinence had cleared up.

The initial physical setbacks engendered by the subarachnoid haemorrhage I dealt with quite positively when I returned home. My days were spent trying to make basic improvements to my mobility. I was angry and depressed about it all, but used the energy positively (as I still do) because I did not want to be in wheel chair for the rest of my life. Even during the first year I never gave up on the idea I could make a full recovery and I still haven't!

During my time in the wheel chair I felt transparent again and frustrated because people in shops, etc., generally talked to the person pushing me, or talked to me as though I was 'simple' which, with a degree in business finance, I knew I wasn't! People even spoke loudly to me in single syllables, and this I felt was almost more crushing than the disability itself!

Nowadays I rarely feel sorry for myself, but during the early days of recovery I used to think 'Why me?', but I never dwelled on it. It has made me realise that this can happen to anyone at any age, anytime. I am now acutely aware of the fragility of human health.

Previously, I had worked as a Group Facilitator for the charity Mind, successfully setting up and running four drop-in centres for people with mental health problems.

Table 1.4   *(Continued)*

Therefore, I was aware of the danger of becoming depressed. To this day, I believe that it was my tendency to turn any anger outwards, directing the energy into my recovery that enabled me to avoid becoming overly depressed.

Paradoxically, although my movement is still limited on my right-hand side (I still define myself as hemiplegic), I am in some ways healthier than I was before the subarachnoid haemorrhage. My diet and fitness regime is now much more important to me. I do not take my health for granted.

I would rather be dealing with this disability than a mental health problem which is invisible to the outside world. I want to get to the stage where my physical disability fades and is not noticeable.

Between the subarachnoid haemorrhage and complete recovery I work toward manageable goals, some small ones, for example, getting to the gym regularly and sticking to a healthy eating programme. Larger ones included visiting my son (unassisted) in Australia last Christmas and my best friend in Canada this June. Something a couple of years ago I would not have even considered. I am also having refresher lessons in an adapted car as I have now had my driving license returned from the DVLA. I remain very focused. Prior to the subarachnoid haemorrhage I was a slender, energetic woman who loved to skate, ski and dance, I am determined to do these things again.

The medication and the loss of mobility made me put on three stones. I have taken control of this by joining a slimming club and have lost over two stone which has improved my mobility. I have made additional friends by doing this and it's made me realise that even people who have not survived major trauma still have mobility and health issues from such everyday things as obesity/and or other eating disorders. The whole experience has radically altered the nature of my 'friendship' groups. This sort of thing really sorts out the 'wheat' from the 'chaff'. I have always had a large cross section of friends. It was quite strange because many friends who were ever present when I was in hospital disappeared when I was discharged. Good friends who I had shared holidays and life experience with simply vanished. Some remained consistent, seeing me as much as they ever did. In a way this is good because it is not patronising but sometimes I feel certain close friends and family try to ignore my disability and this has its own set of problems. For example in practical terms I cannot cope with late nights as well as before.

Other people, like my original and continual life saver Lesley, and close friend Dagmar, did not feature heavily as friends before my subarachnoid haemorrhage. They were not in my social set. They are now indispensable, and I value their friendship. It's made me realise qualities in people perhaps I wouldn't have done without the stroke. In addition I have met a completely new set of people of all ages and social backgrounds. I have a male personal assistant, Chris, who has a wicked sense of humour who says, I quote, 'this job is like the Hotel California you check out but you never leave!' I have become close to a fitness trainer, Brigid, who has encouraged me in the gym and swimming pool. She even entered me for a Concept 2 (stationary rowing machine) series of Rowathlon challenges over six months in which I was competing against nondisabled rowers. I beat many of them!

(continued)

Table 1.4   (*Continued*)

When I am out and about now people tend not to realise I am disabled, thinking only that I have sprained my ankle or something as I wear a leg splint. This can be difficult. For example, when I am in the supermarket people can get impatient with me. My right hand has limited movement which makes payment and packing at the checkout impossible to do unaided.

Since losing weight and gaining more mobility, my self-image has improved and I am beginning to feel more like me! I try to make my recovery and not my disability define me. I use my hatred of being disabled to spur me on! I have also used various cognitive techniques to enhance recovery, for example, hypnotherapy, positive visualization, etc.

The experience has activated me toward helping other survivors of brain trauma. I'm a Stroke Patient, Carer and Public (PCIP) Involvement volunteer for the Avon, Gloucester, Wiltshire and Somerset (AGWS) Cardiac and Stroke Network. I am also being used in a drug trail HPS2-THRIVE. I am a volunteer for Salisbury Hospital for Functional Electrical Stimulation (FES). I am open to trying any new technique that will aid recovery. I have taken up swimming (I was never very confident in the water before) and am conquering my fear of 'going under' both in and out of the pool!

I am looking forward to the future.

The effects of stroke: the professionals' perspective

Models of disability

The tangible, observable effects of stroke can be conceptualised according to a model developed by the World Health Organisation (WHO), the International Classification of Functioning, Disability and Health (ICF; WHO, 2001). This model can assist in understanding the relationship between the early effects of stroke and the subsequent outcomes.

- Functioning refers to the physiological functioning of body systems and structures. Thus the functioning of the brain is affected by stroke. Impairments are problems in body function, occurring as a significant deviation from or loss of former functioning. The loss of motor ability, sensory ability and memory, as a result of damage to the brain, are impairments.
- Disability involves both activity limitation and participation.
  - o Activity is the execution of a task or an action by an individual. Activity limitations are difficulties in executing activities. For example, if someone is unable to get dressed, this is an activity limitation.
  - o Participation is the involvement in a life situation. Participation restrictions are problems in fulfilling life roles, such as the inability to work or to go out socially. (WHO, 2001, pp. 212–13)

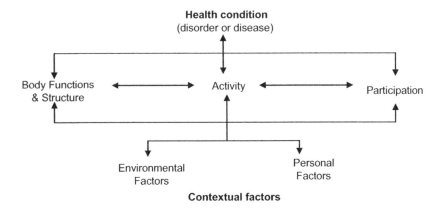

Figure 1.1 International classification of functioning, disability and health. Reproduced with permission from World Health Organization. (World Health Organization. 2001. *International classification of functioning, disability and health (ICF)*, p. 26. Geneva: World Health Organization.)

The ICF highlights how a person's health condition interacts dynamically with contextual factors to create problems with functioning, activity and participation, as shown in Figure 1.1.

For someone with a stroke, there may be loss of movement in one arm, an impairment; problems with personal self-care, an activity limitation; and a desire not to engage in social occasions, a restriction in participation. Further contextual factors may include the attitude of a partner, living in a geographically isolated place and lack of availability of alternative support.

Impairments after stroke

Strokes lead to a broad range of impairments, which depend on the blood vessels involved and the parts of the brain affected, as discussed further in chapter 3. The relation between the lesion and the final outcome is a reflection of treatment, management and natural recovery, as well as individual patient factors. It is therefore perhaps unsurprising that stroke confers a wide spectrum of effects. The most prominent impairments are motor and sensory deficits, aphasia and visual field problems (Bogousslavsky & Caplan, 2001). Symptoms that are less prominent, but nevertheless important for understanding the psychological effects of stroke, include cognitive, behavioural and emotional problems (Bogousslavsky, 2003). The impact of these, for both the people affected and their families, could be viewed as an inevitable consequence of the lesion; they will, however, be influenced by the success (or failure) of acute treatment, rehabilitation and the support provided after stroke. Whilst many with stroke have similar symptoms, very few will have all of the same symptoms. It is, in part, this heterogeneity of symptoms, and the resultant problems in daily life, which necessitates a comprehensive and individual in-depth assessment of every stroke patient, and subsequently, the development of individualised treatment and management plans. In addition, those with stroke frequently have substantial comorbidity, such as diabetes, osteoarthritis, myocardial infarction, heart failure, osteoarthritis and generalised cerebrovascular disease, all of which compound the effects of stroke (Sturm, Donnan, Dewey, Macdonell, Gilligan & Thrift, 2004).

Disabilities after stroke

Disabilities, according to the WHO ICF model, include both the loss of activities and the effect on participation. Loss of activities includes the loss of ability to carry out activities of daily living. These are often classified into personal self care activities, such as washing, dressing and bathing, and instrumental activities of daily living, those needed to be independent on the home, such as making a hot drink, cooking a meal and cleaning the house. Loss of participation covers much wider roles, such as the ability to work, engage in leisure activities and have a social life. The latter is also affected by the environment and patients' lifestyle, and not just the direct consequences of the stroke.

Models of need

It is also helpful, particularly when planning the development of services relevant to stroke survivors and their carers, to consider not just problems and their consequences, but also needs and, perhaps most importantly, unmet needs (French, Leathley, Radford, Dey, McAdam, Marsden, Sutton *et al.*, 2009). These are defined (French *et al.*, 2009, p.13) as:

- '**Problem:** a condition, impairment or functional limitation acquired as a consequence of stroke;
- **Need:** an ability or aspect of life where support for either the stroke survivor or carer may be required to promote health and well-being, or to maximise activity and participation;
- **Unmet:** need: an area of need which is perceived by the user to be unmet, or which does not meet specified standards'.

French *et al.* (2009) conducted an extensive mapping study of the available literature and consulted with user groups of stroke survivors and carers to identify categories of need. These included everyday living needs, physical needs, emotional and well-being needs, social needs, communication and cognition needs, financial, legal and care needs, re-enablement needs and carer needs. A framework of needs was produced, which is shown in Figure 1.2 and demonstrates the breadth of issues identified.

Further work is needed to explore, not just the aetiology and time course of particular problems, but also the nature of the complex relationships between

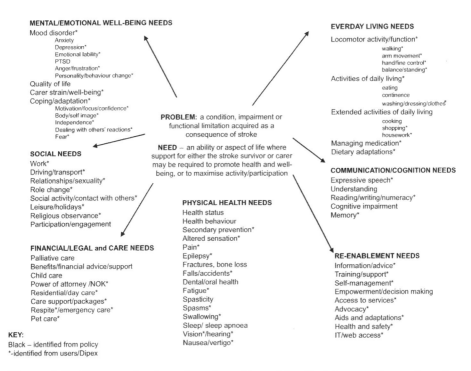

MENTAL/EMOTIONAL WELL-BEING NEEDS
Mood disorder*
    Anxiety
    Depression*
    Emotional lability*
    PTSD
    Anger/frustration*
    Personality/behaviour change*
Quality of life
Carer strain/well-being*
Coping/adaptation*
    Motivation/focus/confidence*
    Body/self image*
    Independence*
    Dealing with others' reactions*
    Fear*

SOCIAL NEEDS
Work*
Driving/transport*
Relationships/sexuality*
Role change*
Social activity/contact with others*
Leisure/holidays*
Religious observance*
Participation/engagement

FINANCIAL/LEGAL and CARE NEEDS
Palliative care
Benefits/financial advice/support
Child care
Power of attorney /NOK*
Residential/day care*
Care support/packages*
Respite*/emergency care*
Pet care*

KEY:
Black – identified from policy
*-identified from users/Dipex

PROBLEM: a condition, impairment or
functional limitation acquired as a
consequence of stroke

NEED – an ability or aspect of life where
support for either the stroke survivor or carer
may be required to promote health and well-
being, or to maximise activity/participation

PHYSICAL HEALTH NEEDS
Health status
Health behaviour
Secondary prevention*
Altered sensation*
Pain*
Epilepsy*
Fractures, bone loss
Falls/accidents*
Dental/oral health
Fatigue*
Spasticity
Spasms*
Swallowing*
Sleep/ sleep apnoea
Vision*/hearing*
Nausea/vertigo*

EVERDAY LIVING NEEDS
Locomotor activity/function*
    walking*
    arm movement*
    hand/fine control*
    balance/standing*
Activities of daily living*
    eating
    continence
    washing/dressing/clothes
Extended activities of daily living
    cooking
    shopping*
    housework*
Managing medication*
Dietary adaptations*

COMMUNICATION/COGNITION NEEDS
Expressive speech*
Understanding
Reading/writing/numeracy*
Cognitive impairment
Memory*

RE-ENABLEMENT NEEDS
Information/advice*
Training/support*
Self-management*
Empowerment/decision making
Access to services*
Advocacy*
Aids and adaptations*
Health and safety*
IT/web access*

Figure 1.2 Framework of needs and problems identified from policy and stroke survivors and carers. Reproduced with permission from French, B., Leathley, M. J., Radford, K., Dey, M. P., McAdam, J., Marsden, J., *et al.* (2009). UK Stroke Survivor Needs Survey Information Mapping Exercise. Report to the Stroke Association. © University of Central Lancashire 2008.

these different categories of need. It is the understanding of these relationships that will give greater insight into how to ensure mental and emotional well-being, to provide prevention and treatment strategies that are tailored to individual patient needs and circumstances; and to deliver patient-orientated services in the future.

Conclusions

There is a broad range of effects of a stroke across a wide range of domains, subjective as well as physical. Both the patients' perspective and the professionals' perspectives need to be understood to gain a comprehensive awareness of the psychological effects of stroke. Identification of the full range of problems, the needs that arise in the patient and family and the extent to which any unmet needs can be met will facilitate the development of a comprehensive plan for the management of the effects of a stroke.

Chapter 2

Clinical Stroke Services

Global and national dimensions

Stroke is a global issue. The World Health Organisation (2006) estimated that stroke accounted for 5.7 million deaths worldwide in 2005, 9.9% of all deaths, and it was found to be the second most common cause of mortality worldwide in 1990 (Murray & Lopez, 1997). Patterns of stroke incidence are changing worldwide; in high-income countries there has been a 42% decrease in stroke incidence 1970 to 2008, but in middle- to low-income countries this trend has been reversed and there has been an increase in stroke incidence of over 100%. By 2008 the incidence rate for stroke in both high- and low-income countries was about 70 per 100,000, but the rate for haemorrhagic stroke was 10 per 100,000 in high-income countries and 22 per 100,000 in low-income countries (Feigin, Lawes, Bennett, Barker-Collo & Parag, 2009). During the early years of the twenty-first century in the United Kingdom, the prevalence of stroke was between 2% and 3% across all age groups, but prevalence increased with age to about 12% in the over 75s. Estimates of annual incidence rates over this period varied widely, depending on the region, but generally were within the range of 100–200 per 100,000 overall, with rates for women being somewhat higher than men, and older groups (over 75 years) having much higher rates of over 1000 per 100,000. Stroke accounted for 9% of all deaths and was the second biggest single cause of death after heart disease, and it caused about 5% of premature deaths in the under 75s. In line with other developed countries, rates of death from stroke in the United Kingdom fell to about one third of their level in 1968 in the early years of the twenty-first century, but stroke mortality remained considerably higher in people from lower socioeconomic groups. The total cost of stroke to the United Kingdom economy was £4.5 billion in 2006/2007 with 56% of this being for health and social care, 21% in lost production and 22% for informal care (Stroke Association/British Heart Association, 2009). An estimate for 2009 put the total cost of stroke to the

Psychological Management of Stroke, First Edition. Nadina B. Lincoln, Ian I. Kneebone, Jamie A.B. Macniven and Reg C. Morris.
© 2012 John Wiley & Sons, Ltd. Published 2012 by John Wiley & Sons, Ltd.

United Kingdom as £8.9 billion with 49% spent on formal care, 15% due to lost productivity and 27% accounted for by informal care (Saka, McGuire & Wolfe, 2009).

Health services and treatment protocols for stroke are organised country by country, each with its own particular approach and emphasis. This plurality of approaches can underpin differences in the process of care and in outcomes, such as those identified between England, Northern Ireland and Wales (Rudd, Irwin, Rutledge, Lowe, Wade & Pearson, 2001). It also has the potential to enable comparisons and contrasts that signpost ways of improving stroke services (Markus, 2007). However, variation across nations may be caused by many factors, such as the prevalence of risk factors, access to care, quality of care and the ways in which outcomes are recorded (Giroud, Czlonkowska, Ryglewicz & Wolfe, 2002), and consequently the comparison of raw outcome data can be misleading in the absence of adjustment for confounding factors (Tilling, Kunze & Beech, 2002). Despite national differences in the implementation of stroke services, there have been attempts by a number of bodies, notably the International Stroke Society, the European Stroke Council and the World Health Organisation, to foster international cooperation and develop international guidelines. One very encouraging outcome of international collaborations was the Helsingborg Declaration which signified an agreement to pursue a nine-year strategic plan to develop and improve stroke services across Europe (Kjellström, Norrving & Shatchkute, 2006). The domains addressed by the plan were

- organization of stroke services,
- management of acute stroke,
- prevention,
- rehabilitation after stroke, and
- evaluation of stroke outcome and quality assessment.

Reading this document in the light of the stroke strategies for developed countries underscores the high degree of international concordance that exists, at least within the concourse of the developed countries of the Western hemisphere. This congruence is largely thanks to underpinning by the international pool of research knowledge, and to databases, such as the Cochrane Library, which publish influential systematic reviews of research into assessment methods, treatments and service configurations. An example of such a review is one that examined the benefit of psychotherapy in the prevention of depression after stroke (Hackett, Anderson, House & Halteh, 2008a). It was encouraging to see that psychological and social care were important facets of the Helsingborg declaration. Psychological and neuropsychological expertise were identified as vital components of multidisciplinary stroke rehabilitation teams, and psychological research into cognitive rehabilitation was highlighted as a priority area. There was also a recommendation that voluntary associations of stroke survivors and carers should be encouraged, as well as self-help groups supported by professionals. The declaration noted that the impact of self-help groups extends beyond providing support, information and counselling; they have the potential to contribute to the coordination of local, regional and national efforts to promote better stroke care and social support for people with stroke, and may also encourage social recognition and even provide a source of financial compensation for caregivers.

Despite the significant degree of international consensus, the implementation of stroke services within national boundaries exhibits a degree of diversity that makes the task of writing a chapter on stroke services a daunting one. The approach here is to take the service structures, policies and relevant legislation applicable to the four home countries of the United Kingdom as exemplars of the wider international efforts to specify and improve stroke care. Even this is a somewhat complex task due to devolved health ministries and legislature (for Scotland), but fortunately the four countries have developed approaches to stroke that have much in common. Recently they have agreed to work collaboratively to develop a Stroke-Specific Education Framework (Department of Health, 2009a) through the United Kingdom Forum for Stroke Training (UK-FST), which has been established to work towards the achievement of recognised, quality-assured and transferable education programmes in stroke. Training and education, workforce competences, professional development and career pathways will be linked across the United Kingdom.

The service frameworks of countries from outside of the United Kingdom have not been included in detail since this would risk confusion. However, much of the evidence base underpinning treatments and service organisation is derived from studies conducted across a number of developed nations, and for this reason the reviews of this evidence and guidelines included in this chapter will be relevant to those from outside the United Kingdom. Moreover, especially well-developed or forward looking national services or policies, such as the Dutch policy for supporting stroke carers (van Heugten, Visser-Meily, Post & Lindeman, 2006), are included in the relevant chapters below.

The United Kingdom National Health Service

Stroke care in Britain is principally accomplished within the National Health Service (NHS), the world's largest publically funded health service. In 2006/ 2007, 175,000 inpatient stroke cases were treated in England, about 1% of all inpatients (Stroke Association/British Heart Foundation, 2009). The years between 2000 and 2010 witnessed profound changes as the NHS Plan unfolded (Department of Health, 2000). The programme of reform and modernisation is set to continue for the next ten years with the publication of the 'Next Stage Review for England' (Darzi, 2007) and a new NHS Constitution for England (Department of Health, 2009b). Meanwhile parallel development programmes are being designed and implemented by devolved governments in the home nations of Wales, Scotland and Northern Ireland.

Throughout the reforms, the NHS has retained the core principle of delivering a universal, comprehensive, needs-based service that is free at the point of delivery; but little else has remained unchanged. The new NHS has national blueprints outlining services for many population groups and conditions (National Service Frameworks), while national guidelines for the treatment of major conditions, based on research evidence, are collated and published by the National Institute for Health and Clinical Excellence (NICE) and by bodies such as the Royal College of Physicians and the Scottish Intercollegiate Guidelines Network. There is less central control; healthcare providers enjoy greater freedom to commission locally relevant services within a central framework for commissioning. This framework promotes a set of principles or 'competencies', such as public involvement, an evidence base and collaboration with clinicians. It maintains a clinical governance framework embodying standards for excellence and safe practice and ensures that outcomes are monitored and performance is evaluated. However, all healthcare agencies are expected to be transparent in their decision making and operation, and the World Wide Web has been harnessed to make knowledge, policy and performance indicators more accessible. The NHS is becoming more accountable, and the inclusion of the views of patients and carers in planning, implementing and monitoring services now has legal force through Section 11 of the Health and Social Care Act, 2001 (Her Majesty's Government, 2001) and Part 14 of the Local Government and Public Involvement in Health Act, 2007 (Her Majesty's Government, 2007a).

From a psychological perspective, it is gratifying that the psychological benefits of personal control and choice in promoting satisfaction, well-being and physical health (Kunzman, Little & Smith, 2002; Rodin, 1986) have been guiding principles in framing new policies and guidelines. At an individual level, personal preferences are to be more fully considered when planning treatment and care, and patients and their carers are to be given more choice, involvement and control over what happens to them and to health services (Department of Health, 2007b; Secretary of State for Health, 2007a). Inequities in health and healthcare continue to be addressed, and fairness has become a major principle as healthcare services strive to become more universally accessible and equitable. Traditional treatment delivery by professionals will be increasingly supplemented with self-help and self-care schemes within 'expert patient' programmes, some specific to stroke, and health service users and their carers will become involved in shaping stroke services (National Stroke Strategy for England; see Department of Health, 2007a). Organisational boundaries are becoming more permeable; joint planning and working between the health services, social services, third sector charitable organisations and the private sector are becoming the norm. At the same time, regulation of the health professions has been reformed and strengthened by the inception of new uni- and multiprofessional regulatory bodies. Clinical psychology has been included under the auspices of the Health and Care Professions' Council since 2009, along with 12–20 other health professions. There is an increased emphasis on independent, lay membership of these regulatory bodies (Secretary of State for Health, 2007b). Traditional professional demarcations may become much more flexible with the advent of new training approaches to promulgate and quality-assure knowledge and competencies for specific conditions. One such development is the United Kingdom Stroke-Specific Education Framework which has been implemented since 2010 (UK Forum for Stroke Training, 2009).

Mental health and mental capacity legislation

Two important pieces of United Kingdom health legislation have set out principles and practice for working with people with psychological impairments, including many that occur in people with stroke. The Adults with Incapacity (Scotland) Act 2000 (The Scottish Government, 2000) and the Mental Capacity Act 2005/2007 (England and Wales; Her Majesty's Government 2005, 2007b) and their associated codes of practice represent a comprehensive, unified and systematic approach to decision making by people with cognitive impairments, their carers and healthcare workers (see Decision Making and Mental Capacity, chapter 9). The Amendments to the Mental Health Act 2007 for England and Wales (Her Majesty's Government, 2007b) and the Mental Health (Care and Treatment) (Scotland) Act 2003 (The Scottish Government, 2003), have clarified the definition of mental illness and include consideration of public safety while sharing many basic principles with the mental capacity legislation:

- Respect for patients' past and present wishes and feelings
- Respect for diversity generally including, in particular, diversity of religion, culture and sexual orientation
- Minimising restrictions on liberty
- Involvement of patients in planning, developing and delivering care and treatment appropriate to them
- Avoidance of unlawful discrimination
- Effectiveness of treatment
- Consideration of the views of carers and other interested parties
- Patient well-being and safety

These major changes and reforms, and the planned developments over the next ten years, provide an exciting backdrop for psychologists entering health professions. There will be opportunities to become involved in shaping new, responsive services that use the best of modern technology while retaining the core principles of the NHS and consideration for fundamental human values.

Stroke-specific guidelines and service blueprints

Direct stroke services cost about £3 billion per annum in England and Wales in the early part of the twenty-first century (National Audit Office, 2005, 2010). With such large expenditure at stake, it is important that services are accessible, acceptable and cost-effective. The development of clinical practice guidelines, based on systematic reviews of the evidence for treatment effectiveness and on expert opinion, helps to translate the evidence base into clinical practice. At the same time, such guidelines harmonise service provision and promote consistency and quality standards across geographically and organisationally separate services. Guidelines, especially if available in plain language versions, can empower patients by enabling them to make informed choices and provide a basis for influencing public policy through identification of omissions or shortfalls in care. They assist clinicians in making treatment choices and can be used to sieve out ineffective treatments, and as the basis for the systematic audit of services. They also serve to identify gaps in the evidence base and thereby stimulate new and specifically targeted research. Finally, healthcare organisations and professions rely on guidelines to standardise care and as a benchmark of quality and good practice. The benefits of guidelines have been well established, and it has been shown that that adherence improves patient satisfaction (Reker, Duncan, Horner, Hoenig, Samsa, Hamilton *et al.*, 2002), and outcome (Duncan, Horner, Reker, Samsa, Hoenig, Hamilton *et al.*, 2002).

However, the development of guidelines also carries risks (Woolf, Grol, Hutchinson, Eccles & Grimshaw, 1999). The consequences of errors in guidelines will be multiplied many times by their widespread application; the evidence base is often complex, containing gaps and contradictions which require value-based subjective judgements; the composition of guideline development groups may skew recommendations; and decisions may be influenced by factors, such as cost saving or professional convenience, which run counter to patients' priorities. Guidelines may encourage the inflexible application of treatments which do not take account of patients' individual needs and circumstances, and may therefore reduce choice and shared decision making. They may also be misused to influence public opinion by advocacy groups with particular political agendas. Their proliferation and increasing detail increase the information load on practitioners and the time they need away from patients to review and update their knowledge and skills. If guidelines are not carefully drafted and harmonised across related conditions, they can become contradictory and confusing. They may also undermine professional competence by presenting oversimplified choices and restricting the use of clinical judgement and intuition ('cook-book practice'), and may encourage defensive practice to avoid possible litigation, even when the treatments provided are not in the best interests of patients. Finally, many guidelines do not include consideration of the cost or relative cost-effectiveness of treatments, and may therefore encourage the squandering of scarce resources.

The importance and widespread adoption of guidelines have spurred endeavours to improve their quality and avoid some of the pitfalls identified above. The AGREE collaboration (2003) developed a framework for assessing the quality of the guideline development process (Table 2.1) with 23 individual elements organised around six domains. These were applied by Hurdowar, Graham, Bayley, Harrison, Wood-Dauphinee and Bhogal (2007) to eight

Table 2.1   The AGREE Framework. Reproduced from Quality and Safety, The AGREE collaboration, 12, 18–23, 2003 with permission from BMJ Publishing Group Ltd.

The AGREE framework for clinical practice guideline development

Domain 1. Scope and purpose
1. The overall objective of the guideline is specifically described.
2. The clinical question covered by the guideline is specifically described.
3. The patients to whom the guideline is meant to apply are specifically described.

Domain 2. Stakeholder involvement
4. The guideline development group includes individuals from all the prevalent professional groups.
5. The patient's views and preferences have been sought.
6. The target users of the guideline are clearly described.
7. The guideline has been piloted among target users.

Domain 3. Rigour of development
8. Systematic methods were used to search for evidence.
9. The criteria for selecting the evidence are clearly described.
10. The methods used for formulating the recommendations are clearly described.
11. The health benefits, side effects and risks have been considered in formulating the recommendations.
12. There is an explicit link between the recommendations and the supporting evidence.
13. The guideline has been externally reviewed by experts prior to its publication.
14. A procedure for updating the guideline is provided.

Domain 4. Clarity and presentation
15. The recommendations are specific and unambiguous.
16. The different options for management of condition are clearly presented.
17. Key recommendations are easily identifiable.
18. The guideline is supported with tools for application.

Domain 5. Applicability
19. The potential organizational barriers in applying the recommendations have been discussed.
20. The potential cost implications of applying the recommendations have been considered.
21. The guideline is supported with tools for application.

Domain 6. Editorial independence
22. The guideline is editorially independent from the funding body.
23. Conflicts of interest of guideline development members have been recorded.

national and pan-national stroke guidelines focussing on different aspects of stroke care (prevention to discharge). The Scottish Intercollegiate Guideline Network (SIGN) Guidelines for Management of Patients with Stroke (Scottish Intercollegiate Guideline Network, 2003) and the Royal College of Physicians Intercollegiate National Clinical Guidelines for Stroke (Royal College of Physicians, 2002a) both scored highly. Problem areas common to most of the guidelines were consideration of cost-effectiveness, absence of piloting, lack of support for application and poor recording of the perspectives and interests of the guideline developers.

The United Kingdom's National Service Frameworks

A number of the United Kingdom's guidelines have been particularly influential in shaping stroke services over the past decade. The Older Peoples' National Service Framework for England (Department of Health, 2001) has a separate chapter for stroke with an emphasis on prevention and specialist stroke care pathways from admission to life after discharge from hospital. There is a blueprint for a specialist service model built around multidisciplinary teams, including clinical psychologists, working primarily within designated stroke units. The publication of this framework in England, and its counterparts in Wales, Scotland and Northern Ireland, prompted a major expansion of specialist stroke units across Britain which in turn produced major improvements in outcomes for stroke survivors (Alawneh, Clatworthy, Morris & Warburton, 2010). There was also much of relevance to stroke in the National Service Framework for Long Term Neurological Conditions (Department of Health, 2005) which sets 11 quality standards:

- A person-centred service
- Early recognition and prompt diagnosis and treatment
- Emergency and acute management
- Early and specialist rehabilitation
- Community rehabilitation and support
- Vocational rehabilitation
- Providing equipment and accommodation
- Providing personal care and support
- Palliative care
- Supporting family and carers
- Caring for people in hospital or other health and social care settings

The United Kingdom's Clinical Guidelines for Stroke

Detailed and specific guidance on the care of stroke survivors and support for their carers is contained in the 'National Clinical Guidelines for Stroke'. These guidelines were developed by an interprofessional group under the aegis of the Royal College of Physicians and revisions have appeared at four-yearly intervals since the first edition in 2000 (Royal College of Physicians, 2000). Other indicators of service provision and performance have been collected and published at regular intervals in Stroke Sentinel Audits at local, regional and national levels (Royal College of Physicians, 2002b, 2005, 2007, 2008b, 2008c). More recently, additional guidelines for the management of the initial, acute phase, of stroke have been developed in collaboration with NICE (National Collaborating Centre for Chronic Conditions 2008). At the time of writing, NICE is also developing new generic 'quality standards' for stroke incorporating the National Clinical Guidelines and the Initial Management Guidelines (NICE, 2009b), and is developing guidelines for 'rehabilitation after stroke'.

Children fall outside of the generic stroke guidelines. Although uncommon, the incidence of stroke in childhood may exceed 3.3 per 100,000 (Lynch, Hirtz, DeVeber & Nelson, 2002). It affects several hundred children each year in the United Kingdom, and strokes were in the top ten causes of death in childhood. Special guidelines for childhood stroke have been developed in the United Kingdom (Paediatric Stroke Working Group Royal College of Physicians, 2004) and the United States (Roach, Golomb, Adams, Biller, Daniels, DeVeber *et al.*, 2008). The treatment of children with stroke in the United Kingdom is an exception in that it utilises paediatric services, ideally tertiary paediatric neurology services, rather than specialist stroke services. The paediatric services have special expertise in meeting the particular needs of children in relation to parenting, education and the longer term impact of a serious medical condition early in life. They are also conversant with the special legal framework for consent to treatment that applies to children and their parents. In addition, they are well placed to network with wider children's services within local authorities and third sector organisations. Because of their special characteristics and separateness, children's stroke services and strokes in childhood fit more comfortably into the domain of childhood illness and paediatrics, and have not been covered in this book.

The United Kingdom's home nations' stroke strategies

Comprehensive plans for stroke services are contained within the National Stroke Strategy for England (Department of Health, 2007a). This strategy, together with similar strategies for Wales, Scotland (Chest, Heart and Stroke Scotland, 2003b) and Northern Ireland (Department of Health, Social Services and Public Safety, 2008), aims to improve the prevention and treatment of stroke by articulating a series of 20 quality markers targeting aspects of stroke treatment as well as service configuration and service development. These stroke strategies also specify greater public and user involvement in service planning, delivery and monitoring and more user and carer involvement in planning their own treatment. A key feature is to raise public and professional awareness of stroke to the level achieved for coronary heart disease. Stroke is to be seen as a medical emergency, and a new slogan 'time is brain' is underpinned by an awareness that 1.9 million neurons may die for each minute that a new stroke goes untreated. This provides the rationale for the development of services to permit the rapid treatment of stroke within specialist acute units. There is considerable enthusiasm for 'clot-busting' (thrombolysis) treatment within the first hours after stroke onset for at least some of the strokes caused by clots, because there is good evidence that if given quickly it reduces rates of death and dependency (Wardlaw, del Zoppo, Yamaguchi & Berge, 2009). The NICE guidelines for the diagnosis and management of the acute phase of stroke (National Collaborating Centre for Chronic Conditions, 2008) will undoubtedly encourage more widespread application of thrombolysis for stroke.

However, even timely thrombolysis leaves a significant proportion of survivors with major impairments and dependency, and it is salutary to note that the 2008 sentinel audit found less than 1% of all stroke survivors in the United Kingdom received thrombolysis (Royal College of Physicians, 2008b). Moreover, a significant proportion of stroke survivors cannot receive thrombolysis due to exclusion criteria, such as concurrent health conditions, seizures and haemorrhagic aetiology, or due to missing the four and a half-hour maximum treatment 'window' because of uncertainty about time of onset, having a stroke while sleeping, delays in transfer to hospital and delays in brain imaging. Even people with seemingly mild symptoms, or no obvious residual deficits, can be adversely affected with significantly reduced quality of life and emotional, social and mental health problems (Duncan, Samsa, Weinberger, Goldstein, Bonito, Witter, Enarson & Matchar, 1997). For these reasons, it is important that medium-term rehabilitation and long-term care in the community are not neglected, and that psychological approaches to helping those with major long-term stroke-related disabilities continue to be developed and applied.

With this in mind, the stroke strategy was not limited to acute treatments, and it provides a framework for rehabilitation and long-term services, stipulating close monitoring through regular audits against the quality markers. The strategy seeks to improve services through better integration within service networks and by proactive workforce planning and enhanced staff training. Psychological needs of survivors and carers are also considered. Quality Marker 2 is concerned with managing lifestyle risks such as diet, smoking and alcohol. Quality Marker 3 emphasises the need for survivors, carers and relatives to have information, advice, emotional support and advocacy throughout the stroke care pathway and lifelong. Quality Marker 8 recommends immediate structured assessment including screening for cognitive and perceptual problems. Quality Markers 15 and 16 are concerned with community integration and return to work, respectively, and Quality Marker 20 reinforces the need for research and audit into all aspects of care to increase the scope and quality of the evidence base.

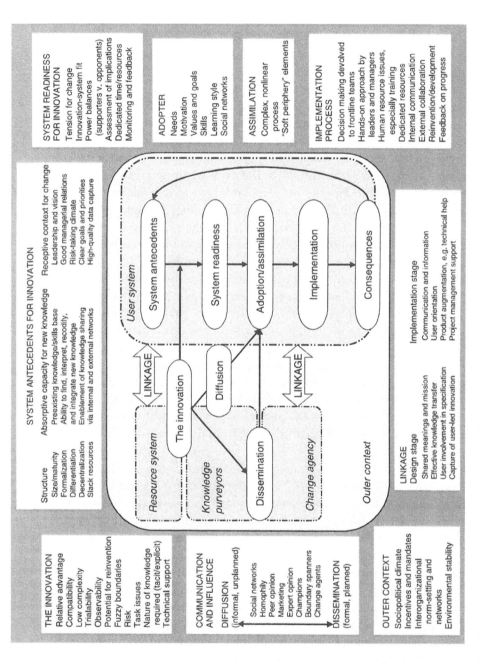

Figure 2.1 Conceptual model for the adoption of innovations. From Greenhalgh, T., Robert, G., Macfarlane, F., Bate, P., & Kyriakidou, O. (2004). Diffusion of innovations in service organizations: Systematic review and recommendations. *Milbank Quarterly*, 82, 581–629. © Milbank Memorial Fund.

The strategy provides a blueprint, but the degree of specificity and the clarity of its recommendations vary considerably from the very specific and concrete guidelines for aspects of acute medical care, to less well-articulated, general aspirations for many aspects of psychological relevance, such as the provision of 'emotional support' and 'psychological care'. Nevertheless, it provides a framework with considerable potential for the development and enhancement of psychological care for stroke survivors and their families. The changes in service organisation and delivery between 2006 and 2010 stemming from the National Stroke Strategy for England, coupled with the development of performance indicators, audits and additional funding, have reduced the chances of dying from a stroke within 10 years from 71% to 67%. At the same time, the average number of quality-adjusted life years (QALYs) per patient has increased from 2.3 to 2.5 with a modest increase in per-patient cost of only 7% in real terms (National Audit Office, 2010).

The United Kingdom Stroke-Specific Education Framework

The National Strategy for Stroke has already stimulated and informed the development of a United Kingdom Stroke-Specific Education Framework (UK Forum for Stroke Training, 2009) which specifies the service requirements, knowledge, skills and competencies needed for 16 elements of care within the stroke pathway. These 16 elements are closely linked to the first 16 Quality Markers of the Strategy which relate to the direct care and follow-up of stroke survivors. The final four quality markers are concerned with service aspects and are not included in the education framework.

Knowledge translation, implementation of guidelines and audit

The formulation of guidelines is only part of the endeavour aimed at improving services. The second part is the translation of guidelines into practice. Greenhalgh, Robert, Macfarlane, Bate and Kyriakidou (2004) summarised the outcome of a comprehensive review of research and theory relevant to implementation of innovations in healthcare that was commissioned by the United Kingdom's Department of Health. The conclusions are summarised in Figure 2.1 and demonstrate that the adoption of new practices depend on a large number of interdependent elements, many of which interact in a complex and recursive fashion. The elements include attributes of the innovation itself, the manner in which it is disseminated, the characteristics of adopting individuals and the organisation, the process used for implementation and finally the overarching context and climate. The processes involved in adoption may be even more multifaceted than implied by the model of Greenhalgh *et al.* (2004), and Grol, Bosch, Hulscher, Eccles and Wensing (2007) discussed over 20 relevant theoretical perspectives encompassing the process of change itself, the individual professional, the social setting, the organizational context, the political context and the economic context. Moreover, none of the analyses above incorporates consideration of the impact of service user characteristics and the influence of service user organisations.

The method used for dissemination is one crucial factor in successful implementation. Bero, Grilli, Grimshaw, Harvey, Oxman and Thomson (1998) reviewed the knowledge translation literature and identified four effective dissemination strategies:

- Educational outreach visits
- Reminders, manual or computerised
- Multifaceted interventions, combining two or more of the following:
    o Audit and feedback
    o Reminders
    o Local consensus processes
    o Marketing
- Interactive educational meetings (e.g. participation of staff in workshops)

Bero *et al.* (1998) concluded that several approaches, which were generally considered to be effective, were in fact unreliable in improving compliance with guidelines. These were audit and feedback alone, local champions, local discussion and patient-mediated interventions. They also concluded that there was a lack of evidence for the effectiveness of both the distribution guidelines and of didactic teaching in changing practice. These conclusions were broadly echoed by Grol and Grimshaw (2003) following a review of studies on changing practice for hand hygiene, but they added the caveat that dissemination efforts may need to be tailored to the particular treatment or practice involved, and adapted according to the nature of the evidence and the target organisation or service.

Despite the evidence that audit alone does not improve adherence to guidelines, audit against the standards set by the National Clinical Guidelines for Stroke (Stroke Sentinel Audits) have been the main approach to monitoring stroke guidelines in the United Kingdom, and have occurred at regular intervals since 2002. The results have indicated the proportion of stroke survivors who were able to access specialist services, and the proportion that were treated in particular ways known to improve outcomes. They have also revealed service shortfalls, and were helpful in identifying lack of psychological services and low rates of screening for depression (see the 'Psychological Services for Stroke' section of this chapter). The results were broken down into regions and individual services, to identify precisely where changes in organisation or practice were required. Once areas of noncompliance have been identified, psychological approaches may be of value in understanding why individual staff comply or fail to comply with guidelines and in formulating interventions to improve compliance (Grol, Bosch, Hulscher, Eccles & Wensing, 2007). The theory of planned behaviour (Ajzen, 1985) holds that behaviour is determined by behavioural intention, which is itself determined by the evaluation of a course of action (is it effective?), perceptions of others' views about the action (do colleagues think it is worthwhile?) and belief in personal control over performing the action (is it possible for me to perform it?). Elements of the model were associated with adherence to stroke care guidelines (Hart & Morris, 2008), and the approach could potentially be harnessed to inform interventions aimed at increasing compliance, as it has in domains other than stroke (Elliott & Armitage, 2009). Several elements of the theory of planned behaviour were also reflected in the outcome of a study by that used panels of healthcare 'experts' to arrive at a consensus about the factors underpinning change in individual practice (Michie, Johnston, Abraham, Lawton, Parker, Walker *et al.*, 2005). Twelve influences were identified: (1) knowledge, (2) skills, (3) social and professional role and identity, (4) beliefs about capabilities, (5) beliefs about consequences, (6) motivation and goals, (7) memory, attention and decision processes, (8) environmental context and resources, (9) social influences, (10) emotion regulation, (11) behavioural regulation and (12) nature of the behaviour. Once again, interventions targeting these domains for individual staff may improve implementation of guidelines, but other factors, such as organisational and contextual influences, also require consideration (Greenhalgh *et al.*, 2004). An approach that shows promise is the engagement of facilitators, individuals who assist those adopting the innovation to achieve the goals of implementation by providing them with practical help or more general 'enabling' assistance (Rycroft-Malone, Kitson, Harvey, McCormack, Seers, Titchen *et al.*, 2002). Facilitators are able to assess and respond to events and influences from a variety of sources and may proactively defend the intervention effort from derailment by barriers and capitalise on any beneficial events that occur.

Unfortunately, achieving significant change in the practices used in stroke services through the implementation of guidelines faces considerable obstacles. Korner-Bitensky, Menon-Nair, Thomas, Boutin and Arafah (2007) surveyed 243 stroke practitioners (physiotherapists and occupational therapists) and found that over half preferred to base their practice on considerations of workload demands, patient flow and patient satisfaction rather than evidence of treatment efficacy. The most frequent reason for using a treatment was that the practitioner had learnt it in college (and half the sample had trained more than ten years earlier!). Less than 10% of the staff were classified as seeking evidence about treatment effectiveness, and this compared with 3% reported in similar studies of medical practitioners.

Despite these obstacles, there is evidence that adherence to stroke guidelines can be improved. Schwamm, Fonarow, Reeves, Pan, Frankel, Smith, Ellrodt, Cannon, Liang, Peterson and LaBresh (2009) found significant improvements in the adherence to guidelines for the provision of six medical stroke treatments, and for smoking cessation over a five-year period. A composite performance measure improved from 83.52% to 93.97% during the intervention period which encompassed over 300,000 patients in nearly 800 hospitals in the United States. The intervention itself was a multifaceted intervention package 'get with the guidelines' (Labresh & Tyler, 2003) that included organizational-level stakeholder meeting, local champions, opinion leader meetings, an internet-based guideline tool, training sessions with follow-up, continuous audit cycles with rapid dissemination of outcomes and an accreditation system for participating hospitals that required staff attendance at national events.

Psychological services for stroke

During their treatment and aftercare, stroke survivors will experience several services: ambulance, accident and emergency, acute medical unit, rehabilitation ward, a specialist community stroke team or generic community healthcare team and possibly also support through stroke clubs and voluntary sector organisations such as Different Strokes and the Stroke Association. Psychological problems may arise at any stage, and psychological expertise may be required for one or more of several problems that commonly occur after stroke. Cognition may be affected from time of the stroke, and early multidisciplinary assessment has been recommended (Department of Health, 2007a; Duncan, Zorowitz, Bates, Choi, Glasberg, Graham, Katz, Lamberty & Reker, 2005). Neuropsychological assessment by a psychologist can be especially useful in identifying hidden, complex and high-level impairments. Mood disorders may occur at any time after a stroke, and affect about a third of all survivors at some stage (Hackett, Yapa, Parag & Anderson, 2005). Consequently survivors require regular monitoring of mood, and a proportion of them require specialist treatment for depression. Stroke survivors and carers experience a range of transitional psychosocial issues soon after discharge, and the trend towards earlier discharge may present increasingly complex challenges (Pringle, Hendry & McLafferty, 2008) that require psychological interventions. Some stroke survivors may experience problems with community reintegration, especially with retuning to work, and others may experience mental health difficulties that affect treatment adherence or recovery. In view of the number and salience of psychological issues facing stroke survivors, access to a psychologist, as part of the core post-acute rehabilitation team, has been recommended in the United Kingdom (Department of Health, 2001; Royal College of Physicians, 2008a) and in the United States (American Heart Association/American Stroke Association Endorsed Practice Guidelines; Duncan *et al.*, 2005).

A list of the major psychological needs of stroke survivors and their carers was presented in the revised British Psychological Society 'Guidelines for Stroke' (Division of Clinical Psychology/Division of Neuropsychology, 2010). This document also reviewed the evidence base for assessments and psychological interventions designed to address the needs that were identified:

- Cognitive impairments
- Reactions to disability and dependency
- Depression and emotional lability
- Anxiety and trauma; assessment and treatment
- Post-stroke pain
- Post-stroke fatigue
- Adjustment difficulties and challenging behaviour
- Carer support
- Improving service delivery

Because psychological needs arise at different stages and encompass many different areas, psychological services require a commensurate degree of flexibility to enable assessments and interventions to take place. Interventions for needs such as depression and anxiety have been developed and evaluated in the mental health sphere and are included in NICE guidelines for mental health conditions (NICE, 2009a, 2011). In selecting psychological treatments it will be important to establish that mental-health derived treatments for anxiety, depression and trauma are effective in stroke and not to rely only on evidence from mentally ill populations. Generic, mental health interventions will need to be sensitively adapted when used in the stroke arena, and this may require input from a psychologist or psychiatrist with knowledge and experience of stroke and the particular treatment.

The aim of the British Psychological Society, Division of Neuropsychology/Division of Clinical Psychology guidance was to brief service managers when planning stroke services. They recommended staffing levels for an average general hospital catchment area of 500,000 as two whole-time-equivalent qualified clinical psychologists and one whole-time-equivalent psychology assistant. *At least* one of the qualified posts should be *additional* to the provision recommended for older adult services. At the present time this remains an aspiration rather than a reality, since the advent of specialist hospital-based stroke units has unfortunately not produced a commensurate increase in psychological care. Successive sentinel audits have recorded little improvement, the most recent revealing that only one third of stroke units had access to clinical psychology services, and that even where psychologists were present, the whole time equivalent per bed was low (Royal College of Physicians, 2008b). There were no comparable figures for community services, but the lack of psychology is likely to be as marked, or even greater. This state of affairs has come about despite the recommendations of the National Service Framework and the National Clinical Guidelines for Stroke which both highlight the need for clinical psychology service input and the vital role of clinical psychologists in the stroke team.

> The most striking observations are the dire shortage of psychology services (needed to define cognitive deficits, to work with other professionals to maximise rehabilitation potential, to help with the management of mood disorders and provide

support to patients and carers dealing with a major life event). (Royal College of Physicians, 2008b, p.13)

One psychologically relevant standard for stroke care (Royal College of Physicians, 2008a) that has consistently been poorly met and shown little improvement over successive sentinel audits is screening for mood; only a little over half of survivors (55%) had their mood screened in 2006 (Royal College of Physicians, 2007), and this figure rose by only 10% in the next two years to 65% (Royal College of Physicians, 2008c). Compliance with screening requires staff awareness of its need and purpose, relevant knowledge and skill, belief in its efficacy, organisational support and a sense that it is part of their role (Hart & Morris, 2008). Therefore, it is unsurprising that standards of psychological significance, such as mood screening, mirrored the standard for psychology service input and were not achieved when psychological services were absent or severely limited. The lack of clinical psychology services was also reflected in the results of studies of experiences of stroke care; psychological aspects of care were often reported as the most problematic areas by carers and survivors (see below).

The scarcity of psychologists in stroke services means that assessment and treatment of psychological issues must often be provided by other healthcare professions, and the psychologist's role may be to provide training, supervision and support to those involved in direct care, rather than providing it themselves (Division of Clinical Psychology, 2007). Some specific therapies that have traditionally been practised by psychologists, such as cognitive-behavioural therapy, are increasingly being taught to other professions and generic mental health workers (Department of Health, 2008b). Consequently, some services employ therapists to deliver evidence-based therapies, such as cognitive-behavioural therapy for depression (despite limited evidence for its effectiveness after stroke), with a psychologist providing support and supervision as required. An intervention based on motivational interviewing has shown promise in both preventing and treating depression post stroke (Watkins, Auton, Deans, Dickinson, Jack, Lightbody et al., 2008). This intervention was delivered by nurses and psychology graduates, with specific training and supervised by a clinical psychologist. It is also feasible that some of the shortfall in psychologists could be offset by other professions, such as psychiatrists with a specific remit for input into mental health issues arising from physical health conditions (liaison psychiatrists), and this may be the case in some countries. However, in the United Kingdom most psychiatrists for working-age adults are based in mental health services with strict criteria for inclusion, such as psychosis, substance abuse and severe depression; they do not normally become involved with depressed stroke survivors unless the condition is severe and resistant to treatment by conventional antidepressants. Acceptance for treatment by mental health teams is often considered but rejected due to the presence of stroke as a comorbidity. For older stroke survivors, psycho-geriatric services may become involved, but normally only when there is severe cognitive impairment combined with challenging behaviour. This paucity of mental health services for stroke survivors highlights the need for psychologists to be available within stroke services, as recommended by UK and US guidelines.

The subsequent chapters of this book will help to remind service leaders of the evidence for the importance of psychological factors, such as depression and anxiety, in directly determining outcomes, the role of cognition and behaviour in determining the level of care and supervision required and finally the place of personality, culture, beliefs and attitudes in shaping orientation towards care and perceptions of its acceptability. It is hoped this may help to engender services that consider and meet the many and varied psychological needs of stroke survivors and carers.

Improving psychological outcomes through service organisation

This section will consider service provisions that are relevant to psychological well-being, but are not specifically psychological interventions; for example, the implementation of goal setting, the provision of particular (nonpsychology) therapists or family support workers. Specific psychology interventions, such as cognitive rehabilitation or psychotherapies for depression and anxiety, will be considered in the relevant chapters. When considering the evidence, it is important to distinguish three key elements that determine the success of healthcare intervention (Donabedian, 1993). The first is efficacy, the improvement that the intervention brings in ideal conditions which is normally assessed in randomised controlled trials. The second element is effectiveness, or the improvement realised when the intervention is used in normal practice, and the third is efficiency, or the reduction in the cost afforded by the intervention. For the interventions described below, the research deals principally with efficacy, and effectiveness and efficiency data are available only for specialist stroke unit care.

Specialist stroke units

There is ample evidence from randomised controlled trials, and other sources, that treatment in specialist stroke units and special stroke care pathways reduces death and dependency, and that many of the specific treatments used within specialist stroke services are effective (Alawneh *et al.*, 2010). A large-scale systematic review (Stroke Unit Trialists' Collaboration, 2007), included nearly 7000 stroke survivors in over 25 trials. Despite variability across trials and a number of neutral results, this meta-analysis found that treatment in organised stroke units produced a small, but significant reduction in death rate and larger improvements in the combined outcomes of death plus dependency and death plus institutionalisation. The benefits were maintained at five years post stroke and were found across the age range and in males and females. Length of stay was also shorter in organised stroke units than in general wards or other types of care. Two of the three trials that collected survivor satisfaction data showed survivors favoured stroke unit care, but one found no difference in satisfaction. Stroke unit care was superior to care in general wards or less specialist units, but effects for individual outcome measures, such as dependency, institutionalisation and death rates, were modest or nonsignificant, and the benefits of stroke unit care were robust only for combined measures (e.g. death and dependency, or death and institutionalisation). Unfortunately, the psychological measures used in some of the studies were not included in the meta-analysis, so information about the psychological benefits of stroke units is absent. Seenan, Long and Langhorne (2007) conducted a review of observational studies of stroke care and concluded that the benefits of specialist stroke care were replicated in normal practice, outside of clinical trials. While the evidence for improvement in combined outcome measures is important, the lack of consistent effects on individual outcome measures makes it harder to determine which components of care, or combinations of components, promote the observed benefits. Morris, Payne and Lambert (2007), using qualitative methods to explore the perceptions of staff, found that stroke unit staff valued specialisation, it improved their sense of efficacy and morale and it also fostered a sense of sharing and camaraderie between survivors. However, staff reported that specialisation could also engender service fragmentation and conflict. Survivors' with comorbid conditions, such as heart disease or dementia, require careful consideration, since specialist stroke unit staff may lack some of the generic skills of staff on general medical wards. It is important that such survivors receive the best care, and feel that they are receiving the best care, for all their significant conditions.

Goal setting

A number of studies have considered specific organisational aspects of stroke teams that may impact on a range of outcomes, including those of psychological significance. In a series of articles in 1999, Wade (1999a, 1999b) addressed goal setting in stroke care. Evidence was sparse, but Wade found 13 randomised trials and two controlled clinical trials; none were specific to stroke, but four involved brain-damaged individuals. The results pointed to the benefits of goals setting at team and individual therapist level. Benefits were maximised when goal setting involved survivors and set reachable, but challenging, long- and short-term targets. Wade concluded that the planning of individual, patient-centred goals was vital for the proper coordination of therapy within multidisciplinary stroke teams. However, goal planning required careful implementation and monitoring; goals could be vague and specificity differed between rehabilitation professions, there was sometimes a lack of survivor involvement in goal setting, and there was a risk that goals focused on service needs rather than the survivor's needs (Wressle, Oberg & Henriksson, 1999). A study of rehabilitation professionals using the Delphi technique (Playford, Siegert, Levack & Freeman, 2009) showed consensus about the importance of goal setting and that goals should be specific, relevant to survivors, time limited, ambitious and incremental. Goal setting was also seen as a central aspect of the relationship between survivor and professional. There was less agreement about the balance between the ambitiousness and achievability of goals, and the extent to which patient-centred goals could be realised.

Multidisciplinary coordination

Stroke teams typically communicate and coordinate their activity and set goals in weekly multidisciplinary meetings where stroke survivors are discussed, but usually not present. However, another model for team coordination is the multidisciplinary ward round, where the different professions meet with each other and then with each survivor in turn (Monaghan, Channell, McDowell & Sharma, 2005). Using this model, Monaghan *et al.* (2005) showed improvements in meeting the standards for stroke set by the National Service Framework for Older People, number of survivors' needs considered, appropriate goal setting and survivor involvement. There was also a more positive team climate. The ward-round was the third phase of the study, coming after a phase that used multi-disciplinary team meetings, so greater practice in achieving standards, rather than the different model of team coordination, may have underpinned the improvement. Despite this, the approach shows promise and merits further evaluation.

Early supported discharge

Early supported discharge home, where survivors return home early to complete their rehabilitation with continuing care and therapy from a multidisciplinary team, is a service-based approach that has been found to improve outcome. A meta analysis of 11 randomised controlled trials including 1597 survivors (Langhorne, Taylor, Murray, Dennis, Anderson, Bautz-Holter *et al.*, 2005) comparing early supported discharge with conventional hospital care found a reduced risk of death or dependency combined, but no significant improvement in death rates alone, a shorter hospital stay by eight days on average, an increased probability of returning home and greater reported satisfaction with services. The effect on independence in activities of daily living was not consistent across measures; the extended activities of daily living scales showed an improvement, but not the personal activities of daily living scales. Benefits were greatest when survivors were supported by a specialist multidisciplinary team comprised of physiotherapy, occupational therapy and speech and language therapy staff with medical, nursing, and social work support, whose work was coordinated through regular meetings (Langhorne *et al.*, 2005). Larsen, Olsen and Sorensen (2006) reviewed the outcome of seven randomised controlled trials and concluded that institutionalisation and length of stay were improved by early supported discharge, but death rates were unaffected. The effect of early discharge on functioning as measured by the Barthel Index (Collin, Wade, Davies & Horne 1988; Mahoney & Barthel, 1965) differed between the studies reviewed, and the authors concluded that the psychological skills of the multidisciplinary support team were determinants of outcome. A systematic review (Langhorne & Widen-Holmqvist, 2007) discussed the trials included in the earlier meta-analysis (Langhorne *et al.*, 2005) and one additional randomised controlled trial. The conclusions were similar to the earlier review; there was no overall effect of early supported discharge on survivors' death rates, independence as measured by the personal activities in daily living scales, subjective health status or mood scores, or on carer outcomes. However, survivors who received this intervention were more likely to be able to live at home and were more satisfied. This last finding may reflect the concordance of this approach with many survivors' desire to return home as soon as possible. The effects were consistently observed across trials and statistically significant, but relatively small. As expected, hospital stays were reduced significantly. In addition, the only model of care that was found to be effective was the inclusion of a specialist stroke coordinator in addition to a multidisciplinary team. Stroke unit treatment with early supported discharge has also been found to be more cost-effective than stroke unit treatment alone (Saka, Serra, Samyshkin, McGuire & Wolfe, 2009). In conclusion, the studies included in the reviews highlighted the complex nature of early supported discharge services and the importance of staff skills and partnership working with survivors and carers. Despite the modest improvements in outcomes, the reduction in hospital stay was an important factor to many survivors since it enabled them to start their community re-integration sooner.

Family support workers

Another intervention that has been studied systematically using randomised controlled trials is the provision of post-discharge support to survivors and their carers. In a meta-analysis of 16 studies employing stroke liaison workers, Ellis (2006, 2007) concluded that the only dependable result was an increase in survivor and carer satisfaction. Visser-Meily, van Heugten, Post, Schepers and Lindeman (2005), in a review of interventions for caregivers, identified ten studies that used support interventions after discharge. The results of these studies were mixed, improvements in carer function were found in only four of ten studies, and even in these studies effects across the major outcome measures were not consistent. This approach will be considered in greater detail in chapter 20, which focuses on the carers and families of stroke survivors.

Input from professions

Some studies have looked at the benefits to community-living stroke survivors of having input from a particular profession. Three systematic reviews of the benefits of occupational therapy (Legg, Drummond & Langhorne, 2006; Legg, Drummond, Leonardi-Bee, Gladman, Corr, Donkervoort *et al.*, 2007; Walker, Leonardi-Bee, Bath, Langhorne, Dewey, Corr *et al.*, 2004) all concluded that occupational therapy for survivors after discharge from hospital was beneficial. In contrast, several large-scale trials produced nonsignificant results including Parker, Gladman, Drummond, Dewey, Lincoln, Barer *et al.* (2001), and benefits may have been restricted to the particular target of the therapy. For example, occupation therapy focussed upon activities of daily living improved a range of activities of daily living, but did not improve leisure activities. Conversely, leisure-focussed occupational therapy improved leisure activities, but not activities of daily living (Walker *et al.*, 2004). However, occupational therapy targeted on personal activities of daily living did increase performance in these activities and also had a significant impact on combined outcome measures which included dependency (Legg *et al.*, 2007).

Information provision

Finally, information provision has been consistently identified as a prominent concern of stroke survivors and carers in large-scale surveys (Healthcare Commission 2005; Kelson, Ford & Rigge, 1998; Stroke Association, 2001) and is a central quality marker in the stroke strategy for England (Department of Health 2007a). Good-quality information is of profound psychological importance. It underpins peoples' ability to understand and predict events, to put their current predicament into perspective and to manage their anxiety about the future, and it influences their capacity to behave in ways that reduce risks and enhance well-being through treatment adherence. Stroke is a condition that affects the ability to assimilate information due to the shock of its sudden and unexpected onset and its effect on information processing and memory. Consequently, effective communication may require services to adopt special strategies for information provision. Smith, Forster, House, Knapp, Wright and Young (2008) reviewed 17 randomised controlled trials of the provision of information to stroke survivors and carers. They concluded that interventions to enhance information provision improved knowledge, increased satisfaction with aspects of information provision and reduced depression but did not have a measureable impact on anxiety, survival or other functional outcomes. Active involvement of survivors in obtaining information was superior to simply giving out information. These results provide compelling evidence for the role of information in recovery from stroke, and may even underestimate its importance, since a lack of comparable measures across studies meant that many outcome measures were not evaluated using data from all the trials, and this reduced the statistical power to detect positive effects.

Swain, Ellins, Coulter, Heron, Howell, Magee *et al.* (2007) reported a study of focus groups of service users with a variety of conditions that used probes to test the adequacy of the information services that they accessed. They found that information was frequently available, but was not well presented, signposted or coordinated across organisations and sectors. Service users most frequently wanted information about:

- voluntary sector support groups,
- support for the family or carer(s),
- condition-specific services,
- the financial benefits available and how to claim them, and
- how to comment on or complain about services.

   The report made a number of recommendations, including the development of centralised information resources to signpost available information sources, staffed by people who seek out and disseminate information.

Satisfaction with services

The gathering of information about service recipients' experiences of services by interviews, focus groups or questionnaires, is perhaps the most intrinsically psychological approach to evaluating services, since it relies on peoples' perceptions and judgements. It also provides a route to establishing what people think about services and how they are likely to behave towards them. Patients' and carers' views about their healthcare have typically been assessed by patient 'satisfaction' measures. There is evidence that satisfaction does reflect differences in care received by stroke survivors (Pound, Tilling, Rudd & Wolfe, 1999) and that survivors' perceptions of their unmet care needs accurately reflect their health needs (Scholte op Reimer, de Haan, Limburg & van den Bos, 1996). Moreover, satisfaction has been shown to be related to compliance with treatment (Harris, Luft, Rudy & Tierney, 1995) and with willingness to return for further treatment (Meterko, Nelson & Rubin, 1990). Some studies have even found improvement in satisfaction to be the main beneficial outcome attributable to new treatments (Dennis, O'Rourke, Slattery, Staniforth & Warlow, 1997). Ellis (2006) also reached the conclusion that increased satisfaction was the main dependable improvement across studies of the effects of providing stroke liaison workers.

   However, satisfaction is a complex concept with many determinants that are unrelated to the quality of care received (Fitzpatrick, 1990), and its measurement may foster an illusory sense of objectivity that masks a failure to capture important aspects of service users' experiences and perceptions (Williams, 1994). The determinants of satisfaction include age, perceived health and mental health (Cleary, Edgmanlevitan, Roberts, Moloney, McMullen, Walker & Delbanco, 1991; Rahmqvist, 2001) and expectations (Sitzia & Wood, 1997). Because of this, global satisfaction ratings are unlikely to reflect the adequacy, appropriateness or efficacy of care received. Recipients of treatments may find it particularly difficult to evaluate them and make satisfaction ratings when the treatments are complex, technical or delivered when the person is not fully alert (Fitzpatrick, 1990). Scholte op Reimer *et al.* (1996) provided a good example of how satisfaction ratings may fail to capture important aspects of care. In their questionnaire study of the relationship between satisfaction and aspects of stroke care in 23 hospitals in the Netherlands, two important objective quality markers, continuity of care and secondary prevention of stroke, were unrelated to satisfaction. However, two factors of psychological significance, perceived unmet needs and emotional distress, were associated with satisfaction. The issues described above have raised questions about the usefulness of patient satisfaction as a general approach to gauging service quality (Haas, 1999).

The measurement of patient satisfaction is also fraught with difficulties (Carrhill, 1992), with many questionnaires being poorly constructed and inadequately validated (Sitzia, 1999). Specific criticisms include the observation that measures are professionally determined and do not measure things of importance to care recipients; they are based upon expectations and preferences rather than experience, and take an over-simplified perspective of the relationship between satisfaction and dissatisfaction. A series of in-depth interviews with patients demonstrated that patients' evaluation of healthcare was biased towards positive judgements and an avoidance of complaining (Staniszewska & Henderson, 2005). Factors predisposing to positive evaluations include loyalty, luck, gratitude, faith and comparison with the less fortunate. Further evidence for the limitations of satisfaction as an index of the quality of care comes from a large-scale study which found that over half of the patients rating inpatient care as 'excellent' actually had problems with 10% of the aspects of healthcare included in the questionnaire (Jenkinson, Coulter, Bruster, Richards & Chandola, 2002). Similarly, 97% of stroke survivors and 92% of carers were satisfied with acute stroke care, despite 46% of the survivors and 66% of carers being dissatisfied with at least one aspect of care (Wellwood, Dennis & Warlow, 1995).

Stroke survivor experience in services

Because of these shortcomings, recent large-scale approaches to the assessment of the quality of care have eschewed patient satisfaction in favour of obtaining information about specific, concrete experiences within the care system (Jenkinson *et al.*, 2002). This approach was adopted by the Healthcare Commission and has been used in national studies of patient experience during inpatient and community stroke care (Healthcare Commission, 2005, 2006).

Studies of stroke survivors' views and experience have told us much about services. The Stroke Association (2001) carried out a questionnaire survey of stroke survivors that included carer experiences and provided opportunities for individualised comments. They obtained 2252 responses from members of the association and from advertisements, but the date of the hospital admission and the time since the stroke were highly variable. At the time of the survey, which predated the implementation of the Older People's NSF and the widespread availability of specialist stroke care, survivors and carers reported very significant problems with services. These highlighted the omission of important aspects of care, delays, poor service quality, lack of information and deficient support for carers. Kelson *et al.* (1998) conducted a study using focus groups and individual interviews with stroke survivors and carers recruited through the Stroke Association and Different Strokes in England. This study was also conducted before the Older People's NSF and the widespread availability of specialist stroke units. They found that experiences were highly variable: many survivors and carers felt that the services offered were of a high quality, while others had experienced significant shortcomings. The issues resembled those found by the Stroke Association (2001), but other issues emerged as well: lack of acknowledgement of symptoms on admission, lack of understanding of needs by staff, lack of staff knowledge and skills relevant to stroke care, poor communication with survivors, mismanagement of pre-existing or comorbid conditions and pessimistic predictions about recovery. A study of wards and units in Southampton in the United Kingdom included an audit against good practice guidelines and a brief survivor survey which drew 55 responses. One third of survivors were dissatisfied with their hospital care, particularly the lack of therapy and information, staff shortages and poor knowledge and awareness of stroke amongst staff (Tyson & Turner, 1999).

A more recent and systematic survey, after the introduction of specialist stroke units, was conducted by the Healthcare Commission in 2004 (Healthcare Commission, 2005). This surveyed the hospital and immediate post-discharge experiences of more than 1700 stroke survivors in 51 acute hospital Trusts in England over a three-month period. It used a questionnaire with 54 questions that focussed on the survivors' experiences, but a significant limitation was that it did not ask about the experiences of carers. There was an opportunity to comment at the end under two headings, 'Was there anything especially good about your care?' and 'Could anything have been improved?', and the questions themselves were framed after consultations with stroke survivors to ensure their relevance. The study found a high level of satisfaction with inpatient care (69% rated it as 'excellent' or 'very good'), and the ratings were more positive when survivors were cared for in specialist stroke units than in general wards. However, there were also unmet needs. Identified problem areas were lack of information, poor preparation for discharge and inadequate post-discharge support, lack of involvement in decisions and few opportunities to ask questions about care. Survivors also felt that there was a lack of specific therapies, inadequate help with personal care (especially toileting) and too little attention to emotional problems. In this context, it is disappointing that the questionnaire included cognitive difficulties (confusion) along with depression and crying in a single question on 'emotional issues', thus making it impossible to separate out these important aspects of psychological care. The Health Care Commission (2006) followed up

875 of these survivors for a year into the community care phase. While the survivors were generally positive about care received from GPs, the overall evaluation of care was much lower than during the hospital phase, and only 22% reported 'excellent' or 'good' care (27% fewer than in the hospital phase). However, those treated in specialist stroke units generally made better evaluations of their care. From a psychological perspective, one of the most frequently reported shortfalls was lack of emotional care, with 49% of participants finding this to be the case. Information about stroke and stroke services and involvement in decision making were other important shortfalls of psychological importance, as was perceived lack of support for carers. Carers were not included in the survey, so the results were based on the perceptions of the survivors alone. The survivors also experienced difficulties with obtaining practical support for everyday living.

A study of a hospital stroke service using focus groups (Morris *et al.*, 2007) included carers as well as survivors and found that both these groups highlighted four areas as important determinants of their experience: information, the attitudes of staff, the availability of therapies and being treated as a complete person with a history and wider interests and needs than only their recovery from stroke. The carers additionally highlighted the importance of attention to the survivors' individual needs and the impact of the burden of care.

Taken together, these findings suggest that survivors' experience of stroke care has improved markedly with the advent of specialist care. In contrast, needs of a primarily psychological nature, such as support for emotional and cognitive difficulties, information, being treated as a complete person and empowerment through inclusion in decision making, are still often unmet. Once again, these findings point up the severe shortage of psychological input to these services. The literature also demonstrates that carers' experience of services is a relatively neglected area. No large-scale recent surveys included carers, other than one in Scotland that included carers and survivors (Chest Heart and Stroke Scotland, 2003a), and many of the small-scale studies of carers used unstandardised questionnaires that focussed on global satisfaction (Low, Payne & Roderick, 1999).

Stroke services: staff, the neglected dimension

Many of the shortfalls in service provision stem from organisational and staff factors within stroke teams rather than any lack of suitable treatments or assessments. Screening for mood is one such example; several potentially suitable screening instruments exist, but they are not used consistently. It is a truism to say that 'any service is just as good as its staff', and studies in mixed hospital wards have demonstrated the importance of staff factors. Staff satisfaction and morale were associated with patients' satisfaction (Weisman & Nathanson, 1985; Fosbinder, 1994; Tzeng, Ketefian & Redman, 2002) and good doctor–nurse collaboration was also related to patients' satisfaction (Larrabee, Ostrow, Withrow, Janney, Hobbs & Burant, 2004). Despite this evidence, there has been remarkably little research into the perceptions, experiences and functioning of staff in stroke services.

Tyson and Turner (1999) included an 'open-ended' staff question asking for explanations of service shortfalls. They found that many staff were not aware of omissions in care, but did acknowledge lack of knowledge and skills in some areas and that staffing levels were too low to perform all their roles adequately. Hart and Morris (2008) found further evidence for shortfalls in knowledge in one specific area; only 8% of multidisciplinary staff reported being conversant with mood screening guidelines. Bennett (1996) interviewed stroke rehabilitation nurses about caring for stroke survivors with depression, and found that lack of training, time and skills were perceived as barriers to effective care for this condition. Burton (2000b) interviewed nurses in stroke rehabilitation and delineated three aspects of their role: caregiver, facilitator of personal recovery and care manager. Time restrictions limited their engagement in the second role. Bendz (2003) examined the reactions and feelings of younger stroke survivors (under 65) in the first year after stroke and compared these with the written notes of staff. The results suggested that staff ignored important subjective reactions such as loss of control, fatigue and fear of relapse, and instead took a more goal-focussed approach with an emphasis on functions and training. Morris *et al.* (2007) conducted focus groups with staff and identified a number of salient areas, several of which have psychological significance and resonate with the finding of the previous studies.

- The benefits of a specialist stroke service
- The drawbacks of service fragmentation (around professions, specialties or locations)
- Frustration with lack of resources to provide 'complete care' and opportunities to use advanced skills
- Difficulties with providing consistent care
- Poor morale
- But, despite everything, a will to fight for positive change

The special skills of psychologists (Division of Clinical Psychology, 2007) are particularly suited to the context of stroke care, and may help in ameliorating some of the issues identified above and promoting more effective care:

- A broad knowledge base
- The ability to conduct and review research
- A range of approaches or modalities
- Skills in supervision
- The ability to deal with complex presentations
- The ability to work with teams, supporting service and organisational development
- The ability to offer oversight and 'umbrella', or consultancy

Psychologists' training equips them with an understanding of organisational processes and team dynamics, as well as the skills to intervene at an organisational level to support and enhance team functioning (British Psychological Society, 2007; Onyett, 2007). The key to successful stroke rehabilitation is the effective functioning of the multidisciplinary team (Department of Health, 2001; Royal College of Physicians, 2008a). Therefore, it will be vital to have a team member who appreciates and has skills in team building, training and teaching methods, consultancy, leadership and management as well as expertise in helping teams to adopt new practices and in supporting team members.

Diversity and stroke services

People from some ethnic groups are over-represented in stroke services due to major differences in the incidence of stroke. The stroke mortality rates for Bangladeshi men, Jamaican men and women and West African men was two or three times higher than the rates for the corresponding UK-born groups (Stewart, Dundas, Howard, Rudd & Wolfe, 1999; Stroke Association/British Heart Foundation, 2009). Moreover, the ageing population profile for black people in the United Kingdom may further inflate the number of black people having strokes.

Therefore, it is concerning that older people from ethnic minority backgrounds in the United Kingdom experience inequities in access to health services, and may encounter discrimination or a lack of cultural awareness within services (Ebrahim, 1996). Different ethnic groups have markedly different patterns of help seeking and service uptake which may also affect access to services (Aspinall & Jacobson, 2004). Mold, McKevitt and Wolfe (2003) reviewed studies of stroke survivors' and professionals' beliefs and assumptions about stroke and stroke services. They considered studies of a range of social factors that might influence the equity of stroke care; age, income, class, identity and ethnicity. The review concluded that psychological factors related to how survivors and professionals viewed themselves and each other were crucial determinants of both the delivery and the demand for services, and also underpinned service equity. This review also highlighted how important it is that health workers avoid incorrect assumptions about other cultures based on stereotypes that may have been inculcated during childhood. One common assumption that requires challenging is the notion that 'they look after their own' (Murray, 1998). These kinds of assumptions are often unconsciously held and may create unwitting biases. Those working with diverse groups should be alert to these issues when reflecting on practice and in supervision. Preferably, special training should be sought that involves members of the ethnic groups involved.

It is important to expand knowledge about how different populations understand stroke, its causes and prevention, and about their beliefs regarding recovery and their expectations of services (Pratt, Ha, Levine & Pratt, 2003). Such knowledge will help in finding means to overcome barriers to service uptake and delivery. The beliefs and expectations of carers about their roles are also vital, and helpful guidelines for working with carers from some ethnic groups have been produced, although none are specific to stroke (Afiya Trust and the National Black Carers and Carers' Workers Network, 2002).

The role of religion is important in shaping beliefs about stroke and expectations of treatment (Bham & Ross, 2005), and professionals should be sensitive to the fact that the most efficacious treatment, as defined by NICE, may not always be the most acceptable or appropriate. Ethnic carers also find solace and meaning for their caring role in religion and spirituality (Pierce, 2001), and this challenges heath care professionals to blend their practical knowledge and expertise with sensitive cultural awareness when supporting those with very different belief systems.

Future directions

People in professions relevant to stroke, especially those starting out in clinical, health or neuro-psychology, or experienced professionals moving specialty to fill positions in stroke services, will find exciting opportunities to develop psychological approaches in the second decade of the twenty-first century. General trends for the next decade are already mapped out; the stroke strategies of developed nations set relevant targets and define quality markers which will help to shape services and improve practice. In the United Kingdom the NHS plan will continue to unfold and there is a background of new, person-centred health legislation to support good practice. The guidelines and strategies include much of psychological relevance: identification and treatment of depression, screening and interventions for cognitive impairments and greater involvement and empowerment of survivors and carers in decisions about their own treatment and about service development. The National Stroke Guidelines and the new stroke strategies all provide a framework for delivering and monitoring service objectives and quality. However, the delivery of psychological interventions is lagging well behind the development of guidelines, and consequently psychological assessments and treatments are not reliably accomplished, and psychological therapists are absent from many services. One future direction, therefore, is to address these shortfalls. The way forward may well be through psychologists working within teams to train, support and supervise other professionals to deliver interventions, while taking on only the most complex cases themselves (Onyett, 2007).

The stepped-care service model advocated by NICE for the common mental health disorders of anxiety, depression and obsessive-compulsive disorder (NICE, 2007) offers a promising service framework to accomplish improved access to psychological care for hospitalised and community stroke survivors.

Stepped-care services are organised to help survivors, carers and healthcare professionals to identify and access the most effective, but least intrusive, intervention appropriate to a person's needs. Stepped-care systems need to ensure a smooth transition between steps so that survivor experience is not disjointed. The various steps are often referred to as ranging from 'low intensity' to 'high intensity'. Relatively brief interventions provided at steps 1 and 2 are often described as low-intensity treatment. Treatment provided at step 3 and beyond for survivors with more severe symptoms, or those who have not responded to low-intensity treatment, is known as 'high intensity'. Most survivors receive treatments on lower steps before receiving treatments from higher steps. Starting treatments on lower steps reduces the burden of more intensive treatment on the survivor, service providers and commissioners. The stepped care models proposed for mental health will require adapting for stroke, and will need different configurations when applied to community and hospital settings. A suggested model is shown below, with progression depending on response at each step:

1. Recognition of psychological needs by frontline staff in hospital or primary care. Assessment by a psychologist who determines the next level of intervention (two to five).
2. Referral to a group facilitated by low-intensity workers and including peer supporters (experienced, trained and professionally supported survivors recruited from former patients and funded by health or social care); emotional support, information exchange, linking to further support and information services. This might require 'in-reach' into hospitals by peer supporters.
3. Individual support from low intensity workers and befrienders or peer supporters with specialist training combined with group support as for step 2.
4. Support from a trained and supervised professional with psychological expertise (psychologist, mental health nurse or psychiatrist) to supplement steps 2 to 4. Specialist psychological therapy. Medication if required.
5. Inpatient treatment for mental health needs. Second-line medications if required. Intensive psychotherapy. Milieu therapy.

This approach might also be adapted to meet the needs of carers suffering from significant psychological difficulties.

The engagement of peer supporters, usually survivors and carers who have long-term experience of a condition, is increasing in acute healthcare. Although there are currently no studies of the use of this approach with stroke survivors, the basis for its benefits has been elucidated (Dennis, 2003). It has been used with apparent success in other neurological conditions (Schultz, 1994; Schwartzberg, 1994). There is also a growing pool of studies investigating the effectiveness of the approach across a range of conditions that is due to be summarised in a systematic Cochrane review (Doull, O'Connor, Welch, Tugwell & Wells, 2005).

One specific issue of psychological relevance emerging from the recent guidelines and strategies is whether stroke services should continue to be included under the aegis of the Older Peoples' National Service Framework. Age is a major risk factor for stroke, but strokes can happen at any age, and as a neurological condition it has much in common with other long-term neurological conditions. This has been acknowledged in the National Stroke Strategy for England which makes explicit links to the 11 quality requirements of the Long-Term Conditions National Service Framework. Any move to reduce the association between stroke and old age would be welcomed by young stroke survivors who may feel out of place in services designed around the needs of older people, and find that having a disease associated with old age threatens their self-image and identity as 'young' (see chapter 21).

While the overarching service framework for stroke is mapped out, there remain several areas where information is sparse and research is required. Wolfe, Rudd, McKevitt, Heuschmann and Kalra (2008) included a number of projects of psychological significance in the 'top ten' identified in their report on research issues emerging from the new Stroke Strategy for England.

- Research into the effectiveness of the public awareness campaigns aimed at reducing delays in hospitalisation
- Patient- and carer-centred methods for identifying the long-term needs and long-term adjustment of patients and carers
- Identification of the relationship between patient numbers, dependency and staffing requirements with a view to providing more specific guidance on appropriate staffing numbers and skills
- Exploration of how to identify and meet the training needs of stroke professionals, especially with regard to patients' and carers' long-term needs
- The development of a comprehensive outcome measure that has broad acceptance and patient and carer relevance

A systematic study of research priorities was conducted in Canada with a multiprofessional panel of researchers, clinicians and a service user (Bayley, Hurdowar, Teasell, Wood-Dauphinee, Korner-Bitensky, Richards *et al.*, 2007). The study used a Delphi technique to develop a consensus about priorities for research. Five priority areas were identified including two of psychological significance: community reintegration after stroke and cognitive rehabilitation. The first, community reintegration, overlaps with Wolfe *et al.*'s aim to research long-term needs, but interestingly there are no other points of concordance about psychological research priorities. The poor representation of psychologists on the panels may account for this lack of consistency.

Much remains to be done in developing more specifically psychological standards for care and adapting services to meet the needs of minority groups, but the basic infrastructure is in place and, perhaps more importantly, there is a will and determination to improve stroke care and enable services to become more responsive to survivors' and carers' needs over the whole course of their lives after stroke.

Chapter 3

Neurological Basis of Stroke and Related Vascular Disorders

Introduction

Any evaluation of the psychological effects of stroke requires a clear understanding of the neuroanatomical context in which the sudden and often devastating brain damage occurs. Even a basic knowledge of the vascular system and functional neuroanatomy of the brain can add considerable depth to a clinician's hypotheses. Any assessment which takes into account the mechanism of the stroke is more likely to be focused, efficient and ultimately meaningful for the patient, the patient's family and health professionals. There is considerable heterogeneity in the presentation of patients with stroke. It is therefore vital that any neuropsychological formulation takes account of the aetiology, the acute and longer term cognitive and emotional sequelae and the other numerous and complex medical and psychological factors associated with a stroke.

This chapter will introduce the principal functional and anatomical areas of the brain and explore the relationship between neurological lesion and cognitive function. Stroke is a term used to describe a sudden disruption to the blood supply in the brain. The definition provided by the World Health Organisation (WHO, 1980) is that of 'rapidly developing clinical signs of focal (at times global) disturbance of cerebral function, lasting more than 24 hours or leading to death with no apparent cause other than that of vascular origin'. Neurological symptoms must persist for longer than 24 hours and often include a combination of lateralised upper or lower limb weakness, speech and language problems, and cognitive impairment. The clinical diagnosis of stroke will typically be made by physicians or neurologists,

Psychological Management of Stroke, First Edition. Nadina B. Lincoln, Ian I. Kneebone, Jamie A.B. Macniven and Reg C. Morris.
© 2012 John Wiley & Sons, Ltd. Published 2012 by John Wiley & Sons, Ltd.

often with subsequent confirmation from neuroradiological investigations, using magnetic resonance imaging (MRI) or computed tomography (CT). There are two types of stroke, according to whether the disruption of the blood supply is due to ischaemic infarction, a loss of blood supply to the brain, or intracerebral haemorrhage, bleeding within the brain. The area of brain that is deprived of an adequate blood supply, and its interconnections, determine the characteristics of the stroke.

Neuroanatomy of stroke

The main regions of the brain include the cortex, subcortical structures and cerebellum. The gross anatomy of the brain is illustrated in Figures 3.1 and 3.2. The brain is typically subdivided into the cerebrum, the cerebellum and the brainstem. The cerebrum comprises the two cerebral hemispheres, the diencephalon, comprising the epithalamus, thalamus, hypothalamus and subthalamic zone, and the midbrain. The cerebellum, or 'small brain', is a compact, densely cell-populated structure located underneath the cerebral hemispheres. The brainstem forms the central axis of the brain and includes the pons and the medulla oblongata.

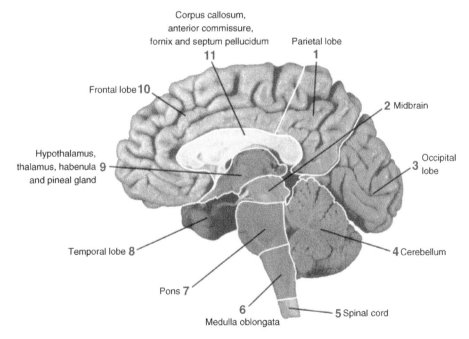

Figure 3.1 Gross anatomy: midsaggital aspect. Reproduced with permission of John Wiley & Sons, Inc., from Woolsey, T. A., Hanaway, J., & Mokhtar, H. G. (2008). *The Brain Atlas* (3rd ed.), p. 9. Hoboken, New Jersey: John Wiley & Sons.

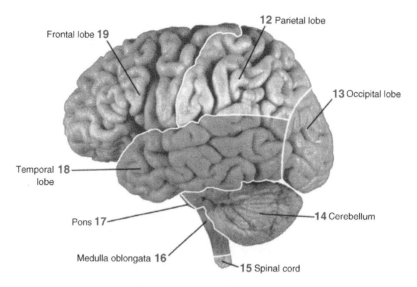

Figure 3.2 Gross anatomy: lateral aspect. Reproduced with permission of John Wiley & Sons, Inc., from Woolsey, T. A., Hanaway, J., & Mokhtar, H. G. (2008). *The Brain Atlas* (3rd ed.), p. 9. Hoboken, New Jersey: John Wiley & Sons.

The cortex

Most brain regions are described as either 'grey matter' or 'white matter' structures. The cerebral cortex, the outer layer of the brain, is grey matter, comprised of tightly packed neurons and neuroglia. The surface of the brain is contoured with gyri (convolutions) and sulci (fissures). Several major sulci such as the central sulcus (Sylvian Fissure) and lateral sulcus (Rolandic Fissure) define the regions of the cortex, referred to as lobes; these are the frontal lobe, temporal lobe, parietal lobe and occipital lobe. Debate continues over the value and validity of defining a further constellation of cortical and subcortical structures within the brain as the limbic lobe (Heimer & Van Hoesen, 2006). The cortex is protected by the skull and by the meninges; three layers of connective tissue comprising the strong, thick dura mater which is firmly attached to the skull; the web-like arachnoid, which is separated by cerebro-spinal fluid (CSF) from the thin, loose pia mater, which closely follows the contours of the brain surface.

Subcortical regions

There are several subcortical (literally meaning 'below the cortex') grey matter structures. These include the thalamus, and basal ganglia structures, such as the putamen, caudate nucleus and globus pallidus. The bulk of the remaining subcortical brain tissue is largely composed of white matter; long myelinated axonal tracts through which cortical and subcortical structures are linked. Large

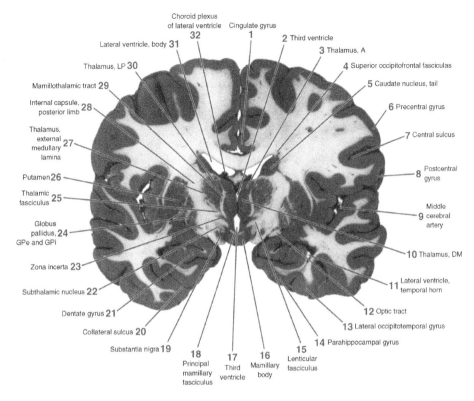

Choroid plexus
of lateral ventricle   Cingulate gyrus
32   1   2 Third ventricle
Lateral ventricle, body 31   3 Thalamus, A
Thalamus, LP 30   4 Superior occipitofrontal fasciculas
Mamillothalamic tract 29   5 Caudate nucleus, tail
Internal capsule, 28   6 Precentral gyrus
posterior limb
Thalamus,   7 Central sulcus
external 27
medullary
lamina
Putamen 26   8 Postcentral
                                               gyrus
Thalamic 25
fasciculus   Middle
                                             9 cerebral
Globus   artery
pallidus, 24
GPe and GPi
Zona incerta 23   10 Thalamus, DM
Subthalamic nucleus 22   11 Lateral ventricle,
                                               temporal horn
Dentate gyrus 21   12 Optic tract
Collateral sulcus 20   13 Lateral occipitotemporal gyrus
Substantia nigra 19   14 Parahippocampal gyrus
                    18   17   16   15
                 Principal Third Mamillary Lenticular
                 mamillary ventricle body fasciculus
                 fasciculus

Figure 3.3   Coronal section revealing subcortical structures. Reproduced with permission of John Wiley & Sons, Inc., from Woolsey, T. A., Hanaway, J., & Mokhtar, H. G. (2008). *The Brain Atlas* (3rd ed.), p. 68. Hoboken, New Jersey: John Wiley & Sons.

strokes will often damage both grey and white matter structures. Small, focal, cortical strokes may have relatively limited effects, whereas even tiny lesions to subcortical structures can cause significant disability or, in the case of some brainstem lesions, death (Jaster, 2001). The most relevant subcortical structures affected by stroke include the basal ganglia, especially the caudate nucleus, putamen and globus pallidus, together with the thalamus, the internal capsule and brainstem structures such as the medulla oblongata. Figure 3.3 is a coronal section of the brain illustrating the location of some of these important subcortical regions.

The vascular system

Stroke is the consequence of disruption or damage to the blood supply of the brain. It is therefore useful for clinicians to have some understanding of neurovascular geography. The survival of brain tissue is dependent on an adequate supply of oxygenated blood, which is provided by a complex system of intracerebral arteries, veins and capillaries. Figure 3.4 illustrates the main

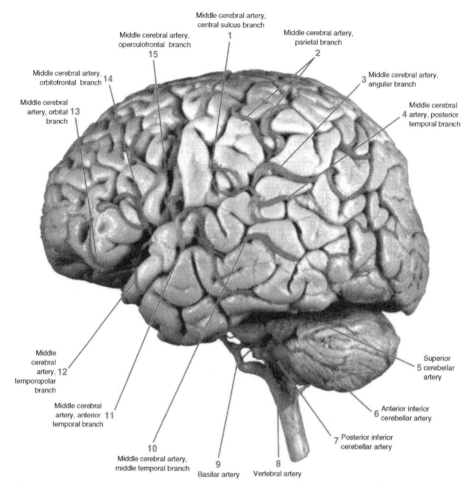

Middle cerebral artery, central sulcus branch 1

Middle cerebral artery, operculofrontal branch 15

Middle cerebral artery, parietal branch 2

Middle cerebral artery, orbitofrontal branch 14

Middle cerebral artery, orbital 13 branch

Middle cerebral artery, angular branch 3

Middle cerebral artery, posterior temporal branch 4

Middle cerebral artery, 12 temporopolar branch

Superior cerebellar artery 5

Middle cerebral artery, anterior 11 temporal branch

Anterior inferior cerebellar artery 6

Middle cerebral artery, middle temporal branch 10

Posterior inferior cerebellar artery 7

Basilar artery 9

Vertebral artery 8

Figure 3.4 Main cerebral hemisphere and brainstem arteries. Reproduced with permission of John Wiley & Sons, Inc., from Woolsey, T. A., Hanaway, J., & Mokhtar, H. G. (2008). *The Brain Atlas* (3rd ed.), p. 22. Hoboken, New Jersey: John Wiley & Sons.

cerebral hemisphere and brainstem arteries. Figure 3.5 illustrates the arteries of the insula and lateral sulcus. Figure 3.6 illustrates the lateral aspect of the arterial territories, and Figure 3.7 illustrates the inferior aspect of the arterial territories.

Although there is considerable heterogeneity in neurovascular geography with cerebral asymmetries of the vascular system frequently observed, some key vascular landmarks are generally true across most patients. In each hemisphere, the three main cerebral arteries are the anterior cerebral artery (ACA), the middle cerebral artery (MCA) and the posterior cerebral artery (PCA). These cerebral arteries originate from the internal carotid and vertebral arteries of the neck. The anterior and middle cerebral arteries of both hemispheres and the vertebrobasilar system are interconnected via a system of communicating arteries at the

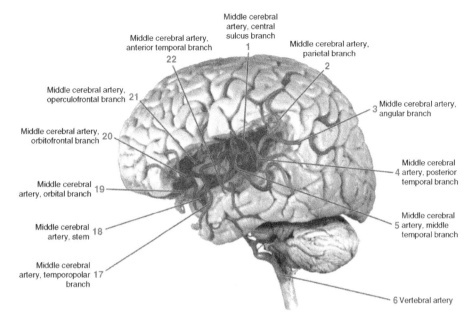

Figure 3.5 Arteries of the insula and lateral sulcus. Reproduced with permission of John Wiley & Sons, Inc., from Woolsey, T. A., Hanaway, J., & Mokhtar, H. G. (2008). *The Brain Atlas* (3rd ed.), p. 23. Hoboken, New Jersey: John Wiley & Sons.

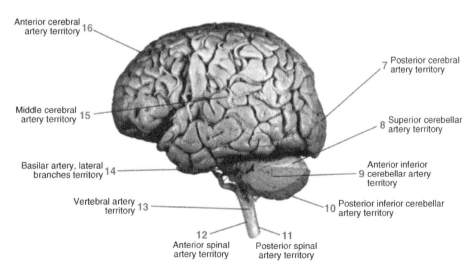

Figure 3.6 Lateral aspect of the arterial territories. Reproduced with permission of John Wiley & Sons, Inc., from Woolsey, T. A., Hanaway, J., & Mokhtar, H. G. (2008). *The Brain Atlas* (3rd ed.), p. 23. Hoboken, New Jersey: John Wiley & Sons.

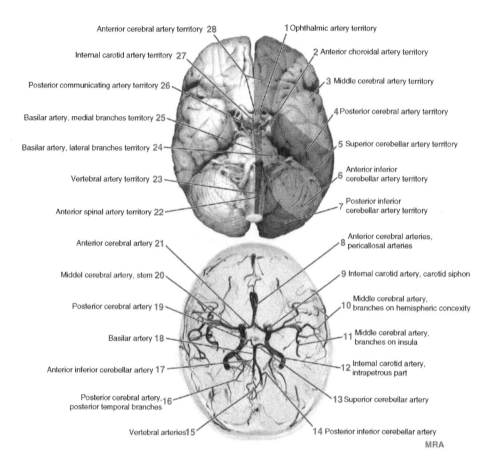

Anterrior cerebral artery territory 28

Internal carotid artery territory 27

Posterior communicating artery territory 26

Basilar artery, medial branches territory 25

Basilar artery, lateral branches territory 24

Vertebral artery territory 23

Anterior spinal artery territory 22

Anterior cerebral artery 21

Middel cerebral artery, stem 20

Posterior cerebral artery 19

Basilar artery 18

Anterior inferior cerebellar artery 17

Posterior cerebral artery, 16 posterior temporal branches

Vertebral arteries 15

1 Ophthalmic artery territory

2 Anterior choroidal artery territory

3 Middle cerebral artery territory

4 Posterior cerebral artery territory

5 Superior cerebellar artery territory

6 Anterior inferior cerebellar artery territory

7 Posterior inferior cerebellar artery territory

8 Anterior cerebral arteries, pericallosal arteries

9 Internal carotid artery, carotid siphon

10 Middle cerebral artery, branches on hemispheric concexity

11 Middle cerebral artery, branches on insula

12 Internal carotid artery, intrapetrous part

13 Superior cerebellar artery

14 Posterior inferior cerebellar artery

MRA

Figure 3.7   Inferior aspect of the arterial territories, and axial magnetic resonance angiography (MRA) image revealing Circle of Willis. Reproduced with permission of John Wiley & Sons, Inc., from Woolsey, T. A., Hanaway, J., & Mokhtar, H. G. (2008). *The Brain Atlas* (3rd ed.), p. 39. Hoboken, New Jersey: John Wiley & Sons.

base of the brain known as the Circle of Willis, shown in Figure 3.7. However, some people do not have complete interconnection via a Circle of Willis (Krabbe-Hartkamp, van der Grond, de Leeuw, de Groot, Algra, Hillen *et al.*, 1998) and morphological variation of the Circle of Willis has been implicated as a factor in carotid artery disease.

   By far the most common locus of ischaemic stroke is in the territory of the middle cerebral artery. This artery serves the largest proportion of the cerebral hemisphere, as can be seen from Figure 3.5. The middle cerebral artery supplies blood to perisylvian cortical regions, the basal ganglia and white matter structures, such as the internal capsule. Middle cerebral artery stroke typically results in motor impairment in the contralateral side of the body due to involvement of the motor strip of the frontal lobe or the internal capsule. In addition, sensory problems are common because of the involvement of the sensory strip in the adjacent parietal cortex. The anterior cerebral arteries supply the medial regions of the anterior cerebral hemispheres, as well as some basal ganglia structures and orbital frontal lobe regions. The anterior cerebral arteries are interconnected via the anterior communicating artery. The posterior cerebral arteries supply the brainstem, spinal cord, midbrain, thalamus and medial aspects of the temporal and occipital lobes.

Each main cerebral artery also has many branches which form smaller arteries, arterioles and capillaries. Together these continually supply brain tissue with essential oxygen and glucose, which are not stored in the brain. If the cerebral blood flow is interrupted, even for just a few minutes, permanent neuronal damage occurs. The vascular system can compensate for interrupted blood flow by compensatory mechanisms, often through the Circle of Willis. For example, blood flow may be rerouted via the anterior or posterior communicating arteries. The brain also utilises a vasodilation mechanism, which increases the blood flow to areas affected by restricted blood flow. Ultimately, failure or exhaustion of these compensatory mechanisms will result in ischaemia, the interruption of blood supply to the brain, and then infarction, the necrosis of brain tissue, leading to an ischaemic stroke. In any ischaemic stroke, there will be an area of infarction in which there is irretrievable tissue loss. However, surrounding this is an area known as the ischaemic penumbra in which function is disrupted but can be restored when reperfusion of blood occurs.

The drainage of blood from the cerebrovascular system occurs through a network of cerebral veins. It is relatively uncommon for stroke to arise from occlusion or damage to these veins. However, if this does occur then the consequences can be just as devastating as an arterial stroke (Filley, 2008).

Neuropathological mechanisms

Stroke may be due to cerebral infarction or cerebral haemorrhage. In addition, transient ischaemic attack (TIA) and vascular dementias share much in common with focal stroke. However, the neuropathological aetiology is complex. Although the distinction between ischaemic and haemorrhagic stroke is perhaps of most relevance, for any given patient there will also be considerable nuance in the underlying neuropathology that can meaningfully inform prognosis, prevention, medical treatment and rehabilitation. If, for example, a haemorrhagic stroke in a given patient has resulted from a primary neuropathological mechanism related to hypertension (raised blood pressure), this will prompt specific medical treatment and preventative management. For another patient, the knowledge that an ischaemic stroke has resulted from very recent thrombosis (obstruction of blood flow due to a blood clot) may precipitate a completely alternative medical treatment, such as thombolysis – the rapid pharmacological breakdown of a blood clot. For these patients, expectations for rehabilitation and recovery may be radically different. For example, the aim of thrombolysis will be to minimise or even eliminate the long-term sequelae of stroke. In contrast, a patient with a significant haemorrhagic stroke will be likely to have to adapt to substantial permanent deficits, and longer term rehabilitation will focus on compensation rather than restitution of function.

Ischaemic stroke

By far the most common aetiology for stroke involves an ischaemic mechanism, such as atherothrombosis, embolism or small vessel disease. A thrombus can develop where the walls of the blood vessel have hardened and accumulated fatty deposits such as cholesterol (atherosclerosis), progressively reducing the flow of blood, which ultimately coagulates and blocks the blood vessel. Embolism is the obstruction of blood flow due to a blockage by an embolus, which is a loose blood clot, air bubble or other particle. This occlusion of the blood vessel always originates from outside the intracerebral vascular system. The thrombosis may be associated with heart disease or due to disease or injury in other regions of the body. Other sources of embolism include bacteria, tumour cells and material from injected drugs (Festa, Lazar & Marshall, 2008). The circulatory system carries the embolus into the intracerebral vascular system, where it becomes lodged and causes an ischaemic stroke. One of the most common sites of embolism is the middle cerebral artery territory (Bogousslavsky, Vanmelle & Regli, 1988).

Another source of embolism leading to stroke is from carotid stenosis, a narrowing of the carotid arteries (Blaser, Hofmann, Buerger, Effenberger, Wallesch & Goertier, 2002). Atherosclerosis can significantly reduce the blood flow to the brain, and the site of carotid artery stenosis can be a major source of emboli. From a medical perspective, it is therefore important to identify carotid artery stenosis as early as possible; early treatment with carotid endarterectomy or endovascular treatment can significantly reduce the risk of stroke (Coward, Featherstone & Brown, 2005). Early signs of carotid stenosis include TIA.

Small vessel ischaemic disease accounts for approximately 25% of first-episode ischaemic strokes (Bamford, Sandercock, Jones & Warlow, 1987). Hypertension is a risk factor for small vessel ischaemia, although a significant proportion of patients with this condition are normotensive (Lammie, 2002). The neuropathology of small vessel ischaemia is often, somewhat controversially, referred to as lacunar stroke. Lacunes are small cavities located deep within the brain (Lammie, 2002). Most lacunes are Type I, irregular cavities of 1–20 mm in diameter, representing old, small infarcts, and occur in the putamen, caudate, thalamus, pons, internal capsule and hemispheric white matter (Lammie, 2002). Type II lacunes are haemorrhagic; Type III lacunes are associated with dilated

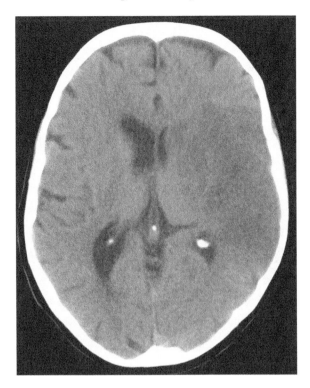

Figure 3.8 Unenhanced CT image of an ischaemic stroke in the left middle cerebral artery territory. Reproduced with permission from Dr Rob Dineen, University of Nottingham.

perivascular spaces (Poirier & Derouesne, 1984). The majority of lacunar strokes are nevertheless associated with atherosclerosis or fibrinoid necrosis, tissue death in the walls of blood vessels (Lammie, 2000).

Figure 3.8 is an unenhanced CT scan showing low attenuation and swelling in the left middle cerebral artery territory in keeping with acute infarction. Figure 3.9 is a T2-weighted MRI scan showing hyperintensity and swelling of the left middle cerebral artery territory in the same patient. Figure 3.10 is a diffusion weighted image of the same patient showing hyperintensity (representing diffusion restriction), in keeping with acute infarction.

Haemorrhagic stroke

Primary intracerebral haemorrhage (ICH) accounts for the large majority of haemorrhagic stroke. This usually involves the sudden rupture of small blood vessels, damaged by chronic hypertension or amyloid angiopathy, the deposition of amyloid-β in the arteries (Chakrabarty & Shivane, 2008). Secondary mechanisms for intracerebral haemorrhage include trauma, tumours, impaired coagulation, ruptured aneurysms, vascular malformations, vasculitis and mechanisms

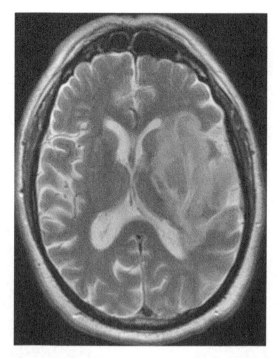

Figure 3.9   T2-weighted MR image of ischaemic stroke in the left middle cerebral artery territory. Reproduced with permission from Dr Rob Dineen, University of Nottingham.

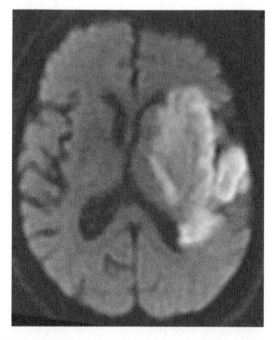

Figure 3.10   Diffusion weighted image of ischaemic stroke in the left middle cerebral artery territory. Reproduced with permission from Dr Rob Dineen, University of Nottingham.

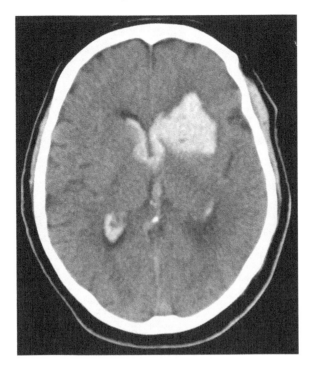

Figure 3.11   Unenhanced CT image of an intracerebral haemorrhagic stroke in the left anterior striatum, with extension of the haemorrhage into the ventricular system. Reproduced with permission from Dr Rob Dineen, University of Nottingham.

associated with drug and alcohol abuse (Chakrabarty & Shivane, 2008). ICH is no longer viewed as a relatively simple bleeding event which ends rapidly through clotting; imaging evidence now demonstrates that the process of ICH is complex, often with expansion of the haematoma, the localised collection of blood, over several hours following initial onset of symptoms (Chakrabarty & Shivane, 2008). Continued bleeding can worsen the inflammation of the parenchyma, causing oedema and secondary brain damage due to breakdown of the blood–brain barrier and direct cytotoxicity (Mayer & Rincon, 2005). Acute bleeding into the brain (intracerebral haemorrhage), the ventricles or the subarachnoid space (subarachnoid haemorrhage) is associated with high morbidity and mortality (Chakrabarty & Shivane, 2008).

Figure 3.11 is an unenhanced CT scan demonstrating an acute left anterior striatal intracerebral haemorrhage, with extension of the haemorrhage into the ventricular system. Figure 3.12 is a T2-weighted MRI scan of the same patient showing the haematoma (low signal) with surrounding oedema (high signal), with blood also visible in the ventricular system.

Intracerebral haemorrhages may occur due to rupture of an arteriovenous malformation (AVM). AVMs are vascular abnormalities that are typically present

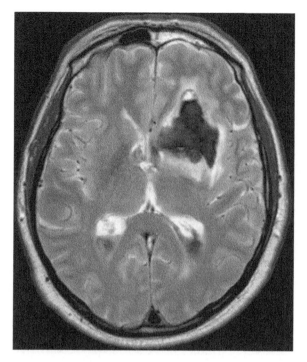

Figure 3.12   T2-weighted MR image of an intracerebral haemorrhagic stroke in the left anterior striatum, with extension of the haemorrhage into the ventricular system. Reproduced with permission from Dr Rob Dineen, University of Nottingham.

from birth and occur anywhere in the brain (Lantz & Meyers, 2008). AVMs can cause both hypertension and hypotension in adjacent blood vessels. For many people with AVM, there are no discernable neurological symptoms. However, a proportion of people with AVM have haemorrhages associated with ruptured AVM blood vessels. It is typically the leakage of blood from the AVM and associated brain damage which is thought to cause neuropsychological impairment, as opposed to there being any direct effect of the AVM on neuropsychological functioning. Approximately 12% of AVMs are estimated to become symptomatic (Hashimoto, Iida, Kawaguchi & Sakaki, 2004).

About 5% of strokes involve a subarachnoid haemorrhage (SAH; Bederson, Connolly, Batjer, Dacey, Dion, Dirinjer *et al.*, 2009), in which blood is released onto the surface of the brain via a burst blood vessel just below the arachnoid membrane and just above the pia mater. There are several mechanisms by which the brain is damaged in a SAH, including direct toxic effects of blood on brain tissue. Most seriously, an SAH can cause profound reductions in cerebral blood flow, reduced cerebral autoregulation and acute cerebral ischaemia (Bederson *et al.*, 2009). The mortality rate is particularly high in SAH, estimated at 45–50% in some studies (Broderick, Brott, Duldner, Tomsick & Leach, 1994). Recurrent haemorrhage can occur with aneurysmal

SAH, and this is associated with higher rates of mortality or severe disability (Bederson *et al.*, 2009).

Stroke syndromes

The brain damage associated with stroke is typically focal and circumscribed. While there are well-established clusters of neurological symptoms following stroke, related to the neuroanatomical location, there are always individual differences between patients even with apparently very similar damage. Broad classification systems such as the Oxfordshire Community Stroke Project Classification (OCSP), as shown in Table 3.1, are useful to describe the clinical

Table 3.1 Oxfordshire Community Stroke Project (OCSP) Classification of Stroke (Mead, G.E., Lewis, S.C., Wardlaw, J.M., Dennis, M.S., & Warlow, C.P., 2000. How well does the Oxfordshire Community Stroke Project classification predict the site and size of the infarct on brain imaging? *Journal of Neurology, Neurosurgery and Psychiatry*, 68, 559, with permission from BMJ Publishing Group Ltd).

CT or MRI Appearance	*Clinical Syndrome*	*Abbreviation*
Large cortical MCA infarct (whole of the cortex supplied by the MCA plus adjacent white matter and part or all of the ipsilateral basal ganglia) or more than half of the MCA territory plus ACA or PCA territory	Total anterior circulation infarction	TACI
Medium-sized cortical infarct (about half the MCA territory)	Partial or total anterior circulation infarction	PACI or TACI
Small cortical infarct (less than a quarter of the MCA territory) or any of the ACA territory	Partial anterior circulation infarction	PACI
Border zone cortical infarct between ACA and MCA or PCA and MCA territories	Partial anterior circulation infarction	PACI
Large (>1.5 cm) subcortical infarct (striatocapsular)	Total or partial anterior circulation infarction	TACI or PACI
Small (<1.5 cm) subcortical infarct (lacunar) (including centrum semiovale infarcts)	Lacunar infarction	LACI
Cortical infarct in PCA territory	Posterior circulation infarction	POCI
Brainstem or cerebellar infarct (including small infarcts in the pons)	Posterior circulation infarction	POCI

MCA = middle cerebral artery; ACA = anterior cerebral artery; PCA = posterior cerebral artery.

presentation. Patients will often be diagnosed according to these criteria; in acute rehabilitation settings, judgements regarding likely prognosis and length of stay may be made with reference to known clinical syndromes.

It is also worth considering the heterogeneity of the structure of the brain across individuals. The localisation of a lesion by imaging is informative, but it is not uncommon for lesions on imaging to be theoretically incongruent with a patient's apparent clinical symptoms (Hand, Kwan, Lindley, Dennis & Wardlaw, 2006). Cerebral infarctions are also not always visible on imaging (Brazzelli, Sandercock, Chappell, Celani, Righetti, Arestis *et al.*, 2009).

According to the OCSP classification system, the majority of acute strokes can be usefully categorised by clinical symptomatology, often confirmed by subsequent brain imaging. Syndromes (S) (or infarcts [I] when imaging has confirmed an ischaemic stroke) identified by this system are

- Lacunar syndrome (LACS), including pure motor stroke, pure sensory stroke, sensorimotor stroke and ataxic hemiparesis.
- Posterior circulation syndrome (POCS), including brainstem or cerebellar signs, and/or isolated homonymous hemianopia.
- Total anterior circulation syndrome (TACS), including a triad of hemiparesis or hemisensory loss, dysphasia or other new higher cortical dysfunction, and homonymous hemianopia.
- Partial anterior circulation syndrome (PACS), including only two of the features of TACS, or isolated dysphasia or parietal lobe signs.

One of the key defining features of anterior circulation syndromes is the presence of higher cortical dysfunction. In left hemisphere strokes, this is often aphasia or apraxia; in right hemisphere strokes, this is often impairment of visuospatial abilities and, in addition, may include impairment of attention, executive abilities and speed of information processing. These focal lesions will produce characteristic patterns of cognitive impairments as illustrated in Table 3.3.

Lacunar strokes result from small infarcts due to the occlusion of a single perforating artery. Although the definition of lacunar stroke syndromes exclude the cognitive dysfunction associated with cortical lesions, such as aphasia, visual inattention and hemianopia (Bamford *et al.*, 1987), recent evidence suggests that a significant proportion of patients with lacunar stokes do have cognitive impairments. Grau-Olivares, Arboix, Bartres-Faz and Junque (2007) prospectively studied 40 patients with lacunar infarction and found that 23 of the patients (58%) had evidence of mild cognitive impairment, particularly impairment of executive function. Table 3.2 describes the generally agreed classification of lacunar stroke syndromes. In contrast with other stroke subtypes, there is a relatively low mortality rate associated with lacunar stroke (Bamford *et al.*, 1987).

Table 3.2 Specific Subcortical Stroke Syndromes (Adapted from Donnan *et al.* 2002. Table on Specific Subortical Stroke Syndromes (pp. 30–4) from chapter "Classification of Subcortical Infarcts" by Geoffrey Donnan *et al.* "By Permission of Oxford University Press").

Presumed single perforator artery territory infarcts (lacunar infarcts)
Location: commonly internal capsule, striatum, or thalamus.
Mechanism: small vessel disease, the precise nature of which remains uncertain since few cases have been studied pathologically. Described phenomena include lipohyalinosis secondary to the effects of hypertension, *in situ* atheroma either at the mouth or along the length of the penetrating vessel. Emboli from large vessels of heart thought to be uncommon, but frequency is uncertain.
Clinical Features: there are five recognised classical (lacunar) syndromes:

1. Pure motor hemiparesis.
2. Sensorimotor stroke.
3. Pure sensory stroke.
4. Dysarthria, clumsy hand syndrome.
5. Ataxic hemiparesis. Face, arm and leg involvement are characteristic for a, b and c. The most important clinical feature is the absence of cognitive symptoms or signs (except in the case of thalamic infarcts). Other clinical presentations have been described but are less specific for single perforator territory infarction *per se.*

CT/MRI appearance: small circular or oval changes <1.5 cm diameter (approximately). In a substantial proportion of cases, CT may be negative which may suggest the presence of a brainstem lacunar infarct.

Striatocapsular infarcts
Location: caudate, anterior limb of internal capsule, putamen.
Mechanism: middle cerebral artery origin occlusion due to embolus (cardiac or internal carotid artery origin), middle cerebral artery pathology (atheroma, arteritis, dissection), other mechanisms uncertain.
Clinical features: hemiparesis with neuropsychological dysfunction, arm weakness greater than face or leg. Occasionally cortical signs may be minimum or absent.
Subtypes:

1. Caudate head.
2. Caudatocapsular.
3. Putamental.
4. Putamentocapsular.

CT/MRI appearances: comma-shaped changes in the striatum.

Internal borderzone infarcts (subcortical junctional infarcts)
Location: paraventricular region, high internal capsule.
Mechanism: distal middle cerebral artery occlusion (beyond perforating vessels and before bifurcation), severe extracranial carotid occlusive disease. Anterior and posterior subtypes may be due to occlusion of superior or inferior divisional branches of the middle cerebral artery, but this remains to be proven.

(continued)

Table 3.2   (*Continued*)

Clinical features: usually varying degrees of hemiparesis with hemisphere-specific neuropsychological dysfunction.
Subtypes:

1. Confluent internal borderzone infarct:
    i)   anterior
    ii) posterior
    iii) total
2. Partial internal borderzone infarct (nonconfluent):
    i)   anterior
    ii) posterior
    iii) total

CT/MRI appearances: confluent or nonconfluent hypodensity in periventricular region.

Anterior choroidal arterial territory infarcts

Location: low internal capsule, medial globus pallidus.
Mechanism: uncertain. Perhaps *in situ* disease of vessel (smaller infarcts), or embolism (larger infarcts).
Clinical features: hemiparesis, hemianaesthesia, hemianopia, or a combination of these. Neuropsychological dysfunction may be a feature of larger infarcts.
CT/MRI appearances: changes of oval shape in low internal capsule encompassing the territory of more than a single perforator territory.

Thalamic infarcts

Location: thalamic regions.
Mechanism: in situ disease of small vessel or mouth of parent artery, cardioembolism (paramedian territory), other causes are rare.
Clinical features: a variety of syndromes with moderate motor and sensory signs, memory impairment, dysphasia if the left thalamus is involved, neglect if the right thalamus is involved. Additional distinguishing features include: confusion, behavioural changes, and eye movement disorders (posterior-thalao-subthalamic paramedian artery); contralateral ataxia (thalamogeniculate pedical). Posterior choroidal artery infarcts may produce an isolated homonymous horizontal sectoranopia.
Subtypes (dependent on arterial territory): tuberothalamic, posterior thalamo-subthalamic paramedian, thalamogeniculate pedicle, posterior choroidal
MRI appearances: small circular or oval-shaped changes in the thalamus.

White matter medullary infarcts

Location: centrum semiovale, external/extreme capsule (territory of the medullary penetrators from the pial middle cerebral artery system).
Mechanism: uncertain, but most probably larger infarcts due to embolism (heart to artery, or artery to artery) and smaller infarcts due to *in situ* small vessel disease.
Clinical features: small infarcts may cause a partial hemiparesis including single limb involvement. Larger infarcts have similar clinical expressions to pial middle cerebral artery territory infarcts.
CT/MRI appearances: circular/oval shape in the centrum semiovale/external extreme capsular region.

Table 3.2 (*Continued*)

Extended large subcortical infarcts

Location: hemispheric white matter/internal capsule/basal ganglia.

Mechanism: large vessel disease (internal carotid and/or middle cerebral artery occlusion).

Clinical features: same as large middle cerebral artery territory infarct with dense hemiplegia and neuropsychological dysfunction appropriate to the affected hemisphere.

CT/MRI appearances: extended involvement of hemispheric white matter and basal ganglia with cortical sparing.

Leukoaraiosis

Location: periventricular region (lateral ventricles) and centrum semiovale.

Mechanism: uncertain. Hypertensive mechanisms may be involved.

Clinical features: presumed cognitive decline or asymptomatic.

CT/MRI appearances: involvement of periventricular and central core of hemispheric white matter.

Subcortical stroke classification

Lesions involving subcortical regions can be classified clinically, clinico-radiologically or clinico-pathologically, and the classification of such strokes has been the source of some controversy for many years (Donnan, Norrving, Bamford & Bogousslavsky, 2002). In practice, many stroke physicians advocate a clinico-radiological approach to the classification of subcortical cerebral infarction (Donnan *et al.*, 2002), as outlined in Table 3.2. This approach is more detailed and refined than that typically adopted for the general classification of cortical and subcortical infarct syndromes, such as the OCSP system.

The subcortical stroke classification system by Donnan *et al.*, (2002) is useful as it provides a framework for explaining combinations of symptoms, which tend not to occur following cortical lesions. Haemorrhagic subcortical strokes associated with hypertension typically occur in the basal ganglia and thalamus, due to the proximity of these structures to the relatively high pressure Circle of Willis (Sutherland & Auer, 2006). Most subtypes of subcortical stroke will also cause some degree of cognitive impairment. For example, posterior choroidal thalamic lesions can mimic transient global amnesia (Gorelick, Amico, Ganellen & Beneveto, 1988), with anterograde amnesia, attentional or executive dysfunction also reported in the literature (Van der Werf, Weerts, Jolles, Witter, Lindeboom & Scheltens, 1999). Thalamic strokes are possibly the smallest lesions that can lead to amnesia (de Freitas & Bogousslavsky, 2002), and are thought by some to be associated with a disconnection mechanism corresponding to interruption of the Papez loop (de Freitas & Bogousslavsky, 2002). Recovery of the neuropsychological impairment associated with such lesions can be quite rapid, with only moderate selective verbal or nonverbal memory difficulties evident a few months post stroke in many cases (Rousseaux, Cabaret, Lesoin, Devos, Dubois & Petit, 1986).

Rare syndromes associated with subcortical lesions can explain apparently unusual constellations of symptoms. Most cortical strokes result in symptoms affecting the opposite side of the body, the contralateral side. However, some strokes can affect the same side of the body, the ipsilateral side. For example, Marchetti, Carey and Della Sala (2005) described a case of 'crossed right hemisphere syndrome' following an isolated left thalamic haemorrhagic lesion. This patient showed neuropsychological symptoms typically associated with right hemisphere damage, such as impaired visuospatial processing, visuospatial memory, motor impersistence, dysprosody and apathy. There were no signs of any contralateral visual inattention, and language, verbal memory and praxis were intact.

Other stroke syndromes

Other rare syndromes can involve a combination of contralateral and ipsilateral symptoms. The best known of these are Wallenberg's syndrome and Horner's syndrome. Wallenberg's syndrome is characterised by vertigo, hoarseness and dysphagia, and is usually associated with lateral medullary lesions (Marx & Thömke, 2009). Horner's syndrome is characterised by ptosis (a drooping upper eyelid), ipsilateral cerebellar ataxia and loss of pain and temperature sensation on the face, with similar loss of pain and temperature sensation on the trunk and limbs of the contralateral side (Zhang, Liu, Wan & Zheng, 2008). These crossed sensory symptoms can be misinterpreted, and some patients with these conditions can in extreme circumstances be suspected of feigning symptoms, due to the perceived incongruence of contralateral and ipsilateral symptoms resulting from the same stroke. In fact, the neuroanatomical location of such strokes explains the combination of ipsilateral and contralateral symptoms, due to the involvement of the inferior cerebellar peduncle and vestibular nuclei (causing dizziness, cerebellar ataxia and nystagmus), together with the spinal trigeminal tract and its nucleus (causing ipsilateral loss of pain and temperature sensation in the face) and the nucleus ambiguus (causing paralysis of the muscles of the soft palate, pharynx and larynx on the ipsilateral side) (Kiernan, 2008). The symptoms of Horner's syndrome are thought to be caused by the involvement of the descending pathway to the intermediolateral cell column of the spinal cord (Kiernan, 2008).

Cerebral autosomal dominant arteriopathy with subcortical infarcts and leukoencephalopathy (CADASIL) is a rare disease associated with genetic linkage to chromosome 19 (notch 3 mutation), with pathological findings involving small vessel arteriopathy with granular osmiophilic material (Davous, 1998). According to Davous (1998), probable CADASIL can be diagnosed clinically if there is young age of onset (below the age of 50) with at least two of the following signs: stroke-like episodes with permanent neurological signs, migraine, major mood disturbance and subcortical dementia. In addition, there should be no vascular risk factor aetiologically related to the deficit, evidence of an inherited autosomal dominant transmission and abnormal MR imaging of the white matter without cortical infarcts. Possible CADASIL can also be diagnosed (Davous, 1998) when there is a later age of onset, above the age of 50, with multiple stroke-like episodes without permanent neurological signs (i.e. TIA-like episodes). Although relatively rare as compared with nonhereditary stroke, patients with CADASIL may occasionally be seen by stroke services, but patients with this diagnosis may require a different management approach, given the neurodegenerative nature of the condition.

Transient ischaemic attack (TIA)

A transient ischaemic attack is a temporary neurological event with stroke-like symptoms that by definition lasts less than 24 hours. The mechanism of TIA is thought to typically be associated with arterial stenosis (Fisher, 2002). Although the neurological symptoms resolve, often within minutes or hours, there can be significant distress and anxiety associated with the experience of having a TIA. The medical assessment and prophylactic treatment of patients with this condition is vital as TIA is a significant risk factor for stroke. Many clinicians advocate the view that a TIA is essentially the same as a stroke, in that it is a neurological event in the progressive course of generalised vascular disease (Daffertshofer, Mielke, Pullwitt, Felsenstein & Hennerici, 2004), and that both conditions should be treated with equal seriousness.

Vascular dementias

Cerebrovascular disease can give rise to various forms of dementia. It is recognised that in 25–30% of people with dementia, the dementia is of vascular origin (O'Brien, Erkinjuntti, Reisberg, Roman, Sawada, Pantoni *et al.*, 2003). There is, however, considerable controversy about the classification of vascular dementias (Roman, Sachdev, Royall, Bullock, Orgogozo, Lopez-Pousa *et al.*, 2004). O'Brien *et al.*, (2003) produced a useful classification of vascular dementias highlighting the pathological mechanisms by which they are linked, as illustrated in Figure 3.13. The most well known vascular dementia is multi-infarct dementia, which comprises multiple large cortical infarcts occurring over time. This leads to a progressive deterioration in cognitive function, which typically occurs in a stepwise pattern. Subcortical ischaemic vascular dementia comprises small vessel disease and ischaemic white matter lesions. The diagnostic criteria require the onset of the dementia

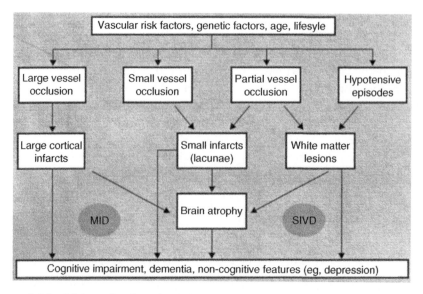

Figure 3.13 Main pathophysiological mechanisms in vascular cognitive impairment. Reproduced with permission from O'Brien *et al.* (2003). (Preprinted from *Lancet Neurology*, 2, O'Brien, J. T., Erkinjuntti, T., Reisberg, B., Roman, G., Sawada, T., Pantoni, L., *et al.*, 2003. Vascular cognitive impairment. *Lancet Neurology*, 89–98, with permission from Elsevier.) [MID=multi-infarct dementia; SIVD=subcortical ischaemic vascular dementia]

to be related to cerebrovascular disease. In addition, cognitive changes may precede the development of vascular dementia by a few years, as a result of disturbances in the cerebral blood supply (Bäckman & Small, 2007; Laukka, MacDonald & Backman, 2008). Vascular dementia may also occur in conjunction with Alzheimer's dementia (O'Brien *et al.*, 2003; Sellal, Wolff & Marescaux, 2004).

Patterns of cognitive impairment following stroke

The nature of cognitive problems is described more fully in chapter 4, but the broad overall pattern of impairments according to the neuroanatomical basis of the stroke is summarised in Table 3.3. Damage to each lobe can produce characteristic impairments according to the lobe affected. So, parietal lobe lesions tend to be associated with visuoperceptual disorders and apraxias, temporal lobe lesions with memory problems, occipital lesions with visual agnosias and frontal lobe lesions with executive impairments. However, because stroke is due to disruption of the vascular supply to the brain, it is more useful to consider cognitive impairments according to the territories supplied by the various blood vessels, than use the traditional classification based on the lobes of the cortex.

Table 3.3 Typical Patterns of Cognitive Impairment following Stroke

Type of stroke	Primary cognitive impairments	Other associated impairments
Right hemisphere middle cerebral artery	Visuoperceptual	Left-sided motor
		Left-sided sensory
		Left hemianopia
Left hemisphere middle cerebral artery	Aphasias	Right-sided motor
	Apraxias	Right-sided sensory
		Right hemianopia
Anterior cerebral artery	Executive function	
Posterior cerebral artery stroke	Visual agnosias	Cortical blindness
Subcortical stroke	Executive	
	Attention	
	Speed of information processing	
Thalamic infarction	Memory	
	Attention	
	Executive	
Vascular dementia	Executive	Language
	Attention	
	Speed of information processing	
Multi-infarct dementia	Aphasias	Dysarthria
	Apraxias	
	Agnosias	
	Memory	
Subcortical ischaemic vascular dementia	Executive	Motor problems
	Speed of information processing	Mood changes
	Memory problems (recall)	

Stroke in the territory of the middle cerebral artery produces cognitive impairments which vary according to the hemisphere affected and the degree of cerebral dominance for language. In those who are left-hemisphere dominant for language, the majority of the population, left MCA stroke will typically produce language problems and right MCA stroke visuospatial problems. However, in those who are left-handed for writing, cerebral lateralisation is less marked and there may be a lesser degree of lateralisation of cognitive functioning. There are also a few people who are left-hand dominant for writing who have language abilities lateralised to the right hemisphere. Posterior cerebral artery strokes may produce visual agnosias.

Patients with vascular dementia typically present with impairments in executive function, attention and speed of information processing. Language impairments can also occur. Although episodic memory impairments may be present they are less marked than in Alzheimer's dementia. Cognitive impairments may also precede vascular dementia and include impairments in episodic memory (Bäckmann, 2008) and executive abilities (Sellal *et al.*, 2004).

Changes over time

Multiple mechanisms are involved in the improvement in function that is observed over time following focal stroke. Early changes may be due to reduction in cerebral oedema and reperfusion. In the area surrounding the infarction, there are structural changes which may account for some improvement over time in the early weeks after stoke (Benowitz & Carmichael, 2010), including structural changes in axons, dendrites and synapses. In addition, neurochemical changes occur, suggesting potential options for salvaging areas of brain damage through drug treatments (Chavez, Hurko, Barone & Feuerstein, 2009). MRI studies have indicated that there are changes in cortical maps during recovery after stroke, suggesting that different areas of the brain can become involved in functions originally subserved by the damaged area. Increased activity in areas of the brain distant from the lesions and reduction in lateralisation due to increased activity of the contralesional hemisphere are observed in the early weeks after stroke (Cramer, 2008). Diaschisis is the mechanism by which a focal stroke can produce areas of reduced cerebral blood flow and metabolism distant from the location of the stroke itself (Carmichael, Tatsukawa, Katsman, Tsuyuguchi & Kornblum, 2004). It is thought that this mechanism might impair functional recovery, or alternatively may promote structural reorganisation after a stroke, with some evidence of the formation of new cortical and subcortical connections having been reported in animal studies (Carmichael *et al.*, 2004). These processes therefore substantially account for changes in the effects of stroke over time. Additionally, rehabilitation aims to increase connectivity within the brain through repeated activation (Robertson & Murre, 1999). There are also behavioural and compensatory processes which may account for late recovery (Kwakkel, Kollen & Lindeman, 2004). This means that stroke is not a static event but one which is evolving over time, with increasing importance of environmental factors in the later stages of recovery. In small vessel disease and vascular dementia there is deterioration over time, comparable to that seen in Alzheimer's disease, though this may be modifiable by control of vascular risk factors (O'Brien *et al.*, 2003).

  From the perspective of psychologists working with stroke patients, it is important to anticipate that neuropsychological deficits after a stroke may not be entirely explained by the area of focal stroke damage, and that some deficits evident in the initial weeks and months post stroke may resolve rapidly, as several mechanisms improve wider cortical and subcortical connections. Cognitive deficits are also likely to recover later after stroke than motor deficits (Cramer,

2008). At present these mechanisms are not fully understood, but they may be an important source of future research that could influence treatment and rehabilitation strategies.

Conclusions

Psychologists will often have a wealth of information about the patient available to them, especially within an inpatient hospital setting, including the opinions of the medical staff and other members of the multidisciplinary team. Imaging evidence is often informative, and the psychologist should be familiar with the technology and terminology used by neuroradiologists. It is also helpful to have an appreciation of the potential fallibility of medical investigation, and to adopt a respectfully inquisitive approach to the often contradictory opinions expressed within multidisciplinary teams. The clinical neuropsychologist will aim to derive a neuropsychological formulation based on not only the specific neurological symptoms of the stroke but also the contribution of premorbid patient characteristics, the patient's history of cognitive or mental health problems, the current social context and the patient's personal attitudes towards illness and brain injury.

Section 2

Cognitive Effects of Stroke

Chapter 4

Neuropsychological Symptoms of Stroke

Introduction

Stroke can affect any cognitive function, and so a description of the neuropsychological symptoms of stroke could, in theory, comprise a list of all known neuropsychological phenomena. However, there are several commonly encountered patterns of cognitive impairment after stroke. The most common cognitive impairment is an impairment of language, aphasia, which is dealt with separately in chapter 7. Other common cognitive impairments are apraxia, visuoperceptual and visuospatial problems, memory impairment, disorders of executive function, impairment of attention and problems with social and emotional perception. Each of these will be reviewed to describe the nature of the impairment, the associated lesion location, the pattern of change over time and the effect on daily life. Rehabilitation of cognitive impairments is considered in chapter 11.

Apraxias

Apraxia is a loss of ability to execute skilled movement, which cannot be accounted for by 'weakness, incoordination, sensory loss, poor comprehension or inattention to command' (Geschwind, 1975). Apraxias are cognitive impairments that affect limb movement and speech. As with the aphasia–dysphasia distinction, in clinical practice the terms apraxia and dyspraxia are often used interchangeably, although originally apraxia was considered to be a loss of movement and dyspraxia an acquired disorder of movement. The classic example of apraxia is the patient who is unable to demonstrate waving goodbye to request but waves goodbye as the examiner leaves the room. Automatic behaviours are retained, but movements are not under volitional control.

Patients do not usually complain of apraxia, but they present in clinical practice as clumsy and lacking dexterity in their unaffected hand. They may be

Psychological Management of Stroke, First Edition. Nadina B. Lincoln, Ian I. Kneebone,
Jamie A.B. Macniven and Reg C. Morris.
© 2012 John Wiley & Sons, Ltd. Published 2012 by John Wiley & Sons, Ltd.

observed during rehabilitation to have difficulty following instructions in physiotherapy, as they cannot perform activities they are requested to do, even though they have the physical capability, or are unable to copy demonstrations. They may be slow to perform daily life tasks, such as washing and dressing. Although they can complete the tasks, these are carried out in a laborious manner, and problems are particularly apparent on those activities which have to be done with the unaffected hand, due to the presence of a hemiplegia. Observations of mealtime behaviour (Foundas, Macauley, Raymer, Maher, Heilman & Gonzalez, 1995) and reports of using eating implements (Sunderland, 2000) indicate that patients are clumsy in their use of utensils. Patients demonstrate difficulty in dressing; for example, Goldenberg and Hagman (1998) found patients made errors putting on and taking off a T-shirt, even though they were able to complete the task, and Walker, Sunderland, Sharma and Walker (2004) observed that patients with left hemisphere stroke dressed the nonparetic arm first, instead of dressing the paretic arm first, or showed a disorganised dressing strategy, which they attributed to impaired action control due to apraxia. As Sunderland and Shinner (2007) pointed out, one reason patients do not report difficulties is because they ascribe them to the use of the nondominant hand for activities for which they would previously have used their dominant hand.

There is some debate and inconsistency over the classification of the apraxias. Early studies by Liepmann in 1908 (Goldenberg, 2003; Koski, Iacoboni & Mazziotta, 2002; Sunderland & Shinner, 2007) proposed two types of limb apraxia: ideomotor and ideational. Ideomotor apraxia is defined as the inability to pantomime object use or to imitate gesture, whereas ideational apraxia is thought to involve the loss of the actual concept of an action. However, most of the research concerns ideomotor apraxia and the notion of ideational apraxia has been questioned (Hermsdorfer, Hentze & Goldenberg, 2006; Sunderland & Shinner, 2007). Most clinicians and researchers accept the validity of a distinction between ideomotor and ideational apraxia when considering limb apraxia. The distinction rests on the type of errors made, in that a patient with ideomotor apraxia may be expected to show temporal or spatial errors with appropriate movements, such as a clumsily executed demonstration of tooth brushing; the patient with ideational apraxia will show inappropriate movements, such as demonstrating brushing their teeth using a combing action, with impaired action content (Sunderland & Shinner, 2007). However, the differentiation between inaccurate performance and content errors is difficult. Sunderland and Shinner (2007) gave the example of a patient who makes chopping movements instead of slicing movements when asked to pantomime slicing bread, which could be due to inaccurate control of the arm or loss of knowledge of how bread is cut. Thus, although De Renzi and Lucchelli (1988) supported the distinction between these two types of apraxia in a few patients, they can co-occur and the distinction probably does not contribute to our understanding of the nature of apraxic difficulties. In addition, various other subtypes of apraxia have been put forward (Koski *et al.*, 2002), including limb-kinetic, buccofacial, conceptual, optical and tactile. It is accepted that apraxia of speech can occur independently of limb apraxia and this is covered in chapter 7. Although some classifications have emphasised the functional deficits associated with the apraxic condition, for example dressing apraxia and gait apraxia, this probably adds little to our understanding of the problem. In addition, constructional apraxia has been defined as an inability to construct a complex object by arranging its components in their correct spatial relationships. This has been found to occur due to both right and left hemisphere lesions with similar incidence. These tasks involve complex skills, including spatial, executive and motor. It had been suggested that this disorder can result from the impairment of two different types of 'dorsal' perceptual processing (Laeng, 2006). Rather than being a disorder of movement, this is a visuospatial disorder, which can arise from left hemisphere damage producing 'categorical' errors (i.e. displacement of an object's position or inversion of parts) or the right hemisphere giving rise to 'coordinate' errors (i.e. errors in distance and angle) (Laeng, 2006). On the basis of this theory, either route can produce functionally similar disruption of visuospatial constructional ability, but neither is due to an apraxia.

Estimates of the prevalence of limb apraxia range from 28% to 57% in patients with left hemisphere stroke and from 0% to 34% in patients with right hemisphere strokes (Donkervoort, Dekker, van den Ende, Stehmann-Saris & Deelman, 2000). As with other prevalence studies, there are large variations in estimates according to the method of recruitment of participants and the choice of measures used to identify impairment. For example, Pedersen, Jorgensen, Kammersgaard, Nakayama, Raaschou and Olsen (2001) reviewed 618 stroke patients admitted to hospital within seven days of stroke onset and asked them to point, wave and salute as a measure of limb apraxia. Impairment was found in only 7% of patients (10% left hemisphere, 4% right hemisphere), but this was a relatively insensitive measure of apraxia. In contrast, Donkervoort *et al.* (2000) reviewed all patients with first left hemisphere stroke in 14 rehabilitation centres and 34 nursing homes in the Netherlands. They found 28% of those in rehabilitation centres and 34% in nursing homes had apraxia, using a clinical diagnosis of apraxia by occupational therapists. More formal testing has led to higher estimates. For example, De Renzi, Motti and Nichelli (1980) suggested that up to 50% of patients with left hemisphere stroke and 20% of patients with right hemisphere stroke show symptoms of ideomotor apraxia. Similarly, Sunderland, Bowers, Sluman, Wilcock and Ardron (1999) assessed ipsilateral dexterity in patients within a month of a first unilateral middle cerebral artery stroke and found characteristic patterns of errors on a bean spooning task, such that those with left hemisphere stroke adopted atypical postures, whereas those with right hemisphere strokes showed visual errors, such as missing an object and going back to collect it later. The frequency of apraxia in these patients was high, with two thirds of left hemisphere patients performing lower than any control on an action imitation task.

There is some evidence of recovery from apraxia over time (Basso, Capitani, Della Sala, Laiacona & Spinnler, 1987; Donkervoort, Dekker & Deelman, 2006), but the problem may persist for more than six months. Thus, although Sunderland (2000) observed improvements in ipsilateral dexterity, five of the 12 (42%) left hemisphere stroke patients remained impaired on action imitation tasks six months later, indicating a persisting apraxia. Donkervoort *et al.* (2006) also found patients improved on an apraxia test over time, but that about 90% remained apraxic for at least six months after stroke.

The relationship between apraxia and independence in functional activities of daily living remains complex. Some studies have found no significant relationships between apraxia and functional abilities (Hanna-Pladdy, Heilman & Foundas, 2003; Pederson *et al.*, 2001; Walker & Lincoln, 1991). However, generally these have used relatively insensitive measures, so for example Pederson *et al.* (2001) found that limb apraxia was not associated with functional abilities, as assessed on the Barthel Index. However, the Barthel is predominantly a measure of personal self-care, with items rated as dependent or independent, and it includes few items which require hand use. Walker and Lincoln (1991) and Hanna-Pladdy *et al.* (2003) both used a global measure of dressing. As highlighted by Sunderland *et al.* (1999), it is not that patients are unable to do tasks, but that they cannot do them as well as they did prior to the stoke, particularly if the task has to be carried out using the unaffected arm on its own, rather than being able to use both arms. Studies which have included detailed analysis of apraxic errors on specific activities of daily living have shown that apraxia affects the ability to perform activities in everyday life (Foundas *et al.*, 1995; Goldenberg & Hagmann, 1998; Walker *et al.*, 2004a). In addition the inclusion of patients with varying degrees of hemiparesis may also mask the effect of apraxia, as those who are able to carry out tasks as they would have done before the stroke are not disabled by the apraxia, but those who have to learn new compensatory skills are disabled (Sunderland & Shinner, 2007).

The underlying cognitive deficit and location of lesions responsible for apraxia remains unclear with conflicting evidence for both the cognitive processes and the brain areas involved. Ideomotor apraxia is defined as the inability to pantomime object use or to imitate gesture. Although it had long been believed that ideomotor apraxia has little impact on actual object use and naturalistic action (Heilman, Rothi & Valenstein, 1982), there is evidence that the effect is greater than previously thought (Sunderland & Shinner, 2007). The classical view is that apraxia is a disorder of motor programming, whereas recent theories of apraxia recognise that perceptual, conceptual and motor aspects are all involved. Gesture production requires access to stored information about how to perform a symbolic gesture and also a direct route which enables copying of meaningless gestures. This direct route probably requires spatiomotor representations of the relative position of body parts (Sunderland, 2007). These differences have led to the suggestion that left hemisphere stroke patients have difficulty with conceptual mediation, that is, using knowledge about the human body in the transition from visual perception to motor execution, whereas right hemisphere stroke patients have problems with the visuospatial analysis of gestures (Goldenberg, 1996).

Ideomotor apraxia is usually associated with damage to focal left parietal or frontal cortical regions (Sunderland & Sluman, 2000). In one study (Roy, Heath, Westwood, Schweizer, Dixon, Black *et al.*, 2000) patients with left hemisphere lesions were more often impaired in pantomiming the use of an object to verbal command, whereas an equal proportion of right and left hemisphere lesioned patients were impaired on imitating a pantomime performed by the experimenter. Haaland, Harrington and Knight (2000) examined this further by comparing stroke patients with and without ideomotor limb apraxia following left hemisphere strokes. They found that those who made errors imitating gestures had damage of the left hemisphere, involving the middle frontal gyrus and intraparietal sulcus. Support for the role of the right hemisphere in the visuospatial analysis of gestures comes from other studies (Goldenberg, 1999; Goldenberg, 1996; Heath, Roy, Westwood & Black, 2001). The discrepancies may be partly due to the nature of the errors made as well as the tasks involved (Pazzaglia, Smania, Corato & Aglioti, 2008).

Thus, apraxia is common problem, particularly after left hemisphere stroke, and may co-occur with aphasia. It produces impairment in the ability to manipulate objects with the unaffected hand and may delay progress in rehabilitation.

Visuoperceptual and visuospatial disorders

The most frequently encountered visual problem after stroke is homonymous hemianopia, defined as impaired visual perception or blindness for one half of the visual field (Zihl, 1995). For about 70% of patients, less than 5 degrees of the affected visual hemi-space is spared (Zihl, 1989). The condition is often confused with visual inattention, and hemianopia and visual inattention often co-occur (Rowe, Brand, Jackson, Price, Walker, Harrison *et al.*, 2009). In clinical practice, differentiation between the two conditions is often made by using bedside methods, such as alternating and simultaneous visual confrontation to both sides of visual space (Stone, Halligan & Greenwood, 1993). However, this is not always reliable and specialist field testing may be needed (Walker, Findlay, Young & Welch, 1991). Even within the hemi-field, blindness may not be complete and patients may be able to respond to objects they are unaware of seeing (Sahraie, Trevethan, Weiskrantz, Olson, MacLeod, Murray *et al.*, 2003). Bilateral posterior lesions will produce cortical blindness, in which patients are unaware of seeing but yet are able to respond to some visual stimuli. For example, a patient, Viv, was observed during physiotherapy sessions to avoid bumping into objects in her path even though she reported being unable to see them.

Visuoperceptual and visuospatial disorders include disorders of visual recognition (agnosias), disorders of visuospatial abilities and visual neglect (inattention). Visual perceptual disorders are common after right hemisphere stroke, though they may also occur following left hemisphere stroke (Edmans & Lincoln, 1987). They also occur following posterior cerebral artery strokes, causing lesions in the occipital and posterior parietal lobes. They comprise a collection of problems without a clear theoretical framework to link them all together, either using models derived from cognitive psychology or through an understanding of the anatomical basis.

Visual agnosias

Visual agnosia is a failure to recognise objects through vision, though patients may be able to describe some features of objects they cannot recognise. Lissauer (1890) distinguished two main types of visual agnosia: apperceptive and associative agnosias. In apperceptive agnosia patients are unable to assemble perceptual information. In associative agnosia they fail to retrieve stored knowledge about an object despite intact perception. The difficulty is not due to a naming problem because they can provide the name if given as a description, such as 'it is the fruit that is round and red and grown in greenhouses'.

Patients with apperceptive visual agnosia are unable to recognise objects presented visually. This may occur despite their ability to describe core features, such as light and dark or straight lines, and they may report that they can see the object. This is also evident because they may be able to copy the object, trace their finger round the outline and match it with an identical copy. However, they are unable to extract its global structure. Warrington and James (1988) reported three patients with right posterior parietal lesions. All had average verbal abilities as assessed using the WAIS Verbal IQ, National Adult Reading test and Recognition Memory Test Words. They were able to differentiate figure ground (Visual Object and Space Perception [VOSP] screening), judge whether shapes were squares or rectangles (Effron squares) and form a coherent shape. However, they failed on VOSP Fragmented Letters, Silhouettes and Unusual Views. The deficit was not due to loss of knowledge about the object as they were able to sort pictures into categories, such as objects in the kitchen and dangerous animals, and were able to match pictures by function. These deficits in the ability to identify objects through vision produced no impairments in daily life.

Karnath, Ruter, Mandler and Himmelbach (2009) described patient JA, a 74-year-old, right-handed man, who suffered from an ischaemic stroke during a coronary angiography. The patient complained about an inability to 'see' objects, watch TV or read newspapers. He could manage to dress himself provided he knew where items of clothing were, but he could not identify them from vision. He also reported difficulties in recognizing relatives and close friends from their faces and had to rely on their voices. Despite this he was able to go for walks and to go shopping, using a written shopping list which he gave to the shop assistants. He moved around safely and never collided with potential obstacles. He was able to shake hands and looked straight at the examiner as well as correctly looking at objects on the table in front of him. On testing he showed disturbed visual perception of shape and orientation and an inability to recognise objects through vision. He was able to perceive colour and movement, and he was able to reach for objects. His difficulties were therefore fairly circumscribed to problems with visual perception.

Riddoch and Humphreys (1987) identified another type of apperceptive agnosia in which the problem lay in integrating visual information to form a whole; integrative agnosia. They reported patient HJA who had visual recognition problems following a stroke after a heart operation. HJA had bilateral occipital damage, extending into the temporal lobes. His problem was specific to visual recognition as he was able to name common objects through touch (visual naming 62% correct, tactile naming 86% correct). He was able to see the objects, as he was able to copy complex drawings, but he performed the task very slowly, line by line. As a result of this copying strategy there were some errors in his copies. On an object decision task (real/not real), he performed at chance level (58% correct). However, when asked to provide definitions from memory he showed a clear knowledge of what objects were. For example, in describing a lettuce he called it 'a quick growing annual plant cultivated for human consumption of its crisp green succulent leaves which grow in the young state of the plant tightly formed together in a ball-shaped mass'. HJA had problems in picture naming, identification of figures that overlap and in object decision. He was however good on tactile naming, copying, drawing from memory and giving definitions from memory. The problem lay in the integration of visual information to identify a whole object.

Patients with associative agnosia can recognise the key features but cannot access the name. They are able to see whole form of shape, have no problem copying figures but are unable to recognize the objects. They have a selective visual naming impairment, given that perceptual function and spontaneous speech are normal, and they are able to name from description. Assessment may include miming the use of visually presented objects or the examiner pretending to use objects with the patient indicating whether or not the movement is correct (e.g. hammer); both can elicit impairment. In addition semantic categorisation is poor, for example patients have difficulty grouping pictures into semantic categories (e.g. fruit or tools). They also show poor knowledge of semantic attributes and cannot accurately respond to questions, such as 'Is it a real animal? Is it wild? Does it hop?' Most patients with associative agnosia are poor at recalling visual characteristics of objects, such as 'Does it have stripes? Does it have a furry tail?', because they are unable to retrieve stored visual and perceptual information.

The classification of visual agnosias varies between authors, but the broad concepts of apperceptive and associative remain at the extremes of the spectrum. The lesion locations of these two types are different with apperceptive agnosia due to right inferior parietal lobe damage, an area supplied by the middle cerebral artery, and associative agnosia due to left occipitotemporal damage.

Prosopagnosia

Prosopagnosia is a selective inability to visually recognize faces. This may be so severe that even a spouse's face does not seem familiar and patients may not recognise their own face in mirror. They know it is a face, can usually differentiate race, sex and age and can interpret emotional expression but do not recognise who it is. There are two types, which parallel the types of visual object agnosia. Patients with apperceptive prosopagnosia have a visual processing deficit. They are unable to match two views of the same face as being the same person. Those with an associative prosopagnosia are unable to recognize familiar faces, even though they retain knowledge about the people. For example, they may not recognize a picture of David Cameron's face, but if asked who the present Prime Minister of the United Kingdom is and what he looks like they can tell you. They may retain implicit knowledge, as they take longer to learn incorrect names of people from their photographs than correct ones. The deficit seems specific to faces, as patients can still recognise other people by their silhouette, clothing, gait, mannerisms and voice.

Patients with prosopagnosia can often describe the facial features, but have no sense of familiarity. This seems to be a specific deficit in face processing and it is not simply that faces are difficult objects to discriminate. Prosopagnosia has been described following lesions in several locations, although it seems to be predominantly due to right hemisphere lesions. The range of lesion locations led Fox, Iaria and Barton (2008) to suggest that face recognition requires a distributed network within the brain. They also suggested that prosopagnosia may be due to disconnections between processes and regions rather than as a result of damage to specific areas of the brain.

Visuospatial disorders

Visuospatial disorders include problems with route finding, visual localisation, visuospatial imagery and visuoconstructional tasks. Patients with impairment of route finding ability tend to get lost. In hospital, they may lose their way from their bed to the bathroom and present as if they are confused. Those at home may fail to find their way around a familiar neighbourhood. All places appear unfamiliar. This topographical agnosia occurs because the patient fails to recognise localities and their landmarks with their unique orienting value. Patients can describe a route from memory, and can follow a route using a map, but if relying only on visual cues, they have difficulty. Topographical agnosia is a form of visual agnosia, and often associated with colour agnosia and prosopagnosia, although it may occur in isolation. It is generally due to right medial occipital lesions. Topographical agnosia needs to be differentiated from topographical amnesia, which is an inability to remember topographical relation-ships between landmarks, although they can be identified individually. So patients can identify buildings but are unable to describe routes or to use maps. Patient will know they have a stove, a fridge, a washing machine, a table and chairs in their kitchen but are unable to describe their relative positions or draw the room layout. Some cope by learning a visual sequence of locations. For example, Helen got lost one day on her way from the occupational therapy department to the psychology department and ended up in the ward instead. On questioning she said she knew the route involved going through the green door to the gate, then to the hollyhocks and then up the ramp. It turned out that the gardeners had cut down the hollyhocks, so she lost her cue to enable her to recognise the route.

Specific difficulties in visual localisation may also occur following bilateral lesions in the occipito-parietal boundary. These present as distortions in judge-ment of distance and depth. Patients misreach as they cannot judge where things are in space, and they bump into objects due to misjudging distance. They may also report that everything looks unusually large (macropsia), small (micropsia) or far away (teleopsia). For example, Hazel became very distressed during a physiotherapy session because she was being asked to walk 'so far', even though the distance was in reality quite short and well within her capabilities; her perceptual deficit made things look very far away, and hence gave her the impression she was being asked to do an impossible task.

Working memory includes a visuospatial sketchpad. This is used for naviga-tion in space. To remember a route you need to know what you have just seen and its topographical relationship to other items. Impairments occur following right frontal lesions. In addition remembering where things are in space, memory for location, occurs following right temporal lesions (hippocampus). Selective disturbances in perception also produce corresponding problems in imagery. Patients who cannot remember spatial locations can also have difficulty manip-ulating images in space. For example they have problems with mental rotations. Visuoconstructional deficits produce problems in drawing that can be detected on tests such as copying the Rey complex figure, cube counting (VOSP) and in pattern construction in both two dimensions, such as WAIS Block Design, or three dimensions, such as the Rivermead Perceptual Assessment Battery 3D copy.

Body perception disorders

There are a collection of perceptual disorders which relate to the awareness of one's body and the relationship between body and space. These include body orientation problems, anosagnosia and somatoparaphrenia. Body orientation problems cause difficulties in practical daily tasks as patients are not aware of the relative position of their body parts. This has been associated with right/left confusion. Gerstmann (1940) reported that in 1924 he had noted that finger agnosia, R-L disorientation, acalculia and agraphia (peripheral) tended to co-occur and this combination of symptoms, subsequently labelled Gerstmann's syndrome, was considered to be a feature of left parietal lesions. However, although this combination of symptoms can occasionally occur together (Rusconi, Pinel, Dehaene & Kleinschmidt, 2010), it is much rarer than originally believed and is probably not a useful description for the majority of stroke patients. The main problems which occur after stroke are in the perception of the position of body parts and changes in position of the body in relation to the external world.

Anosagnosia is the unawareness or denial of a disorder, including denial of hemiplegia, hemianopia, or hemianaesthesia (Vallar & Ronchi, 2006). It may be difficult to distinguish these problems from visual inattention, in that patients are not aware of their problems across these conditions. However, in anosagnosia there is more active denial as compared with inattention. For example, in the acute stage patients may be unaware of any weakness to the extent that they try to get out of bed despite having a severe hemiplegia and may deny the inability to use a hemiplegic arm. This can cause significant distress as they fail to understand why they need to be in hospital and why people consider that they will not be able to cope with activities of daily living. There seems to be some implicit awareness of the deficit as, when asked to report what they are able to do, patients will report no problems but when asked what the examiner would be able to do if he were in the patients' present state, they will report limitations (Marcel, Tegner & Nimmo-Smith, 2004).

Estimates of the frequency of anosagnosia depend on the method and timing of assessment. Stone *et al.* (1993) examined patients within 3 days of stroke and found anosagnosia in 28% of right hemisphere and 5% of left hemisphere stroke patients. Baier and Karnath (2005) assessed 128 stroke patients in hospital within 156 days of stroke using a four-point rating scale (Bisiach, Vallar, Perani, Papagno & Berti, 1986). Eight patients (6%) had a denial grade of 2, recognising their paresis only after demonstration, and four (3%) had a denial grade of 3, remaining unaware of their deficit even after demonstration. In a subsequent study, Baier and Karnath (2008) assessed 75 consecutive acute right hemisphere stroke patients using the same scale and found 12 (15%) with anosagnosia. Systematic reviews (Jehkonen, Laihosalo & Kettunen, 2006a; Orfei, Robinson, Prigatano, Starkstein, Rusch, Bria *et al.*, 2007) found that the frequency of anosagnosia varied across studies; with Jehkonen *et al.* (2006a) reporting estimates ranging between 11% and 60% in right hemisphere stroke patients and between 6% and 24% in left hemisphere patients. Orfei *et al.* (2007) reported estimates between 7% and 77%. The variation has been attributed to differences in recruitment, sample size and timing of initial assessment. However, from a practical perspective it is clearly a significant problem for many stoke patients, particularly those with right hemisphere strokes.

Magnetic resonance imaging of these patients (Karnath, Baier & Nagele, 2005) has indicated that the right posterior insula seems to be crucial in the sense of limb ownership and awareness or beliefs about limb movement. However, Orfei *et al.* (2007) also identified studies suggesting that anosagnosia occurs following lesions of the frontal and prefrontal cortex. According to Vallar and Ronchi (2006), anosagnosia usually resolves over time, although there are cases reported in the literature where it has persisted for several years.

Somatoparaphrenia involves delusional beliefs concerning the contralesional side of somatic or extra somatic space. Patients disown their paralysed limbs, claiming that someone else's arm is in bed with them and at times attempting to get rid of the stray limb. Vallar and Ronchi (2009) reviewed the phenomenon and reported that it is usually due to right hemisphere stroke giving rise to a left somatoparaphrenia. It is associated with motor and sensory impairment but can occur without associated anosagnosia for motor deficits or personal neglect. Baier and Karnath (2008) identified 11 out of 79 (14%) acute right hemisphere stroke patients showing abnormal attitudes towards their left affected limbs within three days of the stroke, and six of these had a definite somatoparaphrenia. They concluded that the impairment was due to a deficit in multisensory integration and of spatial representation of the body.

Supernumerary phantom limbs may arise following lesions in either the right or left hemisphere but have been reported more frequently after right hemisphere stroke (Halligan, Marshall & Wade, 1993; Halligan & Marshall, 1995). Srivastava, Taly, Gupta, Murali, Noone, Thirthahalli *et al.* (2008) described a patient who believed she had extra limbs following a stroke, a belief which persisted for seven months. Their interpretation of the phenomenon was that knowledge of the position of a limb is based on integrating motor and sensory feedback. If this information is discrepant, then the perceived body shape is altered, causing the patient to perceive a supernumerary limb to resolve the discrepancy in the information.

Visual neglect

Visual neglect, also known as visual inattention, is a syndrome in which patients do not attend to a proportion of the contralesional visual field (Adair & Barrett 2008; Manly, 2002; Parton, Malhotra & Husain, 2004); the classic example being patients who will eat one half of their plate of food, leaving the other half untouched, who are unaware when people approach them on the left and who are unaware of the left side of their environment. This is distinct from hemianopia in which there is loss of vision to one side of space. Patients with hemianopia are aware of the problem and will often compensate by extra scanning movements and turning their heads. Patients with full visual fields may nevertheless fail to report the contralesional stimulus when it is presented simultaneously with an ipsilesional stimulus, a phenomenon known as 'extinction'. Patients may have extinction but not neglect but patients with neglect may also show extinction. Extinction may also occur in other modalities, such as tactile and auditory.

Visual neglect can occur following stroke to either hemisphere, but is more common and usually more severe following right hemisphere stroke, affecting the left visual hemispace (van Zomeren & Spikman, 2003). In most patients, this is due to a right middle cerebral artery stroke, but it can also occur after posterior cerebral artery stroke (Bird, Malhotra, Parton, Coulthard, Rushworth & Husain, 2006). Ipsilesional visual inattention has also been reported (Kim, Na, Kim, Adair, Lee & Heilman, 1999), but is much less commonly encountered in clinical practice. Although neglect most commonly applies to the visual modality, the condition can also apply to auditory, motor and somatosensory modalities (Guerrini, Berlucchi, Bricolo & Aglioti, 2003; Sinnett, Juncadella, Rafal, Azanon & Soto-Faraco, 2007).

The incidence figures vary widely (12–100%) depending on sampling, timing and methods of assessment (Bowen, McKenna & Tallis, 1999). Studies in the acute stage show the problem occurs frequently in acute stroke and mild neglect occurs in those with left hemisphere lesions. Stone *et al.* (1993) assessed 171 stroke patients within three days of stroke and reported that visual neglect occurred in 82% of assessable right hemisphere patients and 65% of left hemisphere patients. However, it recovers relatively quickly following left hemisphere stroke in comparison with right hemisphere stroke, and severe chronic neglect is usually only seen after right hemisphere damage.

As with other stroke-related impairments, the neuroanatomical underpinning of visual neglect is complex, with damage to several cortical and subcortical structures implicated across various studies (Adair & Barrett, 2008; Committeri, Pitzalis, Galati, Patria, Pelle, Sabatini *et al.*, 2007; Manly, 2002). Husain and Rorden (2003) reported that the right hemisphere cortical regions that are damaged in patients with neglect include both posterior areas (junction of the temporal and parietal lobes, inferior parietal lobe, intraparietal sulcus and the superior temporal gyrus) and frontal areas (inferior frontal gyrus and middle frontal gyrus). Subcortical lesions can sometimes lead to neglect, probably because of indirect effects on the cortex. Committeri *et al.* (2007) examined 52 right hemisphere stroke patients and assessed patients on measures of personal and extra personal neglect and examined the neural basis of these impairments using MRI scans. Awareness of extrapersonal space was based on the integrity of a circuit of right frontal (ventral premotor cortex and middle frontal gyrus) and superior temporal regions, whereas awareness of personal space was dependent on the right inferior parietal regions. Disruption of personal space awareness seemed to be due to a functional disconnection between regions important for coding proprioceptive and somatosensory inputs, and regions coding more abstract egocentric representations of the body in space. However, Hillis, Barker, Beauchamp, Gordon and Wityk (2000) emphasised that the location and extent of the lesion is not always the best predictor of disability and the extent of the ischaemic penumbra is more important.

Visual neglect is probably not a unitary syndrome but a collection of problems which each manifest as a failure to attend to one side of space (Adair & Barrett,

2008). Various theories have been put forward to account for visual neglect, and various types have been identified on the basis of double dissociations. Sensory accounts consider the failure to see objects as due to a visual field defect, such as hemianopia, but it should be noted that hemianopia and neglect are independent problems, although they commonly occur together, and can be differentiated using specialist approaches to visual field testing (Walker *et al.*, 1991). Motor theories account for some patients who seem to have difficulty initiating movements to the left. The suggestion is that part of the failure on cancellation tasks is due to this intentional component. Coulthard, Parton and Husain (2006) reviewed studies of motor control in patients with neglect and concluded that although patients with neglect demonstrate a failure to initiate movements into the left side of space, the pattern of deficits is highly variable. In addition, patients with motor neglect fail to use their contralesional limbs even though they have little or no weakness.

Representational theories of neglect propose that patients have a distorted representation of space and patients are unaware of the left side of space. The classic evidence for this comes from an account by Bisiach and Luzzatti (1978) who asked patients to imagine standing on the steps of the cathedral at one end of the main square in Milan and to describe the buildings and then to imagine standing at the other end of the square and to describe the buildings. In each case they described the buildings on their right. So although they knew all the buildings in the square, as they reported buildings from both sides, when reporting what they could see in their imagination, they only reported the right side of space. Even in severe neglect targets to the left may eventually be found if there are few distractors to the right – so the left does "exist" in the minds of these patients. There are also accounts of patients with an object-based neglect (Chatterjee, 1994; Ota, Fujii, Suzuki, Fukatsu & Yamadori, 2001) in which they fail to report the left side of objects regardless of where they are presented in the visual field. So, for example, patients will copy the right half of objects at various points in the visual field, and not just omit objects on the left.

The dominant theory considers that visual neglect is due to a deficit in directing spatial attention. Heilman, Bowers, Coslett, Whelan and Watson (1985) proposed that the right hemisphere is dominant for attentional control and normally directs attention to both sides of space, whereas the left hemisphere only controls attention to the right. Right hemisphere damage therefore results in an imbalance in the direction of attention. Kinsbourne (1993) proposed an attentional gradient in which each hemisphere pushes attention to the contralateral side. The left hemisphere has a more powerful effect, therefore left neglect is more common than right. Posner, Walker, Friedrich and Rafal (1984) suggested damage to right posterior parietal areas results in an inability to disengage attentional focus from a left-sided target.

These accounts capture the fluctuating, attentional nature of neglect. Impaired spatial working memory has also been proposed to account for some of the impairments seen. Husain and Rorden (2003) investigated search patterns in patients with neglect and showed that these are chaotic and patients fail to remember that they have already found targets. The severity of neglect correlated with performance on a nonlateralised spatial working memory task (Husain, Mannon, Mort, Hodgson, Driver & Kennard, 2002) and recovery of both neglect and spatial working memory occurred at similar rates.

Various types of visual neglect occur including motor neglect, object-based neglect and visual inattention. Neglect may also cause problems with specific tasks, such as reading, which gives rise to a neglect dyslexia. In addition, neglect occurs in personal, peripersonal and far space (Adair & Barrett 2008). For example, Halligan and Marshall (1991) reported a patient who had severe neglect in peripersonal space yet was accurately able to throw darts and demonstrated no neglect in far space. Visual neglect comprises a collection of syndromes rather than one underlying deficit. These lead to several dissociable forms which can occur independently, but often coexist due to either overlapping cognitive skills or the proximity of the lesions which cause them. The most prominent theoretical account suggests that neglect is due to impairment of attentional control interacting with impaired spatial working memory.

Memory impairment

Memory impairment is a frequently reported cognitive symptom after stroke (Aben, Kessel, Duivenvoorden, Busschbach, Eling, Bogert *et al.*, 2009; Doornhein & de Haan, 1998). In a systematic review of memory problems in stroke patients without dementia (Snaphaan & de Leeuw, 2007), the prevalence of memory impairment ranged from 23% to 55% three months after stroke, and from 11% to 31% a year after stroke. There are several subtypes of memory impairment, with some evidence of a relationship between the location of the stroke and the resulting memory deficits (Lim & Alexander, 2009). Brain lesions resulting from stroke can directly affect memory by damaging areas and pathways associated with known memory processes, such as the limbic system, or indirectly by affecting other brain regions associated with cognitive functions upon which memory depends, such as perceptual or attentional systems.

Episodic memory

Episodic memory refers to the ability to remember personal events and the temporal-spatial relations among these events (Tulving, 1972). Originally Tulving conceptualised episodic memory as distinct from semantic memory, which he described as a parallel and overlapping memory system representing organised knowledge about the world (Tulving, 1972). Episodic memory can be further classified according to memory for events prior to the stroke (retrograde memory) or memory for events after the stroke (anterograde memory, i.e. the ability to lay down new memories). Both anterograde and retrograde amnesic syndromes can result from a stroke, although retrograde amnesia is more common following bilateral stroke (Della Sala, Laiacona, Spinnler & Trivelli, 1993), and where present following unilateral stroke tends to involve less significant impairment (Batchelor, Thompson & Miller, 2008).

Lim and Alexander (2009) provided an excellent review of episodic memory impairment after stroke. Table 4.1 summarises the various episodic memory difficulties that can occur, with their neuroanatomical correlates (Lim & Alexander, 2009). It should be emphasised, however, that individual strokes rarely selectively affect one memory system. Just as individual memory tests cannot isolate individual memory systems, so in reality the picture is more complex than Table 4.1 might suggest.

It is a widely held view that episodic memory impairment caused by focal unilateral stroke tends to be restricted to either verbal or nonverbal material; right hemisphere stroke is associated with nonverbal memory impairment, whereas left hemisphere stroke is associated with verbal memory impairment. However, a clear distinction between memory for verbal and nonverbal material is rarely evident in clinical practice, with memory-impaired stroke patients often demonstrating a combination of verbal and nonverbal memory impairment on testing (Frisk & Milner, 1990). Gillespie, Bowen and Foster (2006), in a meta-analytic and narrative review of the literature, found mixed evidence regarding the performance of right hemisphere and left hemisphere stroke patients on verbal memory tests, although there was a trend for right hemisphere stroke patients to show superior performance on tests of verbal recall and recognition as compared with the left hemisphere stroke patients. It is generally accepted that bilateral lesions are necessary for a patient to present with permanent global episodic memory impairment (Lim & Alexander, 2009). The stroke sub-types giving rise to memory disorders are shown in Table 4.1.

Other memory problems

Working memory impairment, the inability to retain and manipulate information for a short time, is frequently encountered after stroke (Jaillard, Naegele, Trabucco-Miguel, LeBas & Hommel, 2009) and can have a significant effect on a patient's ability to engage in rehabilitation (Malouin, Belleville, Richards, Desrosiers & Doyon, 2004). However, working memory may be conceptualised as an executive or attentional function, rather than as a memory function *per se* (Alexander, Stuss & Fansabedian, 2003; Kane, Conway, Miura & Colflesh, 2007). Stroke patients may present with working memory impairment as a direct result of a lesion to any of a number of neuroanatomical locations, or as an indirect consequence of other symptoms, such as fatigue, pain, and depression, which have an impact on general attentional resources.

Table 4.1   Summary of Stroke Subtypes Causing Memory Disorders. (Lim, C., & Alexander, M.P., 2009. Stroke and episodic memory disorders, *Neuropsychologia, 47,* 3048, with permission from Elsevier).

Location/vascular territory	Anatomy	Memory deficits	Associated deficits
Left posterior cerebral artery (PCA)	Hippocampus Medial temporal lobe Collateral isthmus	Verbal memory	Visual field deficits Colour agnosia Alexia without agraphia Anomia
Right PCA	Hippocampus Medial temporal lobe Collateral isthmus	Visuospatial memory	Visual field deficits Prosopagnosia
Bilateral PCA	Hippocampus Medial temporal lobe Collateral isthmus	Explicit memory Retrograde memory	Cortical blindness Apperceptive agnosia Associative agnosia
Left anterior thalamus	Anterior thalamus Mammillothalamic tract Internal medullary lamina	Verbal memory Visuospatial memory	Executive dysfunction Mixed transcortical aphasia
Right anterior thalamus	Anterior thalamus Mammillothalamic tract Internal medullary lamina	Visuospatial memory	Executive dysfunction Visuoperceptual deficits
Left genu internal capsule	Anterior thalamic peduncle Inferior thalamic peduncle	Verbal memory	Frontal lobe system
Right genu internal capsule	Anterior thalamic peduncle Inferior thalamic peduncle	Visuospatial memory	Frontal lobe system
Medial thalamic	Dorsomedial nucleus Centromedian nucleus Internal medullary lamina	Verbal memory Visuospatial memory Retrograde memory	Hypersomnolence Attentional deficits Ocular motility
Basal Forebrain	Septal nuclei	Verbal memory Visuospatial memory	Confabulation Executive dysfunction Anosognosia for amnesia

Prospective memory, the ability to carry out a planned action at a future time, can be impaired after stroke. Kim, Craik, Luo and Ween (2009) found that a small sample of stroke patients performed less well on tests of prospective and retrospective memory, and executive control. The authors hypothesised that the primary mechanism underlying these patients' prospective memory impairment was the inability to self-initiate effortful cognitive processes, an executive dysfunction.

Autobiographical memory impairment tends to be associated with bilateral hippocampal lesions (Rosenbaum, Moscovitch, Foster, Schnyer, Ga, Kovacevic, *et al.*, 2008), and so profound autobiographical memory loss is relatively rare in single-episode stroke patients. However, some degree of autobiographical memory impairment can occur in unilateral stroke (Batchelor *et al.*, 2008), especially those affecting the right hippocampus. The degree of impairment following unilateral stroke tends to be relatively mild, with patients rarely spontaneously complaining of difficulties in recalling autobiographical events, although this may in some cases be due in part to problems with insight.

Semantic memory impairment can also occur after stroke, but is more likely to be associated with primary acquired language impairment and a different (left temperoparietal and prefrontal) neuroanatomical aetiology than that of the semantic memory impairment associated with semantic dementia (bilateral atrophy of the anterior temporal lobes) (Jeffries & Lambon-Ralph, 2006).

Even in patients with profound episodic memory impairment, some memory functions can remain intact. For example, patients may be able to acquire new motor, perceptual or cognitive skills. In essence, non-declarative memory, such as implicit learning, priming and classical conditioning, may remain intact, even for example in patients with bilateral stroke resulting in profound impairment of anterograde and retrograde declarative memory (Gold & Squire, 2006).

Executive dysfunction

The term 'executive functioning' describes a constellation of cognitive domains, such as conceptual reasoning, cognitive flexibility, planning and problem solving, which have long been associated with damage to the frontal lobes (Stuss & Knight, 2002). However, the picture is highly complex, as executive functions have been shown to occur following damage to regions other than the frontal lobes, and conversely it is quite possible for a patient to have no discernable cognitive impairments on testing following an isolated frontal lobe lesion. Frontal lobe stroke usually occurs in the context of additional cortical and subcortical involvement (Vataja, Pohjasvaara, Mäntyla, Ylikoski, Leppävuori, Leskela *et al.*, 2003). This is perhaps unsurprising, given that stroke is a vascular disorder. In any major stroke, the blood supply to a large portion of the brain is likely to be affected. The nature of the vascular geography of the brain is such that a stroke affecting a frontal cortical region of the brain is likely to additionally affect nonfrontal and subcortical regions. For example, a stroke in the anterior cerebral artery territory may affect some or all of the medial regions of the frontal and parietal lobes, and anterior parts of the corpus callosum, internal capsule and basal ganglia (Nieuwenhuys, Voogd & van Huijzen, 2008). Other regions of the frontal lobes are supplied by the middle cerebral artery, such as the lateral surfaces of the frontal lobes (Nieuwenhuys *et al.*, 2008). Even posterior cerebral artery strokes may affect executive functioning through involvement of the thalamus (Van der Werf, Scheltens, Lindeboom, Witter, Uylings & Jolles, 2003).

Vataja *et al.* (2003) investigated MRI correlates of executive dysfunction in patients with ischaemic stroke and found executive dysfunction to be present in 34% of their sample of 214 elderly patients three months after stroke. The authors found a preponderance of patients with executive dysfunction whose stroke affected the frontal-subcortical pathways. They also found that left-sided lesions predisposed to executive dysfunction more than right-sided lesions. Perhaps most intriguingly, they also found that pontine stroke lesions were associated with a higher rate of executive dysfunction, which they argued could either reflect the effects of more severe vascular brain disease or a possible direct effect of brainstem lesions on executive functioning.

It is evident from recent research that there are neuroanatomical correlates for several subtypes of executive functioning, for example 'energization' associated with the superior medial, 'task setting' associated with the left lateral and 'monitoring' associated with the right lateral frontal lobe regions (Stuss & Alexander, 2007). Depending on the specific focal lesion location, it is therefore quite possible for patients to have isolated cognitive executive difficulties, or behavioural problems associated with the 'dysexecutive syndrome' without any evidence of executive dysfunction on cognitive tests. More typically, in clinical practice it is a significant challenge to differentiate between the effects of a stroke on executive functioning because of the frequent co-occurrence of language, visuospatial and attentional deficits, which can all affect performance on 'executive' tests (Ballard, Stephens, Kenny, Kalaria, Tovee & O'Brien, 2003). Zinn, Bosworth, Hoenig and Swartzwelder (2007) assessed stroke patients admitted to hospital within a week of stroke on a battery of tests of executive ability. They found that in acute stroke patients impairment occurred on 60% of the tests completed and about half of the patients performed in the impaired range on nearly all of the tests examined. Symbol Digit Modalities, design fluency production and Trail Making switching scores showed the highest frequency of impairment with 75%, 56% and 50% impaired respectively. Executive impairments were also found in those with TIA, affecting 58%, 50% and 40% respectively. The deficits in the TIA patients were attributed to the effects of cerebrovascular disease.

Studies of cognitive impairment in patients with vascular dementia also indicate that impairments of executive function are common (Lafosse, Reed,

Mungas, Sterling, Wahbeh & Jagust, 1997; Padovani, DiPiero, Bragoni, Iacoboni & Gualdi 1995), and often co-occur with impairments of attention and speed of information processing. Stephens, Kenny, Rowan, Allan, Kalaria, Bradbury *et al.* (2004) assessed 384 elderly stroke patients over 75 years old, three months after stroke, on the CAMCOG-R and compared them with 66 healthy controls. Stroke patients were divided into those with no significant cognitive impairment (n = 259), vascular cognitive impairment nondementia (n = 92) and post-stroke dementia (n = 33) on the basis of clinical evaluations. Stroke patients with no significant cognitive impairment performed significantly worse than healthy controls on measures of executive function, speed of information processing and perception. Thus even in the absence of obvious cognitive impairment, as defined using a clinical diagnosis, impairment of executive abilities was present. As the executive problems were not detected by routine clinical diagnostic procedures, it follows that these often go unrecognised in clinical practice.

There is little information on the pattern of recovery in executive functioning over time. Nys, Van Zandvoort, De Kort, Jansen, Van der Worp, Kappelle and De Haan (2005a) reported on the 6–10-month recovery of 111 patients after first-ever stroke. They found that at baseline 32% of patients were impaired on tests of executive functioning, whereas at 6–10-month follow-up approximately 14% of patients were impaired. This is broadly consistent with the recovery shown in other cognitive domains by this sample. However, only a limited number of executive tests were administered at baseline (Brixton Spatial Anticipation Test, Visual Elevator of the TEA, and Letter Fluency). It is also clear that impairments in other domains, such as perception and language, may have affected performance on these tests.

Zinn *et al.* (2007) highlighted the many ways in which executive impairment may affect the ability to engage in rehabilitation. For example, those with deficits in initiation and persistence may have difficulty engaging in a series of exercises; impairments of planning or problem solving may lead to unsafe transfers and increase the risk of falls; deficits of attention or cognitive speed may affect the ability to process complex information and reduced prospective memory, remembering to remember something, and reduced information processing capacity may make it difficult for rehabilitation patients to remember and follow complex treatment regimens. They suggested that patients with impairments of executive function may fail to benefit fully from rehabilitation as a result of these problems. There is also evidence of an association between the presence of executive impairments and worse functional outcomes (McDowd, Filion, Pohl, Richards & Stiers, 2003; Mok, Wong, Lam, Fan, Tang, Kwok *et al.*, 2004; Pohjasvaara, Vataja, Leppavuori, Kaste & Erkinjuntti, 2002).

Executive impairments may be associated with acquired behavioural problems such as disinhibition, impaired self-regulation and poor social functioning. Behavioural difficulties after stroke are discussed in Chapter 12.

Social and emotion perception

The ability to recognise emotion, either through the visual or auditory modality, is a complex perceptual task which underpins many impairments of social functioning and behavioural disturbances. Impairments occur in the ability to recognise emotion from facial expression. For example, patients may be unable to report whether someone is sad, anxious or afraid. In addition, some will also not be able to detect mood from the tone of a speaker's voice. Deficits in recognising emotion from faces is more common following right hemisphere lesions than left, whereas deficits in the ability to detect emotion in voices occurs following both right and left hemisphere lesions (Kucharska-Pietura, Phillips, Gernand & David, 2003). Positive mood states, such as happy and excited, are more easily recognised than negative states, such as sad, angry and afraid. The deficits are illustrated in Figure 4.1.

Impairment in these skills can lead to misinterpretation of social situations and may account for some behavioural problems and difficulties in interpersonal relationships. Flaherty-Craig, Barrett and Eslinger (2002, p. 310) described a patient who showed loss of emotion perception following a right parietal-occipital haemorrhage. Although he could recognise when his wife was happy,

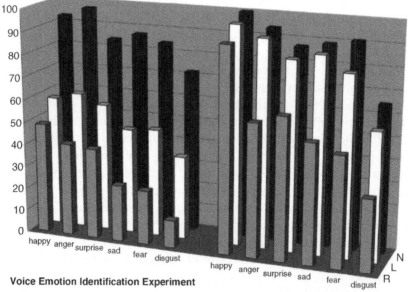

Voice Emotion Identification Experiment

Face Emotion Recognition Experiment

R: right hemisphere stroke patients;   L: left hemisphere stroke patients;
N: healthy control participants.

Figure 4.1   Emotion recognition after stroke. (Kucharska-Pietura K., Phillips M. L., Gernand W., David A.S., 2003, Perception of emotions from faces and voices following unilateral brain damage, *Neuropsychologia, 41*, 1082–90, with permission from Elsevier.)

he was not able to discriminate between pleasant surprise, joy or excitement. He perceived all expressions of disappointment, sadness, fear and anger, as anger. This led to him responding inappropriately in interactions with his wife and he presented as if lacking empathy. He had to learn to use verbal reasoning skills to compensate for his inability to recognise emotion in faces.

In addition, the expression of emotion may also be affected by stroke (Nakhutina, Borod & Zgaljardic, 2006). Left and right hemisphere stroke patients and healthy controls were assessed on two occasions about a year apart. The task was to say a sentence using one of eight randomly presented emotions: three positive or pleasant (happiness, pleasant surprise, and interest) and five negative or unpleasant (sadness, disgust, unpleasant surprise, fear, and anger). Stroke patients were impaired relative to healthy controls at baseline, approximately 1–2 years after stroke. In addition, right hemisphere patients with frontal lesions were more impaired than right hemisphere stroke patients without frontal lesions. Left hemisphere stroke patients showed the opposite effect with patients with frontal lesions performing better than left hemisphere stoke patients without frontal lesions. There was also a difference in the pattern of recovery over time. Right hemisphere stroke patients showed deterioration in performance over time whereas those with left hemisphere lesions improved.

Attentional impairments

Attentional deficits are very common after stoke. Within the acute phase, estimates range between 46% and 92% (Stapleton, Ashburn & Stack, 2001). At discharge from hospital estimates suggest a prevalence of 24% and 51% (Hyndman, Pickering & Ashburn, 2008) and prevalence estimates suggest that between 20% and 43% of patients continue to have some form of attentional impairment at four years after stroke (Hyndman & Ashburn, 2003). Again, depending on one's theoretical perspective, attentional impairments may be described as largely 'executive'. For example, Norman and Shallice's (1986) Supervisory Attentional System is a theoretical account of executive functioning which, as the name suggests, describes the allocation of attentional resources as central to the process of executive functioning. There is a clear practical overlap between deficits in working memory, information processing, executive functioning and various subtypes of attention, such as divided, switching, sustained and selective attention. As discussed above, visual neglect is also a disorder of attention.

Sustained attention (concentration) is clearly an important prerequisite for many complex cognitive functions. Motor recovery has been shown to be dependent on intact sustained attention, since sufficient sustained attention is a prerequisite for learning (Robertson, Ridgeway, Greenfield & Parr, 1997). Other specific attentional disorders, such as auditory and visual selective attention, and divided attention, will also affect functional recovery, although there is currently insufficient evidence of the direct influence of specific attentional disorders on longer-term functional outcome after stroke (Hyndman *et al.*, 2008).

Speed of information processing can be impaired following a stroke (Ballard *et al.*, 2003; Gerritsen, Berg, Deelman, Visser-Keizer & Meyboom-de Jong, 2003; Rasquin, Lodder, Ponds, Winkens, Jolles & Verhey, 2004). Estimates of prevalence have varied between 50% and 70% (Hochstenbach, Mulder, van Limbeek, Donders & Schoonderwaldt, 1998; Rasquin *et al.*, 2004). Patients also report problems themselves (Visser-Keizer, Meyboom-De Jong, Deelman, Berg & Gerritsen, 2002; Winkel *et al.*, 2006). Qualitative interviews with patients with slowed speed of information processing (Winkens, Van Heughten, Fasotti, Duits & Wade, 2006) indicated that these difficulties had widespread effects on daily life. The majority of participants complained that they were not able to process incoming information, when for example having a conversation, speaking on the telephone, speaking during meetings, listening to the radio or watching television. Gerritsen *et al.* (2003) demonstrated that the effect of a stroke on information processing speed depended to some extent on which hemisphere was damaged. In their study, patients with right hemisphere stroke were slower than controls on all information processing tasks, and slower than left hemisphere stroke patients on visuomotor tasks. Left hemisphere stroke patients were slower than controls only on more complex categorisation tasks (Gerritsen *et al.*, 2003).

Conclusions

Stroke can lead to complex and disabling cognitive symptoms, the combination of which can be difficult to delineate. Prominent symptoms include apraxia, aphasia and visual inattention. However, the entire range of known neuropsychological impairment is possible. While brain imaging and neuropathological data are very relevant, there is often relatively little correlation between these investigations and the apparent clinical neuropsychological profile. The neuropsychological assessment is therefore central in quantifying the functional deficits after stroke, in predicting recovery, and in targeting limited rehabilitation resources (Nys *et al.*, 2005). After a first ever stroke, patients can expect a period of natural recovery, which may be enhanced by rehabilitation. It is incumbent upon the neuropsychologist to assess the extent and nature of cognitive impairment evident after stroke accurately in order to inform intervention.

Chapter 5

Screening for Cognitive Problems after Stroke

Introduction

The majority of stroke patients have cognitive impairments (Lesniak, Bak, Czepiel, Seniow & Czlonkowska, 2008; Nys, van Zandvoort, De Kort, Jansen, De Haan & Kappelle, 2007). This includes impairments in all cognitive domains, including attention, memory, language, visuospatial and executive abilities. These affect rehabilitation outcome (Hochstenbach, Anderson, van Limbeek & Mulder, 2001; Hommel, Miguel, Naegele Gonnet & Jaillard, 2009; Lesniak *et al.*, 2008; Nys, van Zandvoort, De Kort, van der Worp, Jansen, Algra *et al.*, 2005b). Therefore, cognitive problems need to be identified so that they can be taken into account when planning rehabilitation, determining discharge plans and discussing problems that people are likely to encounter in the future. In addition, some patients have a dementia after stroke, usually vascular, which produces a progressive decline in cognitive abilities over time. This needs to be recognised, as it has implications for the clinical management of the patients. However, the definition of dementia is not always consistent, and different systems of classifying dementias produce different categories (Pohjasvaara, Mäntylä, Ylikoski, Kaste & Erkinjuntti, 2000).

Many guidelines for stroke services (Division of Clinical Psychology/Clinical Neuropsychology, 2010; Department of Health, 2007a; Royal College of Physicians, 2008a) recommend screening for cognitive problems early after stroke, which may be used to predict functional outcome (Nys *et al.*, 2005b; Paolucci, Antonucci, Gialoreti Traballesi, Lubich, Pratesi *et al.*, 1996; Tatemichi, Desmond, Stern, Paik, Sano & Bagiella, 1994). Screening may improve discharge planning, rehabilitation treatment, and the long-term outcome of people with stroke (Edwards, Hahn, Baum, Perlmutter, Sheedy & Dromerick, 2006b). Early identification of cognitive impairments is seen as a quality marker

Psychological Management of Stroke, First Edition. Nadina B. Lincoln, Ian I. Kneebone, Jamie A.B. Macniven and Reg C. Morris.
© 2012 John Wiley & Sons, Ltd. Published 2012 by John Wiley & Sons, Ltd.

for stroke services (Department of Health, 2007a). In clinical practice, the ideal would be to have a short screening measure to identify those with cognitive problems who may then be referred for further evaluation. However, in many clinical services the screening measures are the only assessment of cognitive function that takes place. It is therefore important that measures used to screen for cognitive problems are sensitive i.e. they detect all those who have cognitive problems. Given that most stroke patients, approximately 70%, have cognitive problems (Lesniak *et al.*, 2008; Nys *et al.*, 2007), screening measures need to be more efficient than simply classifying all stroke patients as cognitively impaired. They also need to detect impairment in different cognitive domains, such as language, attention, perception, memory and executive abilities, as this will change rehabilitation planning.

A test used for screening should have good criterion validity, i.e. the ability to accurately detect the presence of impairment in a given population. This requires high levels of sensitivity and high levels of specificity (Loong, 2003). Sensitivity refers to the ability of a test to identify correctly those people in a population who have the impairment (i.e. the proportion of true positives identified by the test). Specificity refers to the ability to identify correctly those people who do not have the impairment (i.e. the proportion of true negatives). Sensitivity and specificity are statistically linked and trade off with each other. Increasing the sensitivity of a test by lowering the cut-off scores decreases the specificity. Screening measures should generally have a sensitivity of greater than 80% and a specificity of greater than 60% (Dewey, personal communication). The 'area under the curve' (AUC) statistic is used to summarise the combined sensitivity and specificity of a test. An AUC of 1.0 is a perfect screening test (100% sensitivity and 100% specificity), 0.80 or more is good and below 0.70 is poor. A positive predictive value describes the chance of a positive test result being correct and a negative predictive value the chance of a negative result being correct. Predictive power statistics take into account not only the diagnostic accuracy (sensitivity and specificity) but also the natural prevalence (base rate) of impairment in a population. This is important because base rates can affect the likelihood of a true positive or true negative result, over and above the accuracy of the particular test being used. For example, in a population where there is high prevalence of impairment, a positive test result is more likely to be correct compared to a positive test result using the same test in a population with a low prevalence rate, regardless of the accuracy of the test. In an acute stroke population, high base rates of cognitive impairment of around 70% (Nys *et al.*, 2005a) will naturally contribute towards high positive predictive power and low negative predictive power. It might therefore be assumed that there is little clinical value to using a screening measure with stroke patients which has a PPV of less than 70% or a NPV of less than 30%. Unfortunately, as highlighted by Cullen, O'Neill, Evans, Coen and Lawlor (2007), these values are rarely reported, and even if they are the base rates used are those of the setting in which the test was applied.

One criticism of many of the measures used in clinical practice is that they lack sensitivity. Many, such as the Mini-Mental State Examination (MMSE) (Folstein, Folstein & McHugh, 1975), Abbreviated Mental Test (AMT) (Hodgkinson, 1972), Addenbrooke's Cognitive Examination-Revised (ACE-R) (Mioshi, Dawson, Mitchell, Arnold & Hodges, 2006) and Cambridge Cognitive Examination (CAMCOG) (Huppert, Brayne, Gill, Paykel & Beardsall, 1995), were developed for the identification of people with dementia, and are therefore sensitive to impairments of memory but do not take account of the more frequent problems after stroke, such as attention, executive and visuospatial difficulties. Evidence is needed for their validity in stroke related cognitive impairment and vascular dementia, which occurs in about 30% of stroke patients (Henon, Durieu, Guerouaou, Lebert, Pasquier and Leys, 2001; Pohjasvaara, Erkinjuntti, Ylikoski, Hietanen, Vataja & Kaste, 1998). As the pattern of cognitive impairment may differ (see chapter 4), the choice of cognitive screening measures may differ, but relatively few studies have made a clear distinction between post-stroke cognitive impairment and post-stroke dementia. For stroke related cognitive impairment the best approach may be to use a battery of short tests, which are sensitive to the range of cognitive problems following stroke, as opposed to those which are common in people with dementia. The ideal would be to develop a stroke specific screening measure, but until this is available existing measures will be used in clinical practice and it is important that those using them are aware of their strengths and limitations in the context of screening for cognitive impairments after stroke.

Screening for post-stroke dementia

There are many short cognitive tests used to detect dementia (Cullen *et al.*, 2007), and several are used in clinical practice to detect those with dementia following stroke. However, caution should be exercised as the criteria used for classifying patients with dementia are not always consistent with each other (Pohjasvaara *et al.*, 2000). The most commonly used test is the MMSE, but others, such as the ACE-R and CAMCOG, have been used in some centres. These are usually used by doctors as part of their clinical examination of the patient.

The MMSE (Folstein *et al.*, 1975) was developed as a diagnostic tool for people with early signs of dementia. It comprises 20 items in two sections, one covering the cognitive domains of orientation, memory and attention, and the second addressing language and perception. It has been criticised (Husband & Tarbuck, 1994; Mathuranath, Nestor, Berrios, Rakowicz & Hodges, 2000) for including limited assessment of visuospatial and executive abilities. It relies on intact language ability and therefore is not appropriate for the 30% of stroke patients who have communication problems. It has established reliability, with high internal consistency, test–retest reliability and interrater reliability (Strauss, Sherman & Spreen, 2006, p.180). It has been validated against a clinical diagnosis of dementia and a standardised version (S-MMSE) is available (Molloy, Alemayehu & Roberts, 1991). Desmond, Tatemichi and Hanzawa (1994) evaluated 36 stroke patients, six with dementia. The sensitivity and specificity of the MMSE (sensitivity 83%, specificity 87%) were satisfactory, but it was a small sample and patients were assessed after discharge from hospital. Srikanth, Thrift, Fryer, Saling, Dewey, Sturm *et al.* (2006) evaluated 79 patients a year after a first-ever stroke. Cognitive impairment not dementia (CIND) and dementia were diagnosed independently using a comprehensive cognitive battery and DSM-IV criteria. Eight patients were diagnosed with post stroke dementia. The sensitivity of the S-MMSE for identifying dementia at cut-off 23/24 was poor (50%, specificity 94%, PPV 50%, NPV 94%) suggesting it was of little value. Tang, Mok, Chan, Chiu, Wong, Kwok and Lam (2005) compared the performance of the MMSE and the Initiation-Perseveration subtest of the Mattis Dementia Rating Scale (MDRS-IP) in screening for dementia in 83 patients with lacunar infarcts admitted to a stroke unit. Dementia was diagnosed in ten patients (12%) by a psychiatrist, blind to the MDRS-IP and MMSE scores. Although the MMSE was found to be sensitive (93%) to dementia, it was probably because they used a cut-off of 18/19. The MMSE was specific (80%) but also had a low PPV (PPV 36%, NPV 98%). They suggested the low PPV was due to the low prevalence of dementia, and the results also indicated that the MDRS-IP seemed to have little advantage over the MMSE.

The Addenbrookes Cognitive Examination (ACE) was developed because of the lack of sensitivity of the MMSE to dementia (Mathuranath, Nestor, Berrios, Rakowicz & Hodges, 2000). The ACE comprises the MMSE plus additional items, which expanded on memory, language and visuospatial components. The ACE has been found to be more sensitive than the MMSE for detecting dementia (Mathuranath *et al.*, 2000). A revised version, the ACE-R, with modifications designed to make it easier and quicker to administer, to increase the sensitivity and to facilitate cross-cultural usage, has superseded the ACE in clinical practice (Mioshi *et al.*, 2006). There are five subscales; attention and orientation, memory, fluency, language and visuospatial and the test takes between 12 and 20 minutes to administer. The validation of the ACE-R (Mioshi *et al.*, 2006) was similar to that of the original ACE (Mathuranath *et al.*, 2000). Two cut-off scores were identified (88 and 82). At a cut-off of 88, the ACE-R gave excellent sensitivity (94%) and good specificity (89%) for the detection of dementia, whereas using a cut-off score of 82 reduced sensitivity (84%) whilst increasing specificity (100%). Whilst Mioshi *et al.*'s (2006) findings were promising, they acknowledged that the ACE-R was developed within a specialised setting and recommended that the ACE-R also be studied in community samples where disease characteristics and prevalence rates may be different. Larner (2007) examined the ability of the ACE-R to identify patients with a dementia (types included dementia of the Alzheimer's type, fronto-temporal dementia, vascular dementia and dementia with Lewy bodies) in a community sample and found good sensitivity but the specificity rates were lower. However, the ACE-R has not been validated as a screening measure for post-stroke dementia.

The CAMCOG (Huppert *et al.*, 1995) forms part of the Cambridge Mental Disorders of the Elderly Examination (CAMDEX) (Roth, Huppert, Mountjoy & Tym, 1999) and was designed to assess the range of cognitive functions required for a diagnosis of dementia. The CAMCOG comprises the MMSE plus additional questions, yielding scores for several cognitive domains, orientation, language, memory, praxis, calculation, abstraction and perception, for analysis of impairments in specific areas. In a validation study in stroke patients (De-Koning, van Kooten, Dippel, van Harskamp, Grobbee, Kluft *et al.*, 1998), a CAMCOG total cut-off score of 79/80 was optimal for the discrimination of patients with dementia (dementia of the Alzheimer's type, vascular dementia or other dementias) from those without (sensitivity 92%, specificity 96%), whereas the MMSE gave poorer specificity (85%). A revised version, the CAMCOG-R, incorporates two tests of executive function, ideational fluency and a visual reasoning task. Leeds, Meara, Woods and Hobson (2001) compared these two tasks with existing measures of executive abilities in 83 stroke patients. Although the new CAMCOG-R executive functioning tests showed moderate correlation with the Weigl and Raven tests, which are both measures of reasoning ability ($p < 0.01$), the authors concluded that the extra time taken to administer the tests may not be justified. The new executive function tests were also vulnerable to the effects of depression.

The CAMCOG and CAMCOG-R are both lengthy and relatively complex to administer for screening purposes. De-Koning, Dippel, van Kooten and Koudastaal (2000) developed a shortened version, the 'Rotterdam-CAMCOG' (R-CAMCOG), for use with stroke patients. This assesses orientation, remote memory, recent memory, recall, recognition, perception and abstraction. It takes ten minutes to administer, with the reduction in length achieved by removing items with floor and ceiling effects and items with poor diagnostic validity. An optimal cut-off score of 33/34 was recommended for the detection of post-stroke dementia (de Koning *et al.*, 2000). De-Koning, van Kooten, Koudastaal and Dippel (2005) conducted an independent validation study with 121 stroke patients who were between three and nine months post stroke. They reported the R-CAMCOG to have good validity for the detection of dementia post stroke, as defined by neuropsychological assessments, information from carers and DSM-IV criteria. At the recommended cut-off of 34/34, the sensitivity was 66% and specificity 94% with positive and negative predictive values of 82% and 87% respectively. However, the optimum cut-off of 36/37 yielded higher sensitivity (83%) but lower specificity (78%) (PPV 76%, NPV 92%). The authors questioned whether the lack of executive items in the R-CAMCOG was a drawback in using the test to screen for post stroke dementia.

The Abbreviated Mental Test (AMT) (Hodgkinson, 1972) is a ten-item screening measure involving memory and orientation questions. Barber and Stott (2004) used the AMT to identify dementia in 67 stroke patients. The area under the ROC curve for the AMT for dementia diagnosis was 0.87. A cut-off of 8/9 produced the best balance with a sensitivity of 76% and a specificity of 77%. However, the criterion for classifying patients as having post-stroke dementia was the RCAMCOG, which itself had not been well validated.

Some dementia screening tests, such as the Informant Questionnaire for Cognitive Decline in the Elderly (IQCODE), Checklist for Cognitive and Emotional consequences following stroke (CLCE-24) and Telephone Interview for Cognitive Status (TICS) (Brandt, Spencer & Folstein, 1988), are based on standardisation of carer reports. These have also been evaluated in stroke patients. Srikanth *et al.* (2006) evaluated the 16-item IQCODE in detecting dementia in a community-based sample of 79 first-ever stroke patients. Patients were diagnosed independently using a comprehensive cognitive battery and DSM-IV criteria. The IQCODE ≥ 3.30 was sensitive (88%) but not specific (63%). ROC curves showed that obtaining high scores on either the IQCODE (≥ 3.7) or low scores on the S-MMSE (≤ 21) produced an acceptable balance between sensitivity (88%) and specificity (87%), but the positive predictive value remained low (44%).

The Checklist for Cognitive and Emotional Consequences following Stroke (CLCE-24) was evaluated in 69 stroke patients (van Heugten, Rasquin, Winkens, Beusmans & Verhey, 2007) by comparison with the MMSE and CAM-COG. Patients with complaints on the CLCE-24 also showed problems on the MMSE and the CAMCOG ($p < 0.05$). The CLCE-24 was a predictor of the MMSE and CAMCOG (adj. $R^2 = 0.13$ and 0.16, respectively) at 12 months post stroke. It was suggested that the CLCE-24 was a usable and valid instrument for cognitive screening by health care professionals in the stroke service in the chronic phase after stroke. However, no cut-off points were provided so it is left up to the individual assessor to decide which patients need further evaluation.

Another measure which can be administered by proxy is the Telephone Interview for Cognitive Status (TICS) (Brandt *et al.*, 1988). Desmond *et al.* (1994) investigated its use in a sample of 36 people with stroke, 6 of whom had dementia, and found it to be sensitive for picking up cognitive difficulties. The optimum cut-off for detecting dementia was 24/25 on the TICS, which had 100% sensitivity and 83% specificity. Barber and Stott (2004) tested the validity of the TICS with 64 stroke patients in the community, 24 (38%) of whom had post-stroke dementia, as defined using the R-CAMCOG, using cut-off 32/33. They examined both the 11-item TICS and a 13-item modified version, the TICSm, which included additional delayed recall items. The area under the ROC curve for both the TICS and TICSm was 0.94 indicating good screening power. The optimum cut-off of 28/29 on the TICS produced a sensitivity of 88% and a specificity of 85% for the diagnosis of post-stroke dementia. For the TICSm, a cut-off of 20/21 produced a sensitivity of 92% and a specificity of 80%.

They concluded that the TICS and TICSm telephone questionnaires were suitable for assessing cognitive function in community stroke patients. However, it should be noted that this was in relation to post-stroke dementia, defined using the R-CAMCOG rather than a comprehensive clinical assessment. It is possible that some of these patients had post-stroke cognitive impairment rather than dementia and were missed by the R-CAMCOG.

Cognitive screening measures are needed when cognitive impairment is not obvious. Therefore, measures have been developed for the detection of mild cognitive impairment, which often precedes dementia. The Montreal Cognitive Assessment (MOCA) (Nasreddine, Phillips, Bedirian, Charbonneau, White-head, Collin *et al.*, 2005) was developed to detect mild cognitive impairment, in a memory clinic setting, in those who performed within the normal range on the MMSE. It comprises 12 subtests assessing eight cognitive domains, giving results on a 30-point scale. Items are differentially weighted according to their ability to discriminate those with mild cognitive impairment from healthy controls. A cut-off of 25/26 was the optimum for differentiating those with mild cognitive impairment and mild Alzheimer's disease from healthy controls. The advantage of the MOCA is that it includes more emphasis on visuospatial and executive abilities than several of the earlier screening tests. Although it has been reported to be useful for screening stroke patients (Cummings, personal communication; Dale, personal communication), no formal evaluations have yet been identified comparing MOCA with comprehensive cognitive assessment in stroke patients to detect post-stroke dementia.

Screening for post-stroke dementia therefore remains problematic. The standard measures used, such as the MMSE and AMT, have low sensitivity. The positive predictive values are not high, and therefore many patients will need further evaluation. There are several potentially appropriate tests, but all require further validation in stroke patients.

Screening for cognitive impairment after stroke

Most stroke patients suffer from cognitive impairment as a result of the stroke lesion, which does not lead to a progressive dementia, but affects their progress in rehabilitation. For this reason, stroke-related cognitive impairments need to be identified in the acute stroke setting in order to identify those who need further evaluation and to assist in rehabilitation planning.

The MMSE is widely used in clinical practice for detecting cognitive impairment after stroke in addition to post-stroke dementia. However, the validity for detecting cognitive impairment after stroke is doubtful and using the MMSE for this purpose probably does little more than to tick the audit box that cognitive screening has been carried out. A positive result almost certainly indicates that there is cognitive impairment, but a negative result has little clinical value. Blake, McKinney, Treece, Lee and Lincoln (2002) compared performance on the MMSE with performance on a detailed neuropsychological assessment in a group of 112 stroke patients admitted to stroke rehabilitation units. The sensitivity of the MMSE, when applying a cut-off value of 24/25, was found to be moderate (62%, specificity 88%). However, the neuropsychological assessment was always administered after the MMSE and in some cases as long as three months after the screening assessment. Therefore, the sensitivity may be an overestimate, as patients may have recovered between administration of the MMSE and comprehensive assessment and thus milder deficits, which were missed by the MMSE, were no longer present when the full assessment was completed. Nys, van Zand-voort, de Kort, Jansen, Kappelle and de Haan (2005c) improved on this study by administering the comprehensive neuropsychological assessment in the same session as the MMSE. Using this same cut-off of 24/25, Nys *et al.* (2005c) classified 53% of a sample of 38 acute stroke patients as cognitively impaired whereas comprehensive neuropsychological assessment identified cognitive impairments in 70% of the sample (Nys *et al.*, 2005c). A cut-off of 24/25 had moderate specificity (60%) but poor sensitivity (57%). In particular patients with reasoning disturbances (69%) were misclassified as cognitively intact by the MMSE, as were 64% of those with executive disorders, and 57% with visual perceptual impairments. Memory disorders were better detected but 20% of those with verbal memory problems were missed and so were 50% of those with visual memory problems.

This lack of sensitivity has also been reported by others (Fure, Wyller, Engedal & Thommessen, 2006; Mysiw, Beegan & Gatens, 1989; Pendlebury, Cuth-bertson, Welch, Mehta & Rothwell, 2010; Srikanth *et al.*, 2006). Mysiw *et al.* (1989) compared the MMSE and Neurobehavioral Cognitive Status examina-tion in 38 stroke patients. The MMSE detected cognitive impairments in 14 patients (37%), whereas the Neurobehavioral Cognitive Status examination identified impairments in 35 (92%), with increased sensitivity most apparent on tests of orientation and memory. Fure *et al.* (2006) examined the MMSE in 71 patients in the first week after an acute lacunar stroke. 41 of the 71 (58%) patients had cognitive impairments on a neuropsychological test battery, but only 19% of these were identified using the conventional cut-off of 24/25 on the MMSE (specificity 92%, PPV 78%). Raising the cut-off to 28/29 increased the sensitivity to 69% (specificity 67%, PPV 74%), but even then the MMSE failed to identify 30% of patients with cognitive problems. Srikanth *et al.* (2006) also found the S-MMSE to have very low sensitivity in 69 community stroke patients a year after first-ever stoke. Cognitive impairments were identified using a comprehensive battery of neuropsychological tests in 29 patients. The S-MMSE only detected 14% of those with cognitive impairment but not dementia (specificity 100%, PPV 100%). The MMSE therefore seems to have very little value in screening for cognitive problems after stroke. For the majority of those patients identified as impaired using the MMSE, this will be evident from their clinical presentation. Knowing a stroke patient has cognitive problems detected by the MMSE does not indicate the cognitive domains affected, and it is this information that is needed for planning rehabilitation.

The ACE-R may be more sensitive to cognitive impairment than the MMSE, as it includes additional tests of visuospatial abilities. It has also been shown to be superior to the MMSE in brain-injured patients (Gaber, 2008). Morris, Hacker and Lincoln (2010) found the ACE-R to be more sensitive then than MMSE, in detecting cognitive impairment in 101 acute stroke patients. There were 50% who scored below the cut-off of 24 on the MMSE; in contrast, using a cut-off of 82 on the ACE-R, 75% were impaired. In a subgroup of 60 patients, the ACE-R was found to be more sensitive and specific than the MMSE in relation to a brief neuropsychological test battery. The optimum cut-off was 82, which gave good sensitivity (80%) but unsatisfactory specificity (40%). The positive predictive value was 87% indicating accuracy for positive results, but the negative predictive value was only 28%, indicating that many of those with high scores did have cognitive impairment. The area under the curve indicated that, overall, the ACE-R performed no better than chance (ACE-R AUC = 0.53, $p > 0.05$).

The Montreal Cognitive Assesment (MoCA) (Naserddine *et al.*, 2005) has been compared with the MMSE for detecting cognitive impairment after stroke. Pendlebury *et al.* (2010) assessed 413 patients with stroke or TIA at a six-month or five-year follow-up visit. There were 167 (40%) who had cognitive impairment on the MMSE, as compared with 291 (70%) on the MoCA, supporting the lack of sensitivity of the MMSE. A similar study by Dong, Sharma, Chan, Venketasubramanian, Teoh, Seet *et al.* (2010) compared the MoCA and MMSE in 100 patients within two weeks of stroke. There were 59% impaired on the MoCA as compared with 43% on the MMSE.

Although research by de Koning *et al.* (2005) indicated the R-CAMCOG was probably a good screening measure for post-stroke dementia, they did not look at ability to detect post-stroke cognitive impairment. Te Winkel–Witlox, Post, Visser-Meily and Lindeman (2008) directly compared the CAMCOG, R-CAMCOG, MMSE and Functional Independence Measure-Cognition score in 169 stroke patients who completed the measures after admission to rehabilitation. Spearman correlations between the tests were high, but there was no direct comparison of the sensitivity and specificity of the tests. The authors concluded that the R-CAMCOG was an efficient alternative to the CAMCOG as a screening tool for cognitive dysfunction of stroke patients, but there was limited evidence to support this claim.

Most of the above tests have been developed in psychiatric services with the aim of diagnosing dementia and tend to be used by medical staff in conjunction with their clinical examination. Several short batteries of cognitive tests have been created from comprehensive neuropsychological assessment to screen for cognitive problems. In clinical practice, these tend to be used by psychologists and occupational therapists, rather than the medical teams. These screening batteries include the Repeatable Battery for Assessment of Neuropsychological Status (RBANS) (Randolph, 1998), Middlesex Elderly

Assessment of Mental State (MEAMS) (Golding, 1989) and Comprehensive Cognitive Neurological Assessment in Stroke (Coconuts) (Hoffmann, Schmitt & Bromley, 2009).

The Repeatable Battery for Assessment of Neuropsychological Status (RBANS) (Randolph, 1998) was developed as a neuropsychological screening battery that covers the cognitive domains of immediate memory, delayed recall, language, visuospatial abilities and attention/executive. Four of the domain indices were demonstrated to have good convergent validity with other measures of cognitive function in 158 stroke patients admitted to hospital for rehabilitation (Larson, Kirschner, Bode, Heinemann & Goodman, 2005). The attention/executive index was only moderately correlated with other measures, which may reflect the lack of construct validity for the concept of executive function (see chapter 4) rather than inadequacies with the assessment. Wilde (2006) assessed 210 ischaemic stroke patients admitted to a rehabilitation unit. They completed the RBANS, Visual Form Discrimination, Controlled Word Association, MMSE, Line Bisection and Complex Ideational Material tests. Two factors were identified (language/verbal memory and visuospatial/visual memory) which accounted for 61% of the variance. The utility of the RBANS as a screening measure in stroke patients in comparison to comprehensive neuropsychological assessment remains yet to be undertaken.

The Middlesex Elderly Assessment of Mental State (MEAMS) (Golding, 1989) is a battery of 12 short cognitive tests designed to detect cognitive impairment in elderly people with dementia. Cartoni and Lincoln (2005) evaluated the MEAMS as a cognitive screening measure in 30 stroke patients. They found that in relation to a more comprehensive assessment, the MEAMS had low sensitivity (52%) but high specificity (100%), using a cut-off score of 3 or more fails to indicate impairment. An advantage of the MEAMS is that separate subtests can be considered. Cartoni and Lincoln (2005) evaluated the MEAMS in relation to four cognitive domains (memory, language, perception and executive) and found that the sensitivity of the MEAMS subtests ranged from 11% to 100% and the specificity ranged from 69% to 100%. Only the language screening subtest, Naming, showed both good sensitivity and specificity in relation to further cognitive assessment. Bunton (2008), examined the MEAMS in relation to assessment on the RBANS in 91 acute stroke patients. The MEAMS was less sensitive than the RBANS (sensitivity 56%), suggesting the RBANS to be more suitable for screening purposes than the MEAMS.

There have been some attempts to develop stroke specific screening measures by using a battery of tests. The Comprehensive Cognitive Neurological Assessment in Stroke (Coconuts) (Hoffmann *et al.*, 2009) was designed to assess the full spectrum of cognitive disorders after stroke including both mild cognitive impairment of the vascular type and vascular dementia. The Coconuts comprises 60 items in five cognitive domains. It was administered to 1796 stroke patients within the first month of stroke. Cognitive impairment was identified in

1569/1796 (87%) of stroke patients. The sensitivity to lesions assessed by MRI was high (91%) but specificity was low (35%) indicating that only a few patients with no detectable cognitive impairment on the Coconuts had no lesions on MRI. This low specificity is likely to have arisen because some silent brain lesions may not be associated with cognitive impairment. The subscales were examined in relation to other established neuropsychological tests assessing frontal, language, visuospatial, visual processing and memory abilities. Correlation coefficients were high and there were many patients identified with impairments in each domain, but there was no indication of the sensitivity and specificity of the subscale scores in relation to comprehensive neuropsychological assessment. The authors also recognised the limitations of combining ordinal and nominal values to give a total score, but justified it by the fact that this approach is used in the standardisation of many other scales. They also suggested that the Coconuts should be used more qualitatively to determine whether full neuropsychological assessment is needed. However, given the high proportion of patients with cognitive problems, this would indicate that most patients should have a comprehensive neuropsychological assessment. The Coconuts is also lengthy to administer and it may be better to spend the time on assessments with greater sensitivity to impairments in specific cognitive domains.

Kitching, Salthouse and Hopkins (2007) also used this approach and compiled a stroke screen, targeted predominantly at memory and executive function. This battery included Matrix Reasoning, Name and address recall, Controlled Oral Word Association, BADS Rule shift, Digit Span and MEAMS Remembering pictures. Validation was carried out with 31 stroke patients within 2 weeks of stroke. However, validity was established in relation to the presence of memory and executive impairment as inferred from CT scan reports rather than a comprehensive neuropsychological assessment. The sensitivity of subtest scores ranged from 11% to 78%, with auditory recall and COWAT having the highest positive predictive values. Given that visuospatial problems are common consequences of stroke, the lack of visuospatial measures means the battery will not provide a comprehensive cognitive screen.

Cognistat (a modification of the Neurobehavioral Cognitive Status Examination) (Keirnan, Mueller, Langston & Vandyke, 1987) comprises 10 subtests to assess ten cognitive domains; orientation, attention, understanding of simple commands, repetition of sentences, naming, visuoconstruction, verbal memory, calculation, similarities/verbal abstraction and every-day/concrete judgement. Nøkleby, Boland, Bergersen, Schanke, Farner, Wagle *et al.* (2008) evaluated Cognistat, together with an 18 item functionally oriented assessment, the Screening Instrument for Neuropsychological Impairment in Stroke (SINS) and clock drawing with 49 stroke patients. Cognitive impairments were identified on a comprehensive battery of neuropsychological tests in six cognitive domains: language, visuospatial function, attention and neglect, apraxia, speed in unaffected arm and memory.

Patients were classified as 'definitely impaired' or 'not definitely impaired' in each of these domains. Although the overall scores of both Cognistat and SINS had adequate sensitivity to detect impairment in any cognitive domain (82% for the Cognistat composite score, 71% for the SINS composite score), the specificity was low (50% and 67% respectively). Clock drawing performed no better than chance and did not provide any useful information about visuospatial function, attention or neglect.

Although there are other screening test in clinical use, such as the Neuro-psychological Assessment Battery (Stern & White, 2003) and the Cognitive Assessment of Minnesota (Rustad, DeGroot, Jungkunz, Freeberg, Borowick & Wanttie, 1993), no validation studies have been identified to determine their screening properties in stroke patients. Of the short tests batteries which have evidence of validity for screening purposes, the RBANS seems to have the best potential to be used as a screening measure after stroke. However, there are concerns about the ability to detect cognitive impairment in all domains. Further validation is needed before it is adopted in routine clinical practice. The screening properties of measures to screen for both dementia and cognitive impairment after stroke are summarised in Table 5.1. The results overall indicate that in the acute stage none of the screening measures has adequate sensitivity and specificity to detect either cognitive impairment or dementia. The Rotterdam CAMCOG has best supporting evidence in patients recruited more than three months after stroke but the two studies of the Rotterdam CAMCOG are both from the same centre and therefore would benefit from independent validation.

Screening in cognitive domains

In rehabilitation settings, there tends to be a greater need for the identification of impairment in specific cognitive domains. Measures have been developed to detect impairment in the main domains affected by stroke. Theoretically, if all these measures were combined into a single battery it would be possible to detect any aspect of cognitive impairment, which could then be evaluated further.

Language

Historically language screening is the best established. Language problems affect about a third of stroke patients (see chapter 7), and screening is used to identify those who need specialist evaluation by a speech and language therapist. There are several measures available, the most commonly used in clinical practice being the Whurr Aphasia Screening Test (Whurr, 1996), Sheffield Screening Test for Acquired Language Disorders (SSTALD) (Syder, Body, Parker & Boddy, 1993) and Frenchay Aphasia Screening Test (FAST) (Enderby, Wood & Wade, 1997).

Table 5.1 Screening Properties of Measures to Screen for Dementia or Overall Cognitive Impairment after Stroke

Screening measure	Study	Stroke sample	Criterion measure	Cut-off	Sens[y] %	Spec[y] %	PPV %	NPV %
ACE-R	Morris, Hacker & Lincoln, 2010	n = 61 inpatients in acute stroke ward	Cognitive assessment battery	81/82	80	40	87	28
AMT	Barber & Stott, 2004	n = 64 Outpatients within 6 mpo	R-CAMCOG	87/88	90	20	85	28
				8/9	76	77		
CAMCOG	de Koning et al., 2000	n = 284 hospital patients assessed 3 to 9 mpo	Cognitive tests and DSM-II-R criteria for dementia	77/78	91	88	64	98
COCONUTS	Hoffmann et al., 2009	n = 1796 consecutive patients within 1 mpo	Stroke lesions on MRI	3.4/3.5	91	35	88	41
COGNISTAT	Nokleby et al., 2008	n = 49 patients on rehabilitation wards	Cognitive assessment battery	8/9	81	67		
MEAMS	Cartoni & Lincoln, 2005	n = 30 rehabilitation patients in hospital	Cognitive assessment battery	2/3	52	100	100	19
	Bunton (2008)	n = 91 acute patients in hospital	RBANS	2/3	51	93	90	78
MMSE	Desmond et al., 1994	n = 36 outpatients	Diagnosis of dementia	23/24	83	87	56	96
	Blake et al., 2002	n = 112 inpatients on stroke rehabilitation wards	Cognitive assessment battery	24/25	62	88		
	Nys et al., 2005c	n = 34 acute inpatients	Cognitive assessment battery	24/25	64	60	78	50
	Fure et al., 2006	n = 71 one week after lacunar stroke	Cognitive test battery	24/25	19	92	78	45
				28/29	69	65	74	61

(Continued)

Table 5.1 (*Continued*)

Screening measure	Study	Stroke sample	Criterion measure	Cut-off	Sens[y] %	Spec[y] %	PPV %	NPV %
	Tang et al., 2005	n = 83 Lacunar infarction within 7 days	Psychiatric diagnosis of dementia	18/19	93	80	36	98
	Srikanth et al., 2006	n = 79 community patients with first stroke 12mpo	Cognitive impairment on cognitive test battery	23/24	14	100	100	63
IQCODE	Srikanth et al., 2006	n = 79 community patients with first stroke 12mpo	DSM-IV dementia	23/24	50	94	50	94
			Cognitive impairment on cognitive test battery	3.2/3.3	41	67	46	62
R- CAMCOG	De Koning et al., 2000	n = 284 hospital patients assessed 3 to 9 mpo	DSM-IV dementia	3.2/3.3	88	63	21	98
			Cognitive tests and DSM-II-R criteria for dementia	33/34	91	90	68	98
	De Koning et al., 2005	n = 121 stroke patients between 3 and 9 mpo	Cognitive tests and DSM-IV criteria for dementia	33/34	66	94	82	87
TICS	Desmond et al., 1994	n = 36 outpatients	Diagnosis of dementia	36/37	83	78	76	92
				24/25	100	83	55	100
	Barber & Stott, 2004	n = 64 Outpatients within 6 mpo	R-CAMCOG	27/28	88	85	78	92
TICSm	Barber & Stott, 2004	n = 64 Outpatients within 6 mpo	R-CAMCOG	20/21	92	80	74	94

They were all designed to detect aphasia rather than dysarthria, and also detect oral apraxias, though this has rarely been considered in validation studies. The FAST is very brief and designed to be easy to administer on acute medical wards. It requires only a set of cards and provides an assessment of spoken language, understanding, reading and writing. In many clinical situations it is only the spoken language and understanding sections that are used, despite the fact that clinically it would be useful for a nurse or doctor to know whether a patient is better at communication through visual rather than oral modalities. The criticism of the FAST is that it is not sensitive to mild language impairment and therefore does not identify everyone who would need to be referred to a speech and language therapist.

Salter, Jutai, Foley, Hellings and Teasell (2006) reviewed six aphasia screening tools. One problem they identified was that information pertaining to the measurement properties and clinical utility of the tests was limited. On the basis of their review they concluded that the FAST appeared to be the most widely used and thoroughly evaluated tool found within the stroke research literature. It has been found to have good sensitivity to language impairment but the specificity is affected by other factors and it may perform no better than careful clinical examination (O'Neill, Cheadle, Wyatt, McGuffog & Fullerton, 1990). However, the requirement to conduct the FAST may ensure that a careful examination takes place, which is not always the case in routine clinical practice. Edwards, Hahn, Baum, Perlmutter, Sheedy and Dromerick (2006b) found that the FAST detected 19 (36%) patients with language problems in a sample of 53, of which only 4 (8%) had been detected according to their case records. The FAST was more sensitive than the Ulleval Aphasia Screening test (UAS) (Thommessen, Thoresen, Bautz-Holter & Laake, 1999) (87% as compared with 75%) but less specific (80% vs. 90%). Further evaluation of the measurement properties and clinical utility of these screening tools is needed.

The Sheffield Screening test for Acquired Language Disorders (SSTALD) (Syder *et al.*, 1993) covers a higher level of language abilities than the FAST and is short, taking about ten minutes to administer, but some of the more complex items may involve a memory component as well as language. The test includes assessment of spoken language and understanding but there are no reading and writing items. It has been validated in stroke patients and been shown to be both sensitive and specific to language problems (Blake *et al.*, 2002). Al Khawaja, Wade and Collin (1996) compared the FAST and SSTALD in 50 consecutive patients with suspected aphasia. The two measures were highly correlated. Comparison of their ability to identify aphasia in comparison with a speech and language therapists' assessment showed that the SSTALD was more accurate (FAST sensitivity 87%, specificity 80% and accuracy 86%; SSTALD sensitivity 89%, specificity 100% and accuracy 90%). Both were short and simple to administer. However, the SSTALD is now out of print and therefore no longer easily available.

Visuospatial

Screening for visuospatial problems requires both screening for visual neglect and spatial problems, the former being much better established as part of routine clinical practice. Menon and Korner-Bitensky (2004) identified 62 tests for visual neglect, so choosing the appropriate one is not easy. The most commonly used and best validated screening assessments for visual neglect include Albert's test, line bisection, Behavioural Inattention Test (BIT) Star Cancellation, Ravens Coloured Progressive Matrices and the Rey figure copy.

Albert's test or line cancellation is probably the longest established but lacks sensitivity (Halligan, Marshall & Wade, 1989) and patients with mild visual inattention may compensate for their difficulties. In contrast BIT Star Cancellation, which has both an irregular layout of targets and varied stimuli, is more sensitive. Halligan *et al.* (1989) showed that 57% of stroke patients with visual inattention were correctly identified (sensitivity) using Line Crossing as compared with 100% using Star cancellation. Jehkonen, Ahonen, Dastidar, Koivisto, Laippala & Vilkki*et al.* (1998) in a similar study on the BIT, supported the evidence that Star Cancellation was the most sensitive test of the BIT (sensitivity 80%, specificity 91%, PPV 84% and NPV 88%) but suggested that a three-test combination of line crossing, letter cancellation and line bisection was sufficient to detect neglect in the acute phase (sensitivity 95%, specificity 97%, PPV 95% and NPV 97%). However, these tasks take about five minutes to complete, whereas line bisection only takes a few seconds. Line bisection will miss many patients with visual inattention (Halligan *et al.*, 1989; Jehkonen *et al.*, 1998) and has been shown to have poor test–retest reliability (Lezak, Howieson, Loring, Hannay & Fischer, 2004). However, Bailey, Riddoch and Crome (2000) found star cancellation and line bisection to be equivalent in their ability to detect neglect in 107 stroke patients, with a sensitivity of 76%, and more sensitive than the Baking Tray Test (67%) or draw a daisy (56%), but the specificity and predictive values were not reported. In a comprehensive study of screening measures for neglect, Azouvi, Samuel, Louis-Dreyfus, Bernati, Bartolomeo, Beis *et al.* (2002) assessed 206 right hemisphere stoke patients on a battery of neglect measures. 177 patients (86%) demonstrated neglect on at least one measure, but the individual tests only identified neglect in between 19% (bisection of 5 cm line) and 51% (starting position on the Bells test) of patients, thus the individual tests were all much less sensitive than the entire battery. Line bisection and cancellation tasks may produce differing results due to differences in the location of lesions which give rise to them (Rorden, Berger & Karnath, 2006), so patients who fail on one type of test will not necessarily fail the other, unless they have severe problems.

Ravens Coloured Progressive Matrices (RCPM) may also be used as an indicator of visual neglect. Blake *et al.* (2002) identified that a cut-off of 18/19 on the total score had a sensitivity of 91% and specificity of 72% for the detection of visual neglect. In addition, qualitatively the pattern of responding may suggest neglect, when patients give disproportionately more answers of 3 and 6, indicating they are responding mainly to stimuli on the right. Blake *et al.* (2002) calculated a laterality index which was based on the proportion of errors to one side. Using a cut-off of 24%/25% lateralised had a sensitivity of 76% and specificity 78% for detecting neglect but had little benefit over using the total score. However, when this pattern of responding occurs it can be very striking.

Thus, it seems that BIT Star Cancellation is probably the most useful individual test for detecting visual neglect in the acute stage after stroke, but more than one test should be administered as there are inconsistencies in performance on different measures of visual neglect. Using standardised measures, such as BIT Star Cancellation, is likely to lead to improved identification of neglect as Edwards *et al.* (2006b) found that the BIT Star Cancellation detected 28 (52%) patients with inattention in a sample of 53 stroke patients, of which only 11 (21%) had been detected according to their case records.

There have been fewer investigations of screening measures for spatial problems. The Rey Figure copy is an easily administered short test of visuospatial abilities, which will identify both visual neglect and spatial difficulties. The scoring system is however designed to detect the spatial components of the task, and although qualitatively visual neglect will be apparent from the copies, this is not reflected using the standard scoring systems. Lincoln, Drummond, Edmans, Yeo and Willis (1998) compared the Rey figure copy with a comprehensive assessment on the Rivermead Perceptual Assessment Battery (RPAB) administered by an occupational therapist in 61 stroke patients receiving rehabilitation. The Rey copy detected perceptual impairments in 31 of the 32 patients who were impaired on the RPAB (sensitivity 97%) but specificity was low (48%), in that many failed the Rey copy but did not have perceptual problems, as identified on the Rivermead Perceptual Assessment Battery. This may be because the Rey was also picking up impairments in planning (Strauss *et al.*, 2006) which would not be detected by the RPAB.

Some subtests of the Visual Object and Space Perception (VOSP) battery (Warrington & James, 1991), such as fragmented letters, number location, position discrimination and cube analysis, are used in clinical practice and are potentially appropriate as screening measures. People who fail the tasks are considered to have problems with visuospatial perception but there are no formal evaluations of their sensitivity and specificity as screening measures.

Other cognitive abilities

Tests of executive ability have been examined as measures to identify vascular cognitive impairment. O'Sullivan, Morris and Markus (2005) assessed

32 patients with ischaemic leukoaraiosis and 17 age and education matched controls. They used a brief battery comprising the MMSE, Digit symbol, FAS verbal fluency, Backward digit span and Trail making B-A and compared the findings with a comprehensive battery which included the WAIS-R, Wisconsin Card Sorting Test and Wechsler Memory Scale. Trail Making B-A and Digit symbol were both sensitive and specific tests to detect patients with ischaemic leukoaraiosis (Trail Making B-A sensitivity 88% specificity 76%; Digit Symbol sensitivity 91% specificity 76%), whereas the MMSE performed less well (sensitivity 63%, specificity 76%). Even when only those with MMSE >27 were considered, that is those who did not have an identified dementia, the battery was able to discriminate between the two groups. The brief battery also discriminated the groups as well as the full neuropsychological tests battery and the authors therefore suggested that Trail Making and Digit Symbol tests could be used for screening in clinical practice, but this requires further verification. Oral Trail Making has been suggested (Abraham, Axelrod & Ricker, 1996; Ricker, Axelrod & Houtler, 1996), but Bunton (2008) found little evidence to support its use.

There has been little evaluation of the screening properties of measures of apraxia, attention and memory. Some brief measures are used in clinical practice, but their sensitivity relative to comprehensive evaluation has not been assessed. One reason for this is that potential screening measures tend to be administered as the preliminary part of a comprehensive neuropsychological assessment rather than on their own. The information on sensitivity and specificity is not needed in this context. However, it would be beneficial to know about their screening properties, as it would indicate the amount of additional information gained by administering a comprehensive assessment. An example of the use of a cognitive screening test in clinical practice is shown in Table 5.2.

Conclusions

The advantage of routine screening for cognitive problems is that impairments are detected which otherwise go unnoticed by the clinical team (Edwards *et al.*, 2006b). However, there is little point in using measures which are not sensitive to cognitive problems after stroke. It is also important to use measures that will identify impairments in specific domains as these will inform rehabilitation. In addition, it has been shown that providing a brief cognitive assessment may be beneficial for carers. McKinney, Blake, Treece, Lincoln, Playford and Gladman (2002) randomly allocated stroke patients to receive a cognitive assessment by a psychologist as part of their clinical care or not. Carers of those who were assessed for cognitive impairment showed a trend towards less strain than carers of patients who were not assessed (p = 0.06). The authors attributed this to carers understanding the nature

Table 5.2 Case Example of Cognitive Screening

Dermot was a 70-year-old married man who was admitted to an acute stroke ward with a mild right-sided weakness following a stroke. He lived with his wife and had two married daughters and two grandchildren. He left school at 16 and had worked as a butcher, postman and bus driver until he retired 6 years previously.

On the stroke ward he was mobile and had no obvious cognitive problems. Four days after his stroke, he was screened on the MoCA test by an occupational therapist as part of routine cognitive screening. The results are shown in Figure 5.1.

On the MoCA test he was able to name pictures of animals but had problems on visuospatial, executive and memory tasks. The occupational therapist noted there was severe cognitive impairment, even though it had not been apparent on the ward, and referred him to a clinical psychologist for further assessment.

He was pleasant and cooperative throughout the assessment. There was no evidence of either anxiety or depression. On formal cognitive testing, his probable premorbid level of functioning as estimated from the Schonell Graded Word Reading Test and National Adult Reading Test was average, which is consistent with his education and occupational history. His current level of general intellectual function, as assessed on Raven Progressive Matrices, was below average suggesting cognitive deterioration. His language abilities, as assessed on the Graded Naming Test and Token Test were average. On tests of perception he showed some impairment of visuospatial abilities. He failed two subtests of the Visual and Object Space Perception Battery, Silhouette Recognition and Object Decision. His Rey figure copy was also impaired. Memory testing on the Doors and People test and California Verbal Learning Tests indicted severe impairment of both visual and verbal memory. In addition he was impaired on tests of executive abilities, the Stroop and Brixton Spatial Anticipation Test.

Overall the results indicated impairment of visuospatial abilities, memory and executive functioning. As he had a long history of heavy drinking, it was possible that this cognitive impairment was due to the effects of alcohol, or it could be due to a dementia. He was therefore referred back to the medical team for further evaluation.

This case example highlights how cognitive screening picked up problems which would not otherwise have been detected by the clinical teams on an acute stroke ward.

of patients' difficulties. The challenge in clinical practice is how to provide this level of cognitive screening for the large numbers of stroke patients in clinical services. This focus on specific cognitive domains is more likely to provide information to the clinical team about potential cognitive problems. The optimum strategy is therefore likely to be to collate these measures into a composite battery.

Overall the most practical measures to use in an acute stroke setting seem to be the MoCA and the ACE-R. The MoCA is freely available, is quick and easy to administer and is much more sensitive to cognitive impairment than the MMSE. Similarly, the ACE-R is short and has significant advantages over the MMSE. In rehabilitation settings, the RBANS seems to be the most useful, though these are concerns that it may miss some patients with impairment. This can be supple-

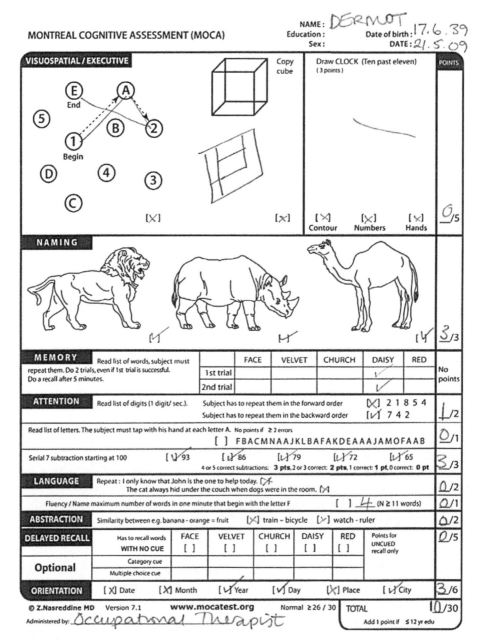

Figure 5.1 MoCA Test completed by Dermot. Copyright Z. Nasreddine MD. Reproduced with permission. Copies are available at www.mocatest.org.

mented by specific measures of neglect (Star Cancellation), visuospatial problems (Rey figure copy), executive function (Trail Making, verbal fluency) and apraxia to ensure that mild impairments are not missed. However, it could be argued that all patients should receive a comprehensive neuropsychological assessment, as none of the screening measures has been shown to be entirely satisfactory. A more practical strategy is to use a brief screening measure, such as the MoCA or ACE-R on all patients in the acute stage. Thos who pass these assessments should then be assessed for domain specific impairments using slightly longer batteries, such as the RBANS, or tests of specific cognitive functions. For those stroke patients who are expected to resume an active lifestyle, those who are not progressing in rehabilitation and those who wish to return to work, comprehensive neuropsychological assessment is essential to identify cognitive impairments.

Chapter 6

Neuropsychological Assessment after Stroke

Introduction

As with the assessment of most other clinical populations, the structure of neuropsychological assessment in stroke depends very much on the specific purpose and context of the assessment. Within hyper-acute settings, for example, detailed neuropsychological assessment is rarely appropriate or genuinely informative, as the patient being assessed is likely to be subject to rapid fluctuations of several important factors, such as level of consciousness, medical status, pain, fatigue and distress. Thus, the usual necessary prerequisites for reliable neuropsychological assessment, such as adequate effort and sustained attention, are rarely achievable. However, basic cognitive screening within this phase of a patient's recovery can be crucial in highlighting potential barriers to early rehabilitation, and can explain functional impairments or perceived motivational or behavioural difficulties.

Neuropsychological assessment within the acute phase of post-stroke recovery is often justifiable, even in the context of spontaneous recovery of functioning. Typically the purpose of cognitive assessment within this phase will be to explain specific functional deficits and, most importantly, to identify strategies or design rehabilitation programmes. Testing will often involve the selection of only a few measures in order to evaluate clinical hypotheses regarding the underlying cognitive deficits associated with a patient's functional disabilities. The process of assessment within this phase is most successful when undertaken in collaboration with other healthcare professionals, such as speech and language therapists and occupational therapists. Collaborative multidisciplinary working within acute rehabilitation settings is often a prerequisite for meaningful neuropsychological assessment.

Psychological Management of Stroke, First Edition. Nadina B. Lincoln, Ian I. Kneebone, Jamie A.B. Macniven and Reg C. Morris.
© 2012 John Wiley & Sons, Ltd. Published 2012 by John Wiley & Sons, Ltd.

Within the rehabilitation phase of recovery from stroke, the purpose of neuropsychological assessment shifts to an emphasis on determining the likely longer term residual neuropsychological deficits. Testing is more likely to focus on the social and occupational impact of neuropsychological deficits, and therefore involve more detailed and comprehensive battery-based assessment. Rehabilitation goals in the first year after stroke are still very much the focus of multidisciplinary input, but the approach taken to intervention will often shift from facilitating recovery from impairment to devising compensatory strategies to circumvent underlying neuropsychological deficits.

Barriers to meaningful neuropsychological assessment

Depending on the timing of the assessment, there can be significant barriers to meaningful post-stroke neuropsychological testing. The majority of patients will have symptoms of language, visuospatial or attentional impairment (Tatemichi, Desmond, Stern, Paik, Sano & Bagiella, 1994). These deficits can affect the choice of tests with which the neuropsychologist can reliably assess other cognitive domains, such as memory and executive functioning. For example, a patient with receptive language impairment may not be able to understand the instructions to some tests, and so the results of such tests, if attempted, cannot be interpreted using standardised normative data. However, even if the data cannot be interpreted formally, meaningful information can be gleaned from the manner in which a patient attempts a task. As with all neuropsychological assessment, the qualitative information can in many cases prove to be as useful in planning rehabilitation strategies as the formal test data.

The average age of stroke is 72 years (Williams, Jiang, Matchar & Samsa, 1999); this restricts the choice of tests available, as normative data tend to be more limited for older age bands (Ivnik, Malec, Smith, Tangalos, Peterson, Kokmen *et al.*, 1992). Patients are also more likely to have pre-existing sensory impairments, such as impaired hearing or vision, which may be overlooked in the context of a busy hospital setting in which the overwhelming focus is often, appropriately, on ensuring the patient's survival and in meeting their basic care needs. It is not uncommon for patients to be referred to the neuropsychologist for assessment of cognition without having been screened initially for poor vision or hearing. The provision of a patient's glasses or hearing aid can be a revelation; pre-existing sensory impairment should always be checked prior to undertaking any neuropsychological assessment.

Despite the many challenges faced by the neuropsychologist in stroke services, meaningful assessment of post-stroke cognitive impairment is possible and can contribute significantly to patients' diagnoses, recovery and rehabilitation. This chapter will introduce the reader to the principles of neuropsychological assessment after stroke, and describe methods of conducting a comprehensive neuropsychological assessment in clinical practice. Specific tests will be reviewed with particular emphasis on their appropriateness for use with stroke patients at different stages of their recovery. A case example will highlight the potential benefits and pitfalls of assessment across the patient pathway.

Principles of neuropsychological assessment

As with neuropsychological assessment of patients in other diagnostic groups, the guiding principles of the assessment of stroke patients are derived from generic standards of good practice in psychological investigation. The main textbooks of clinical neuropsychology describe these principles very comprehensively, and the reader is referred to Lezak, Howieson, Loring, Hannay and Fischer (2004) and Morgan and Ricker (2008) for detailed discussion of the issues. Table 6.1 lists some of the key principles which are particularly relevant to neuropsychological assessment after stroke.

In addition to formal neuropsychological testing, the neuropsychologist can utilise other methods of assessment in order to reach a formulation regarding the impact of a stroke on a patient's cognitive, emotional and functional status. Observation is a key approach, especially within inpatient settings. Collaborative working with other professionals, for example observing an occupational therapy kitchen assessment or a physiotherapy session, can elicit crucial information about the patient's cognitive deficits, and may inform potential rehabilitation strategies. Excellent interdisciplinary communication is a fundamental requirement of neuropsychological assessment; poor communication has the potential to lead to misdiagnoses and misunderstandings, and could therefore interfere with a patient's recovery (Morris, Payne & Lambert, 2007). It is also important to take advantage of family and carers' views during assessment using semi-structured interviews or rating scales. Family and carers often have a good understanding of the patient's pre-stroke everyday functional and cognitive functioning; this information can create an excellent context for the interpretation of neuropsychological test results.

Structure of neuropsychological assessment

Ideally, a stroke service neuropsychologist should be responsible for assessment and intervention across the patient pathway from the stroke event until many years after the stroke. The neuropsychologist working within a stroke service should therefore have access to neuropsychological tests appropriate for assessing patients at different stages of their recovery. The test library should include reliable measures with which to assess the key cognitive domains. The purpose of cognitive testing is to determine the patient's probable premorbid level of cognitive functioning and then to assess their abilities in all cognitive domains, thereby identifying impairments in any given domain. This will lead to hypotheses

Table 6.1 Principles of Neuropsychological Assessment

Principle	Rationale
Clearly define the purpose of the assessment.	It may be that functional assessment is sufficient, or that testing is unlikely to produce reliable data.
Select as few tests as possible.	People are typically very susceptible to fatigue after stroke, and so the more tests they complete, the higher the likelihood of finding impairment (which may not reflect a genuine underlying cognitive deficit).
Maximise the patient's performance.	Tests undertaken while the patient is fatigued or in pain are less likely to provide reliable data.
Take a thorough history.	Testing undertaken without knowledge of a patient's history may lead to erroneous conclusions.
Screen for sensory impairment.	Visual and auditory acuity impairments will adversely affect performance on most tests if uncorrected.
Screen for visual inattention, language and visuoperceptual impairment prior to selecting tests for a comprehensive assessment.	If significant language, visuoperceptual impairment or visual inattention is identified, then it is futile to administer tests reliant upon intact functioning in these cognitive domains.
Wherever possible, establish the functional correlates of impaired test performance in collaboration with occupational therapists, speech and language therapists, physiotherapists and nurses.	Neuropsychological assessment and functional assessment are mutually informative; either in isolation may miss significant information gleaned from the other assessment.
Be especially careful in communicating the test results to other health professionals.	The mention of memory impairment in medical notes can often evolve into an erroneous diagnosis of 'dementia' if the clinician does not take care to explain the test results.

about the cognitive domains affected; further testing is conducted to confirm or refute the hypotheses. It is therefore important that the tests are chosen carefully as otherwise the whole process will be unduly long. A suitable test library is discussed below; although these tests are widely used in stroke, the list is far from exhaustive. Screening tests are considered in chapter 5. Many other appropriate and very useful tests are available, and more tests are currently in development.

The discussion below will introduce some key recommended tests which may usefully be included in any stroke service neuropsychological test library. For a detailed discussion of the psychometric properties of the tests described, and for appropriate normative data, the reader is referred to Strauss, Sherman and Spreen (2006), Lezak *et al.* (2004) and Mitrushina, Boone, Razani and D'Elia (2005).

Orientation and alertness

Simple tests of orientation and concentration help to determine the potential value of further, more detailed assessment. Orientation questions should assess the patient's awareness of:

- Time, including time of day, date, month and year
- Person, including date of birth, home address and body orientation
- Place, including name of the building/hospital, town/city and county/ region
- Recent news or personal events (e.g. the name of the Prime Minister or President, current affairs or recent plot lines from regularly watched tele- vision programmes)

The clinician can rely on questions incorporated into other tests, such as the Wechsler Memory Scale-III orientation questions (Wechsler, 1997a), or use a semi-structured interview which includes orientation questions. Interpretation is qualitative, but is necessary in the context of any assessment; a patient who is completely disoriented to time, place, person and recent events is unlikely to fare well in a comprehensive neuropsychological assessment. In such circumstances, basic screening tests may be sufficient to raise suspicion of dementia or a serious medical condition other than the stroke, which may be affecting the patient's level of alertness.

Premorbid intellectual functioning

Estimates of premorbid intellectual functioning are possible using reading tests, such as the National Adult Reading Test-2 (NART-2; Nelson & Willison, 1991) and Wechsler Test of Adult Reading (WTAR; Wechsler, 2001), but only if acquired language impairment, visual inattention and dysarthria are taken into account. In these tests, patients are asked to read aloud irregular words; the accuracy of their pronunciation is used to estimate premorbid intelligence. The high prevalence of language, perceptual and speech problems is such that these tests are not reliable for all patients in the hyper-acute and acute stages following a stroke. An alternative is to use the Spot-the-Word (STW) subtest of the Speed and Capacity of Language Processing test (SCOLP; Baddeley, Emslie & Nimmo-Smith, 1992). The test is a brief untimed lexical decision task in which the patient places ticks beside the genuine words in 60 pairs of genuine words and pseudo-words. Although this subtest was designed primarily to aid in the interpretation of the Silly Sentences Test (see the 'Information Processing Speed' section below), Spot-the-Word may be used as a broad estimate of premorbid ability (Baddeley *et al.*, 1992). Normative data exist which demonstrate the high correlation of Spot-the-Word score to IQ (Strauss *et al.*, 2006). The advantage of using the Spot-the-Word with stroke patients is that there is no requirement to respond orally.

Where patients are unable to undertake formal tests, the clinician must rely on other markers of premorbid functioning, such as educational and occupational achievement. However, the reliability of estimates based on demographics alone is questionable (Basso, Bornstein, Roper & McCoy, 2000) and should only be used with caution due to the susceptibility of such methods to regression towards the mean; overestimation of premorbid ability at the lower end and underestimation of premorbid ability at the upper end of the range.

General intellectual functioning

Tests of general intellectual functioning are an important component of any comprehensive neuropsychological assessment. Within rehabilitation settings, information regarding a patient's general intellectual ability may inform the choice of treatment strategies, and can help significantly in questions of differential diagnosis, such as the extent to which deficits on testing may represent the effects of either a stroke or of a suspected dementing illness. However, within the acute stage of recovery from stroke (i.e. the first three months), many patients are unlikely to be able to tolerate lengthy testing sessions, and so tests such as the Wechsler Adult Intelligence Scale-IV (Wechsler, 2008) are unsuitable. Although short-forms of such tests may be used, considerable caution must be exercised in the interpretation of any short-form assessment results (Kulas & Axelrod, 2002).

The main tests which should be considered in the assessment of general intelligence after stroke include the following:

- The Wechsler Adult Intelligence Scales are perhaps the most commonly used tests with which psychologists assess general intelligence (Lichtenberger & Kaufman, 2009). The scale has undergone a recent revision (WAIS-IV; Wechsler, 2008). Clinicians working in stroke services, especially acute settings, are unlikely to routinely rely on the complete WAIS, which is lengthy to administer. Short forms, comprising a few selected subtests or the Wechsler Abbreviated Scale of Intelligence (WASI; Wechsler, 1999) (see below), are probably most often used. The WAIS-IV comprises 15 subtests, assessing aspects of verbal comprehension, working memory, perceptual reasoning and processing speed. Individual subtests have the advantage of substantial normative reference groups, and an age range of 16–89 (with the exceptions of supplemental subscales Figure Weights and Cancellation, for which normative data are provided for ages 16–69 only). There is a huge literature on the scale's predecessor, the WAIS-III, and the reader is referred to Strauss *et al.* (2006) for a detailed discussion of normative data, reliability and validity of this version. Key changes to the WAIS-IV include the decision to abandon the traditional Verbal IQ (VIQ) and Performance IQ (PIQ) scores, and replace these with a Verbal Comprehension Index (VCI) and a Perceptual Reasoning Index (PRI). A composite score derived from all of the core subtests is still referred to as a Full Scale IQ (FSIQ). Components of the test will be useful in the assessment of most stroke patients, although in order to obtain meaningful measures of the core indices, such as working memory, two or more subtests must be administered. This can reduce the practical utility of the test within some stroke services, given the typical time constraints for assessment, but this version is a definite improvement from previous versions which required several subtests per index score. The WAIS-IV complete battery is shorter to administer than its predecessors, and several discontinuation rules have been introduced. Although the complete battery is likely to remain too long to administer with most stroke patients, especially within acute settings, it is feasible with those who are younger and those with more subtle deficits. The utility of the test within stroke services is yet to be fully evaluated.

- The Wechsler Abbreviated Scale of Intelligence (WASI; Wechsler, 1999) is a screening measure ideal for estimating general intellectual functioning when time is short. Derived from the WAIS-III Vocabulary, Block Design, Similarities and Matrix Reasoning subtests, the composite score correlates highly with Full Scale IQ scores derived from the full WAIS-III (Wechsler, 1997b). It is also possible to administer only the Vocabulary and Matrix Reasoning subtests to generate a full-scale IQ estimate. Unlike the Raven's Progressive Matrices, the WASI includes both verbal and nonverbal subtests.

- The Raven's Progressive Matrices (RPM; Raven, 1958, 1998) is a test of visual inductive reasoning that has the advantage of not relying on verbalisation or motor skill. Stroke patients with language or motor impairment are therefore often able to understand and attempt this test. Verbal instructions for the test are minimal, and it is possible to present the test without verbal instruction. The two most commonly used versions of the test are the Standard Progressive Matrices (SPM) and the Coloured Progressive Matrices (CPM) (Raven, Raven & Court, 1956). The shorter CPM is more appropriate for use with older adults, especially within the acute phase of post-stroke recovery. The RPM in either format is a valuable test with which to assess a patient's general intellectual functioning. It is non language-based, and is therefore useful in the assessment of stroke patients whose first language is not English, although cultural factors must always be taken into account. If the purpose of the assessment is to establish whether there is any evidence of acquired general intellectual functioning impairment, then the RPM is an excellent choice of test. However, given the reliance on visual reasoning in this test, any patient with impaired visual acuity, visuoperceptual, visuospatial or motor functioning or visual inattention should not have their general intellectual level assessed using the RPM, as their performance is likely to be affected by their primary visual, perceptual or motor deficits. However, the test remains useful in measuring impairments in specific cognitive domains with such patients.

Language

A detailed discussion of language impairment and language assessments is provided in chapter 7. However, some basic language tests which can form part of a more general neuropsychological assessment are outlined below.

Within most rehabilitation settings, stroke patients should have access to speech and language therapy. Speech and language therapists are experts in assessing language functioning, and neuropsychologists will typically defer to their speech and language therapy colleagues in language assessment. In the absence of formal language assessment, several tests exist with which the neuropsychologist can assess subtle language disorders. Impaired performance on language tests may preclude the administration of other tests reliant upon intact language functioning, and so it is often sensible to include some tests of language functioning in the early stages of an assessment. Commonly used tests include the following:

- The Graded Naming Test (GNT; McKenna and Warrington, 1983; Warrington, 1997) is used to assess object naming. Thirty items of increasing difficulty are presented in a confrontation naming task. Impaired performance can occur in aphasia, and also in the early stages of some dementias (Graham, Emery & Hodges, 2004).
- The Boston Naming Test-3 (BNT-3; Goodglass, Kaplan & Barresi, 2000) is a confrontation naming test similar to the Graded Naming Test, with a 60-item version and a short 15-item version.
- The Token Test (TT; De Renzi and Vignolo, 1962) is used to assess comprehension of increasingly complex verbal commands. The patient is presented with an array of coloured tokens and asked to select target tokens on the basis of increasingly complex instructions. The test was originally used to discriminate between aphasic and non-aphasic brain-damaged patients

(De Renzi & Faglioni, 1978) but is now more often used as a measure of verbal comprehension. The test only takes approximately ten minutes to administer. However, the normative data are fairly old and the test materials are fairly abstract, and so to some extent the test lacks ecological validity. Nevertheless, as a preliminary measure of impaired comprehension, the test can be informative.

- The Controlled Oral Word Association Test (COWAT; Benton & Hamsher, 1983; Benton, Hamsher & Sivan, 1994) is a test of phonemic fluency which typically requires patients to generate as many words beginning with F, A and S as they can, with one minute allowed per letter. Normative data exist for other combinations of first letters, such as C, F and L. Phonemic fluency is often impaired in patients with aphasia (Spreen & Benton, 1977). Although the test is also used as an index of executive functioning, impaired performance is only a valid indicator of executive dysfunction in the context of a pattern of deficits in fluency across other tests (Strauss *et al.*, 2006), and in the absence of an acquired language disorder.

Visual inattention (neglect)

It is important when testing for visual inattention to use more than one test, as the nature of the condition varies considerably between patients; many patients will pass one test and yet fail another (Lezak *et al.*, 2004). The patient with visual inattention is also more likely to exhibit the phenomenon when fatigued (Fleet & Heilman, 1986); the assessor must take account of the patient's general level of alertness when trying to establish evidence of visual inattention. If the patient demonstrates visual inattention, this must be taken into account in the interpretation of impaired performance on any tests relying on intact visual perception. For example, the patient with visual inattention may perform poorly on the Raven's Progressive Matrices; obviously this should not be taken as evidence of impaired reasoning or general intellectual functioning, as the patient is unlikely to have adequately attended to the test material.

If visual inattention is identified, tests relying on an intact field of vision or visual perception should be interpreted with caution. It is often sensible to administer tests of visual inattention early in the testing battery, in order to allow meaningful interpretation of impaired performance on subsequent tests.

Commonly used tests to assess visual inattention include the following:

- The Behavioural Inattention Test (BIT; Wilson, Cockburn & Halligan, 1987) is a battery of subtests designed to assess visual inattention. The test includes six conventional subtests and nine behavioural subtests with naturalistic paradigms, such as menu reading, telling the time and map navigation. Some patients compensate for their impairment on more conventional subtests, but make errors on the apparently simpler behavioural tasks. Typically, assessors rely on two subtests in particular:

o The Star Cancellation subtest involves the patient identifying target stimuli of small stars amongst a jumble of words, letters and larger stars. Healthy control participants rarely miss any targets, and missing 2–3 stars constitutes an impaired performance. This subtest is generally considered to be one of the most sensitive to visual inattention (Marsh & Kersel, 1993). Manly, Dove, Blows, George, Noonan, Teasdale *et al.* (2009) suggested that the conventional scoring can be enhanced by evaluating videotaped performance, including factors such as location of first cancellation, overall slowness, variability in speed, systematic slowing with time on task, search organization and tendency to recancel targets.

o The Line Crossing subtest involves the patient 'crossing out' multiple small lines scattered across a sheet of paper. Patients with visual inattention will fail to cross lines to the far left or right of the sheet.

o Line bisection is a variation of tests which typically involve the patient marking lines with an 'X' to indicate the centre point on each of a selection of lines. The patient with visual inattention to the left caused by a right hemisphere lesion will mark the line with considerable deviation to the right. It is recommended that several trials are presented, as patients often perform inconsistently on this test (Lezak *et al.*, 2004). According to Committeri, Pitzalis, Galati, Patria, Pelle, Sabatini *et al.* (2007), line bisection tasks should not be used for diagnostic purposes as elderly healthy patients may show a deviation of up to 3% to the right of the true midline (Halligan, Manning & Marshall, 1990). As Committeri *et al.* (2007) argued, performance on this test does not correlate with visual inattention in everyday life (Ferber & Karnath, 2001), and it is not uncommon for patients with visual inattention on other tests to have no deviation in line bisection tasks (Mort, Malhotra, Mannan, Rorden, Pambakian, Kennard *et al.*, 2003).

• The Balloon's Test (Edgeworth, Robertson & McMillan, 1998) was designed specifically to differentiate between hemianopia and visual inattention in stroke patients. The patient is presented with two subtests; the first involves a simple cancellation task of target 'balloons', that is, circles with short vertical lines underneath, which 'pop out' from distracter circles, due to the perceptual phenomenon described by Treisman and Gelade (1980). The second subtest is more demanding of attentional resources, requiring the patient to cancel out target circles from distracter 'balloons'. The normative data are derived from the performance of older adults, with a mean age of 64. Those with visual field deficits have difficulty on both tasks A and B, whereas those with inattention have selective difficulty on test B. The test has good face validity in the assessment of visual inattention (Menon & Korner-Bitensky, 2004), but as yet there are no published studies examining its psychometric properties. The data provided in the manual only relate to right hemisphere lesions and left visual inattention; no data are provided regarding patients with the opposite pattern of visual inattention (i.e. left hemisphere lesion resulting in right visual inattention), although the test can still be used qualitatively with these patients.

Visuospatial and visuoperceptual functioning

Tests specifically designed to assess visuospatial and visuoperceptual functioning include:

- The Rey-Osterreith Complex Figure Copy test (Osterreith, 1944; Rey, 1959) is used to assess perceptual functioning. The task is simply to copy a complex drawing, as illustrated in Figure 6.1. Scoring can be complex, and various scoring systems exist. The most commonly used scoring system is probably the original version in which the figure is split into 18 components, with scores out of two, one for accuracy and one for correct placement (Lezak *et al.*, 2004). Other scoring systems are available, the most compre-hensive of which is probably the Boston Qualitative Scoring System (Stern, Javorsky, Singer, Harris, Somerville, Duke *et al.*, 1999). Administration is relatively straightforward and parallel forms are available. Although those

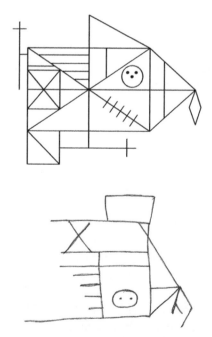

Figure 6.1   Rey Figure Copy by patient with visual neglect. Original Complex Figure reproduced from "Le Test de Copie d'Une Figure Complexe" by P. A. Osterrieth, 1944, *Archives de Psychologie, 30.* In the public domain.

with a hemiplegia may need to use their nondominant hand for writing, there is some evidence that this has a minimal impact on copy scores (Yamashita, 2010). As the name implies, the test material is complex and can be slightly daunting and anxiety provoking for older adults especially within the acute phase of recovery. The figure should not therefore be presented to stroke patients with suspected visuoperceptual impairment prior to more basic screening with simpler line drawing tests. However, most patients find that they are able to complete the copy task if they attempt it.

- The Visual Object and Space Perception battery (VOSP; Warrington & James, 1991) is a battery of eight visuospatial and visuoperceptual subtests designed to discriminate between patients with impaired object perception and those with impaired space perception. The test battery is based on research evidence for separate neuroanatomical pathways responsible for object and space perception tasks (Mishkin, Ungerleider & Macko, 1983). The test remains useful in the discrimination of gross object perception and space perception deficits, although in healthy controls several subtests have ceiling effects and so the ability of the battery to detect subtle impairments may be limited (Strauss *et al.*, 2006). In stroke settings, the VOSP remains one of the few tests available with which the clinician can investigate object and space perception. The test requires minimal motor skills and therefore is useful in those with apraxia or bilateral weakness. However, interpretation should be cautious given that performance declines in healthy controls after the age of 50 (Warrington & James, 1991), and further evidence suggests that some but not all of the subtests are subject to further decline in healthy adults over the age of 70 (Herrera-Guzman, Pena-Casanova, Lara, Gudayol-Ferre & Bohm, 2004).

- The Birmingham Object Recognition Battery (BORB; Riddoch & Humphreys, 1993) is a test battery designed to assess disorders of visual object recognition. There are 14 subtests including size, length and orientation matching, overlapping figures, foreshortened view, picture naming and an associative matching task. The test is perhaps best used when standard screening tests have identified an object recognition deficit, and more detailed analysis is necessary. One of the key advantages of the test battery is that it can be used to determine whether an object recognition impairment is due to apperceptive agnosia, impaired precategorical visual processing or associative agnosia (an impairment of stored knowledge about objects). However, within most clinical settings, the test is perhaps too focused to be appropriate to administer routinely as part of a core assessment battery.

- The Judgement of Line Orientation test (Benton, Varney & Hamsher, 1978) was designed to assess visuospatial perception and derives from research demonstrating right hemisphere superiority in identifying line direction (Benton *et al.*, 1978). Although gross visual inattention will significantly impair performance on this test, other deficits in those patients without visual inattention may also be elicited by the test (Strauss *et al.*, 2006). The test is also relatively brief to administer, requires very little language mediation and minimal motor functioning, and is reliable (Strauss *et al.*, 2006). However, as with many of the VOSP subtests, there is a ceiling effect with healthy controls, and so intact performance on this test does not necessarily exclude subtle visuospatial impairment. The Repeatable Battery for the Assessment of Neuropsychological Status (RBANS; Randolph, 1998) also contains a line orientation task.

- The Rivermead Perceptual Assessment Battery (Whiting, Lincoln, Bhavnani & Cockburn, 1985) is more commonly used by occupational therapists than neuropsychologists as it is a standardised version of tasks used in clinical rehabilitation practice, and is not based on any theoretical model of perceptual abilities. The battery comprises 16 tasks ranging in difficulty from simple picture matching to copying a complex three-dimensional model. It is useful for therapists in helping to identify perceptual impairments, particularly visuospatial difficulties, as it has normative data for elderly people (Cockburn, Bhavnani, Whiting & Lincoln, 1982; Lincoln & Clarke 1987) and evidence of reliability and validity in stroke populations (Bhavnani, Cockburn, Whiting & Lincoln, 1983; Lincoln & Clarke, 1987).

- The Facial Recognition Test (FRT; Benton, Sivan, Hamsher, Varney & Spreen, 1994a) is designed to assess the ability to recognise unfamiliar faces. The test involves matching of identical front-view photographs, matching front view to three-quarter view photographs and matching front-view photographs under different lighting conditions. The test has been shown to be sensitive to cognitive problems following right posterior stroke (Trahan, 1997) and left visual inattention (Strauss *et al.*, 2006). However, language impairment caused by left hemisphere stroke has also been implicated as contributing to poor performance on the Facial Recognition Test (Hamsher, Levin & Benton, 1979). The test is useful for evaluating patients' ability to recognise faces, but there are some psychometric issues, and Strauss *et al.* (2006) recommended that diagnostic decisions using the Facial Recognition Test should be avoided unless supported by other measures with stronger psychometric properties.

Attention

Although visual inattention (neglect) is an attentional disorder, tests of visual neglect are described within the section on visual inattention. Other tests of specific attentional functions which may be useful in assessing stroke patients include the following:

- The Test of Everyday Attention (TEA; Robertson, Ward, Ridgeway & Nimmo-Smith, 1994) assesses selective, switching, sustained and divided attention. The authors argued that the subtests are ecologically valid and therefore of particular value in rehabilitation settings (Robertson *et al.*, 1994). Parallel versions of the subtests are provided, and the test is sensitive to the effects of stroke for older (65+) and younger (50–64) patients (Strauss *et al.*, 2006). An advantage of this test is that subtests can be administered in isolation, as normative data are provided for each subtest. Within rehabilitation settings, the test therefore lends itself well to hypothesis-led neuropsychological assessment. However, as Strauss *et al.* (2006) discussed, the test has some psychometric limitations such as poor test–retest reliability and ceiling and floor effects for some subtests, which can limit interpretation. Some tests, such as the visual search tasks, will be affected by visual inattention.

- The Trail Making Test (TMT; Reitan, 1955) is widely used as a measure of attention, speed and flexible thinking. The original version was a pencil-and-paper task requiring the patient to connect alternating letters and numbers as quickly as possible. Alternative versions include an oral version (Ricker & Axelrod, 1994) which is useful for patients with motor impairment, and a colour version (D'Elia, Satz, Uchiyama & White, 1996) which was designed to be culture-fair. The test is generally considered to be a very sensitive measure of neurological impairment although interpretation of impaired performance can be problematic (Strauss *et al.*, 2006). Of particular note are data suggesting that older adults' performance can fluctuate significantly depending on the time of day the test is administered (May & Hasher, 1998). Clinicians should therefore consider whether this test is appropriate for use with older stroke patients within acute hospital or rehabilitation settings; at the very least, caution must be exercised in interpreting impaired performance.

- The Delis-Kaplan Executive Function System (D-KEFS; Delis, Kaplan & Kramer, 2001) includes a subtest derived from the original Trail Making Test. Obvious advantages of using this version of the test include the excellent normative data, the discrimination between visual scanning, number sequencing, letter sequencing, number–letter sequencing and motor speed and the ability to directly compare performance on this subtest to other D-KEFS subtests.

Memory

The complex memory deficits that can arise from a stroke present a challenge to the neuropsychologist. It can be difficult to decide which specific memory functions should be assessed, especially within a time-limited acute or early rehabilitation setting. It can be helpful to establish some preliminary hypotheses based on the observations of multi-disciplinary staff; careful selection of tests can then verify or disprove these hypotheses. In some services, occupational therapists may undertake some basic memory testing with patients, using for example the Rivermead Behavioural Memory Test-II (Wilson, Cockburn & Baddeley, 2003). This can be helpful, so long as the interpretation of results is undertaken with supervision by, or collaboration with, neuropsychology colleagues. It is vital that memory testing within such services is coordinated, in order to avoid over-testing of patients, or the unethical misuse of tests.

Some commonly used memory tests include the following:

- The Wechsler Memory Scale-IV (WMS-IV; Wechsler, 2009) and its predecessors are perhaps the most widely used set of memory subtests. The seven subtests included in the latest version, the WMS-IV, measure auditory and visual declarative memory and auditory and visual working memory. The battery has the advantage of having been co-developed with the WAIS-IV, and has extensive normative data. Five primary index scores can be derived from the subtest scores: auditory and visual memory, visual working memory, immediate memory and delayed memory. Two key changes are particularly relevant to the assessment of stroke patients. First, the test now has two versions, an Adult battery for patients aged 16–69 and a shorter Older Adult battery for patients aged 65–90. Either version can be used for patients aged 65–69. This addresses one of the key limitations of the WMS-III, the relatively long administration time which was a particular issue in assessing older adults in acute medical settings. Secondly, the WMS-IV includes an optional subtest, the Brief Cognitive Status Exam, which can be used to provide an overall screen of general cognitive functioning. This may prove useful in acute medical settings when assessing older adults and provides a very well-normed alternative to other brief screening measures such as the MMSE. An additional advantage of the WMS-IV is that one subtest, the Verbal Paired Associates, can be omitted and substituted with the California Verbal Learning Test-II in the index score calculation. Having been published relatively recently, there are currently insufficient studies evaluating the potential value of the WMS-IV in the assessment of stroke patients. However, several limitations identified in the WMS-III appear to have been addressed. For example the Faces and Family Pictures subtests, which were reported to have questionable validity (Strauss *et al.*, 2006), have been replaced. The replacement subtests, Spatial Addition, Visual Reproduction (which in the WMS-III was an optional subtest), Symbol Span and Designs, appear to have greater potential clinical value in the assessment of stroke patients, but this is yet to be confirmed by independent research.
- The Doors and People Test (D&P; Baddeley, Emslie & Nimmo-Smith, 1994) is used to assess visual and verbal recall and recognition memory, and is particularly useful in the assessment of stroke patients due to its ability to discriminate between visual and verbal memory impairment. The visual memory components of the test have minimal language requirements and are therefore useful for the assessment of patients with aphasia. The test is also well tolerated by patients, especially the recognition subtests. It is important to take into account a patient's premorbid intellectual level, as Doors and People scores correlate significantly with scores on the National

Adult Reading Test. Davis, Bradshaw and Szabadi (1999) provided correction formulae for this purpose; these are also reproduced in Strauss *et al.* (2006).

- The California Verbal Learning Test-II (CVLT-II; Delis, Kaplan, Kramer, & Ober, 2000) measures verbal learning and memory using a list-learning task. Verbal recall and recognition index scores can be derived from the data, as can information regarding learning strategies, which can be useful in planning rehabilitation, primacy and recency effects, vulnerability to pro-active and retroactive interference, and test-taking effort, amongst other parameters. Normative data are extensive (Delis *et al.*, 2000), and a computerised scoring system is provided with the test.

- The Rey-Osterreith Complex Figure Test (see above) (ROCF; Osterreith, 1944; Rey, 1959; Corwin & Bylsma, 1993) is used to assess episodic memory as well as perceptual functioning. It can also be used qualitatively to assess planning, organisational, problem solving and psychomotor functioning. The test involves the patient copying a complex figure, producing an immediate recall drawing and then producing a further recall drawing three minutes later. Exact procedures vary, with some clinicians varying the duration of delay. Although those with a hemiplegia may need to use their nondominant hand for writing, the evidence suggests that recall accuracy is lower when the nondominant hand is used in the copy trial (Yamashita, 2010). Patients with stroke may have difficulty on this task because of one or more distinct cognitive impairments, and so the data must be carefully interpreted. For example, a poor copy trial may be due to perceptual, psychomotor or executive deficits, and a subsequent poor recall trial in this situation will not necessarily reflect a recall deficit *per se*. However, if well utilised, this test can prove a valuable tool in neuropsychological assessment across acute and rehabilitation settings.

- The Autobiographical Memory Interview (AMI; Kopelman, Wilson & Baddeley, 1990) is a semistructured interview used to assess patients' remote memory, allowing discrimination between deficits in personal semantic and episodic memories. Any significant symptoms of dysphasia may prevent the use of this test. However, in those patients without language impairment, this test can usefully establish the extent of any retrograde memory deficit.

- The Benton Visual Retention Test (BVRT-5; Sivan, 1992) is used to assess visual memory, visual perception and visuospatial abilities. Various simple shapes are presented for the patient to either draw from memory or select from multiple choices. This is a particular advantage in assessing stroke patients, in that those with significant motor impairment can still complete the multiple-choice version. Other advantages include the short administration time (5–10 minutes), parallel forms, and the ability to discriminate between perceptual, motor and memory deficits. More recent normative data are available from Mitrushina *et al.* (2005).

- The Rivermead Behavioural Memory Test-II/Extended (RBMT-II/ RBMT-E; Wilson *et al.*, 2003; Wilson, Clare, Baddeley, Watson & Tate, 1998) is used to assess impairments in everyday memory functioning. Accordingly, this ecologically valid test is focused on function rather than impairment and can be a very useful adjunct to impairment-level based tests. A combination of both forms of memory assessment can be the most informative approach. In practice, it is often used by occupational therapists in order to inform a more comprehensive neuropsychological assessment by the psychologist. This test is one of very few which can be used to assess prospective memory; this can be particularly helpful in assessing older patients, given that prospective memory impairment can be an early indicator of dementia. However, there is some controversy regarding the extent to which the Message subtest is a measure of prospective memory (Strauss *et al.*, 2006). Impaired performance on this subtest may not necessarily represent impaired prospective memory. Towle and Wilsher (1989) recommended that immobile patients could undertake the route learning subtest by moving a small figure around a drawing of a room. Evans, Wilson and Emslie (1996) suggested the use of a model car to move around a ground plan of an area laid out with model trees, houses, a bridge and a garage.

Executive functioning

Assessment of executive functioning in stroke settings is particularly challenging, due to the necessary reliance of most executive functioning tests on several primary cognitive domains. Although the theoretical basis for the concept of the 'dysexecutive syndrome' is beyond the scope of the current chapter, it is important for the clinician to maintain a healthy scepticism regarding the validity and utility of this term, given the varied cluster of functions encompassed by this description. Patients with executive dysfunction may present with one or more of many behavioural difficulties, one or more of many specific cognitive 'executive' difficulties or an idiosyncratic combination of behavioural and cognitive symptoms. The conceptual debates around executive functioning are discussed more fully in chapter 4.

It is perhaps most important in many stroke rehabilitation settings to identify the specific deficits evident in any given patient's cognitive profile in order to target rehabilitation accordingly. For this reason, it is often necessary to administer a wide range of executive functioning tests. Behavioural observation in combination with formal psychometric assessment is particularly important in the assessment of executive functioning in stroke settings. The clinician must reflect on the conceptual ambiguity of executive functioning and the frequent discordance of observed dysexecutive behaviour and performance on formal executive assessments. Patients with average performance on individual executive tests may nevertheless have significant executive dysfunction. Tests specifically designed to assess executive functioning include the following:

- The Behavioural Assessment of the Dysexecutive Syndrome (BADS; Wilson, Alderman, Burgess, Emslie & Evans, 1996) was designed to predict everyday problems that might arise from impaired executive functioning. The subtests are far more akin to functional tasks than the traditional impairment-based executive functioning tests, such as the Stroop. For this reason, stroke patients may see more relevance to the testing process when assessed with the BADS. Subtests of the BADS include the Action Program Test, which requires the patient to solve a problem using some apparatus, and by adhering to some rules. The Key Search Task requires patients to plan how they would search a field in order to find some lost keys, and to draw the route they would take in searching the field. The Zoo Map subtest involves the patient drawing their route around a zoo, showing how they would visit various locations without breaking the stated rules. Two versions are completed: a high demand planning version and a low demand step-by-step rule-following version. The Modified Six Elements subtest requires the patient to follow rules in order to undertake six subtasks within a ten-minute timescale. The test assesses self-monitoring and planning skills, and has considerable face validity in terms of occupational relevance.

  The BADS is a widely used executive functioning battery, and has greater ecological validity than most other executive functioning tests (Norris & Tate, 2000). However, there are no age-based norms for the individual subtests; the whole battery must be administered in order to derive a standardised score. This is often impractical or inappropriate in acute stroke rehabilitation settings. Although test-retest reliability is poor (Strauss *et al.*, 2006), Wilson *et al.*, (1996) explained that this is because at retest many of the subtests have lost their novelty. For example, once the Action Program test solution has been revealed, patients without significant memory impairment will quickly complete the task without errors on retest. Bennett, Ong and Ponsford (2005) suggested that the Modified Six Elements subtest and the Action Program subtest are just as sensitive to executive dysfunction as the BADS composite score (based on neuropsychologist and occupational therapist ratings of executive dysfunction using the Dysexecutive Questionnaire (DEX; Wilson *et al.*, 1996). However, they argued that multiple tests, together with questionnaires, such as the DEX, are necessary to detect executive dysfunction in clinical populations.

- The Delis-Kaplan Executive Function System (D-KEFS; Delis *et al.*, 2001) comprises nine subtests assessing various executive functions; most subtests are derived from pre-existing executive functioning tests, such as the Wisconsin Card Sorting Test (WCST; Heaton, Chelune, Talley, Kay & Curtiss, 1993), the Controlled Oral Word Association test (COWAT; Benton *et al.*, 1994) and the Trail-Making Test (TMT; Reitan, 1955). The test has a very large normative sample of 1750 people aged 8 to 89 years, and three subtests (Sorting, Verbal Fluency and 20 Questions) have parallel forms, normed on a sample of 286 people aged 16–89 years. Individual subtest normative data are reported, and each subtest has a combination of primary and optional measures for detailed analysis of test performance. This is a significant advantage when choosing only a few subtests due to time constraints or if other factors, such as patient fatigue, limit the assessment. Detailed analysis of just a few subtests can help the clinician to interpret impaired performance as being due to executive dysfunction or other factors, such as impaired visual scanning, speed of information processing or motor speed. As the D-KEFS subtests are based on pre-existing, very widely used, tests it could be argued that there is an advantage inherent in administering the D-KEFS versions instead of the original versions. Direct comparison between relative performance on the D-KEFS subtests is theoretically more reliable. The normative data for each of the subtests is derived from the same large sample, and so the clinician can be more confident in comparing relative performance on each of the subtests. Similar comparisons between the original versions of the tests such as the MWCST and COWA typically involve analysis of relative performance on the basis of different normative samples. As with most other tests of executive functioning, the theoretical rationale behind the authors' choice of specific subtests comprising the D-KEFS is not entirely clear, other than that the tests from which they are derived are commonly used to assess executive functioning. For this reason, the clinician should carefully consider the specific deficits revealed by impairment on each of the subtests when planning rehabilitation strategies.

- The Brixton Spatial Anticipation test (BSAT; Burgess & Shallice, 1997) is a rule attainment and following task based on the WCST, which involves 56 pages of the same array of 10 circles, one of which is coloured blue on each page. The patient is required to anticipate where the blue circle will be on the following page as the test proceeds, according to various rules which change without warning. The test does not require a verbal response, so is particularly useful in patients with expressive dysphasia. Van den Berg, Nys, Brands, Ruis, van Zandvoort and Kessels (2009) presented additional normative data for healthy older adults and a stroke reference group. The authors argued that the test has the additional benefits of not requiring a complex motor response, having a relatively short duration, and good test–retest reliability.

- The Multiple Errands Task–Simplified Version (MET-SV; Alderman, Burgess, Knight & Henman, 2003) is derived from Shallice and Burgess' original Multiple Errands Task (MET; Shallice & Burgess, 1991). The patient is required to undertake a shopping task *in vivo*, under observation by the assessor. The test is an impressive attempt to provide a genuinely ecologically valid, standardised test of direct relevance to a patient's everyday life. A further adapted version, the Multiple Errands Task–Hospital Version (MET-HV; Knight, Alderman & Burgess, 2002), has been shown to elicit 'real-life' executive functioning impairment in patients with focal cerebellar vascular lesions (Manes, Ruiz Villamil, Ameriso, Roca & Torralva, 2009). Within stroke rehabilitation settings, the MET-HV has potentially good utility, assuming that the patient being assessed is sufficiently mobile. The test complements formal neuropsychological assessment, especially if more impairment-based tests fail to elicit executive dysfunction which might nevertheless be qualitatively apparent.

Information processing speed

Qualitative observation of functional performance and of performance on any cognitive test can indicate slowed information processing speed. Where the patient is suspected of having slowed information processing speed, caution should be exercised in the interpretation of any timed test. For example, poor performance on a phonemic fluency task may be due to a general slowed processing speed rather than a specific language or executive dysfunction. Specific tests of information processing speed include the following:

- The Digit Symbol and Symbol Search subtests of the WAIS-III/IV together provide an index of information processing speed. As with the other subtests of the WAIS-III/IV, the main advantages of these subtests are the excellent normative data and psychometric properties of the scales. The disadvantages of these subtests for stroke patients include the reliance on intact psychomotor, visuoperceptual and language skills. The processing speed index of the WAIS-III is the most sensitive of the WAIS-III indices to brain disorders (Taylor & Heaton, 2001).
- The Speed and Capacity of Language Processing test (SCOLP; Baddeley *et al.*, 1992) involves the patient completing two subtests – the Spot-the-Word (STW) and Silly Sentences (SST) subtests. The STW, a lexical decision making task, provides an estimate of premorbid intellectual functioning. The SST is a timed sentence verification task designed to assess speed of language processing. Although the original normative data only cover ages 16–64, Saxton, Ratcliff, Dodge, Pandav, Baddeley and Ganguli, (2001) presented normative data for older adults aged 75–94 (reproduced in Strauss *et al.*, 2006). In stroke patients without any language impairment, the SCOLP can provide a useful index of language processing speed, and the test is simple and quick to administer.

Motor functioning tests

After stroke many patients will experience impaired motor functioning. Physiotherapists are expert in the assessment of motor functioning, and within rehabilitation or acute medical settings the patient should have access to physiotherapy. In other settings, and especially in the post-acute phase of recovery from stroke, the neuropsychologist may be working without the benefit of recent physiotherapy assessment of the patient. Although gross motor functioning impairment is beyond the scope of a neuropsychological assessment, the assessment of finer, more subtle, motor impairments can be very relevant to the interpretation of the patient's performance on any other tests which rely on fine motor movement. Tests which can inform the clinician as to a patient's residual fine motor functioning impairment include the following:

- The Purdue Pegboard Test (PPT; Tiffin, 1968) was designed to assess uni- and bimanual hand and finger dexterity. The original purpose of the test was to assess individuals within an occupational context. However, its utility as a clinical test has been long established (Reddon, Gill, Gauk & Maerz, 1988). The test requires the patient to pick up pins and insert them into holes on a board as quickly as possible, with 30-second trials alternating between the left and right hand. A more complex fourth trial involves the assembly of pin, washer and collar units. The PPT provides a useful index of motor dexterity, and Strauss *et al.* (2006) suggested that the test also taps the cognitive speed needed for good social or occupational functioning. The test can be a useful within rehabilitation settings and in assessing patients aiming to return to work.
- The Nine Hole Peg Test (Mathiowetz, Weber, Kashman & Volland, 1985) is a simple timed test of motor coordination involving the placement of nine wooden dowels into a 3×3 wooden matrix. There are norms for men and women up to 75 years-old and the test has high interrater reliability and moderate test–retest reliability. The test has been used to evaluate treatments of arm function after stroke (Higgins, Salbach, Wood-Dauphinee, Richards, Côté & Mayo, 2006; Sunderland, Tinson, Bradley, Fletcher, Hewer & Wade, 1992).

Apraxia tests

- The Test for Apraxia (van Heugten, Dekker, Deelman, Stehmann-Saris & Kinebanian, 1999) is one of several which are based on De Renzi and colleagues' substantial body of work on the nature and examination of apraxia (De Renzi, Faglioni & Sorgato, 1982). The Test for Apraxia, as with other similar tests, requires the patient to imitate the examiner's actions, or produce actions to command, both with and without actual objects. Actions assessed include the use of objects (e.g. a toothbrush) or the production of symbolic gestures (e.g. wave goodbye). Various quantitative scoring systems exist. Van Heugten *et al.*'s (1999) study demonstrated sensitivity and specificity above 80% for the Test for Apraxia scoring system in a sample of 44 stroke patients with apraxia, 35 stroke patients without apraxia and

50 healthy controls. Normative data exist for some other scoring systems (Haaland & Flaherty, 1984), but these are usually based on relatively limited normative samples.

- The Apraxia Test (Kertesz & Ferro, 1984) is a short standardised test of 20 items in four categories: facial (e.g. put out your tongue), intransitive upper limb (e.g. scratch your head), transitive (e.g. use a comb) and complex (e.g. pretend to drive a car). Patients are asked to carry out the movement to verbal command, and if this is incorrect or no response is given, the patient is asked to imitate the action. Items are scored on a three-point scale. Cut-off scores are provided for each subscale and the total score to differentiate those with apraxia from those without.

Tests of response bias and suboptimal effort

Within every neuropsychological testing context, the degree to which a patient is able and willing to give their best effort to the testing process will influence the validity of the test results. Discussion of the complex and rapidly developing field of symptom validity is beyond the scope of the present chapter. Indeed, even definitions of the various associated terms 'response bias', 'suboptimal effort', 'symptom validity' and 'malingering' would require at least a chapter. The reader is encouraged to refer to Larrabee (2007), Boone (2007) and Rogers (2008) for comprehensive reviews of the issues. It is perhaps sufficient for the purpose of the present chapter to state that the clinician must always consider whether the results of tests truly reflect the patient's underlying cognitive ability, or whether other factors, such as fatigue, pain, depression, attention and motivation, may have so hindered a patient's performance that the results of administered tests are invalid. Some measures which purport to test the validity of a patient's test performance include the following:

- The Test of Memory Malingering (TOMM; Tombaugh, 1996) is perhaps the most widely used test of feigned or exaggerated memory impairment. The test involves the patient being presented with 50 line drawings, which are then presented in a forced-choice recognition task with 50 non-target drawings. Explicit feedback as to the patient's performance is provided during each of the two learning trials and the retention trial. There is good evidence that the test reliably differentiates between people with genuine memory impairment and those who are not giving their best effort to the memory task. The test appears to be much more challenging than it actually is, and unless someone has significant global cognitive impairment and/or a genuine dementia, they are unlikely to perform below 45/50 on the second learning trial. For those stroke patients who do not show evidence of dementia or global cognitive impairment, premorbid learning disability or significant visuoperceptual impairment, the TOMM has good specificity and sensitivity in the assessment of exaggerated cognitive impairment (Strauss *et al.*, 2006). There is also evidence that patients with aphasia generally achieve high scores on the TOMM (Tombaugh, 1996).

- The Word Memory Test (WMT; Green, 2003) assesses feigned or exaggerated memory impairment using the immediate and delayed recognition of 20 semantically related word pairs. The patient is exposed to the list twice, either by listening to the examiner read the list aloud or by reading the word pairs on a computer screen, and then has to select previously seen words from 40 new pairs of words. As with the TOMM, explicit feedback as to the patient's performance is provided during each trial. A delayed recognition trial is presented without warning after 30 minutes. After these 'effort' tests, further tests of memory are presented, including multiple-choice and paired-associate subtests. Delayed free recall and long delayed free recall can also be assessed. Although the author of the test published evidence suggesting excellent sensitivity and specificity in the detection of suboptimal effort using the WMT (Green, 2003), other researchers have reported evidence that the WMT is more of a test of cognitive ability than of effort (Batt, Shores & Chekaluk, 2008). Batt *et al.* (2008), using a distraction task to evaluate the impact of increased attentional demands on performance on the WMT and TOMM, found an unacceptable level of specificity of the test, with a high rate of false positives, contradicting Green's (2003) findings. The test should therefore be used with considerable caution, especially if attentional difficulties are suspected. Batt *et al.* (2008) found that the TOMM was not as susceptible to increased attentional demands as the WMT, with an acceptable rate of false positives under the increased attentional condition.
- Other measures which form part of standard neuropsychological batteries; these 'embedded' measures are increasingly seen as having the greatest potential in assessing symptom validity. Examples include the WMS-III word list recognition subtest (Hacker & Jones, 2009), and the California Verbal Learning Test–II total recognition discriminability (Wolfe & Scott, 2009).

Assessments of the effect of cognitive impairments on everyday life

In addition to formal testing of cognitive abilities on standardised tests, it is often also useful to assess the effects of cognitive impairment in daily life.

Visual neglect

The behavioural manifestations of visual neglect can be assessed using questionnaires. Towle and Lincoln (1991) developed the Problems in Everyday Living Questionnaire as a subjective measure of visual neglect. The patient has to report how often problems, such as bumping into door frames and making errors when dialling the telephone, have occurred. The Catherine Bergego Scale (Azouvi, Marchal, Samuel, Morin, Renard, Louis-Dreyfus *et al.*, 1996) is a similar scale which contains ten items that the patient has to rate according to their severity. It has been found to have good interrater reliability and validity. Test–retest reliability and sensitivity to change need to be established. Neither scale has been demonstrated to be sensitive to differences between interventions. An alternative approach has been to ask patients to carry out practical tasks and to observe their performance. Zoccolotti, Antonucci and Judica (1992) described a scale which included tasks involving the exploration of external space, dealing cards and serving tea, and others related to the patient's own body, using a comb or razor. The scales were found to have high interrater reliability and internal consistency, and concurrent validity in relation to conventional impairment measures. To assess the effects of domain-specific interventions, tests of neglect for body space, peripersonal space and locomotor space may be used. Robertson *et al.* (1998) used a variant of the Hair Combing Task (Zoccolotti & Judica, 1991) to measure neglect of body space, the Baking Tray Task (Tham & Tegner, 1996) to assess peripersonal space and a tailor-made navigation task to assess locomotor neglect. The Shapes Task (Maddicks, Marzillier, & Parker, 2003), in which the patient has to name 20 shapes on a wall three metres away, has also been used for this purpose. The behavioural subtests of the BIT provide functional measures of neglect, with evidence of construct and predictive validity (Hartman-Maeir & Katz, 1995).

Attention

The Rating Scale of Attentional Behaviour (Ponsford & Kinsella, 1991) consists of 14 items scored on a five-point scale, according to their frequency of occurrence over a week. It showed moderate correlations with neuropsychological measures of attention, good internal consistency and good intrarater reliability, but agreement between raters working in different contexts was less satisfactory. Scores showed change over time with treatment, but the correspondence to neuropsychological measures of attention was low. Discrepancies seemed to occur as a result of emotional factors and expectations of the therapists. This highlights the difficulty of validating such scales, and Ponsford and Kinsella (1991) suggested that more concrete descriptions of scale items might reduce this subjectivity.

Memory

There are several subjective memory questionnaires available which are suitable for identifying daily life memory problems in stroke patients. The Everyday Memory Questionnaire (EMQ) (Sunderland, Harris, & Baddeley, 1983) has several versions: 27 items, 20 items and 13 items. It has been used both for patients to assess their own problems and for relatives to report problems in patients (Tinson & Lincoln, 1987). Five factors, reflecting the underlying memory processes, have been identified on the EMQ in healthy individuals: retrieval, task monitoring, conversational monitoring, spatial memory and memory for activities (Cornish, 2000). The EMQ has concurrent validity in that it correlates moderately with tests of memory, and its reliability is acceptable, though not good. Similar scales include the Subjective Memory Assessment Questionnaire (Davis, Cockburn, Wade & Smith, 1995) which is short and has been validated for stroke patients, and the Memory Failures Questionnaire (Gilewski, Zelinski & Schaie, 1990) which contains more items in four subscales, including one on the use of mnemonics. There is conflicting evidence on the extent to which the Memory Failures Questionnaire correlates with prospective memory (Kinsella, Murtagh, Landry, Honfray, Hammond, O'Beirne *et al.*, 1996; Zelinski, Gilewski & Anthony-Bergstone, 1990). One problem with subjective memory measures is that they are often more highly correlated with mood than with memory abilities (Lincoln & Tinson, 1989).

Executive abilities

The Dysexecutive Questionnaire (DEX; Wilson *et al.*, 1996) comprises 20 items on a Likert scale that describe behaviours related to the dysexecutive syndrome. Patient and carer versions exist. It forms part of the BADS, but has no normative data and does not contribute to the overall BADS composite score. Nevertheless, this can be an important qualitative tool in assessing a patient's dysexecutive symptoms. DEX ratings by professionals have been shown to correlate with patients' performance on the Action Program and Modified Six Elements subtests (Bennett *et al.*, 2005). Reliability has been evaluated by the authors and validity by other small studies (Norris & Tate, 2000). Significant correlations have been reported between executive tests, such as Wisconsin card sorting (0.37) and phonemic fluency (0.35), and ratings on the DEX (Burgess, Alderman, Evans, Emslie & Wilson, 1998), and with the Disability Rating Scale (−0.52) (Hanks, Rapport, Millis & Deshpande, 1999). A rating scale for problem solving behaviours was developed by Von Cramon, Matthes-Von Cramon and Mai (1991) to evaluate the behavioural effects of treatment. Aspects of problem solving behaviour were rated according to the frequency of their occurrence. The scale was found to be reliable and sensitive to improvements.

General cognitive impairment

The Cognitive Failures Questionnaire (CFQ) (Broadbent, Cooper, Fitzgerald & Parkes, 1982) is a five-point self-rating scale that determines the frequency with which cognitive slips, arising from failures in perception, memory and motor functions, have occurred. There are versions for both patients and significant others. The CFQ includes the behavioural consequences of several cognitive deficits and is not specific to any cognitive domain. It has been used as a measure of outcome of treatment, including cognitive assessment in stroke rehabilitation (McKinney, Blake, Treece, Lincoln, Playford & Gladman, 2002).

Neuropsychological formulation

Neuropsychological assessment within stroke services will often form a component of a comprehensive psychological formulation. It is helpful to have a formulatory framework in order to plan the most effective interventions. Diagrammatic formulation is often useful in explaining patterns of strengths and weaknesses to the patient and the multidisciplinary team, although simple descriptive formulations can sometimes suffice. Figure 6.2 is an example of a diagrammatic formulation, based on a formulation framework developed by Evans (2006). This illustrates the neuropsychological formulation diagram used to help explain the experience of a 52-year-old woman who, following a total anterior circulation stroke (TACS), developed depression, anger and anxiety symptoms. In this example, the patient's presenting difficulties, as identified through multidisciplinary assessment incorporating neuropsychological testing, are illustrated with an emphasis on the interaction of insight and cognitive impairment in the development of her depressive symptoms. Neuropsychological assessment revealed a constellation of attention, memory and executive deficits, with possible subtle language deficits. These deficits were hypothesised as impacting upon her insight, which in combination with her experience of loss in the context of premorbid dependent coping style and limited family and social support was exacerbating her emotional difficulties. Although Figure 6.2 is

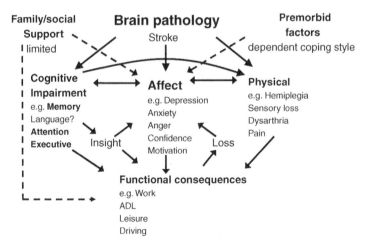

Figure 6.2   Example of a neuropsychological formulation diagram. (Evans, J.J., 2006, Theoretical influences on brain injury rehabilitation. Presented at Oliver Zangwill Centre 10th Anniversary Conference. Available at www.ozc.nhs.uk.)

Table 6.2   Case Example of a Neuropsychological Assessment

Background

Jennifer was a 41-year-old insurance administrator who had sustained a bifrontal intracerebral haemorrhagic stroke one year prior to the assessment. Her subsequent haematoma resolved without surgical intervention over several weeks. Her main symptoms following the stroke included memory problems, difficulties with planning and organising, and anxiety. She had made a good physical recovery and had returned to work about nine months after the stroke. However, at work she had noticed problems with sequencing tasks and fatigue. Her manager was concerned about Jennifer's ability to continue in her previous role. She was referred to the clinical neuropsychologist because of her difficulties at work and in her relationship with her husband. There was no evidence of depression. She scored within the minimal ranges on the Beck Depression Inventory–Fastscreen and on the depression symptoms subscale of the Hospital Anxiety and Depression Scale (HADS). However, she scored within the significant range on a measure of anxiety symptoms (anxiety subscale of the HADS).

At interview, her behaviour was appropriate and she gave a clear account of her difficulties.

Test results

Reading tests were used to determine her estimated premorbid level of functioning:

	Errors	Estimated Premorbid Intellectual Level (Using regression equation)	
Schonell Graded Word Reading Test	5/100		
National Adult Reading Test	22/50		
Combined Score	27/150	70–75th percentile	(High average)

Jennifer's current intellectual level was also assessed:

	Raw Score	Percentile	
Raven's Standard Progressive Matrices	41	65th	(Average)

Her estimated premorbid intellectual level was consistent with what would be expected on the basis of her education and work history. She left school at the age of 17 with several O Levels and initially trained as an administrator. There was no evidence of a significant decline in general intellectual functioning from her estimated premorbid level.

Jennifer's language abilities were assessed as follows:

	Raw Score	Percentile	
Graded Naming Test	21/30	65th	(Average)
Controlled Oral Word Association Test	20	<5th	(Impaired)
Speed and Capacity of Language Processing Test	Scaled Score	Percentile	
Speed of Comprehension	12	75th–90th	(Above average)
Spot the Word	10	50th	(Average)
Discrepancy	−2	>25th	(Average)

These scores indicated some residual impairment of word finding, in the context of average naming and speed of language processing. It was hypothesised that her impaired verbal fluency might reflect an executive functioning deficit rather than a language impairment.

Jennifer's perceptual abilities were assessed using the Visual Object and Space Perception Battery (VOSP), and the Rey Complex Figure copy trial. She passed all VOSP tests, indicating no impairment in visual perception. On the Rey Complex Figure copy trial she obtained a score of 35/36, also indicating no impairment in visuospatial functioning.

Jennifer's memory was assessed using the Wechsler Logical Memory Test, the Doors and People Test, the California Verbal Learning Test-II and the Rey Complex Figure immediate and delayed recall trials.

Wechsler Logical Memory Test	Raw Score	Percentile	
Immediate Recall	14.5	8th	(Borderline impaired)
Delayed Recall	8.0	<5th	(Impaired)

Jennifer's ability to recall meaningful story information immediately was borderline impaired. Her ability to recall the information after a 30-minute delay was impaired.

Doors and People Test	Age Scaled Score	Percentile	
Doors	2	<1st	(Impaired)
Shapes	1	<1st	(Impaired)
Overall Visual Memory	2	<1st	(Impaired)
People	3	<1st	(Impaired)
Names	8	25th	(Low average)
Overall Verbal Memory	4	<5th	(Impaired)

Jennifer's verbal and visual memory were impaired, and were significantly lower than would be expected from her estimated premorbid level of functioning.

California Verbal Learning Test-II	Raw Score	Percentile	
Total Learning Trials 1–5	35	<1st	(Impaired)
Interference Trial	5	25th	(Low average)
Short Delay Free Recall	2	<1st	(Impaired)
Short Delay Cued Recall	4	<1st	(Impaired)
Long Delay Free Recall	3	<1st	(Impaired)
Long Delay Cued Recall	3	<1st	(Impaired)
Yes/No Recognition Hits	14/16	5th–10th	(Borderline impaired)
Forced Choice Recognition	16/16	–	(Average)

Her CVLT leaning ability, recall indices and recognition indices were almost all impaired or borderline impaired.

Rey Complex Figure	Raw Score	Percentile	
Copy Trial	34.5/36	>16th	(Average/low average)
Immediate Recall Trial	15.0/36	8th	(Borderline impaired)
Delayed Recall Trial	13.5/36	<5th	(Impaired)

Her immediate visual recall was borderline impaired, and her delayed visual recall was impaired.

Jennifer's executive abilities were assessed using the D-KEFS Stroop Test, Nelson Modified Card Sorting Test and Brixton Spatial Anticipation Test. Her impaired performance on the Controlled Oral Word Association Test was also taken to reflect a deficit in executive functioning.

(continued)

Table 6.2   (*Continued*)

D-KEFS Stroop Test	Scaled Score	Percentile	
Colour Naming	10	50th	(Average)
Word Reading	10	50th	(Average)
Inhibition	6	9th	(Borderline impaired)
Switching	5	5th	(Impaired)

   Jennifer's performance on this Stroop task was indicative of impaired executive functioning.

Nelson Modified Card Sorting Test	Raw Score	Classification
Categories	6	(Average)
Errors	2	(Average)
Perseverative Errors	0	(Average)

   Jennifer's performance on this test of conceptual shift was within normal limits.

	Scaled Score	Percentile	
Brixton Spatial Anticipation Test	2	<5th	(Impaired)

Note: This test has an average scaled score of 6 and a standard deviation of 2.

   Her performance on this test of rule detection was impaired.

   Overall, there was evidence of executive dysfunction across several tests, although Jennifer scored within normal limits on some tests and subtests of executive functioning.

   A test sensitive to poor effort and feigned cognitive impairment was also administered:

Test of Memory Malingering	Raw Score
Trial 1	47/50
Trial 2	50/50

   There was no evidence of any significant lack of effort or simulated cognitive impairment.

Opinion, formulation, intervention and outcome

On the basis of the tests undertaken for the assessment, there was evidence of significant memory and executive dysfunction, consistent with a large bilateral frontal haemorrhagic stroke. Other functions, such as general intelligence, visuoperceptual and language functioning, appeared to be relatively intact. The profile of deficits revealed by the assessment helped to explain the everyday difficulties Jennifer was experiencing, especially in her work tasks. A formulation was derived from the test results and interview data, and shared with Jennifer and her husband. The clinical neuropsychologist and Jennifer then worked collaboratively to select and adapt several rehabilitation strategies for use in Jennifer's work place and at home. The clinical neuropsychologist also met with Jennifer's employer to discuss potential adaptations to her work tasks and to explain her apparent cognitive difficulties. Her employer was very supportive, and, over the next few months, Jennifer's job role was adapted and she incorporated her rehabilitation strategies into her everyday routine. After a few months, she described feeling less anxious and more able to cope with her acquired cognitive difficulties, and scored significantly lower on a measure of anxiety symptoms (HADS anxiety subscale). Although she had slightly less responsibility at work, this suited her and meant that she could meet all of her targets. She also reported that she and her husband were adapting better to the changes imposed on

Table 6.2 (*Continued*)

them by the stroke. Her husband reported that he could better understand the impact of the stroke on Jennifer's thinking, emotion and behaviour. They both reported that as a result their relationship was improving, and perhaps even becoming stronger than it was prior to the stroke.

---

relatively simple, such formulations can help in explaining the myriad of contributory factors relevant to psychological adjustment to stroke. Formulations can be usefully shared with patients, family members and staff. One key message is that neuropsychological assessment is not simply about measuring deficits, but can be essential in explaining the maintenance of psychological difficulties after a stroke (via a formulation), and therefore inform all concerned as to possible avenues for intervention.

The formal testing of a stroke patient to inform the development of a neuropsychological formulation is not an academic exercise. The testing process must be justifiable; there must be a specific purpose to the assessment and a demonstrable outcome. Otherwise, legitimate ethical questions may be raised. Undertaken appropriately, neuropsychological assessment will inform a meaningful formulation, which can be used to plan effective and collaborative neuropsychological rehabilitation strategies. As with any clinical assessment, there are many pitfalls and the clinician working in stroke settings must be particularly mindful not to allow the pressures of busy acute and rehabilitation environments to prevent adequate neuropsychological assessment, which is always in the patient's best interests. A case example is provided in Table 6.2.

Conclusions

Neuropsychological assessment after stroke must be timed appropriately and should have clear aims and a careful rationale for test selection. Undertaken well the results of an assessment can be pivotal in developing a useful formulation, in designing meaningful interventions and in facilitating a patient's recovery or rehabilitation. It is important to avoid various pitfalls of assessment, for example administering individual tests in isolation without consideration of the patient's history and possible primary sensory or language deficits. If these and other common pitfalls are avoided, and test selection is informed by the latest literature and interpreted using the best normative data, the assessment will be meaningful. With care and as part of a collaborative multidisciplinary approach, the neuropsychological assessment can help to transform a patient's functional potential and ultimately their quality of life.

Chapter 7

Communication Problems after Stroke

Introduction

This chapter will review the major communication problems that occur after stroke and their psychological implications. Approaches to managing the psychological consequences for stroke patients and their carers will be considered.

Communication may be impaired as a result of disorders of motor control (dysarthria and oral dyspraxia) or language (dysphasia). Dysarthria is a disorder of articulation, due to weakness, slowness or lack of coordination of the musculature (Kent, 2000). It occurs following lesions of the cortico-bulbar tract, particularly in the left hemisphere, and cerebellum, within the territory of the superior cerebellar artery (Urban, Rolke, Wicht, Keilmann, Stoeter, Hopf *et al.*, 2006). It is common in the acute stage after stroke but often improves quite rapidly, though persistent problems may occur (Urban *et al.*, 2006). Oral dyspraxia is a disorder of motor control due to impairment of the process of planning or programming the movements involved in speaking (Kent, 2000), though the movements themselves may be unaffected. It has been associated with lesions in the left precentral gyrus of the insula (Dronkers, 1996), but this has been suggested to be a result of studying patients late after stroke who have persistent dyspraxia due to large lesions in the territory of the left middle cerebral artery (Hillis, Work, Barker, Jacobs, Breese & Maure, 2004). Subsequent study has shown apraxia of speech to be associated with lesions of the left posterior inferior frontal gyrus (Broca's area) (Hillis *et al.*, 2004; Ogar, Willock, Baldo, Wilkins, Ludy & Dronkers, 2006). See Figure 7.1.

Dysarthria and dyspraxia of speech are both disorders of speech, the output component of the language system. Dysphasia is a disorder of language, which

Psychological Management of Stroke, First Edition. Nadina B. Lincoln, Ian I. Kneebone, Jamie A.B. Macniven and Reg C. Morris.
© 2012 John Wiley & Sons, Ltd. Published 2012 by John Wiley & Sons, Ltd.

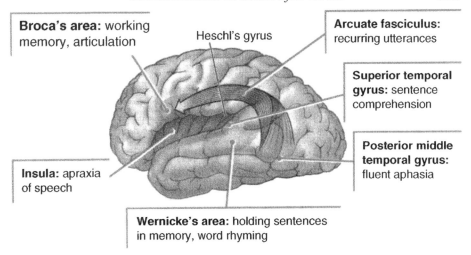

Broca's area: working memory, articulation

Heschl's gyrus

Arcuate fasciculus: recurring utterances

Superior temporal gyrus: sentence comprehension

Posterior middle temporal gyrus: fluent aphasia

Insula: apraxia of speech

Wernicke's area: holding sentences in memory, word rhyming

Figure 7.1 Lesion locations of features of aphasia. Kolb, B., & Whishaw, I. Q. (2003). *Fundamentals of human neuropsychology* (5th edition). New York: Freeman-Worth.

includes impairment of comprehension, reading (dyslexia) and writing (dysgraphia). Dysphagia is a disorder of swallowing also due to impairment of motor control, but generally does not affect communication ability. The prefix 'dys-' is used to indicate impairment, and the prefix 'a-' to indicate a loss of the respective ability; however, in practice complete loss almost never occurs and the two prefixes are used interchangeably.

Aphasia

The classical model of aphasia syndromes is based on clinical observations of links between the characteristic presentation following vascular lesions and results at autopsy. The arrival of modern imaging techniques has shown that while these syndromes remain associated with lesion locations (Yang, Zhao, Wang, Chen & Zhang, 2008), the functional organisation of language processing is more complex than previously suggested. The classical model includes several types of aphasia, each with a distinct lesion location.

Broca's aphasia is characterised by effortful articulation (low fluency and poor initiation) with relatively intact comprehension. Speech is agrammatic, omitting function words and inflections. It is generally associated with damage in the left posterior inferior frontal gyrus. Wernicke's aphasia is characterised by fluent speech with errors in word production, paraphasias and poor comprehension. Paraphasias may be phonemic ('I cooked' becomes 'I koot'), verbal ('house' converted to 'horse'), semantic ('doctor' spoken as 'nurse'), neologisms or jargon. Wernicke's aphasia occurs following damage to the left posterior superior temporal gyrus. Conduction aphasia is characterised by preserved comprehension and fluency but with poor repetition. Although it was interpreted by

Wernicke as due to damage to the arcuate fasiculus, it is now known also to occur with damage to other areas (Hillis, 2007), such as the left supramargional gyrus and temporal cortex (Kreisler, Godefroy, Delmaire, Debachy, Leclercq, Pruvo *et al.*, 2000). Transcortical sensory aphasia features impaired comprehension and production, with fluency and repetition preserved. It usually occurs due to lesions in the angular gyrus of the parietal lobe (Saffran, 2000a) but may also occur following lesions in the left frontal lobe (Kim, Suh, Lee, Park, Ku, Chung *et al.*, 2009). Transcortical motor aphasia involves disturbed initiation or spontaneity of speech, following lesions both in the dorsolateral frontal area and in the supplementary motor cortex of the left hemisphere, as a result of infarction of the anterior cerebral artery (Saffran, 2000a). Anomia (word finding difficulty) is often seen as the endpoint in recovery from the other syndromes, but may be classified as a separate syndrome. Global aphasia follows large lesions and is a combination of both Broca's and Wernicke's aphasia. It is characterised by severely impaired comprehension and very limited verbal output. Reading and writing are also severely affected.

These distinctions between the aphasias are not as robust as originally thought (Godefroy, Dubois, Debachy, Leclerc & Kreisler, 2002; Hillis, 2007; Saffran, 2000a), although they are sufficiently accurate to justify maintaining the classification system for clinical descriptive purposes. Evidence to support the lack of clear association between lesion location and type of aphasia comes from imaging studies. Godefroy *et al.* (2002) examined language abilities in 308 acute stroke patients referred with language difficulties, 14% of those admitted to hospital. Of these, 207 had aphasia. Classical types of aphasia were infrequent (n = 84, 41%) with most patients (n = 107, 52%) having global or nonclassified language impairments. A subgroup of 107 patients was examined with MRI within three months of the stroke (Kreisler *et al.*, 2000). Scans were evaluated blind to the results of the language assessment. Anterior damage was associated with reduced fluency, but only 67% of patients had lesions in the expected locations. Oral comprehension depended mainly on lesions in the posterior part of the temporal region, but only 56% of those with comprehension problems had damage to Wernicke's area. About two thirds (63%) of those with repetition problems had central subcortical damage, and most (83%) of those with mutism had frontal damage. There is also evidence that damage to Broca's area alone leads to transient expressive problems, but a more extensive anterior cortical and subcortical lesion is required for the full aphasic syndrome (Mohr, Pessin, Finkelstein, Funkenstein, Duncan & Davis, 1978; Naeser & Palumbo, 1994). Problems with initiation or sentence generation may reflect an executive rather than linguistic deficit.

Although patients with Broca's aphasia are typically described as having good comprehension, they have been shown to have problems in comprehension related to syntax (Friederici, Fiebach, Schlesewsky, Bornkessel & von Cramon, 2006). Patients with Broca's aphasia have difficulty matching sentences, such as 'the dog was chased by the cat', with the corresponding picture. Functional imaging of healthy participants suggests that the left inferior frontal area probably plays an important role in syntactic analysis (Roder, Stock, Neville, Bien & Rosler, 2002). Syntactic difficulty, as assessed by comparison of responses on easy and difficult sentences, had its strongest effect in the left inferior frontal region, and this was more pronounced for semantic rather than non semantic speech. Meaningful speech elicited more brain activation in the left inferior frontal region than speech containing pseudo-words. Posterior perisylvian centres were also found to be more active with complex sentences than simple sentences, which suggested that a substantial functional overlap exists between brain areas responsible for semantics and those involved in syntax. Further evaluation of this (Friederici *et al.*, 2006) supports the view that separate areas of the left inferior frontal region are responsible for different aspects of language comprehension.

A similar challenge to the traditional model comes from Conduction aphasia, which was thought to arise from a disconnection between Broca's and Wernicke's areas producing a specific difficulty in repetition. However, multiple attempts to correct phonemic errors (*conduite d'approche*) – pretzel, "trep . . . tretzle . . . trethle . . . tredfles . . ." – suggests damage to phonological representations (phonological output lexicon). In some cases a repetition problem may be due to a short-term memory deficit.

In addition, the analysis of meaning in comprehension does not depend just on Wernicke's area. Semantic problems are seen after damage to many areas, including anterior temporal (semantic dementia). In some cases the impairment may be selective to certain semantic categories (e.g. living things) (Saffran, 2000b). Contemporary processing theories suggest multi-attribute semantic representations arising from widespread cortical networks (Hickok & Poeppel, 2000). Similarly, naming problems can arise due to dysfunction in seven cortical areas in the left hemisphere, but there is no direct relationship between the area of activation and different components of the naming task. Each component depends on a number of other functional areas within a network (De Leon, Gottesman, Kleinman, Newhart, Davis, Heidler-Gary *et al.*, 2007). In addition, the right hemisphere is involved in language processing tasks, in particular the control of prosody (Ross, Thompson & Yenkosky, 1997; Ross & Monnot, 2008), in speech perception (Hickok & Poeppel, 2000) and in pragmatics (Beeman, 1993; Martin & McDonald, 2006).

It has been suggested that the patterns of deficit reflect the vascular supply to areas involved in language processing and deficits co-occur because the brain areas are supplied by the same blood vessel rather than because of any underlying functional deficit (Hillis, 2007). So, for example, Broca's aphasia occurs due to infarction of the left middle cerebral artery, which supplies areas responsible for grammatic speech, articulation, verb production and comprehension of grammatically complex sentences. Wernicke's aphasia occurs following infarction of the inferior division of the left middle cerebral artery, which supplies the posterior superior temporal gyrus. In addition, as highlighted by Hillis

(2007), there is individual variability in the pattern, shape and organisation of individual brains, such that localisation of function will only ever be approximate. Deficits may be due to infarction but also to hypoperfusion of the area surrounding an infarction. The evidence to support this is that when blood flow is restored to the hypoperfused areas, language recovery occurs (Croquelois, Wintermark, Reichhart & Meuli, 2003; Hillis, Gold, Kannan, Cloutman, Kleinman, Newhart *et al.*, 2008).

However, from a clinical perspective the location of lesion is of minor importance. The message to be derived from lesion location studies is that multiple components of the language processing system may be impaired and the pattern of deficits is very variable. Assessment of patients therefore requires a comprehensive detailed analysis of the nature of language difficulties, because patterns of impairment cannot be directly inferred from knowledge of lesion location.

Assessment of communication abilities

While lesion location studies help us understand why combinations of language difficulties occur, cognitive models, as illustrated in Figure 7.2, provide a useful framework for the assessment communication ability.

They indicate the processes involved in verbal expression, reading and writing, and are able to incorporate dysarthria and oral apraxia with language processes. Three types of measure are needed in clinical practice. Language screening measures are used to identify the presence of a communication problem. More detailed measures can be administered to characterise and quantify the nature of the communication problem. Measures are also available to assess the effects of communication impairment on daily life.

Language screening measures have been covered in chapter 5.

Language batteries

The aim of a comprehensive language assessment is to characterize the nature of the impairment in order to plan treatment. Several large-scale batteries are available, including 'the Schuell', the Minnesota Test for the Differential Diagnosis of Aphasia (Schuell, 1965), 'the Boston', the Boston Diagnostic Aphasia Examination 3rd edition (the Boston Diagnostic Aphasia Examination–3; Goodglass, Kaplan & Barresi, 2001), and the Western Aphasia Battery–Revised (Kertesz, 2006). These each involve several tasks tapping into the main language domains of expression, comprehension, reading and writing. Following the increasing recognition of the importance of cognitive models in understanding the nature of language impairment, batteries have been developed which are structured around cognitive models of language processing. The Psycholinguistic Assessment of Language Processing Ability (PALPA; Kay, Lesser & Coltheart, 1992) comprises a collection of 60 assessments for the

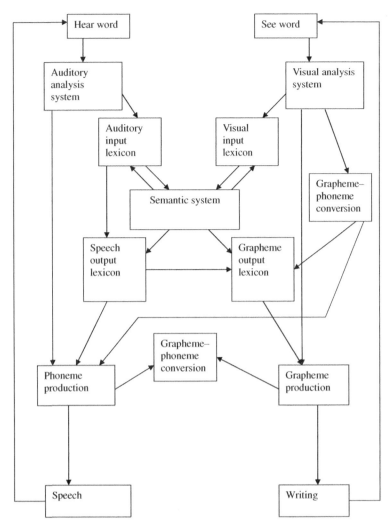

Figure 7.2 Cognitive model of language.

diagnosis of language processing difficulties. The tasks are designed to assess different components of language processing derived from cognitive models of language instead of lesion location studies. The tasks are intended to be used flexibly to explore specific aspects of language impairment in a hypothesis-driven approach. Not all subtests need to be administered, and the assessment can be adjusted according to the patients' difficulties. There are eight modality summary scores and an overall severity score. The Comprehensive Aphasia Test (CAT; Howard, Swinburn & Porter, 2009; Swinburn, Porter & Howard, 2004) comprises 20 tasks to assess language performance, covering a wide range of language functions. It also has eight tests to screen for other neuropsychological deficits (such as inattention, memory and apraxia) which may affect performance on language tests. T scores are obtained for each test and plotted to provide a profile of language abilities. There is evidence of test–retest and interrater reliability. These tests are structured so that not all subtests need to be administered and the assessment can be adjusted according to the patients' difficulties. However, they have very limited normative data and lack of information on reliability and validity. It is generally assumed that people without communication problems will obtain maximum scores on the tasks, which may not necessarily occur, especially when assessing elderly people.

Language measures

There are other language measures developed to be used in the context of a comprehensive neuropsychological assessment.

The Token Test (De Renzi & Vignolo, 1962) is a long-established measure of oral comprehension. Various published versions are available as part of language batteries (Strauss, Sherman & Spreen, 2006) and as a separate assessment (McNeil & Prescott, 1978). It consists of items in five sections graded in difficulty. Section V is also used as a screening measure to assess for the presence of comprehension problems. Although it has established validity as a measure of comprehension, it is affected by other cognitive deficits, such as inattention and memory, and only assesses a limited range of comprehension abilities.

Naming problems are the hallmark of aphasia, and naming tests provide a brief and easy means of quantifying the severity of the expressive language problem. The Boston Naming Test from the Boston Diagnostic Aphasia Examination–3 (Goodglass, Kaplan & Barresi, 2001) is widely used, particularly in research studies. It comprises 60 items and includes a short version (15 items) and a multiple-choice version. There are several studies providing normative data and evidence of reliability and validity (Strauss *et al.*, 2006). In clinical practice the Graded Naming Test (McKenna & Warrington, 1983; Warrington, 1997) provides a shorter alterative with UK norms. It was found to be highly correlated with premorbid intelligence measures (Bird, Papadopoulou, Ricciardelli, Rossor & Cipolotti, 2004) with high reliability over time (Bird & Cippolotti, 2007).

Fluency measures are sensitive to language problems and can assist in the differentiation between language and executive impairment. They are included as part of some test batteries, such as the RBANS (Randolph, 1998) and DKEFS (Delis, Kaplan & Kramer, 2001), and can also be administered independently (Strauss *et al.*, 2006). Aphasic patients have difficulty with both semantic and letter fluency but not design fluency, provided they are able to understand the instructions. Patients with executive problems have difficulty on letter fluency, design fluency and semantic fluency (Henry & Crawford, 2004).

Pyramids and Palm Trees (Howard & Patterson, 1992) is a test of semantic ability. It comprises a set of 52 picture triads and of 52 written word triads which can be used to create six tasks to assess the extent to which patients can access meaning from the spoken word, written words and pictures. Items were chosen that could be accurately completed by 90% of healthy participants, and less than 90% correct is used as the cut-off to indicate impairment.

Apraxia assessment

Apraxia of speech is often assessed informally through the recognition of the speech characteristics, that is, speech sounds being made in an effortful or erratic way in the absence of muscle weakness. Wertz, LaPointe and Rosenbek (1984) referred to effortful, trial and error, groping articulatory movements, dyspro-sody, articulatory inconsistency on repeated productions of the same utterance and obvious difficulty initiating sentences. Apraxia of speech often occurs together with aphasia, which also leads to sound errors as a result of patients selecting the wrong phoneme. Mumby, Bowen and Hesketh (2007) gave the example of a patient with 'phonemic paraphasia', saying 'speat' instead of 'speak', in contrast to one with apraxia of speech, whose attempts to produce the word 'speech' were 'stree stree skee skeech'. These distinctions are usually made on clinical grounds, but this has been demonstrated to be reliable (Mumby *et al.*, 2007). Mumby *et al.* (2007) compared ratings of four speech and language therapists who were given no definition of apraxia of speech, no training and no opportunity for conferring. The therapists rated video clips of 42 people with communication difficulties following stroke, including aphasia, apraxia of speech and dysarthria. The interrater reliability was high for diagnosing both the presence of apraxia of speech (kappa 0.86) and the severity of apraxia of speech (kappa 0.74).

Patients with oral apraxia have intact comprehension and reading, but may have problems with writing due to limb apraxia. Screening for oral apraxia is incorporated in some of the apraxia screening measures. For example, the Apraxia test (Kertesz & Ferro, 1984), includes five items to assess oral apraxia. An apraxia test developed by Van Heughten *et al.* (1999) included two oral items, but one of these, 'blowing out a candle', was shown to have poor interrater reliability (Zwinkels, Geusgens, van de Sande & van Heugten, 2004). A more detailed assessment is the Apraxia Battery for Adults (Dabul, 2000), which comprises six subtests based on the characteristics of apraxia of speech. It can be used for both the diagnosis of apraxia of speech and for rating severity. In the absence of a 'gold standard' for assessment, diagnosis tends to be made by clinical judgement, with reference to checklists of behaviours. Identification of the perceptual, acoustic and physiological characteristics of apraxic speech is required for planning treatment (Ballard & Robin, 2002).

Dysarthria assessment

There are few standardised tests to screen for dysarthria. The Frenchay Dysar-thria Screening test (Enderby, 1983; Enderby & Palmer, 2008) comprises a series of tasks to assess eight aspects of speech production.

Functional assessment

Measures of functional communication are used to assess the effect of communication problems on daily life and as outcome measures for treatment evaluation. Traditionally they have comprised rating scales completed by another person. The Functional Communication Profile (FCP; Taylor, 1965) is a long-established scale which contains 45 items grouped in five sections (movement, speaking, reading, understanding and other). It ranges from simple daily life communication tasks, such as 'attempts to communicate', to more complex, such as 'understands complex verbal instructions'. Similar scales include the Speech Questionnaire (Lincoln, 1982), Edinburgh Functional Communication Profile (Skinner, Wirz, Thompson & Davidson, 1984), Communicative Effectiveness Index (Lomas, Pickard, Bester, Elbard, Finlayson & Zoghaib, 1989), American Speech Hearing Association Functional Assessment of Communications Skills for Adults (Frattali, Thompson, Holland, Wohl & Ferketic, 1995) and Functional Outcome Questionnaire for Aphasia (Glueckauf, Blonder, Ecklund-Johnson, Maher, Crosson & Gonzalez-Rothi, 2003). The Comprehensive Aphasia Test (CAT; Swinburn *et al.*, 2004) includes the Disability Questionnaire, which was designed to explore the disability associated with having aphasia. It includes questions on talking, understanding, reading, writing, intrusion, self-image and emotional consequences. All components loaded onto one factor in a factor analysis, but there is no information on the validity of the subscales.

Many of these scales have the inherent problem of poor interrater reliability, as observers will not see all communication behaviours and the extent to which communication abilities are affected is very subjective and may be as much dependent on characteristics of the observer as the patient. In addition, the extent to which the items are representative of the communication skills used in everyday life has been questioned (Davidson, Worrall & Hickson, 2003). An observational study (O'Halloran, Worrall & Hickson, 2007a) examined the extent to which the behaviours in the FCP corresponded to communication activities which occurred on hospital wards. Most (99%) behaviours observed could be classified into the categories covered by the FCP; however, most observations matched only a few items, in other words, 85% of observations were reflected in 4 of the 45 items (9%). Eighteen (40%) of the FCP items were never observed in a hospital ward setting. This indicates the FCP has redundancy in an inpatient setting and also may not be sensitive to improvements over time. O'Halloran, Worrall, Hickson and Code (2007b) developed the Inpatient Functional Communication Interview for the assessment of functional communication abilities in an acute hospital setting. This comprises 12 items that were likely to be observed in acute hospital settings, could be measured reliably, were rated by doctors and nurses to be important and were of importance to patients. Preliminary evaluation of the reliability indicated it had good interrater and intrarater reliability when administered to ten stroke patients in an acute hospital setting (O'Halloran *et al.*, 2007b). Functional measures therefore need to be selected according to the setting in which they are to be used.

The Communication Outcome after Stroke (COAST) scale (Long, Hesketh, Paszek, Booth & Bowen, 2008) was developed as a patient-centred measure of communication effectiveness in the everyday life, appropriate to people with aphasia or dysarthria. It was developed for use as an outcome measure in intervention studies. The COAST comprises 20 items which reflect everyday communication ability, both verbal and nonverbal, opinions of confidence and improvements, and the impact of functional communication on people's lives. It has evidence of good internal consistency in a sample of 97 patients with communication problems, and high test–retest reliability (α 0.83–92; ICC 0.72–0.88). Convergent validity was established in relation to the Frenchay Aphasia Screening Test and employment status but evidence of its sensitivity to change is not yet available. It is administered to the patient, so that it is the patients' perception that is recorded rather than that of an observer. This potentially limits the extent to which it can be used with all aphasic patients. However, as only five of 102 people in the validation study (Long *et al.*, 2008) were unable to complete more than three items of the COAST and only eight of 100 participants recruited to a randomised trial (Bowen, personal communication) were unable to complete more than three COAST items, this seems to be a minor problem. A carer version is also available (Long, Hesketh & Bowen, 2009).

The Communication Activities of Daily Living (Holland, Frattali & Fromm, 1999) comprises a series of role-play activities which occur in daily life in patients in the community, such as going to the doctors or buying groceries. Responses are scored according to their communication effectiveness regardless of the communication modality used. However, despite being an attempt at simulating naturalistic behaviour, the situations require greater understanding than would be needed in daily life.

The most important functional communication skill is the ability to have a conversation. Although detailed conversation analysis is used in research studies, it is not practical for most clinical purposes. However Hesketh, Long, Patchick, Lee and Bowen (2008) developed a brief conversational assessment that could be used as a measure of functional communication. A ten-minute sample of conversation with an unfamiliar partner was videotaped. Partners were trained research assistants and conversations were facilitated through a framework script. These tapes were rated by speech and language therapists, unfamiliar with the participants, using the activity section of the aphasia–dysarthria scale of the Therapy Outcome Measure (Enderby, John & Petherem, 2006). Intrarater and interrater reliability were high, and the authors suggested the method could be used as an outcome measure in clinical trials, to ensure blinded assessment and thereby reduce the potential bias from familiar raters. Video analysis of conversations has also been used to monitor the effects of treatment (Cunningham & Ward, 2003).

The Dysarthria Impact Profile (DIP; Walshe, Peach & Miller, 2008) consists of 48 statements in five sections: the effect of dysarthria on the speaker as a person, the acceptance of dysarthria, the perception of others' reaction to speech, how dysarthria affects communication with others and dysarthria relative to other worries and concerns. Each section had acceptable internal consistency, with some evidence of reliability and validity in a small sample of people with dysarthria. It is, however, one of the few scales to address the impact of dysarthria specifically rather than communication problems in general.

Language rehabilitation

Language restitution

Early attempts at language rehabilitation relied on restitution approaches. The aim was to provide practice on those tasks which patients found difficult in order to stimulate the recovery process. The effectiveness of this approach remains controversial. Despite several early trials comparing language rehabilitation with no language rehabilitation (Lincoln, McGuirk, Mulley, Lendrem, Jones & Mitchell, 1984; Shewan & Kertesz, 1984; Wertz, Weiss, Aten, Brookshire, Garcia-Bunel, Holland *et al.*, 1986) and with attention placebo controls (David, Enderby & Bainton, 1982; Hartman & Landau, 1987), there was no clear message emerging from the literature. Various meta-analyses have been conducted but are hampered by lack of consistent outcome measures, and data not being available from some of the older trials. Reviews have suggested that language rehabilitation is effective if provided with sufficient intensity. Robey (1994) reviewed 21 studies and by calculating effect sizes concluded that the effect of treatment in the acute stage after stroke was twice that of spontaneous recovery. However, as highlighted by Bowen *et al.* (in press), Robey (1994) freely admitted that once you reject biased evidence the effect sizes reduced to zero. This is supported by a methodologically rigorous evaluation of randomised controlled trials (Kelly, Brady & Enderby, 2010). Analysis of 30 trials showed no overall evidence to support or refute the effectiveness of speech and language therapy.

Intensive therapy

Studies have also been conducted to evaluate the effects of intensity of treatment. Bhogal, Teasell and Speechley (2003) reviewed trials and reported a significant effect if treatment was provided for 8.8 hours per week for 11 weeks, as compared to no effect of providing 2 hours per week for 23 weeks. Overall those studies which had positive results provided 98.4 hours of therapy as compared with the neutral trials which provided 43.6 hours. Those studies which have produced most evidence of benefit have provided treatment intensively. However, this level of provision is not always feasible, particularly early after stroke, when many patients are not able to cope with intensive rehabilitation (Legh-Smith, Denis,

Enderby, Wade & Langton-Hewer, 1987). This is also evidenced by the failure to deliver intensive treatment in a high proportion of patients in a randomised trial in an NHS stroke rehabilitation service (Bakheit, Shaw, Barrett, Wood, Carrington, Griffiths *et al.*, 2007). It is also not representative of the level of provision of language rehabilitation in many centres. A pragmatic trial of UK clinical practice (Bowen *et al.*, in press) compared language rehabilitation provided by NHS speech and language therapists, with an equivalent amount of attention control provided by university-employed part-time visitors. Therapy began in the acute stage after hospital admission and continued, as necessary, after transfer of care into the community, for up to 16 weeks. Results showed little difference between the groups on the COAST or the TOM rating of videotaped conversations. This trial will have important implications for the provision of speech and language therapy services in the acute stage after stroke.

If rehabilitation is to be provided intensively, it may be more appropriate to provide it late after stroke rather than in the acute phase when patients are unable to cope with intensive treatment. Moss and Nicholas (2006) reviewed the evidence to support the provision of language rehabilitation more than a year after stroke. There was no significant relation between time since onset and the percentage improvement. The change in therapy ranged between 28% and 51% of maximum possible improvement, in the groups classified according to years since onset, suggesting that improvements late after stroke are possible. However, there is potential publication bias in that single-case studies of unsuccessful treatments are unlikely to be reported, and so it is not possible to ascertain the overall likelihood of significant change. These conclusions have been supported a Cochrane review (Kelly, Brady & Enderby, 2010) which indicated that those who received intensive treatment had better outcomes than those who received conventional therapy, though more patients dropped out from intensive therapy.

There has also been a suggestion from the literature that the effectiveness of the intervention may be related to the precision with which the impairment can be defined. It is assumed that the more precisely the nature of the deficit can be identified, the more selectively the intervention can be targeted at the underlying deficit. Single-case experimental design studies have illustrated very specific responses to treatment. For example, both semantic and phonologically based treatment have been using for improving naming ability (Nickels, 2002). Leonard, Rochon and Laird (2008) evaluated phonological components analysis, in which patients were prompted to elicit phonological components of a word they could not name, such as what it rhymes with and the sound of the first letter. Treatment was evaluated with ten aphasic patients with naming impairments, using a single-subject multiple baseline design. Seven patients showed improvement in naming treated items and gains were maintained for one-month follow-up. Edmonds, Nadeau and Kiran (2009) evaluated Verb Network Strengthening Treatment, a semantically based treatment strategy, using an ABA design, in four participants with aphasia. Results were positive, indicating improvement in lexical retrieval of nouns and verbs in sentences containing both trained and untrained items. Gains were maintained one month after treatment in three of the four participants, the other was not assessed. There was also generalisation to the production of connected speech.

Functional training

Thus, it seems that intensive language rehabilitation can improve language abilities in those patients who can cope with intensive language rehabilitation. However, there are many stroke patients for whom such intensive treatment is neither appropriate not practical. For these people other approaches are needed, such as a compensation approach, to train people to cope in daily life despite their language problems, rather than attempting to retrain the underlying language deficit. Aphasic patients can be trained in functional communication skills. In addition, conversational partners may be trained so that the burden of communication is shared between the patient and the other person. The non-language-impaired participant is encouraged to use all means possible to assist the communication impaired partner in conveying their message. So, for example, patients are encouraged to use drawings, pictures and finger writing to help to convey a message. Some materials to facilitate this are commercially available through organisations such as Connect, the Aphasia Institute and Winslow Press.

Functional training approaches have been evaluated, though mostly using single-case experimental design methodology. For example, Hopper, Holland and Rewega (2002) evaluated ten sessions of conversational coaching with two patient-partner dyads using a multiple baseline across subject design. Visual analysis of results indicated improvements in the percentage of concepts successfully communicated and one patient showed improvement on the CADL-2. Cunningham and Ward (2003) provided five sessions of training to four partners of severely aphasic patients to support their conversation. All dyads showed an improvement in the use of repair strategies when problems were encountered in conversation, and three of the four dyads showed an increased use of gesture. Statistical analysis did not indicate any significant effects on videoed conversations and mood, but this was partly due to marked individual variability and the trends suggested the treatment strategy was useful. Worrall and Yiu (2000) used a cross-over design with 14 aphasic participants to compare ten sessions of the Speaking Out programme, designed to improve functional communication skills, with ten sessions of recreational activities. Improvements occurred in functional communication skills, but the analysis did not compare the change with the Speaking out programme and recreational activities for all participants, and therefore there may have been insufficient power to detect differences. A review of studies of conversational partner training (Turner & Whitworth, 2006) concluded that most studies reported favourable outcomes, but only one of the studies reviewed was a randomised controlled trial (Kagan, Black, Duchan, Simmons-Mackie & Square, 2001). Kagan *et al.* (2001) randomly allocated volunteer–patient dyads to either receive training in supported communication or not and compared both the skills of the volunteers and the communication abilities of the patients following training of the volunteers. Trained volunteers scored significantly higher on acknowledging competence and revealing competence, and aphasic participants scored significantly higher on social and message exchange skills if their volunteer had been trained. Although results are encouraging, the sample size was small and further evaluation of this approach to treatment is needed.

Rehabilitation of reading and writing

The rehabilitation of reading was the first area to make systematic use of cognitive neuropsychological models to design treatment. Early single-case experimental design studies (Coltheart & Byng, 1989) demonstrated that focussing on very specific reading skills produced improvements in reading in individual patients. Examples of single-case studies continue to be available in the literature and support early studies to indicate training of specific reading and writing skills can improve outcome. For example, Ablinger and Domahs (2009) trained a patient with pure alexia, who read using a letter-by-letter strategy, to read whole words. Assessments completed before, during and after treatment indicated improvement in whole-word reading, in terms of both speed and accuracy. However, despite this, the patient still relied on a letter-by-letter strategy for reading and showed a word length effect. Small, Flores and Noll (1998) treated a patient with phonological dyslexia by teaching phoneme to grapheme correspondences. The patient showed significant improvements, and this was associated with a change in activation pattern on functional magnetic resonance imaging (fMRI) from the main focus of activation in the left angular gyrus to the left lingual gyrus. The results supported the hypothesis that therapy leads to an alteration in brain circuits responsible for language activities. Carlomagno, Pandolfi, Labruna, Colombo and Razzano (2001) compared two model based approaches to writing therapy, lexical therapy, which was intended to stimulate retrieval of whole word spelling, and nonlexical therapy which used a letter by letter approach to spelling. Both treatments produced improvements but lexical treatment produced significant changes in written naming and word writing on dictation, whereas nonlexical treatment produced improvements in writing words and nonwords but not written naming. However, randomised trials are needed to indicate the overall effectiveness of this approach.

Rehabilitation of dysarthria and dyspraxia

Dysarthria

Treatment of dysarthria is based on exercises to improve articulatory function. However, there is little evidence to support the effectiveness of the intervention, and many patients improve over time without specific intervention. A Cochrane review (Sellars, Hughes & Langhorne, 2005) found no randomised trials of rehabilitation for dysarthria, but there are a few small-scale studies suggesting that specific treatments, such as those described below, can improve outcome. Mackenzie and Lowit (2007) treated eight stroke patients with dysarthria using a behavioural approach for 16 sessions over eight weeks. Five participants showed improvement in at least one of the three speech measures, assessing intelligibility and communication effectiveness, which was maintained two months after intervention, and three participants showed no intervention related benefit. Analysis of the group data showed no significant change on three sections of the Dysarthria Impact Profile but there was a significant improvement in acceptance of dysarthria. Wenke, Theodores and Cornwell (2008) evaluated the Lee Silverman Voice Treatment in ten participants with dysarthria, in three of them this was due to stroke. Although a single-case ABA design was used, results were evaluated for the group as a whole. There were significant improvements in vocal loudness in sustained phonation and connected speech, increased vocal frequency range and improved word and sentence intelligibility. There was also significant improvement on ratings of communication initiation and participation and well-being. However, there was no control group so these changes may not be due to the treatment, but participants were all more than six months after onset so spontaneous recovery is unlikely to fully account for the findings, but nonspecific therapist (rather than therapy) effects might, and use of an attention control is required to rule this out. The trial conducted by Bowen *et al.* (in press) is the first to provide evidence from a randomised controlled trial on the effectiveness of therapy for dysarthria as provided in NHS speech and language therapy services. This showed no evidence of benefit of rehabilitation, but the proportion of patients with dysarthria was low and separate data are not yet available for those with dysarthria.

Oral dyspraxia

Similarly, few studies have evaluated the effectiveness of interventions for apraxia of speech (Ballard, Granier & Robin, 2000; Wambaugh, Duffy, McNeil, Robin & Rogers, 2006). A range of treatments have been described (Knollman–Porter, 2008; McNeil, Robin & Schmidt, 1997), mainly based on the principle of practice with feedback, and most of the evaluations have been positive, but most of the studies reported have been case studies or single-case experimental design studies. For example, Wambaugh, Kalinyak-Fliszar, West and Doyle (1998) evaluated a treatment which involved training in minimal pair phoneme contrast at word level. Targeted behaviours were retained six weeks after treatment but generalization to other behaviours was minimal. Ballard *et al.* (2000) based treatment on principles of motor learning and evaluated treatment in two patients with severe apraxia of speech. Although one patient improved on consonant–vowel syllables and the other on consonant–vowel–consonant words, neither demonstrated generalisation to un-trained words. Davis, Farias and Baynes (2009) trained an apraxic patient using implicit phoneme manipulation tasks and demonstrated improved overt speech production and also generalisation to untrained words. Van der Merwe (2007) evaluated the effect of a Speech Motor Learning programme on self corrections in speech using an AB experimental design. Eighteen months of treatment produced reductions in the number of incorrect productions of words and overt attempted self corrections and improvements in the number of successful self-corrections. However, speech errors continued to occur, sug-gesting that the ability to internally monitor speech production remained impaired. Although lack of evidence for effective treatments has been attrib-uted to insufficient understanding of the theoretical basis of apraxia (Ballard *et al.*, 2000) single-case design studies have suggested there are some prom-ising approaches. A systematic review of the literature in 2005 found that there had been no randomised controlled trials (West, Hesketh, Vail & Bowen, 2005).

Psychological effects of communication problems

Communication skills

The effectiveness of daily life communication skills, of both patients and healthcare providers, can have a significant psychological impact on patients. Interview studies of people with communication problems after stroke have shown that healthcare providers lack the knowledge and skills to communicate effectively (O'Halloran, Hickson & Worrall, 2008). Nurses and doctors have been reported to 'talk over' aphasic patients (Parr, Byng & Gilpin, 1997) leaving them feeling shunned and pushed aside. Dickson, Barbour, Brady, Clark and Pato (2008) interviewed 24 stroke patients with dysarthria. Patients reported that their communication difficulties led to changes in self-identity, relation-ships, social and emotional disruptions and feelings of stigmatization or per-ceived stigmatization. The impact of dysarthria was found to be disproportionate to the physiological severity and participants were continually striving to get their speech back to 'normal'. Speech and language therapists were seen as responsible for improvements, not only in communication abilities but also in providing psychological support and promoting well-being.

Training healthcare professionals, families and friends of communication impaired patients can reduce the burden of communication impairment (Turner & Whitworth, 2006). McVicker, Parr, Pound and Duchan (2009) described a communication partner scheme in which volunteers were trained to visit and support people with aphasia in their own homes or in residential settings. The main gain was improvements in confidence in the participants. However, there was no control group for comparison. Similar procedures have been used to train healthcare professionals in supported communication for aphasic patients (Shale, 2004).

Quality of life

Communication problems affect quality of life (Hilari, Byng, Lamping & Smith, 2003; Ross & Wertz, 2003), but it is difficult to determine quality of life using standardised measures, because many require patients to be able to read, understand and respond to complex questions. Specific measures have therefore been developed for assessing quality of life in aphasic patients. The Stroke Specific Quality of Life scale (Williams, Weinberger, Harris, Clark & Biller, 1999) was adapted for people with aphasia (Hilari & Byng, 2001) to create the Stroke and Aphasia Quality of Life Scale. The latter 39-item version was found to have good internal consistency, test–retest reliability and construct validity and to assess four domains: physical, psychosocial, communication and energy (Hilari *et al.*, 2003). Similarly, the Aachen Life Quality Inventory (ALQI), which is based on the Sickness Impact Profile, was modified (Engell, Hutter, Willmes & Huber, 2003) into a picture-based presentation. Engell *et al.* (2003) found good correspondence between the modified version completed by aphasic patients and the ALQI completed by their partners. An alternative approach is to ask relatives to report on behalf of the patient using standard quality of life scales. Sneeuw, Aaronson, de Haan and Limburg (1997) compared stroke patients' reports and reports by relatives on the Sickness Impact Profile. Agreement was higher for the physical dimension (ICC 0.85) than the psychological dimension (ICC 0.61). Evaluation of the correspondence between reports on quality of life by mild to moderate aphasic patients and their partners on a global rating, the SF36, Dartmouth COOP charts and the Ruff Psychological Well-being Scale indicated that relatives could report some domains of quality of life but not others (Cruice, Worrall, Hickson & Murison, 2005) with highest agreement on the SF36. However, relatives tended to rate quality of life lower than patients did themselves. Hilari, Owen and Farrelly (2007) also found lower ratings from relatives than patients themselves on the Stroke and Aphasia Quality of life scale, but the agreement was high enough to suggest proxy measures are acceptable when patients are unable to self-report. Agreement between patients and their relatives was excellent for the overall SAQOL-39 and the physical domain (0.8), acceptable for the psychosocial and communication domains (0.7) but only moderate for the energy domain (0.5). The Burden of Stroke Scale (Doyle, 2002) is a 65-item measure of health status, which covers 12 domains, including three scales to assess physical limitations, six to assess emotional distress and three to assess cognitive limitations. Doyle, McNeil and Hula (2003) evaluated two of these subscales, communication difficulty and communication associated psy- chological distress, in 135 stroke patients with communication impairment and 146 without. They provided evidence for discriminant and construct validity, which suggests they may be useful measures for detecting emotional distress in people with communication problems.

Mood

Patients with communication problems have a high frequency of depression, and estimates of the frequency have generally been higher than in non-aphasic stroke patients. For example, Kauhanen, Korpelainen, Hiltunen, Määttä, Mononen, Brusin *et al.* (2000) found in a small sample of 27 aphasic patients, 70% had depression, on the basis of DSM-III-R diagnosis at three months and 62% at one year after stroke. This compared with 46% and 36% in the non-aphasic sample (n = 74). In addition the severity of depression increased with time as the proportion of aphasic patients with major depression, as compared with minor depression, increased from 11% to 33%, even though the overall rate of depression deceased. In contrast, Damecour and Caplan (1991) observed much lower rates of depression in a sample of 54 aphasic patients (15%), but this may have been due to the method of recruitment, as patients were referred to the study, rather than taking consecutively admitted patients. Both studies relied on psychiatric diagnosis, and the concern is that this is difficult in the presence of communication problems. However, Laska, Martensson, Kahan, von Arbin and Murray (2007) found that in a sample of 89 acute aphasic stroke patients, recruited for a trial of an antidepressant, most (67%) could be assessed by psychiatric interview. Patients with comprehension problems could not be assessed. By including nurse and carer reports and using the MADRS, they managed to assess 76% of patients at baseline and 90% six months later. This suggests that it is possible to use psychiatric interviews and rating scales to diagnose depression in the presence of aphasia, but the accuracy of this diagnosis cannot be ascertained. Measures of the severity of depression generally require higher levels of communication abilities. For a discussion of measures of severity of depression in aphasia, see chapter 14. However, the identification of depression in aphasic patients remains important, as depression has been shown to be a predictor of functional communication skills (Fucetola *et al.*, 2006). In addition to depression, aphasic patients may present with anger and frustration (Kuroda & Kuroda, 2005). Kuroda and Kuroda (2005) found no significant relation between the severity of aphasia and psychological status. This finding is consistent with Bakheit, Barrett and Wood (2004) who found no significant relation between severity of aphasia and self-esteem. Thus, although other psychological variables need to be considered, they are not directly related to the severity of the overall language problem. They may however relate to specific characteristics of the language problems and this remains to be investigated.

Psychologists working with people with communication problems will have to adjust their treatment according to the severity of the patient's language problems. It will also require close collaboration with speech and language

Table 7.1   Case Example of Psychological Intervention in a Patient with Communication Problems

Colin was referred to the clinical psychologist based on a stroke unit because of problems with anger towards his wife, which were causing her considerable distress. He would swear, shout unintelligible words and bang his fists against the chair when she failed to understand his attempts to communicate or when she tried to get him to go outside the home.

Colin was a 56-year-old married man who lived at home with his wife and a dog. He was previously a miner but had retired early because of health problems. Colin had a stroke a year before referral to psychology services, which had left him with a mild right hemiplegia and severe aphasia. He was able to walk short distances with a stick and was independent in personal self-care activities. However, he did not carry out many of his previous social and leisure activities, such as going to the shops, gardening or meeting with friends in the pub. He was assessed on the Sheffield Screening Test for Acquired Language Disorders and scored 6/9 on the receptive scale and 0/11 on the expressive scale. His expressive language was limited to a few words, and even these were not used consistently. He was able to understand simple conversation, but could not cope with long or complex instructions. He read the newspaper on a daily basis, but formal testing indicated he could understand some words but not long or complex sentences. He was also able to write some words, and his written expression was better than his spoken language. His mood was assessed using the Stroke Aphasic Depression Questionnaire 21 (Sutcliffe & Lincoln, 1998) on which he scored 19 indicating low mood. He became very frustrated at his inability to make himself understood and would shout and bang the chair with his hand. He was reluctant to be left on his own, and his wife found it difficult to find time to do domestic tasks, such as shopping. He refused to socialise or go out. He had received individual speech and language therapy for six months but had been discharged as he was no longer making progress. He was offered a group programme for aphasic patients but refused to attend.

Formulation

Colin's problem of anger directed towards his wife was considered to be due to the frustration resulting from his communication problem. This language problem made it difficult for him to socialise, and he was avoiding situations in which he would need to communicate. There was a question about whether he was depressed as a consequence of the communication problems, but he had failed to benefit from antidepressants prescribed by his general practitioner. It was identified that he was distressed by the fact that he could not do activities which he considered he 'should' do as a man, such as fetching in the coal for the fire and buying the drink at the bar in the pub.

Treatment

A behavioural approach was adopted with the aim of increasing Colin's ability to go into situations in which he might need to communicate and increasing activities which he had previously enjoyed, in order to improve his mood. A hierarchy of situations was developed. The initial step was identified which he agreed to try. This involved taking the dog for a walk. At first the route was one on which he would be unlikely to encounter other people. The therapist accompanied him the first few times and then he was encouraged to practice the task on his own on a daily basis. The route was gradually changed to areas where he would be more likely to encounter other people. With guidance from the therapist he practiced nodding and smiling to people and using a

Table 7.1 (*Continued*)

thumbs-up sign instead of words, although occasionally he did manage to say 'hello'. He also carried a card explaining he had communication problems which he could show people if they started up a conversation. From here, he progressed to going to the local shop and taking a shopping list with him. Despite bringing back a few wrong items from the shop, it seemed to improve his confidence in interactions. These activities were then extended to going to the pub with friends, where he had a written drinks order that he could take to the bar. Some tasks that he previously did but were important to him, he could not accomplish due to his mobility problems. Although he wanted to take responsibility for fetching in the coal, he was not able to carry a heavy bucket. Instead he would clean the grate and take the empty coal bucket to the coal shed. His wife would fill it and bring it in, and then he would lay the fire.

Outcome

The outcome of treatment was that Colin was better able to use those communication skills that he had because he did not get so angry and frustrated. He used drawing and writing to assist his verbal communication and he used cards with written messages to cover common situations. He resumed many previous activities, such as walking the dog and gardening. He went out socially, which was also very helpful for his wife. His wife reported that there were no longer episodes of anger even when he got stuck in conveying his meaning. Following psychological intervention he resumed attending a self-help support group for people with communication problems organised by Speakability, a national charity. Despite very marked subjective improvement over time, his scores on the SADQ21 remained very stable. Most responses to questions were 'sometimes', so it is possible that the wife's perception of 'sometimes' was changing as he progressed.

therapists to ensure the approaches are complementary and not conflicting. An example of psychological treatment with an aphasic patient is given in Table 7.1. An example formulation based on the case of Colin is shown in Figure 7.3.

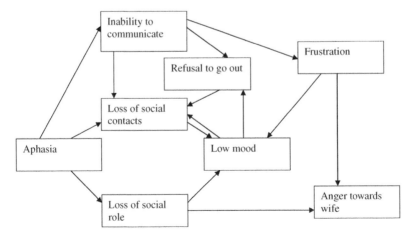

Figure 7.3 Formulation of Colin's mood and communication problems.

Conclusions

Communication problems have important implications for the psychological management of patients after stroke. The assessment and treatment of aphasia are based to a large extent on an understanding of cognitive models of language abilities. In addition, the presence of both aphasia and apraxia will have a direct effect on the ability to assess and treat cognitive problems in other domains. Communication disorders also contribute to problems with low mood. Effective management is therefore likely to involve close collaboration between psychologists and speech and language therapists.

Chapter 8

Driving after Stroke

Introduction

Driving is an important activity of daily living, and many stroke patients who were driving prior to their stroke wish to resume driving (Fisk, Owsley & Pulley, 1997; Klavora, Heslegrave & Young, 2000, Thomas & Hughes, 2009). It increases independence, and loss of driving ability is associated with a poorer quality of life (Hawley, 2010; Legh-Smith, Wade & Hewer, 1986; Marottolli, Mendes de Leon, Glass, Williams, Cooney & Berkman, 2000). Many stroke patients have problems in using public transport (Logan, Dyas & Gladman, 2004), and driving a car may be the most practical way for some people to travel.

Legal aspects, professional judgement and guidelines

The regulations for resuming driving vary between countries. In the United Kingdom, driving licence holders are required to notify the Driver Vehicle and Licensing Authority (DVLA) 'if they have any disability which affects or may in future affect their safety as a driver'. Patients are not allowed to drive in the month after stroke but may resume driving if their 'clinical recovery is judged to be satisfactory'. Patients need only notify the DVLA if there are residual neurological deficits, including impairments of motor function and cognitive abilities or visual field loss. Minor limb weakness requires notification only if adaptations to the vehicle are needed. Greater restrictions are imposed for those driving public transport vehicles and heavy good vehicles. In other European countries, such as Belgium (Akinwuntan, Feys, DeWeerdt, Pauwels, Baten & Strypstein, 2002), all those who wish to resume driving after a stroke are assessed at a specialist driving assessment centre. In addition, in countries where motor

Psychological Management of Stroke, First Edition. Nadina B. Lincoln, Ian I. Kneebone, Jamie A.B. Macniven and Reg C. Morris.

insurance is mandatory, patients will need to declare their stroke to their insurance provider, who may impose an additional premium. Those resuming driving without notifying their insurance company may find their insurance cover invalidated.

McCarron, Loftus and McCarron (2008) reviewed 166 patents referred to a neurovascular clinic in the United Kingdom because of a suspected TIA or minor stroke, finding 42% of patients drove within a month of stroke contrary to national regulations. The UK regulations put the responsibility on patients to notify the DVLA. However, doctors and therapists, who are aware that a patient wishes to resume driving, should notify patients of their responsibilities and the regulations relating to driving. In practice, many patients do not receive this advice (Fisk *et al.*, 1997; Goodyear & Roseveare, 2003; Legh-Smith *et al.*, 1986; Nouri, 1988; Pidikiti & Novack, 1991; Samuelsson, 2005). Hawley (2010) interviewed 140 patients, 60 with stroke, and found that only 28% of stroke patients were offered advice on driving without asking for it. They also found that when advice was given by different members of the multidisciplinary team, it was often conflicting. It is also of concern that some of those who are given advice against driving nevertheless continue to drive and others resume without a valid licence (Devos, Akinwuntan, Nieuwboer, Ringoot, Van Berghen, Tant *et al.*, 2010).

The lack of advice given may be because doctors and therapists are unaware of the guidelines (Goodyear & Roseveare, 2003; Hawley, 2010; Mackenzie & Paton, 2003; Thomas & Hughes, 2009). Hawley (2010) used paper vignettes to determine health care professionals' knowledge of the driving guidelines. The participants were asked to decide whether patients presented in the vignettes were fit, unfit or borderline on the basis of a brief description. The accuracy of doctors was higher than that of allied health professions, but in all cases there were inaccuracies as illustrated in Figure 8.1. In addition, the vignettes were relatively straightforward case examples; in some of the more complex cases encountered in clinical practice, the error rate is likely to be higher.

The National Stroke Strategy for England (Department of Health, 2007a) identified two aspects of driving in the management of stroke. One is that individuals attending primary care following a TIA and those who have had a stroke, need advice about whether and when they may resume driving. In addition, it is recognised that stroke causes a range of difficulties that can prevent people from driving. For those wishing to return to driving, mobility centres across the country can provide an assessment of ability to drive or advice on adaptations required to enable people with physical impairments to resume. These centres also provide advice on modifications to aid access to the vehicle. However, the guidelines in the National Stroke Strategy do not make any recommendations about the timing of such assessments or whether any advice can be given without referral to a specialist mobility centre.

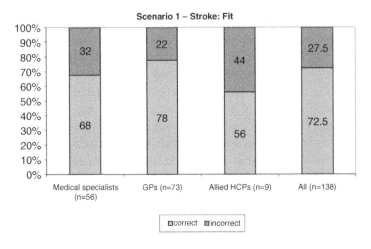

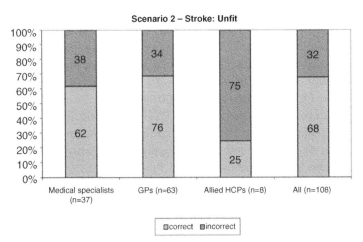

Figure 8.1 Health care professionals' knowledge of the driving guidelines. Professionals were given a vignette to rate as safe or unsafe to drive.
Reproduced from Hawley (2010) with permission.

The National Clinical Guidelines for Stroke (Royal College of Physicians, 2008a, sec. 6.48) presented more specific recommendations. These include the recommendation that that every stroke patient, whether admitted to hospital or not, should be asked whether they drive or wish to drive. The responsible clinician should then identify whether there are any barriers to driving, give accurate advice and document the conclusions. Patients should be told to refrain from driving for at least 12 months in the case of those with a group 2 licence (heavy goods vehicles), or at least four weeks for those with a group 1 licence (cars). However, any return to driving will be dependent on satisfactory recovery and any patients with visual or cognitive problems should be told that they must inform the DVLA and the insurer. In many cases, an on-road assessment will be required if there is any doubt about their safety to drive.

Therefore, it is important that driving is discussed with all stroke patients who were previously driving. This will make patients aware of their legal responsibilities and the fact that their insurance may be invalid if they have not notified the DVLA. It will also provide patients with realistic expectations about their ability to resume driving and enable those who have the required physical and cognitive abilities to retain their driving licences. Screening measures may be appropriate to decide the best time to refer a patient to a specialist driving assessment centre. In a few cases, referring patients for an independent assessment at a specialist driving assessment centre may reduce the conflict caused in those who are advised not to drive, but who nevertheless are convinced they should be allowed to do so.

Crash risk

The evidence for whether stroke produces an increased risk of crashes is conflicting. Haselkorn, Mueller and Rivara (1998) compared the records of drivers before and after hospitalisation for stroke and traumatic brain injury and found no increased risk of crashes 12 months after hospitalisation. In contrast, McGwin, Sims, Pulley and Roseman (2000) interviewed a sample of 447 older drivers (over 65 years) who had crashed (244 at fault and 182 not at fault) and 454 matched controls and recorded their medical characteristics. When compared with drivers not involved in crashes, the drivers who crashed were more likely to have had a stroke (adjusted OR 1.9; 95 percent CI: 1.0, 3.9). 'Not-at-fault' drivers involved in crashes were also more likely to have heart disease, stroke, and arthritis compared with drivers not involved in crashes, but were no different from 'at-fault' drivers in terms of their risk for stroke. These associations were independent of medications. However, the problem with crash data is that the information derived from self-report or police records may be incomplete and minor crashes may not be reported.

Factors affecting ability to drive safely

One way to identify people who are potentially at risk if they resume driving is to investigate factors associated with safety to drive. Lee, Tracy, Bohannon and Ahlquist (2003) examined 101 stroke patients admitted to hospital with acute ischaemic stroke who had driven in the month before admission. Their driving status was established six months later. Those who drove more often before the stroke, were less disabled and were married were more likely to resume driving. This highlights that driving resumption is not entirely a reflection of stroke-related impairments. However, for practical purposes it is the impairments that follow stroke which are likely to provide the most useful indication whether someone is safe to resume driving.

Assessment of fitness to drive

In specialist driving assessment centres the evaluation of fitness to drive is based on assessment of medical, motor, visual, cognitive and emotional factors. Motor impairment after stroke can often be compensated by car adaptations. Patients with hemiplegia can be provided with steering knobs, and the positions of indicators and pedals can be changed. Infrared secondary controls can allow indicators, horn, main dip beam, wipers and washers to be switched without removing the hand from the steering wheel or knob. However, motor impairment presents more of a barrier to driving in those with brain stem stroke or bilateral weakness. Motor function has to be found to be associated with passing a driving assessment (Smith-Arena, Edelstein & Rabadi, 2006), but this may not be entirely due to its direct effect on driving ability, since it may act as a marker of stroke severity and hence other impairments. It might be expected that reaction time would be important; however, simple reaction time, a measure of motor speed, has not generally been found to be an important predictor of safety to drive (Mazer, Korner-Bitensky & Sofer, 1998; Nouri, Tinson & Lincoln, 1987; Ponsford, Viitanen, Lundberg & Johansson, 2008; Soderstrom, Pettersson & Leppert, 2006), although complex reaction time, which includes cognitive decision making processes, has (Lunqvist, Gerdle & Ronnberg, 2000).

Consideration of visual abilities usually involves assessment of visual acuity, visual fields, and visual inattention. There are specific guidelines which apply to all drivers irrespective of the presence of stroke. These are that acuity must be sufficient to be able to read a number plate at 20 metres and a visual field of at least 120° on the horizontal, measured using a target equivalent to the white Goldmann III4e settings, and no significant defect in the binocular field which encroaches within 20° of fixation above or below the horizontal meridian. Studies have examined the relation between acuity and safety to drive after stroke, but this evidence is also contradictory. It has not been an important predictor of driving ability assessed using a road test, in some studies (Mazer *et al.*, 1998; Nouri *et al.*, 1987; Schanke & Sundet, 2000) but has in others (Akinwuntan *et al.*, 2002). However, those without the required level of acuity would not have been assessed on the road. Similarly, visual fields have generally not been found to be important predictors (Akinwuntan *et al.*, 2002, Smith-Arena *et al.*, 2006), but because many studies of stroke patients employing on-road assessment exclude those with visual field deficits (Lundberg, Caneman, Samuelsson & Hakamies-Blomqvist, 2003; Mazer, Sofer, Korner-Bitensky, Gelinas, Hanley & Wood-Dauphinee, 2003; Nouri *et al.*, 1987; Ponsford *et al.*, 2008; Shanke & Sundet, 2000), the specific effect of visual fields has not been assessed in this context. In the study by Akinwiunan *et al.* (2002), four visual tests (monocular vision, binocular vision, stereoscopy and kinetic vision) were carried out with Ergovision equipment. Correlation coefficients between driving ability and all items of the visual test battery were found to be significant. Kinetic vision, the ability to recognize objects in movement, showed the highest association with the decision made by a group of specialist assessors about fitness to drive ($r_s = 0.43$), but acuity was most closely related to assessments of on-road driving ($r_s = 0.44$). Patients with hemianopia are often not given advice about driving. Townend, Sturm, Petsoglou, O'Leary, Whyte and Crimmins (2007a) found that three, of a sample of ten stroke patients with homonymous hemianopia, were driving nine months after stroke. However, Tant, Brouwer, Cornelissen and Kooijman (2002) found that some patients with homonymous hemianopia passed an on-road driving test and the authors suggested that hemianopia should not be an absolute contraindication to fitness to drive.

Several studies have investigated useful field of view (UFOV) as a potential predictor of safety to drive. UFOV is defined as the area in which visual information can be acquired and processed without eye and head movement (Ball, Beard, Roenker, Miller & Griggs, 1988). The UFOV test is a composite measure which includes three aspects of visual attention: visual processing speed, divided attention and selective attention. It therefore combines measures of visual processing and cognitive abilities. Poor scores on the UFOV ($\geq 40\%$ reduction in the area in which visual information can be processed) were found to be associated with an increase in the number of road crashes (Owsley, Ball, McGwin, Sloane, Roenker, White *et al.*, 1998). Akinwuntan *et al.* (2002) assessed the predictive validity of the UFOV in 104 patients with first stroke. The overall UFOV score, the sum of the scores for the three subtests, correlated significantly ($r_s = 0.38$) with on-road driving. However, in a logistic regression it did not emerge as a significant predictor of either the overall team decision about fitness to drive or of on-road driving ability. Mazer *et al.* (2003) examined factors related to driving outcome in a treatment trial of training to increase the UFOV. Using univariate logistic regression they found that that passing the on-road driving evaluation was significantly associated with younger age and with better performance on the Functional Independence Measure, UFOV, reaction time, double cancellation, Charron test and Motor Free Visual Perception Test (MVPT) score and time. However, the amount of variance in outcome accounted for by the different tests was not quoted.

Cognitive abilities and driving

Cognitive abilities, such as visual perception, spatial awareness, attention, speed of information processing and executive abilities, are all involved in driving. In clinical practice neuropsychological tests can assist the on-road assessor to understand the nature of patients' difficulties while driving (Lundqvist *et al.*, 2000). It has also been recognised that although the ideal is to conduct an on-road assessment, this may be costly and impractical

(Klavora *et al.*, 2000) and that cognitive screening tests may detect subtle cognitive impairments which may be missed during an on-road assessment. Cognitive tests may serve two purposes. One is to identify those likely to fail on the road so that a decision can be made to advise them to stop driving without the need for a road test. The other is to identify those who have the cognitive skills required for driving who may then need only an assessment of the physical ability to drive. In many rehabilitation settings, cognitive tests are used to identify those who need on-road evaluation. Several authors have developed batteries of neuropsychological tests which aim to assess each cognitive domain and have explored the relation between these tests and on-road driving ability. Some of these studies have included stroke patients in samples of mixed aetiology (Galski, Bruno & Ehle, 1993; McKenna, Jefferies, Dobson & Frude, 2004; Meyers, Volbrecht & Kaster-Bundgaard, 1999) which makes the findings more difficult to interpret in relation to stroke. Those which have been specific to stroke are summarised in Table 8.1.

Many of the studies have been retrospective analysis of existing data (Akinwuntan *et al.*, 2002; Bitensky, Mazer, Sofer, Gelina, Meyer, Morrison *et al.*, 2000; Mazer *et al.*, 1998; McKenna & Bell, 2007; Ponsford *et al.*, 2008), and therefore road tests or decisions about fitness to drive have not been carried out blind to the predictor variables. This concern also applies to some of the prospective studies (Akinwuntan, Feys, De Weerdt, Baten, Arno & Kiekens. 2006; Klavora *et al.*, 2000) and may lead to inflation of some of the predictive values. However, taken together, the results indicate that cognitive tests may useful to identify people who need an on-road assessment.

Different cognitive tests have been used in these studies. Some have consistently not shown a significant relation with road test performance and are therefore redundant. This includes tests of language and memory (Akinwuntan *et al.*, 2002; Nouri *et al.*, 1987; Ponsford *et al.*, 2008). Other cognitive tests have been shown to be good predictors in more than one geographical centre. Marshall, Molnar, Man-Son-Hing, Blair, Brosseau, Finestone *et al.* (2007) reviewed most of these studies and identified ten studies in which the primary outcome was an on-road driving assessment; the remaining six used driving cessation. They suggested the most useful cognitive screening tests were Trail Making, the Rey Osterreith Complex Figure and the Useful Field of View Test. However, studies of the Stroke Drivers' Screening Assessment (SDSA) (Nouri & Lincoln, 1994) were omitted from the Marshall *et al.* (2007) review and the Rookwood Driving Battery (RDB) (McKenna, 2009) was not available at that time. The UFOV requires equipment which is not available in most clinical settings, and is therefore only likely to be used at specialist driving assessment centres. The cognitive tests which could potentially be used in routine clinical practice, as they have been shown to be useful and have been validated in more than one study, are considered below.

Table 8.1   Studies Evaluating Cognitive Tests as Predictors of Driving Performance on the Road

Study	Study design	Participants	Cognitive abilities tested	Driving outcome	Analysis	Results	Comments
Nouri, Tinson & Lincoln, 1987	Prospective cohort United Kingdom	39 stroke patients who had been driving prior to stroke and wished to resume	Attention, visuospatial, language, executive and memory	Road test blind to cognitive tests results	Comparison between pass, borderline and fail on road test	Cognitive tests showed significant differences between those passing and failing on the road	
Nouri & Lincoln, 1992	Prospective cohort United Kingdom	40 stroke patients who had been driving prior to stroke and wished to resume	Attention, visuospatial, language, executive and memory	Road test blind to cognitive tests results	Comparison between pass, borderline and fail on road test	Cognitive tests showed significant differences between groups on 13/14 measures	Discriminant function analysis was used to generate a predictive equation based on 3 tests
Nouri & Lincoln, 1993	Randomised controlled trial United Kingdom	27 stroke patients assigned to cognitive assessment	Attention and executive	Road test before cognitive testing	Relation between prediction from cognitive tests and road test	SDSA correctly classified 81% of drivers as pass/fail on the road test	
Mazer et al., 1998	Retrospective cohort study Canada	84 stroke patients Mean age 61 years Mean tpo10 months	Reaction time Visual perceptual skills Visual scanning Visual orientation Visuomotor tracking	Road test by same occupational therapist as conducted cognitive testing 39% passed	Logistic regression	Trail Making B and Motor Free Visual Perception test 86% positive predictive value 58% negative predictive value	9% did not take road test because found to have perceptual problems

Korner–Bitensky et al., 2000	Retrospective cohort study Multicentre Canada and United States	269 stroke patients	Motor Free Visual Perception test by OT	54% passed road test	Decision on fitness to drive based on decision of OT and driving instructor	Predictive values PPV 61% NPV 64% MVPT not suitable as sole predictor
Klavora et al., 2000	Prospective cohort study Canada	56 stroke patients, mean age 60.2 years	Cognitive Behavioural Drivers Inventory of visual skills related to driving and Dynavision Performance Assessment Battery	On-road assessment	Accuracy of prediction and multiple regression	CBDI had 66% accuracy, Endurance Dynavision Task 78% accurate Combining the two increased accuracy to 100%
Lundqvist et al., 2000	Prospective case control study Sweden	30 stroke patients 30 healthy controls	Trail Making, Digit Symbol, Colour Word Test, PASAT, Finger tapping, Reaction time, Simultaneous Capacity, WCST	Simulator assessment and road test blind to cognitive test results	50% strokes with low driving skills (20% controls)	Stepwise logistic regression classified 83% with high vs. low driving skills Complex reaction time was most important predictor
Akinwuntan et al., 2002	Retrospective case note review Belgium	104 patients with first stroke referred to driving assessment centre	Rey figure UFOV Fimm-Zimmerman test of attention	Road test and team decision about driving safety	Logistic regression to differentiate between those suitable to drive, not immediately suitable and not suitable	Acuity and Rey figure copy best predictors of road test but only predicted 28% of variance Road test not independent of cognitive test results

(continued)

Table 8.1 (*Continued*)

Study	Study design	Participants	Cognitive abilities tested	Driving outcome	Analysis	Results	Comments
Lundberg *et al.*, 2003	Prospective cohort study Sweden and Norway	97 stroke patients	Nordic SDSA	Road test	Discriminant function analysis	Original equation correctly classified 68%; 78% correctly classified with new equation	
Mazer *et al.*, 2003	Randomised controlled trial Canada	84 stroke patients referred for driving evaluation	UFOV, visual perception, Test of Everyday Attention	Road test by an OT experienced in driving evaluation	Logistic regression as secondary analysis to the RCT	Passing road test associated with FIM, UFOV, RT, double cancellation, Charron and MVPT	
Akinwuntan *et al.*, 2006	Prospective cohort study Belgium	38 patients with first stroke	SDSA	Road test TRIP	Correspondence road test and SDSA classification	Acuity, SDSA dot cancellation, SDSA compass and incompatibility test accounted for 35% variance in road test	
Söderström *et al.*, 2006	Prospective cohort study Sweden	34 stroke unit patients who wished to resume driving (n = 23 on some tests)	Trail Making, Reaction time, finger tapping, Rey, Symbol digit	Road test blind to cognitive tests results	Correlation between cognitive tests and driving (pass/fail) and driving skills (score out of 5)	No significant correlations	

Study	Design	Sample	Cognitive test	Road test	Outcome measure	Results	Comments
McKenna & Bell, 2007	Retrospective Cohort study United Kingdom	n = 129 Referred to driving assessment centre	Rookwood Driving Battery	Road test	Correspondence between Rookwood Driving Battery and road test	Right hemisphere accuracy 77% Left hemisphere accuracy 78%	Road test not blind to cognitive test results
Ponsford *et al.*, 2008	Retrospective cohort study United Kingdom	200 stroke patients median age 62 years	Orientation, praxis, perception, memory, executive abilities	Road test	Correlation between cognitive tests and road test	All cognitive tests significantly correlated with on road tests. Praxis, divided attention and decision time correctly identified 75% of unsafe drivers (PPV 88%)	
George & Crotty, 2010	Prospective cohort study, Australia	43 stroke patients recruited from rehabilitation centres	UFOV SDSA	Road test blind to UFOV and SDSA scores	Correspondence between pass and fail categories using each method	UFOV Divided Attention and Selective Attention and SDSA significantly related to on-road assessment Predictive ability UFOV Divided attention 78%, UFOV Selective Attention 66%, SDSA 75%	

Trail Making B

Trail Making is a test of visual conceptual and visuomotor tracking. It comprises two parts. Trail A requires patients to connect the numbers 1 to 25 in consecutive order. In Trail B, the test sheet contains the numbers 1 to 13 and the letters A to L. The task is to alternate between the series of letters and numbers, 1, A, 2, B and so on. The tasks have to be completed as quickly and as accurately as possible without lifting the pencil from the paper. Mazer *et al.* (1998) used more than three errors on Part B as a cut-off to indicate participants were likely to fail the road test. Trails B had a Positive Predictive Value of 85% (23/27) and Negative Predictive Value 48% (25/52). However, the overlap in the distribution of scores in those who passed and failed was substantial (pass errors mean 1.2, SD 1.9; fail mean errors 5.3, SD 7.0; pass time mean 137.0, SD 64.4; fail mean time 187.4, SD 77.3). Trails B was a better predictor of driving ability in those with left hemisphere lesions than right, but numbers in the subgroups were small. Lundqvist *et al.* (2000) found the time taken to complete Trails B time loaded on to a primary factor assessing attentional processing, which was found to be a significant predictor of on-road performance. Those with high driving skills obtained significantly higher scores than those with low driving skills ($p < 0.01$), but the mean scores of these two groups were not provided. In contrast Söderström *et al.* (2006) found a correlation of only 0.20 ($p = 0.27$, $n = 33$) between Trail Making and driving performance. These findings indicate that performance on Trail Making has been found to be related to diving ability in most studies, and that patients scoring more than three errors on Trails B should be evaluated further. In addition, a meta-analysis of cognitive tests in relation to driving (Devos, Akinwuntan, Nieuwboer, Truijen, Tant & De Weerdt, 2011) found that a cut-off of 90 seconds for Trail Making B classified unsafe drivers with 80%, accuracy (sensitivity for unsafe driving 80%, specificity 62%). The proportion of participants correctly predicted to fail the on-road assessment was 69%, supporting the clinical utility of the Trail Making Test B.

Rey Osterreith complex figure test

The Rey Osterreith complex figure test is a measure of visuospatial perception and visual memory. Patients are required to copy a complex figure and then to draw it from memory. In many driving studies, only the copy stage is conducted. Nouri and Lincoln (1992) found significant differences between those who passed and failed an on-road assessment on both Rey copy and recall (pass copy mean 33.9, SD 2.4, recall 22.4, SD 7.3; fail copy mean 30.0, SD 6.2, recall mean 14.5, SD 7.4), but the overlap in distributions was high. In a discriminant function analysis neither Rey figure copy nor recall emerged as significant predictors of on–road performance. Söderström *et al.* (2006) also reported no significant relationship between Rey figure scores and driving performance. In a retrospective study of stroke patients assessed at a specialist driving assessment centre, Akinwuntan *et al.* (2002) found a significant correlation (r_s 0.48, $p < 0.001$) between the Rey copy and road driving ability and the overall decision about fitness to drive made by a specialist driving assessment team (r_s 0.42, $p < 0.001$). Scores differed significantly ($p < 0.001$) between those who passed, those who needed further evaluation and those deemed unfit to drive, but the actual values were not provided. In a logistic regression, acuity and the Rey copy were the best predictors of on-road driving, accounting for 28% of the variance, of which 24% was from the Rey. Regression analysis to determine overall predictors of the decision about safety to drive did not include the Rey, but in this analysis most of the variance was accounted for by the road test, which in itself reflected scores on the Rey. In a subsequent prospective study (Akinwuntan *et al.*, 2006), the Rey figure emerged as a significant predictor of overall assessment of fitness to drive in conjunction with a measure of neglect and a road test. The implication of this is that visual neglect and visuospatial problems are not easily detected during an on-road assessment because including these measures improved the accuracy of the prediction of the overall decision about fitness to drive. If they had been apparent, the inclusion of the Rey figure and the measure of neglect would not have improved the predictive accuracy over that of the road test alone. The Rey figure may therefore be particularly useful to detect visuospatial problems which may not be apparent during an on-road assessment.

While these results indicate Rey figure copy is an appropriate measure for detecting visuospatial problems which affect safety to drive; there is no clear cut-off point which can be recommended for use in clinical practice to decide that a patient is so unlikely to be safe to drive that a road test is not needed. Akinwuntan, Devos, Feys, Verheyden, Baten, Kiekens *et al.* (2007) suggested a cut-off of 33/34 as part of an algorithm for deciding safety to drive, but the recommendation was that all patients received a road test. The results from Nouri and Lincoln (1992) suggested that anyone scoring less than 32 may be unsafe on the road. However, the use of specific cut-offs on the Rey figure copy requires further evaluation.

Motor Free Visual Perception test

The MVPT is measure of visual perceptual skills in five areas: spatial relations, visual discrimination, figure–ground discrimination, visual closure and visual memory. Mazer *et al.* (1998) used a cut-off of more than 30 (out of 36) to predict passing a road test. In a study with 84 stroke patients, 36 received a score below the cut-off (≤ 30), 31 (PPV 86.1%) of these failed the on-road driving evaluation. Of the 48 who received a score of >30, only 28 passed the driving test, resulting in a negative predictive value of only 58%. The clinical implications of this finding are that those scoring ≤ 30 are likely to fail an on-road evaluation. However, as 42% of those who passed the MVPT test failed on the road, the MVPT cannot be used to indicate a stroke patient is safe to drive.

Even at the highest possible MVPT scores, half of the participants passed and half failed the on-road evaluation. The overlap in distributions of scores was high (pass score mean 32.0, SD 4.1; fail score mean 29.2, SD 4.7), also supporting the limited utility of the MVPT. Age-specific norms are available, but Mazer *et al.* (1998) used the total unadjusted score because driving requires a certain level of function, regardless of age. Korner–Bitensky *et al.* (2000) attempted to replicate these findings in a multicentre retrospective study with 269 stroke patients. They found a positive predictive value of 61% and negative predictive value of 64%, which led them to conclude that the MVPT was not suitable as a screening tool to identify those who were not fit for an on-road assessment. They determined that lowering the cut-off to 25 or less improved the ability of the MVPT to detect people who would fail the road test to 74%, but this needs replication.

In a secondary analysis of data from a treatment trial involving 84 stroke patients, Mazer *et al.* (2003) found, using univariate logistic regression, that passing the on-road driving evaluation was significantly associated with various factors including MVPT score and MVPT time. However, no details of the relative contribution of the MVPT were provided. In all these studies the 1982 version of the test was used (Bouska & Kwatny, 1982), and since then a new version of the MVPT has been published (Colarusso & Hammill, 1996) which does not require the patient to work in the horizontal field. The response options are presented vertically on the page. This eliminates the sensitivity to visual neglect and therefore it is unlikely to be as predictive of driving performance as the original. This unfortunate revision means the MVPT is unlikely to be useful in clinical practice as the 1982 version is no longer easily available.

Stroke Drivers' Screening Assessment

Nouri and Lincoln (1987, 1992) developed the Stroke Drivers' Screening Assessment (SDSA) to screen people with stroke for referral for an on-road assessment. It comprises four tasks, Dot cancellation, Square Matrices Directions, Square Matrices Compass and Road Sign Recognition. In the validation studies (Nouri, Tinson & Lincoln, 1987; Nouri & Lincoln, 1992), stroke patients who wished to resume driving were assessed on a battery of cognitive tests which evaluated abilities thought to be relevant to driving. They then completed an on-road assessment with a driving instructor specialised in the assessment of disabled drivers. This was conducted blind to the results of the cognitive assessment. Discriminant function analysis was conducted on a random sample of 45 patients and validated on the remaining 34. This identified four tests, which correctly classified 82% of drivers in the initial sample and 79% in the validation sample. The weightings derived from these equations were used to provide a score to indicate the likelihood of passing the road test and a score to indicate the likelihood of failing the road test.

The discrepancy between these two scores is used as the basis for any recommendations about cognitive abilities needed for safe driving. The SDSA was shown to have some practice effects (Lincoln & Fanthome, 1994), but no patients improved from fail to pass categories as a result of practice. The predictive value of the SDSA was compared with existing assessment procedures in a randomised controlled trial (Nouri & Lincoln, 1993). The SDSA was significantly better than routine clinical assessments, involving advice from general practitioners and the DVLA, at identifying those who were found to be safe and unsafe to drive on the road (51% vs. 82% correctly classified). A validation study indicated that the SDSA is predominantly a measure of executive abilities (Radford & Lincoln, 2004).

This assessment was further evaluated by Lundberg *et al.* (2003) using a modified version of the SDSA taking into account driving on the right and differences in road signs between the United Kingdom and continental Europe. The Nordic SDSA (NorSDSA) was administered to 97 stroke patients who were also assessed on the road. The SDSA had a sensitivity of 70% and specificity 67% for predicting failing a road test. Lundberg *et al.* (2003) then conducted a discriminant function analysis on 49 stroke patients which was cross-validated on 48 patients. This correctly classified 74% of those who failed and 77% of those who passed giving an overall accuracy of 75%. The cross-validation showed poor sensitivity for failing (36%) but correctly identified all those who passed (100%) and had an overall accuracy of 78% of all patients. This illustrates the problem of deciding whether the aim is to identify safe or unsafe drivers. Lundberg *et al.* (2003) considered the original SDSA as inadequate because it classified some drivers (43 of 64) as likely to fail the road test when in fact they passed. However, if the screening test is to be used to decide who to refer for on-road assessment, these people would be subsequently be given the opportunity to demonstrate they were safe drivers. Missing unsafe drivers by classifying them as likely to be safe may present a more serious consequence. Lundberg *et al.* (2003) added a borderline category on the NorSDSA of -0.49 to $+0.49$, which they suggested could be used to indicate people who need an on-road assessment. Akinwuntan, De Weerdt, Feys, Baten, Arno and Kiekens (2005b) conducted a validation of the road assessment with 38 patients with first stroke. There was 79% agreement between results of a road test and the outcomes (pass/fail) of the SDSA. They suggested this relationship validates the use of on-road assessment but it could also be considered a validation of the SDSA. In addition, George and Crotty (2010) conducted a validation study with 43 stroke patients and found 75% accuracy for predicting road test performance (sensitivity 71%, specificity 78%, PPV 38%, NPV 93%). The test was better able to identify safe drivers than unsafe drivers. The predictive ability was improved by adopted the borderline value of -0.5 to $+0.5$ suggested by Lundberg *et al.* (2003). Although the SDSA was not as accurate as the UFOV test, it is more readily available in clinical settings. In addition, a meta-analysis of cognitive tests in relation to driving (Devos *et al.*, 2011) found that a cut-off of 8.5 points for Road Sign Recognition, 25 points for Square Matrices Compass, classified unsafe drivers with 84% and 85% accuracy respectively (Road Sign Recognition sensitivity for unsafe driving 84%, specificity 54%; compass sensitivity for unsafe driving 85%, specificity 54%) and the proportion of participants correctly predicted to pass the on-road assessment was high (83% and 84% respectively).

Sentinella, Sexton and Inwood (2005) checked the interrater reliability of the SDSA. Three people were videoed, one healthy participant and two stroke patients. One of these stroke patients had severe visual neglect and was therefore not the type of patients who would normally be assessed on the SDSA. Twenty-eight raters scored the videos and the intraclass correlations ranged between 0.88 and 1.00. One source of error was that 8/28 raters miscalculated the equations. The updated manual (Lincoln, Radford & Nouri, 2010) now provides a link to an Excel programme for calculating overall scores. There were some discrepancies in scoring which indicated the use of the test was not as indicated in manual. This has also been addressed in the revised manual by providing a link to a video showing the administration of the SDSA.

Rookwood Driving Battery

The Rookwood Driving Battery (RDB; McKenna, 2009) comprises a collection of 12 tests, to assess those cognitive skills which were considered critical to the ability to move a car in space and to negotiate traffic and road situations. The battery was developed from assessments that had been found useful at a specialist driving assessment centre (McKenna, Jefferies, Dobson & Frude, 2004). The RDB includes measures of visual perception, executive function, attention, praxis and comprehension. On each test patients are recorded as passing or failing the test on the basis of pre-defined cut-off scores. McKenna *et al.* (2004) analysed the results of a series of 142 patients, 62 with stroke, who were referred for assessment of fitness to drive. Using a cut-off score of 11 or more fails to indicate that patients would be predicted to fail the road test; it correctly identified 92% of unsafe drivers (71% sensitivity for passing road assessment, specificity 92%). However, the misclassification was mainly in elderly drivers and the battery was less good at detecting drivers 70 years and over who were safe on the road (sensitivity for passes 37% specificity 85%). As has been noted previously, the agreement between testing and on-road performance is also likely to be high since the assessments were not conducted blind to each other. In the original study, there was no analysis according to diagnosis; however, a replication study (McKenna & Bell, 2007) did analyse subgroups of patients according to diagnosis. They found the sensitivity for detecting fails in right hemisphere stroke patients was 44% and for left hemisphere stroke patients was 39%, although the specificity was much higher (96% for right hemisphere stroke patients and 93% for left hemisphere stroke patients; overall accuracy 77% for right hemisphere stroke patients and 78% for left hemisphere stroke patients).

As with previous research, the ability to detect safe drivers was greater than the ability to detect unsafe drivers.

Summary of screening measures

Cognitive abilities have been shown to be related to on-road driving ability, but the predictive validity of cognitive tests remains uncertain. The best validated test is the SDSA, but this is better at identifying those who are likely to be safe to drive than those who are likely to be unsafe. People who fail the SDSA therefore need to be tested on the road. The Rookwood Driving Battery seems promising but needs independent validation with the road test carried out blind to the results of the RDB. One of the problems with the validation studies is that the predictors identified will depend on what else has been assessed. A test which is predictive in a multiple regression analysis in one study may not be in another if different additional measures have been used. Many of the studies have been retrospective and decisions about driving ability have not been made blind to the results of cognitive assessment. The road assessment or overall team decision has been used as the as gold standard of driving ability, yet information on the accuracy of a single road test in relation to driving ability in daily life is lacking. Also few studies have considered the interrater reliability of the on-road assessor. Standards may vary between on road assessors, particularly those in different centres, and there may also be substantial differences in expected standards between countries. In practice the best use for cognitive screening tests is to determine when to recommend that stroke patients take the on-road assessment. Although it may be possible to identify some drivers who are not going to be safe to drive using cognitive tests, this needs to be done with caution, so as not to unfairly preclude anyone from driving who may be capable of resuming.

Driver retraining programmes

Given that a high proportion of patients are found unsafe to drive after stroke, it is reasonable to consider whether specific interventions could improve their chances of resuming driving. One strategy has been to retrain the specific cognitive deficits involved. For example, Mazer *et al.* (2003) randomised 84 stroke patients referred for driving evaluation to receive 20 sessions of either UFOV training or traditional computerized visual perception retraining. Outcome was assessed by an on-road driving evaluation, visual perception tests and the Test of Everyday Attention, administered by an occupational therapist blind to the intervention received. There were no significant differences between groups on any of the outcome measures, except that those who received training on the UFOV had significantly greater change in UFOV scores (38% vs. 13% reduction). Overall 39% of the UFOV trained group passed the road test as compared with 33% of the control group (p = 0.54). Subgroup analysis revealed that there was a doubling (52% vs. 29%) of the rate of success on the on-road driving evaluation after UFOV training in a subset of participants with right hemisphere lesions, but this was not statistically significant. The main finding was that training on the UFOV improved UFOV but not driving ability. Crotty and George (2009) evaluated training on the Dynavision Light Training board, a device to improve visual scanning and reaction times, in comparison with a waiting list control. They found no significant effects of treatment on either driving ability, scanning or response speed but the sample size was small (n = 26). However, more stroke patients passed the road test following training (n = 10, 77%) than in the waiting list control group (n = 6, 46%).

More encouraging results come from Akinwuntan, De Weerdt, Feys, Pauwels, Baten, Arno *et al.* (2005a) who randomly allocated 83 patients with first stroke to either simulator training or cognitive training for 15 hours over 5 weeks. Treatment was delivered by the same therapist. There was a significant difference in proportion allowed to resume driving; 73% simulator trained as compared with 42% who received cognitive retraining. However, there was a high drop-out rate and only 63% of those randomised were assessed on the road at six months after stroke. Follow-up of these patients five years later (Devos *et al.*, 2010) showed that the benefits of simulator training were maintained, although the difference between the simulator trained and the control group was no longer statistically significant. 60% in the simulator group were considered fit to drive compared to 48% in the control group (p = 0.36).

Given that generalisation of cognitive retraining is known to be a problem (see chapter 11), it would be worth evaluating whether driving lessons would improve patients' performance. Soderstrom *et al.* (2006) gave on-road training to 15 stroke patients who initially failed an on-road assessment. Thirteen of these subsequently passed the road test, but showed no significant improvement in cognitive abilities, suggesting that they learned specific driving skills and the improvement was not simply a result of spontaneous recovery. But the lack of a control group means it is unclear to what extent on road training itself led to the improvements in on-road ability.

Role of simulators

One problem with on-road driving assessment is that it is potentially risky. Therefore simulators have been considered to be useful to test driving behaviour in potentially dangerous situations (Patomella, Tham & Kottorp, 2006). Lundqvist *et al.* (2000) used an advanced simulator in which the participants drove 20 km in a countryside environment. The simulator driving outcome did not predict the on-road driving performance. There are problems with driving simulators in that they may cause motion sickness, cognitively impaired individuals do not respond well to being tested in a completely new environment and they are expensive. Less advanced driving simulators, based on the use of personal computers, have good face validity, but lack validation. Patomella *et al.* (2006) developed the Performance Analysis of Driving Ability (P-Drive), an interval scale measure of driving ability based on Rasch analysis, using an advanced simulator. P-Drive was used to score 101 stroke participants driving in the simulator. It was found to be a valid and stable assessment, but the clinical validity remains to be established in relation to on-road assessment. As the cost of simulators reduces and they become more similar to on-road ability, they have the potential to be used in specialist assessment centres, but the need for screening people prior to referral for specialist assessment will remain.

Recommendations for clinical practice

The use of cognitive assessment in clinical practice is illustrated in Table 8.2, and a suggested care pathway in Figure 8.2.

Patients should be reviewed by members of the multidisciplinary team a month after stroke to determine whether they may wish to return to driving or not. Those who do not plan to return to driving should be reviewed again about three months after discharge from hospital to check they have not changed their views. The reason for this delay is that some people do not anticipate wanting to drive again but after discharge home they change their minds.

Those who wish to drive should be formally assessed by the multidisciplinary team. The first consideration is whether there are medical factors which preclude the patient from driving, such as epilepsy. Visual fields and visual inattention should then be assessed. Driving is not allowed if there is a reduction in visual fields less than 120° on the horizontal. Visual inattention may be assessed using a standardised measure, such as the BIT Star Cancellation. If the patient has adequate vision and no medical contraindications, their cognitive abilities should be assessed. The Rey figure copy and Trail Making tests can be used to indicate people who are unlikely to be safe to drive. The Stroke Drivers' Screening Assessment gives clear guidelines about the score required before patients are likely to be able to drive. If patients pass the SDSA, that is, score more than 0.5 on the discrepancy between the pass and fail equations (i.e. pass equation − fail equation), their motor abilities should be considered. If there are mild motor impairments which do not affect driving safety, the patient should be allowed to resume driving. If they have more marked physical disabilities, then patients should be referred to a specialist driving assessment centre for advice on car adaptations. Patients with borderline scores on the SDSA (-0.5 to $+0.5$) should be referred to a specialist driving assessment centre. For those with fail scores (less than -0.5) or who have mild visual field deficits which may recover, the

Table 8.2 Case Example of a Driving Assessment

David was a 58-year-old man with a partial anterior circulation syndrome stroke due to a left middle cerebral artery infarction. He presented with a right-sided hemiplegia, but was able to walk independently with a stick. He reported difficulties with speech, forgetfulness, fatigue and impulsivity. He was independent in most activities of daily living but his partner had taken over managing the finances. He reported that he was currently driving his car short distances in his local neighbourhood with the support of his wife. He could not recall that he had been given any advice about resuming driving. His goals were to return to driving to the extent that he did before his stroke and to return to work as a flour miller.

David's score on the Beck Depression Inventory was suggestive of severe depression. He also reported experiencing high levels of frustration and frequent anger outbursts. David reported that these anger outbursts felt relatively uncontrollable; although he was confident he could stop himself from hitting others and regretted his outbursts afterwards. Formal cognitive testing was carried out using the Weschler Adult Intelligence Scale–Third edition (WAIS-III), Wechsler Memory Scale (WMS-III), Delis Kaplan Executive Function system (DKEFS), Hayling and Brixton tests and Test of Everyday Attention.

He performed mainly at average level consistent with his probable premorbid level of function. His speed of information processing and working memory were low average (below 25th percentile). On the Wechsler Memory Scale (WMS-III) his ability to recall verbal information after immediate and delayed presentations was also low average. He was impaired on the DKEFS verbal fluency, Trails B and Stroop tests, indicating impairment of executive abilities. There was evidence of impaired attention on the Test of Everyday Attention. These findings led to concern about his safety to drive a car. He was therefore assessed on the Stroke Drivers' Screening Assessment. The overall predictive equation score was 0.3, which is borderline and just in the range of scores of those found safe to drive. He was advised to notify the DVLA of his stroke and was referred for assessment at a Regional Mobility centre. On road assessment identified that DB was safe to drive, although instances of impulsive behaviour were noted. It was felt that these were not sufficient to compromise safety and the recommendation made to the DVLA was that he was fit to drive. His mood improved over this time and he was making plans for returning to work.

Although standard cognitive tests highlighted potential problems with driving, inclusion of the SDSA provided a basis for deciding whether a road test was needed. In some centres where road tests are easily available this stage might not have been necessary, but many centres do not have easy access to specialist on-road assessment.

advice should be to wait for a further three months and then to review their abilities again. Those who fail the SDSA a second time should be advised that their cognitive impairments are such that they are unlikely to be safe to drive.

The Rookwood Driving Battery may be administered as an alternative to the SDSA. However, it should be born in mind that many of the Mobility Assessment centres will use the RDB as part of their assessment procedures and care needs to be taken to avoid duplication of assessments. Although cognitive testing

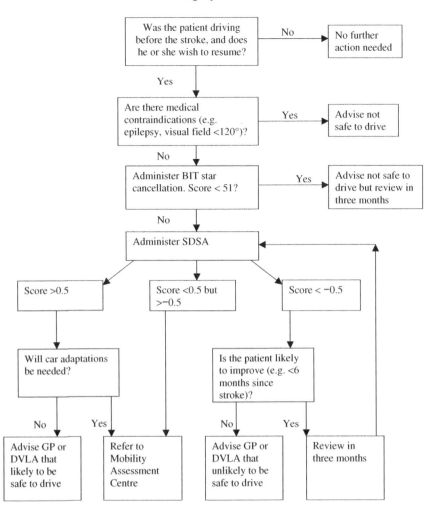

Figure 8.2 Care pathway for initial consideration of fitness to drive.

is likely to be informative, other factors need to be taken into account. Drivers with high level previous driving skills, such as advanced, professional drivers, may be more able to cope with cognitive decline (Lundberg *et al.*, 2003) than those without. Therefore even if these people fail the cognitive tests, they may need to be assessed on the road. Similarly, if a patient is highly distressed by the recommendation that they are not allowed to drive based on cognitive tests, it may be appropriate to refer them to a driving assessment centre, which includes assessment of the road. Used in this way, the cognitive test result may help prepare the patient for the outcome of the road test and provide corroborating evidence to help them accept a negative outcome. In the United Kingdom, the decision about safety to drive rests with the DVLA and the DVLA will contact the patients' GP for an opinion. The GP and consultant should therefore be notified of the results of all assessments in order that they can incorporate these into their recommendations to the driving authorities.

Conclusions

All stroke patients who were driving before their stroke should be advised of the legal requirements for resuming driving and the options available to them should be discussed. For those who wish to resume driving a formal assessment of their potential fitness to drive should be carried out. This assessment will include consideration of relevant medical factors, visual ability, motor function and cognitive impairments. For some patients this will be sufficient to indicate whether they are safe or unsafe to resume driving, and they and the DVLA can be advised accordingly. If there is uncertainty on the basis of the formal evaluation, referral to a specialist driving assessment centre is recommended.

Chapter 9

Decision Making and Mental Capacity

Introduction

There have been few studies of decision making about treatment or discharge in people affected by stroke; much of the research in the area is concerned with mental illness and dementia. This is both surprising and unfortunate since stroke, unlike dementia and other progressive neurological conditions, creates a situation for which most are unprepared, and, unlike many other sudden onset-physical conditions, it often impairs cognitive processes that underpin decision making (Nys, van Zandvoort, de Kort, Jansen, de Haan & Kappelle, 2007). This chapter will consider the legal framework and general literature relevant to decision making in healthcare. Implications for stroke will be considered and stroke-specific research will be included where available. Mental capacity legislation around the world shares many common elements, and its provisions within several jurisdictions will be considered, but the most detailed consideration will be given to the Mental Capacity Act (England and Wales) (2005) (Her Majesty's Government, 2005) and the associated deprivation of liberty statutes contained in the amended Mental Health Act (2007) (Her Majesty's Government, 2007b). The aim is not to provide a concise guide to mental capacity law and practice, since several such guides already exist (Appelbaum, 2007; General Medical Council, 2008; Hardy & Joyce, 2009; Johnston & Liddle, 2007; Joyce, 2008). Instead, the chapter will outline and discuss the principal issues surrounding decision making and mental capacity legislation, with particular reference to stroke.

Decision making

Decision making is an act of judgement that occurs when a person is presented with a choice between two or more alternatives. To make a decision the person must be capable of mental processing that enables them to:

Psychological Management of Stroke, First Edition. Nadina B. Lincoln, Ian I. Kneebone, Jamie A.B. Macniven and Reg C. Morris.
© 2012 John Wiley & Sons, Ltd. Published 2012 by John Wiley & Sons, Ltd.

- assimilate information to enable them to comprehend the circumstances and context of the decision,
- be aware that a decision is possible,
- be motivated to make a decision (even if the decision is not to act),
- understand that at least two alternative choices are available,
- retain the relevant information, and
- consider the possible outcomes of the choices in relation to their individual circumstances.

If a decision requires the cooperation of others, as in most healthcare settings, then the person must also be able to communicate the outcome of their decision. Finally, a person must be able to hold the decision and not change it so frequently that it cannot be enacted.

Legal definitions

In most jurisdictions, there is a presumption that a person has capacity unless it is proven otherwise (Wong, Clare, Gunn & Holland, 1999), and the abilities described above are reflected in the legally prescribed tests of decision making competence used to determine if an individual lacks capacity (see Table 9.1).

In common with most other jurisdictions, both these tests of capacity are *functional* and hinge on whether a person is able to meet the demands presented by a particular decision. They do not depend on diagnosis, deficits in specific cognitive processes or the potential outcome of a decision (Bellhouse, Holland, Clare & Gunn, 2001; Wong *et al.*, 1999). This approach has major

Table 9.1 Elements of the Legal Definition of Decision Making in Two Jurisdictions

Mental Capacity Act 2005 (England and Wales)	*United States (Grisso & Appelbaum, 1998; based upon Section 1(3), of the Uniform Health-Care Decisions Act (National Conference of Commissioners on Uniform State Laws, 1993)*
Understand the information relevant to the decision.	Comprehend the information relevant to the decision.
Retain that information (for as long as necessary to make a decision).	
Use or weight the information in reaching a decision.	Appreciate the significance of the information and outcome for one's own situation.
	Process the information (reason about it) so as to compare and weigh outcomes. *(This requires and implies retention.)*
Communicate the decision.	Express a choice.

implications for the assessment of mental capacity since, construed in this way, capacity is context and time specific and may be enhanced by supportive interventions. Assessments must reflect this by being anchored to particular contexts and times (and therefore may require repeating), and by including education about pertinent facts and issues and aids to decision making where necessary. Another implication of the functional approach is that a *valid* decision requires only that a person possesses all the prerequisite functional abilities in Table 9.1. The outcome of the decision in terms of its 'riskiness', 'reasonableness', 'normality' or 'wisdom' should not influence the judgement about capacity.

The functional approach requires patients to demonstrate a higher standard of ability to meet the demands of more complex decisions, but it does not raise the threshold to reflect the potential risks, seriousness or permanence of the consequences of a decision. The absence of any adjustment for seriousness has led some to propose a 'sliding scale' (Roth, Meisel & Lidz, 1977) where a person would be required to demonstrate a higher level of functioning for a more serious decision. However, this approach leads to an asymmetry that could deprive patients of their autonomy (Berghmans, Dickenson & Ter Meulen, 2004). For example, where the risk of having no treatment is higher than that of having the treatment, a practitioner could deem that a person's level of functioning was insufficient to allow them to refuse the treatment (high risk) but sufficient to allow them to accept the treatment (low risk).

In legal parlance the ability to make a decision about a particular matter is usually referred to as 'capacity' in the United Kingdom, and the lack of such ability as 'incapacity'. In the United States and elsewhere, the term 'competence' is sometimes used in place of capacity; alternatively, 'competence' may be used to denote a legal decision and distinguish it from a clinical judgement of capacity. However, the legal terminology differs between jurisdictions, and there is a lack of consistency in the way these terms are used that can lead to confusion (Bielby, 2005).

In most jurisdictions the legal definition of incapacity includes a 'dual test'; there must be an inability to make a decision combined with an abnormality of mind or brain. The inability to make a decision by itself is not sufficient, and the dual test properly excludes instances of prevarication and vacillation in unimpaired people.

Cognition and decision making

As expected, decision making ability is associated with the size of the stroke lesion (Dani, McCormick & Muir, 2008), and in nonstroke patients components of decision making capacity have been shown to correlate with measures of cognitive abilities including executive functions, memory, comprehension, verbal fluency, mental flexibility, visual and auditory attention and conceptualization (Gurrera, Moye, Karel, Azar & Armesto, 2006; Marson, Chatterjee, Ingram & Harrell, 1996; Moye & Marson, 2007; Okonkwo, Griffith, Belue, Lanza, Zamrini, Harrell *et al.*, 2007). The association with executive functions is especially strong (Dymek, Atchison, Harrell & Marson, 2001). However, decision making ability is multifaceted and context bound, and neither global nor specific measures of cognitive functioning accurately predict decision making capacity for particular decisions (Freedman, Stuss & Gordon, 1991; Murphy & Clare, 2003). A study of 34 stroke patients (Mackenzie, Lincoln & Newby, 2008) illustrated this by demonstrating a lack of association between capacity and cognitive performance measured by a battery of nine tests chosen for sensitivity to cognitive deficits following stroke. Similarly, Vollmann, Kühl, Tilmann, Hartung and Helmchen (2004) found no significant association between neuropsychological test scores of dementia patients and a standard measure of capacity, the MacArthur Competence Assessment Tool–Treatment (MacCAT-T).

Emotion and decision making

The importance of emotional, noncognitive factors in decision making has been noted by several authors (Breden & Vollmann, 2004; Charland, 1998; Owen, Freyenhagen, Richardson & Hotopf, 2009; Vellinga, Smit, van Leeuwen, van Tilburg & Jonker, 2004). Unfortunately, these allusions to the importance of emotional factors in health decision making have not been translated into empirical research. However, clinical experience furnishes several examples of ways in which emotional factors manifest themselves in decision making. For example, it is common to encounter people who do not acknowledge their situation and fail to appreciate that a decision is required. This may be a consequence of the neurological symptom of *anosognosia*, or blindness to impairments. Alternatively, it may be a consequence of the psychological defence mechanism of 'denial', triggered by the trauma of the stroke. In addition, about one third of stroke patients experience depression (Hackett & Anderson, 2005). Since depression distorts reality by exaggerating negative views of a person, their circumstances and their future, it is very likely to impact on a patients' decision making.

Charland (1998) was particularly critical of exclusively cognitive analyses of mental capacity and proposed that emotion is integral to the appraisal of the personal significance of choices, which in turn is a crucial aspect of the appreciation component of capacity (the ability to relate information and consequences to one's own personal situation). He pointed to the occurrence of emotions such as fear, helplessness and embarrassment in healthcare contexts, and their likely impact on choices. However, others have argued that, despite the likely involvement of emotions in decision making, there may be little to be gained by including emotions in the standards for the assessment of capacity (Appelbaum, 1998).

Shared decision making in healthcare

There are a number of domains in which decision making ability is important following stroke, such as the destination after discharge, treatment consent, management of finance, research consent, driving, sexual consent and end of life. For example, immediately following stroke there may be a need to obtain consent for thrombolysis (Akinsanya, Diggory, Heitz & Jones, 2009; White-Bateman, Schumacher, Sacco & Appelbaum, 2007), and at a later stage there may be treatment decisions about artificial hydration, artificial feeding and placement or palliative care.

Ideally, decisions should be taken collaboratively and jointly by the patient and the professional(s). The nature and principles of joint or shared decision making were articulated by Charles, Gafni and Whelan (1997) as involving at least two parties (patient and staff), all parties participating actively, information being shared, and the parties agreeing to the decision. The inclusion of patients (and their carers where appropriate) in decision making has the potential for psychological benefit, and it has been shown to increase sense of agency and control and to promote satisfaction, well-being and physical health (Kunzmann, Little & Smith, 2002; Rodin, 1986). Moreover, Kitwood and Bredin (1992) identified decision making, the 'assertion of desire or will', as one of the 12 indicators of well-being in people with cognitive impairments.

Studies of shared decision making frequently have conceptual and methodological weakness, and evaluations of its efficacy have been mixed (Guadagnoli & Ward, 1998). However, a review by Adams and Drake (2006) concluded that receiving the information required for shared decision making reduced distress and improved functioning; high involvement in decision making improved health outcome, while low involvement increased illness burden. Satisfaction with healthcare was found to increase with shared decision making in some (but not all) of the reviewed studies, and patient involvement in decisions reduced costs by limiting the selection of ineffective treatments. Shared decision making has strong proponents (Elwyn, 2006) who combine ethical and humanitarian arguments with reference to evidence for its efficacy, and the Department of Health (2007b) espoused the shared decision making approach as a preferred method.

Limitations of shared decision making

Despite its advantages, shared decision making has not been universally embraced; Meade (1999) reviewed six studies of cancer treatment that demonstrated some patients did not wish to be actively involved in decision making about their own care. More recent research has echoed this finding (Belcher, Fried, Agostini & Tinetti, 2006; Myron, Gillespie, Swift & William-son, 2008), and the desire to be involved in decision making has been shown to depend on demographic factors, such as age, education, gender, experiences with professionals, diagnosis and type of decision (Say, Murtagh & Thomson,

2006). It seems that patients' view of shared decision making range from feeling 'demeaned, mad, furious, dehumanised, and patronised' when not involved in decisions (Myron *et al.*, 2008) to feeling extremely anxious and uncomfortable when asked to participate in decision making. Clearly, the wishes of patients who request that others make treatment decisions on their behalf should be respected, and this is the recommendation of the General Medical Council (2008). Another area of concern is that patients may make decisions that are incompatible with their own objectives and preferences due to cognitive biases in decision making processes. This may be exacerbated when there are multiple options (Ubel, 2002). Reasons for such errors include the effects short-term emotional reactions to diagnosis, such as denial or anxiety, cognitive errors and the misinterpretation of statistical information about the probability of risks. It is salutary that statistical misinterpretations have been shown to occur in the majority of the population (Schwartz, Woloshin, Black & Welch, 1997). Finally some decisions, like driving (see chapter 8), are governed by legal stipulations that are not conducive to shared decision making in the normal sense.

A fascinating illustration of the considerations discussed above is provided by the case of Mr. Akinsanya, a barrister, who suffered a progressive stroke while remaining alert and conscious. He subsequently recorded and published his experiences (Akinsanya, Diggory, Heitz & Jones, 2009). Mr. Akinsanya was judged as suitable for thrombolysis and was offered the treatment. He initially refused, and his narrative explained the reasons for refusal as not understanding the statistics about benefits and risks, mistakenly believing that thrombolysis treatment was a form of brain surgery, not being able to concentrate on what was being said due to emotional turmoil, preoccupation with contacting work colleagues and difficulty in speaking. He concluded that he lacked capacity to consent and 'it is difficult to see how a patient in my situation could be expected to have the capacity to consent to treatment when going through such emotional turmoil.' The stroke doctors who treated him suggested that the refusal of a beneficial treatment, such as thrombolysis, without a 'long-held or logical reason' is in itself grounds for doubting capacity and for taking the decision for the patient in their 'best interests'. This matter is discussed further in the section on 'best interests' below.

Impaired decision making: mental capacity in health care

Decision making ability, or mental capacity, is defined in the Mental Capacity Act 2005 (England & Wales) with regard to the four elements in the left-hand column of Table 9.1.

In healthcare settings, decision making capacity often becomes relevant when a person needs to make a decision about accepting a treatment or placement. The absence of capacity precludes shared decision making and the advantages that it brings. Even more important, lack of capacity prevents a person from providing informed consent. Since there is a legal requirement that adults must always give consent for treatment or assessment, situations in which people need interventions for which they lack the capacity to consent are particularly problematic. Special legislation is required to deal with this eventuality and protect those who lack capacity and those who act on their behalf without consent. Examples of such legislation are the Uniform Health-Care Decisions Act (National Conference of Commissioners on Uniform State Laws, 1993), the Mental Capacity Act, 2005 (England and Wales) and the Adults with Incapacity Act (Scotland) 2000 (The Scottish Government, 2000). These acts emphasise the principle of personal autonomy, so that a person is presumed capable of a decision until positively shown to be incapable. In their adherence to the principle of personal autonomy, these acts were based on Western philosophical thinking (Owen *et al.*, 2009), but this perspective runs counter to cultural values that endorse collective decision making (Blackhall, Murphy, Frank, Michel & Azen, 1995; Hanssen, 2005), and this may account for the low uptake of some of the acts' provisions in some ethnic groups (see below).

Assessment of mental capacity

Legally and formally, the assessment of mental capacity requires us to establish that a person has the capabilities outlined in Table 9.1 with regard to a specific decision. The assessment is decision specific and time specific, and is typically in the form of a semistructured interview that examines each element of capacity in turn and records a judgement of the probability that the person can perform each function. A proforma of the type often used in practice is included in Tables 9.2 and 9.3. While such assessments are objectively and transparently recorded, and the rationale for decisions is provided, they are nevertheless based on the subjective judgement of practitioners, and the complex nature of capacity renders assessment challenging (Raymont, Buchanan, David, Hayward, Wessely & Hotopf, 2007). Studies of consistency and agreement between the capacity assessments of practitioners produce a mixed picture. Marson, McInturff, Hawkins, Bartolucci and Harrell (1997) found only near-chance agreement (56%) in the competency assessments of five physicians for 29 patients with mild Alzheimer's disease. There were large differences in stringency of judgement (90% to 0% judged incompetent), and the physicians used different cognitive models in their assessments. Fassassi, Bianchi, Stiefel and Waeber (2009) found that specificity for the detection of capacity (the number of patients identified as lacking capacity as a percentage of all those who actually lacked capacity) was 96.5% for judgements made by a senior physician compared with those of a psychiatrist, but the sensitivity (the number identified as having capacity as a proportion of who actually had capacity) was only 57.1%. The sensitivity and specificity cited here are for detection of capacity (positive outcome) and lack of capacity is the negative outcome (Fassassi, personal communication, 2010).

Table 9.2 Stages in the Assessment of Capacity

ASSESSMENT OF CAPACITY

(There is no single method; the method used should suit circumstances.)

STAGES

Trigger: Ascertain validity of the reason for the assessment.
Engagement: Obtain assent to assessment.
Information gathering: About triggers, context, options and consequences.
Education of client: Reasons for assessment, options and consequences.
Assessment: Client's understanding of situation, and their ability to
  • comprehend information
  • remember
  • deliberate and make choices,
  • understand consequences,
  • communicate decision, and
  • maintain decision for a reasonable period.

Action:
1) Person deemed competent: no action, follow their wishes.
2) Person not competent: make best-interests decision or appoint substitute decision maker.

In other words, the physician rarely said someone had capacity when the psychiatrist judged they did not (false positive), but frequently said a person lacked capacity when the psychiatrist said they did in fact possess it (false negative). The agreement with the psychiatric assessment for other members of the healthcare team was even lower. Another problem is that physicians appear to hold different cognitive models about the cognitive functions that are important for capacity. Earnst, Marson and Harrell (2000) found that physicians based their judgements on one or two specific functions, and that the functions differed between physicians. Agreement rates also depend on the nature of the patient sample, and Raymont *et al.* (2007) found 78.5% agreement between practitioners using a heterogeneous sample of 40 consecutively admitted acute general medical patients. This agreement rate is much higher than the near-chance agreement for Alzheimer's patients reported by Marson *et al.* (1997). As well as the patient sample, agreement also depends on staff knowledge and skill, and has been shown to improve with training (Marson, Earnst, Jamil, Bartolucci & Harrell, 2000). Sullivan (2004) reviewed studies of capacity assessment and noted a number of additional difficulties with assessment by healthcare staff. Individual practitioner's assessments showed a lack of agreement with assessments made by multidisciplinary teams, assessment methods used by different physicians were varied and inconsistent and staff assessments were not concordant with standardised assessments. Problems in the assessment of the capacity of stroke patients for making decisions about discharge have also been reported; members of multidisciplinary rehabilitation teams were uncertain about the capacity of around one third of patients on average, and the uncertainly was most

Table 9.3   Example of a Capacity Assessment Form

CAPACITY ASSESSMENT	Date: / /

Name: _____ Dob:_____

Address:_____

Assessment requested by;_____

Reason/trigger for assessment. (Is it valid?)	
Area/target of assessment (the decision that is required).	
Options and choices. (List the alternatives.)	
Consequences; risks and benefits. (What outcomes are associated with each alternative?)	

Function	Clearly able	Probably able	Possibly able	Probably not able	Clearly not able
Able to assimilate and retain relevant information.					
Able to understand problem and context.					
Able to understand choices.					
Able to appreciate consequences.					
Able to relate consequences to own situation and goals.					
Able to express or communicate decision.					

Table 9.3   (*Continued*)

<u>**Methods Used**</u>

Method	Yes	No
Paraphrasing information		
Recalling information		
Describing consequences		
Comparing alternatives provided or self-generated		
Appreciating application to own circumstances		
Communications aids (e.g. drawing, communication book)		

<u>**Decision**</u>

<u>**Comments**</u>

marked for those who were judged to lack capacity by a neuropsychologist (Mackenzie *et al.*, 2008).

In view of the problems with assessment of capacity by staff, it is hardly surprising that attempts have been made to develop standardised procedures and forms to assess capacity. Sullivan (2004) reviews and critiques several such approaches. Some of these are outlined in Table 9.4, which describes five

Table 9.4   Approaches to the Standardised Assessment of Mental Capacity

Approach	*Examples*
General cognitive tests	MMSE (Folstein, Folstein & McHugh 1975); Wechsler series of tests (e.g. WAIS-IV)
Standard neuropsychological tests	Auditory Verbal learning, Controlled Oral Word Association Test, Dementia Rating Scale, Trail Making Test, Wisconsin Card Sorting Test, Wechsler Memory Scale-IV
Independent Living Tests, using realistic materials	Everyday Problem Test (Willis, 1996), Independent Living Scale (Loeb, 1996)
Specific capacity assessment instruments	MacArthur Competence Assessment Tool-Treatment (Grisso *et al.*, 1997)
Vignette-based assessments in which an imaginary situation is presented for the patient to consider	For example, Marson, Cody, Ingram, and Harrell (1995a), and Marson, Ingram, Cody, and Harrell (1995b)

approaches to capacity assessments with examples of each one. The first approach relies on tests of general cognitive functions to determine capacity, the second uses more detailed and specific neuropsychological tests, the third employs realistic materials to assess capacity to make every-day decisions, the fourth approach uses purpose-designed tests of capacity tailored to particular situations and the final approach uses standard vignettes to assess judgement and decision making. Each approach is discussed in more detail below.

General cognitive ability, as measured by the MMSE, has been shown to be associated with capacity in some samples (Pachet, Astner & Brown, 2009; Raymont *et al.*, 2007), and it was noted above that specific cognitive abilities including conceptualisation, semantic memory, attention, verbal recall and word fluency have also been found to be associated with aspects of capacity (Moye & Marson, 2007). However, this association has not been found in stroke patients (Mackenzie *et al.*, 2008), and, depending on the cut-off score used, either the specificity or sensitivity of the MMSE to detect general medical patients who lack capacity has been shown to be poor (Fassassi *et al.*, 2009; Pachet *et al.*, 2009, respectively). Sullivan (2004) noted that the use of neuropsychological tests was frequently recommended when assessing capacity. However, Gurrera *et al.* (2006) demonstrated that the relationship between neuropsychological scores and capacity was complex, and the power of neuropsychological scores to predict capacity varied across the individual components of capacity; understanding (77.8%), reasoning (39.4%), appreciation (24.6%) and expression of choice (10.2%).

There are, moreover, *a priori* grounds to believe that both general and specific cognitive tests alone are unsuited as measures of capacity. First, cognitive and neuropsychological tests were not designed to assess capacity; they do not give specific information about the decision that is the focus of the assessment and most assess fundamental cognitive and perceptual abilities, and not decision making itself. Many tests are lengthy and make much greater demands on a person's attention span than the particular decision for which capacity is being assessed; therefore they set a higher threshold than necessary. Tests also lack material of personal significance to the person, which may further undermine attention and concentration. Finally, the abstract content of these tests is less salient for the person than the personally significant facts and issues surrounding the 'real-life' decision, and therefore the test materials are less likely to be remembered.

Independent living tests such as the Every Day Problem Test (Willis, 1996) use realistic, every-day scenarios, and have good face validity. They assess relevant skills and may yield information relevant to capacity (Sullivan, 2004). But this approach has been sparsely evaluated, and its relevance to capacity for specific decisions about living arrangements after discharge is complex and depends on other, unassessed, individual and contextual factors. These unassessed factors include whether the person would benefit from cognitive rehabilitation, and what support is available to assist their decision making. Vignette-based approaches to capacity assessment may use an imaginary case in which a decision is required. The participant is then interviewed about the vignette to assess whether they can demonstrate the various competencies essential for capacity (understanding, memory, appreciation, expression, etc.). This approach has not been widely evaluated, and what research there is has shown low agreement with other methods of assessment (Sullivan, 2004).

There has been more research into purpose-designed assessments of capacity to consent to treatment (or research) such as the MacArthur Assessment Tool–Treatment (Mac-CAT-T), and there are several reviews, (Dunn, Nowrangi, Palmer, Jeste & Saks, 2006; Sturman, 2005; Sullivan, 2004; Vellinga *et al.*, 2004). The instruments developed may be useful decision aids, and their strength is that they assess the components of capacity included in the legal definition. This makes them specific to given jurisdictions, though the similarity in legislation across different countries (see Table 9.1) affords a degree of generality. Some studies have found that these tests agree well with expert judgements (Bean, Nishisato, Rector & Glancy *et al.*, 1994; Kim, Caine, Currier, Leibovici & Ryan, 2001; Roth, Lidz, Meisel, Soloff, Kaufman, Spiker *et al.*, 1982), but others have found poor agreement (Fassassi *et al.*, 2009), and agreement depends on the domain being assessed (Moye & Marson, 2007).

The Mac-CAT-T will serve to illustrate the nature of these instruments. This uses a semistructured interview lasting 15–30 minutes examining the areas of understanding, appreciation, reasoning and expression of choice. The clinician selects relevant personal information about the patient's condition and discloses it to the patient along with information about treatment options and risks. Throughout the interview, the clinician probes to ascertain understanding, appreciation and reasoning. The interview ends with the patient making a choice. Grisso, Appelbaum and Hill-Fotouhi (1997) claimed it was easy to use this system in a mental health setting; it produced high interrater agreement, gave good discrimination between hospitalised patients and community living people and correlated well with symptom severity. Raymont *et al.* (2007) also reported good interrater reliability for the assessment of capacity in acute general medical patients. In this study transcripts of interviews with patients based on the Mac-CAT-T and one other instrument were rated by five clinicians. They demonstrated high interrater consistency in judgements about whether patients had capacity. The Mac-CAT-T represents something of a 'gold-standard'; it has been tested with more populations than other instruments (Sturman, 2005) and has greater empirical validation than any other similar assessments (Dunn *et al.*, 2006). However, its reliability across a range of conditions has not been fully established. It has also been criticised for being too cognitively oriented, and for neglecting emotional aspects of decision making (Breden & Vollmann, 2004). Finally, the Mac-CAT-T was designed specifically for treatment decisions, and alternative, less well-validated tests, such as the Independent Living Scale (Loeb, 1996), would have to be used for decisions about placement.

It is frequently necessary for professionals to work multiprofessionally when assessing mental capacity. Medical practitioners have a detailed knowledge of the physical risks and benefits of the various treatment options, but may lack specific skills in assessing decision making. For example, where language comprehension or expression is affected, the Mental Capacity Act 2005 recommends the involvement of a speech and language therapist. If cognitive processing or motivation is affected, a clinical psychologist may be able to facilitate decision making. Similarly, decisions about placement after discharge may require the involvement of a social worker working with a speech and language therapist or a psychologist.

A case example is shown in Table 9.5. The case example illustrates that a standardised cognitive screening test (the MMSE), may supplement the assessment of capacity but cannot be the final arbiter of capacity for a particular decision due to the complex and contextual nature of capacity assessment and the limited range of attributes assessed by such tests (Kapp & Mossman, 1996; Moye & Marson, 2007; Pachet *et al.*, 2009; Rutman & Silberfeld, 1992; Vellinga *et al.*, 2004).

Approaches to managing mental incapacity

Patients who lack capacity present serious and frequent difficulties for healthcare practitioners. Moye and Marson (2007) reviewed seven studies demonstrating that rates of incapacity for treatment decisions for older adults in long-term care (in hospitals or nursing homes) ranged between 44% and 69%. In the United Kingdom, Raymont *et al.* (2004) found that 40% of general non-elective acute hospital inpatients did not have the capacity to make decisions, and this rate corresponded closely with the 37% rate found in a Canadian study of general medical patients (Etchells, Darzins, Silberfeld, Singer, McKenny, Naglie *et al.*, 1999). However, a markedly lower rate of 26.7% was reported by Fassassi *et al.* (2009) in a general medical ward in Switzerland. Sugarman, McCrory and Hubal (1998) reviewed 99 studies of consent to treatment in older people and found that age and lower educational standards were commonly associated with impaired ability to consent. Since stroke often causes cognitive impairment (Nys *et al.*, 2007), and occurs most often in older people, the rate of incapacity amongst acute stroke patients may be even higher than that found in the studies above.

When a person lacks the capacity for decisions about their own healthcare, others must usually step in to make the decision for them. This presents a dilemma between the ethical principle of 'personal autonomy' and the principle of 'protection' or 'beneficence'. In order to protect or benefit a person's health, it may be necessary to intervene without their consent, or even in some case without their knowledge. In these circumstances there are three broad strategies available to healthcare staff (see below), and each one was included in the

Table 9.5   Case Example of a Capacity Assessment

Mary was 83, lived in a bungalow in a complex with a warden, and her son and daughter lived nearby. Six weeks prior to her referral to psychology, a blood clot lodged in an artery in the right frontal lobe of her brain causing a stroke, and she became weak down her left side and unable to walk or stand. She made a moderately good recovery; she became fully continent, and could stand and transfer from bed to chair or onto a toilet with a little help, but she could not walk steadily or safely without assistance. Her MMSE score was 18, indicating marked cognitive impairment, and talking with her and examining her MMSE results showed that her orientation to the present and short-term memory for events, pictures and words were very poor. Her son and daughter requested that she be discharged to a nursing home, since they felt she would constantly call on their help if she were to go back to her bungalow. A semistructured interview was employed to assess capacity using the format described in Table 9.3. Her clinical notes were reviewed in advance and the relatives were consulted. During the interview repetition and examples were used to enhance understanding, and prompts for concrete instances were given when responses were vague or nonspecific (e.g. Mary: 'I want to go home'. Therapist: 'Why is that?' Mary: 'I just know I will be happy there'. Therapist: 'Exactly what will make you happy about being at home, tell me three things'). Mary was adamant that she wanted to go back to her bungalow, and appreciated that she needed support and was happy to accept four carer visits each day. She was aware of the context of the decision, the options and the principal risks. She could even articulate (reluctantly) one or two advantages of going to a care home. She could retain the basic facts about the decision and its consequences (indeed she spent much time worrying about the outcome). She was aware of her preferences and remembered vividly that since her husband died 20 years ago she preferred her own company, and had not enjoyed mixing with others. She was able to determine that this preference would be better met by living at home than in a care home. Therefore, she concluded that she would be less content in a care home. The preserved knowledge about her preference for living alone was what Dubler (1985) referred to as a 'sedimented life preference', which, together with a person's maintained value system, should be carefully considered in reaching capacity decisions. Mary's family would have preferred the stroke unit staff to have found that she lacked capacity and discharged her to a nursing home 'in her best interests'. They pointed to her poor memory and possible Alzheimer's disease as the reason for her lack of capacity. However, in terms of the Mental Capacity Act 2005 she had all the attributes necessary for a valid decision. Consequently, she was able to choose her own preferred discharge destination. The family eventually accepted this outcome, and realised that the only route to changing the discharge plan was to persuade her to accept an alternative option.

Mental Capacity Act 2005 (England and Wales), the Adults with Incapacity Act (Scotland) 2000 and the Uniform Healthcare Decisions Act (United States) 1993. The sections below are necessarily brief, and fuller information about the specific provisions of the Mental Capacity Act 2005 (England and Wales) may be found in Hardy and Joyce (2009) and in Johnston and Liddle (2007), and detailed guidance, with case examples, is available in the relevant code of practice (Department for Constitutional Affairs, 2007).

Before discussing particular strategies for managing people who lack capacity, two specific features of the Mental Capacity Act 2005 (England and Wales) should be noted. The first is that it introduced sanctions for those who neglect or mistreat people without capacity, by creating an offence that carries up to five years in prison. The second is that it established an Independent Mental Capacity Advocacy (IMCA) service which must be consulted when serious decision are taken on behalf of people who lack capacity and have no relatives or friends to consult about the options. The IMCA provision provides an important independent check on whether staff abide by the act, and in practice it is a valuable resource that may be consulted about difficult decisions, even in cases where the person has relatives or friends.

Advance directives (living wills)

One option for making decisions on behalf of a person without capacity is to do what the person would have decided if they had capacity. However, the relevant information about a person's past wishes may not be easy to access or to interpret in the current situation. In view of this, the Mental Capacity Act 2005 (England and Wales) has endeavoured to enable people without capacity to influence future decisions about their care through 'Advance Directives' (sometimes called 'living wills') that outline how they would like to be treated in the future if they lack capacity. However, advance directives are limited in scope in the United Kingdom, and can only veto treatments, although in the United States the advance directive is more comprehensive and allows advance approval and specification of some treatments as well as veto (National Conference of Commissioners on Uniform State Laws, 1993). In the event of life sustaining treatments, the Mental Capacity Act 2005 (England and Wales) stipulates that advance directives must be written and witnessed, and healthcare staff should be satisfied that the person anticipated the context and options available at the point of the decision. It is not known what proportion of the population in the United Kingdom make advance directives before the onset of disease. Studies in the United States have produced highly variable rates for the completion of advance directives for cancer patients, ranging from 27% to 65% (Kelley, Lipson, Daly & Douglas, 2009). Age and being white were the only factors consistently associated with having an advance directive across studies. But some of the studies reviewed by Kelley *et al.* (2009) measured rates after diagnosis, and a rate of 22% was obtained in a study that looked at advanced directives prior to diagnosis (Ganti, Lee, Vose, Devetten, Bociek, Armitage *et al.*, 2007). In older adult samples in the United States, advance directive rates varied widely from 2% to 20% (Gillick, 2004), and a very large-scale survey of over 16,000 people who had died in the United States (Hanson & Rodgman, 1996) showed that only 9.8% had made an advance directive.

A UK postal survey (Schiff, Sacares, Snook, Rajkumar & Bulpitt, 2006) found that 454 (56%) of their sample of 811 geriatricians had cared for someone with a living will and that 108 (39%) of these had changed the treatment as a result. Most had found living wills to be helpful in providing insight into patients' wishes and in informing relatives, but concerns were expressed about changes of mind, appreciation of the consequences of decisions and possible coercion.

Advance delegation of decision making

A second approach to decision making in the absence of capacity is proxy decision making by the appointment of a 'surrogate' identified in advance as a person who could make decisions in the event of loss of capacity. In the Mental Capacity Act 2005 (England and Wales), this form of decision making was included in the provision for Lasting Powers of Attorney, in which a person donates the power to make decisions about their property, assets, treatment or welfare to another person (usually a family member). Once the person loses capacity the surrogate acts on their behalf, and their decision carry the same legal weight as the person who lacks capacity. The act stipulates that a surrogate should make decisions in the 'best interests' of the person who lacks capacity (see below). In the United Kingdom such a person can be removed or over-ruled by the Court of Protection if they fail to act in the best interests of the patient. If a person has not donated Lasting Power of Attorney while they retained capacity, and a series of decisions are required over a period of time, another avenue for surrogate decision making in England and Wales is to apply to the Court of Protection to appoint a 'deputy' to make all the relevant decisions for them.

These provisions for proxy decision making are a useful adjunct to individual, informed decision making. But proxy decision makers failed to predict patients' wishes in one third of cases (Shalowitz, Garrett-Mayer & Wendler, 2006) and struggled to contribute effectively, finding it hard to obtain information and support and experiencing high levels of stress (Vig, Starks, Taylor, Hopley & Fryer-Edwards, 2007). Pecchioni (2001) demonstrated that many people in the position to become surrogate decision makers did not discuss the options with their older, vulnerable relatives and were therefore poorly informed about their preferences. In this study 79% of daughters did not discuss caregiving decisions with their mothers, either because they assumed they knew what their mothers would want, or due to denial, not wishing to think about their parent in decline. This finding echoed Sonnenblick, Friedlander and Steinberg (1993), who also found frequent disagreement between siblings about their dying parent's wishes. However, older adults themselves may be partially responsible for this lack of proper discussion. Vandrevala, Hampson, Daly, Arber and Thomas (2006) used focus groups in a study of decisions about cardiopulmonary resuscitation in hospital, and found that a major dilemma for community living older adults was whether to preserve personal autonomy, rely on medical expertise, or to involve the family in the decision. The women in this study were more likely to want family involvement than the men.

Decision taking on behalf of a person without capacity (best interests' decisions)

Finally, and in the absence of either of the above, healthcare staff may act on behalf of a person to 'safeguard or promote their physical or mental health'. In the Mental Capacity Act 2005 (England and Wales) this is referred to as acting in a person's 'best interests', but this term was not used in the Adults with Incapacity Act (Scotland) 2000, although it was implied in the stipulation of how healthcare staff may act on behalf of a person. The Mental Capacity Act 2005 (England and Wales) does not define best interests, but instead makes stipulations about how best interest's decisions should be reached. These were included in a procedural 'best interests checklist' which specifies that staff do not base decisions on stereotypes regarding a person's characteristics or condition; endeavour to involve the person and help them to use any preserved capabilities in making the decision; take account of past wishes, values and preferences; consult with those who know the person; use the least restrictive options; use only restraint which is proportionate to the need to protect the person; and consider the possibility of regaining capacity.

The concept of best interests is complex and multifaceted, and the way in which the act specifies a best interest's checklist, detached from considerations of the relationship between decision taker and patient, has been criticised as impersonal and potentially detracting from personalised care (Dunn, Clare, Holland & Gunn, 2007). The importance accorded to individual, subjective factors in defining best interests means that surrogate decision makers cannot formulate best interests decision in terms of 'best practice' or 'likelihood of greatest benefit'. Instead, decision makers must address the dilemma of whether general notions about what constitutes the 'best course of action' are compatible with a particular individual's 'best interests', taking account of their preferences and beliefs. This is a daunting task for healthcare professionals with little knowledge of an individual and with limited opportunities for obtaining information about a person's preferences or beliefs, such as when the person has no living relatives or in emergencies. In such situations there is a danger that the decision maker's own values, or their stereotypes about the person they are treating, may influence the decision. The position advocated by Akinsanya *et al.* (2009), that those who refuse a beneficial treatment without 'good cause', be deemed to lack capacity and given the treatment in their 'best interests', illustrates this dilemma well.

A further complication is that best interest's decisions entail a tension between stakeholders. They take place within a relationship (healthcare professional–patient or family member–patient), and what constitutes the best interests for the patient may not be the best interests for the other party or parties. Dunn *et al.* (2007) also pointed out that the act's focus on process distracts attention from the moral and ethical dilemmas that underpin best interest's decisions. They noted that many decisions require the balancing of opposing principles, such as autonomy versus risk or long-term benefit versus short-term suffering. The procedural approach embodied in the best interest checklist merely identifies the issues, but does not help to resolve them or facilitate a 'good' decision. Many of these criticisms stem from the act's lack of attention to the nature and definition of best interests. However, some of the problems discussed above have been anticipated by the England and Wales Act. In particular, the inception of the Independent Mental Capacity Advocate scheme, together with the code of practice recommendations about reaching a consensus of all involved, reduce the likelihood that conflicts of interest between staff and patients will result in perverse decisions.

Best interests fallacies

There are some common fallacies about best interests that should be considered in the light of the Mental Capacity Act 2005 (England and Wales).

The first is that a best interest's decision is 'the course of action that the patient would have decided upon'. This perspective privileges the principle of autonomy, but is not entirely concordant with best interests as outlined in the act. According to the act, a decision should have regard to the *outcome* of the course of action. It is the outcome, not the course of action itself, which should determine what is in the person's best interests. Decision takers should consider the outcomes of alternative options with regard to their potential to promote enjoyment and quality of life given a person's particular preferences, values and beliefs. In determining the outcome, the decision taker may well come to a different conclusion to the patient. For one thing, they will normally draw upon different information, based on their individual past experiences and up-to-date facts provided by healthcare staff.

A second fallacy is that best interest's decisions are 'in accordance with the patient's human rights'. The act does not refer to human rights in the context of best interests, and allows decisions that benefit a person whilst restricting their liberty, or, with the 2007 amendments (Office of Public Sector Information, 2007), even depriving them of liberty. Moreover, a best interests' decision may involve declining a course of action or a treatment that a person has a 'right' to receive, if there are grounds for believing they would not have wanted it.

Another misconception is that best interests are 'what I would decide if I were in their place'. This approach patently does not consider the particular wishes and preferences of the individual who lacks capacity, and is clearly not in accordance with the act, despite its benign intent.

Some people believe that best interests decisions embody 'the option that gives the best chance of a good outcome'. As discussed above, this does not consider individual wishes, values and preferences about courses of action and their outcomes. Instead it attempts to base a decision on some universal standard of the 'benefit' of outcomes. This is clearly not appropriate in the context of an act that requires judgements about the benefits of the outcomes of particular decisions for a particular person, taking account of the potential impact on their individual enjoyment and quality of life.

In stroke care it is common to encounter patients who are judged to lack the capacity to make the decision about where they are to be discharged. The discharge decision normally entails a choice between a placement in a nursing or residential home, or returning home. Staff may wrongly assume that if the person lacks the capacity for this decision, then it is in their best interests to be discharged to the place that provides the most care and support. However, this does not necessarily follow. The decision about capacity and the decision about what is in a person's best interests are entirely separate. In a significant proportion of cases a person who lacks capacity for the discharge decision would prefer to go home and could be supported at home with suitable care and supervision. In this case, discharge home would be both in their best interests and the least restrictive option, despite their lack of capacity for the decision.

Aids to improve decision making

Chapter 3 of the Code of Practice for the Mental Capacity Act 2005 (England and Wales) (Department for Constitutional Affairs, 2007) outlines a number of ways in which patients with cognitive or communication impairments may be assisted to make a decision. The proposal includes the provision of concise, relevant information in simplified form using different media (e.g. verbal, nonverbal, written and pictorial). Sign language, translation and specialist speech and language input are recommended where they may help in giving information or in understanding replies to questions. The code suggests that familiar people, such as family and friends, may be engaged to assist in conveying information and interpreting responses.

There is empirical evidence that comprehension, decision making and retention of information can be enhanced by a variety of means. A common procedure is to enhance the written information provided for patients. Jefford and Moore (2008) considered the use of enhanced written materials for improving consent, and reviewed several studies demonstrating that understanding improved with brevity, ease of reading, encouragement to read carefully and allowing time to read forms. However, not all the studies of enhanced forms reviewed by Jefford and Moore produced positive results, and a review of 15 studies of enhanced forms by Flory and Emanuel (2004) found more negative results than positive ones. Despite the mixed results, Jefford and Moore (2008) concluded that plain language should be used in written forms to improve the quality of the decision making process, and that when discussing the decision staff should encourage patients to ask questions and check their understanding.

Other approaches that have had some success in improving understanding are presenting concrete and precise information (Krynski, Tymchuk & Ouslander,

1994), and using multimedia to convey the information. Story books were shown to be effective by Tymchuk, Ouslander, Rahbar and Fitten (1988), and presenting audio and visual material together through video has been shown to improve understanding and decision making (Jeste, Palmer, Golshan, Eyler, Dunn, Meeks *et al.*, 2009; Tymchuk, Ouslander & Rader, 1986). Jeste *et al.* (2009) also used two special techniques that improve multimedia learning; they 'personalised' the information by presenting it in a conversational manner and 'signalled' or 'cued' new information by describing it in advance. However, not all studies of multimedia approaches have demonstrated benefit; Flory and Emanuel (2004) reviewed 12 studies of multimedia interventions to improve informed consent for research and concluded that the evidence for effectiveness was equivocal. However, the negative studies reviewed by Flory and Emanuel did not use the personalisation and signalling techniques incorporated in Jeste *et al.*'s more recent work.

White, Mason, Feehan and Templeton (1995) demonstrated that educating patients in preparation for a decision about whether to accept lung biopsy, and subsequently testing them on their understanding, dramatically improved recall of material on risks of operative procedures; the percentage of people with poor recall was 44% in a group given the standard information but only 13% in a group that received an educational approach. Flory and Emanuel (2004) reviewed five trials of informed consent that used education and testing, all of which showed positive benefits for understanding, although they did note methodological weaknesses in all these studies. Flory and Emanuel (2004) also reviewed five studies of person to person explanation of the information required for consent by a neutral member of the team, and all five studies produced significant or near-significant improvement in understanding. This suggested that individual, personally relevant explication was an important element in promoting understanding and informed decision making.

In addition to the specific aids to improving the knowledge and understanding required for decision making, a qualitative study of service users and carers across a range of services (Myron *et al.*, 2008), found that general factors such as being listened to, the conduciveness of the environment, the friendliness and familiarity of staff, perceived absence of prejudice and being encouraged to develop confidence, were all felt to facilitate decision making.

Finally, Bisson, Hampton, Rosser and Holm (2009) outlined a care pathway with the potential to reduce the high proportion of people with progressive conditions who lose the capacity to make an advance directive before the matter is considered (Fazel, Hope & Jacoby, 1999). Bisson *et al.* (2009) used an approach that required the collaboration of staff and service users to develop a care pathway incorporating education about mental capacity and advance directives. The purpose was to facilitate the consideration of advance directives by people with, or at risk of, Huntington's disease. Although about one third of participants decided not to complete advance directives, all found the process valuable and acceptable, and the rate of completion was far in excess of the average (for the available US samples).

Controversial areas

Deprivation of liberty

The Mental Capacity Act 2005 (England and Wales) requires that decisions taken on behalf of a person lacking capacity minimise the restrictions placed upon the person (the 'least restrictive option') and that any restriction is proportionate to the need to protect them from harm. However, in some circumstances, safeguarding a person may require action that restricts their freedom, either against their express wishes, or without their knowledge and explicit consent. Legally this is termed 'deprivation of liberty', and it was not covered by the Mental Capacity Act 2005 (England and Wales), since this kind of measure requires rights of appeal and review which were not part of the original act.

In the United Kingdom, there are two legal routes to depriving a person of their liberty in healthcare contexts. The first is through the Mental Health Act (1983/2007) (Office of Public Sector Information, 2007) which applies to individuals suffering from a 'disorder or disability of mind' that results in a serious threat to their own health and safety, or that of others. The various sections of the Mental Health Act and its amendments allow for detention in a hospital for assessment or treatment of mental health conditions, compulsory community treatment orders and guardianship. A guardian is a person who may specify where the patient lives, require them to undertake activities or to see health professionals. The act specifies the processes by which a person can be sectioned, the roles and responsibilities of those who care for them subsequently, the ways in which they can appeal, and the use of Mental Health Tribunals to review their condition and any restrictions placed upon them. The Mental Health Act is used infrequently in general hospitals (Richards & Dale, 2009), and in stroke patients it is used only in cases of severe, and usually pre-existing, mental illness, serious and repeated suicide attempts, or cognitive impairment combined with high levels of problem behaviours, such as aggression or attempts to leave when incapable of doing so safely. In a few instances it may be necessary to transfer a stroke patient from a general hospital, or their community residence, to a psychiatric facility for assessment under the Mental Health Act. In addition, two sections of the Mental Health Act (1983), sections 5(2) and 5(4), allow doctors or nurses respectively to hold a voluntary patient in a general hospital for a short period if they consider that the person needs to be detained for their own protection or the protection of others. This is particularly useful in cases of acute, transient behaviour problems.

The second method of protecting stroke patients who exhibit severe problem behaviours and require some form of containment is by the use of the deprivation of liberty provision included in the 2007 Mental Health Act Amendments (Office of Public Sector Information, 2007; Department of Health, 2007c). This provides a detailed template for assessment of a patient leading up to an authorisation order that allows their liberty to be curtailed in their own best interests. The protocol specifies time limits, review procedures and an appeal process. To apply the procedure stroke professionals must complete and submit a detailed proforma which can be used to obtain an urgent authorisation for derivation of liberty for up to seven days. This procedure was implemented only in 2008 and at the time of writing there is little research into its operation or outcomes.

End-of-life decisions in stroke care

End-of-life decision making is a complex and controversial area. The Mental Capacity Act 2005 (England and Wales) specifically disallows 'best interests' decisions motivated by a desire to end a person's life. However, the UK National Clinical Guidelines for stroke (Royal College of Physicians, 2008a) stipulate, 'After stroke all end-of-life decisions to withhold or withdraw life-prolonging treatments (including artificial nutrition and hydration) should be in the best interests of the patient'. The term 'best interests' here is presumably being used in a general sense rather than the legal sense, since many patients who want to end their lives by declining treatments do possess capacity, and do not require 'best interests' decisions in sense specified in the act. The Guidelines for the United States (Adams, del Zoppo, Alberts, Bhatt, Brass, Furlan *et al.*, 2007) are more explicit. They propose, 'Many people would not want to survive if a devastating stroke would lead to a persistent vegetative state or other condition of devastating incapacity'. The US guidelines make reference to respect for advance directives and consulting those with power of attorney or family members about selecting or withholding treatments. They note the importance of giving families clear information about stroke, prognosis and treatment options. Finally, it is recognised that conservative treatment or palliative care may often be the outcome, and that the family should be psychologically supported during decision making and through the terminal phase.

Cases where stroke patients wish to receive treatments to prolong their lives are rarely controversial, but there are some situations, where there has been a devastating stroke, in which families (and patients) may wish to prolong treatments and life against the judgement of the care team (see the LF case in the next paragraph). Conversely, a number of stroke patients request help to end their lives (see Marjory's case in Table 9.6), which presents a serious ethical and legal dilemma, since the Mental Capacity Act 2005 allows a person with capacity to refuse treatments, food or hydration, but it is currently illegal in the United Kingdom for anyone to help a person to terminate their life. A case example to illustrate a wish to end life is given in Table 9.6.

Table 9.6   Case Example of a Wish to End Life

Marjory was 88 and had suffered a moderately severe stroke which had resulted in a left-sided weakness. She had some power in her affected arm and leg, but could not stand unassisted. The physiotherapists thought that she had potential and might eventually be able to transfer with the assistance of one person, and possibly even walk with an aid. Prior to her stroke she had suffered from progressive osteoarthritis and from heart disease over a period of about ten years which caused chronic pain and reduced her mobility. Her husband was in good health and had written a very helpful biography of her life which was in her file. She had obtained an Oxbridge degree and been a senior administrator for aid agencies in Asia, Africa and South America. She had seen much deprivation and suffering and had often been with people at the ends of their lives. She had no children, but was close to nieces and nephews. Latterly her health had prevented her from indulging her passion for gardening, and she had begun to feel that her quality of life was severely diminished. On admission to hospital following her stroke she had told staff that she wished to die and refused all active therapy (physiotherapy and occupational therapy). She was referred to the psychologist for assessment at one week post stroke. When the psychologist arrived, she asked if they had come to help her to die. When he replied this was not possible, she immediately said she did not wish to see him and asked him to leave. It was not clear what previous encounters she had had with medical and other staff on admission, since she was not prepared to talk about anything other than help with dying. There was no opportunity to complete a depression screen or a clinical interview, but her demeanour did not indicate *obvious* depression and was characterised more by anger and frustration. If capacity and depression assessments had been possible, it might have transpired that she had capacity and that her decision was valid. A visit from the staff doctor received a similar response to that given to the psychologist, and they were also unable to complete assessments. The psychologist visited again in a week, after Marjory began to refuse all medication, drink and food. This time she said she was 'dead' and could not talk to anyone. She continued to decline offers to discuss matters with the psychologist and also began to refuse to see her husband who had attempted to discuss her refusal to take medications and nutrition. She was referred to the older adult mental health team for assessment. The psychologist had several meetings to support her husband, who was very distressed by her attitude and her condition. She died about a week later before the mental health team could assess her. This left the unanswered question of what the outcome would have been had she refused to talk to the psychiatrist, as seems likely.

   In this case, a person whom the multiprofessional team deemed to be capable of a reasonable standard of life wished to end her life. She achieved her aim, but it was a moot point whether this was achieved in a manner that minimised suffering and maximised dignity. By contrast, there are instances in which people with very serious strokes, or their families, may wish to prolong life, despite devastating disabilities.

Anderson, Augoustakis, Holmes and Chambers (2009) reported two case studies of young men with brain stem strokes that produced locked-in syndrome. Locked-in syndrome differs from typical stroke in that the person is cognitively unimpaired, despite being unable to move any part of the body other than the eyes. They may survive for ten years or more. Neither of the young patients in Anderson *et al.* (2009) had made advance directives, and neither had discussed end-of-life decisions with their families. One case will be described to illustrate the issues. LF was a 55-year-old school teacher who developed locked-in syndrome following a brainstem stroke resulting from arterial occlusion. He was quadriplegic, but could blink and breathe with ventilator support. He was admitted to an intensive care unit and transferred to a stroke unit two and a half weeks later. Due to his very poor prognosis, the intensive care team raised the possibility of palliative care with his family, but they became distressed and angry, and protective of the patient. The matter of palliative care was raised again by the stroke unit team seven weeks after admission, but the family continued to resist it strongly, and this accentuated the rift between the staff and the family, damaged the family's trust in the staff and prevented further progress with important decision making. LF demonstrated no functional improvement over three and a half months, and was assessed as having no rehabilitation potential and was discharged to a nursing home. However, he did regain capacity to make decisions while in hospital, and was able to communicate choices by blinking. At the time he indicated that he did wish to be given full active treatment. However, three years later he changed his mind and decided to refuse all active medical management and died of pneumonia.

Anderson *et al.* (2009) recommended that families should be asked about the patient's views regarding end of life prior to their stroke, and should then be provided with counselling and education about the condition and its outcome in the early weeks and months so that the implications of any decision they make is clear to them. This approach may allow families time to adjust before end-of-life decisions are fully explored.

Assisted dying and euthanasia

These difficult cases illustrate the dilemma faced by healthcare professionals, patients and families in making end-of-life decisions. In 2004 the Assisted Dying for the Terminally Ill Bill (House of Lords, 2005), designed to allow healthcare professional to prescribe medication to help a person end their lives, was put before the UK parliament, but was blocked by the House of Lords in 2006. The bill proposed that after signing a declaration that they wanted to die, patients could be prescribed medication to end their lives. Only people with less than six months to live, who were suffering unbearably, were deemed to have capacity and were not depressed, would be able to end their life in this way. Relatives, those with powers of attorney, or those acting in best interests would not be able to make this decision for a person who lacked capacity. This procedure is sometimes called 'assisted suicide' and differs from voluntary euthanasia in which a healthcare professional actively brings on the death of a person who wishes to end their life. Despite the absence of active participation in bringing about death, assisted suicide is nonetheless highly controversial. The Royal College of Psychiatrists, the Royal College of Anaesthetists and the Royal College of Physicians of Edinburgh are all neutral on the matter, but the British

Medical Association has vacillated, dropping its opposition to assisted suicide after a debate in 2005, but switching back to opposing it the following year. In 2009, the Royal College of Nursing held a ballot in which the majority of respondents supported assisted suicide. However, the response rate was low (1200 out of 175,000) so they changed their position from opposition to neutrality rather than outright support.

An unresolved psychological issue relevant to this debate is the definition of 'unbearable suffering'. Dees, Vernooij-Dassen, Dekkers and van Weel (2009) reviewed 55 publications on suffering, but found no definition of unbearable suffering in the context of end-of-life decisions. They proposed, 'Unbearable suffering in the context of a request for EAS [euthanasia or physician-assisted suicide] is a profoundly personal experience of an actual or perceived impending threat to the integrity or life of the person, which has a significant duration and a central place in the person's mind'. Interestingly, this definition, and those used in many of the studies reviewed, identified suffering, not as pain or physical impairment, but in psychological terms as loss of function, loss of dignity, loss of control, burden, hopelessness and pointlessness of living. However, this definition has yet to be generally accepted and assessments based upon it will be challenging, especially in conditions such as stroke where there may be cognitive or communication impairments and the possibility of treatable depression.

There are moves to re-introduce the Assisted Dying Bill to the UK parliament in the near future, and a new bill was put before the Scottish parliament in 2010, but in the meantime this approach to dying is available in only a small, but growing, number of countries. Switzerland has permitted physician- and non-physician-assisted suicide since 1941, the Netherlands formally legalised assisted suicide in 2002, but Dutch courts have permitted it since 1984, Belgium legalized it in 2002, and the state of Oregon, United States, legalized assisted suicide in 1994. With the exception of the Netherlands, where it accounts for 1.8% of deaths, the uptake is low and it accounted for less than 0.5% of all deaths in each of the other countries (Dees *et al.*, 2009). Despite its infrequent use, this measure has major psychological implications and will undoubtedly, if introduced in the United Kingdom, be an area requiring psychological expertise.

Implementation of mental capacity policies and legislation

Services and users and carers

Mental capacity legislation across the world aims to promote decision making that is in accordance with people's wishes and preferences, even when they are not able to engage fully with the decision making process. User groups, such as the Alzheimer's Society, have expressed strong support for the Mental Capacity Act 2005 (England and Wales), and carers and service users with experience of mental capacity in decision making also welcomed the principles and provisions of the Act (Manthorpe, Rapaport & Stanley, 2009). There are, however, a number of barriers to the achievement of its principal aims.

First, as noted in the discussion of shared decision making above, a significant proportion of patients prefer to leave the decision to healthcare professionals, and the almost universal desire for information about conditions and their treatment co-exists with ambivalence about participation in decision making itself. In one study of cancer treatment the majority of patients preferred to leave decisions to doctors (Sutherland, Llewellyn-Thomas, Lockwood, Tritchler & Till, 1989). Second, the general population, a proportion of whom will experience the loss of capacity themselves or in a close relative, have poor awareness of mental capacity law (Das, Das & Mulle, 2006; Sayers, Barratt, Gothard, Onnie, Perera & Schulman, 2001; Schiff, Rajkumar & Bulpitt, 2000). Consequently, many people miss opportunities to benefit from advance directives or appointing people with powers of attorney before losing capacity. Third, since the studies of Das, Sayers and Schiff cited above, there has been little mass media publicity for the act in the United Kingdom to improve public awareness. Manthorpe *et al.*'s (2009) sample of service users and carers felt that professionals should publicise the act more comprehensively and provide more specific information about the act's provisions to service users and carers. In the United States, healthcare providers are obliged to inform patients of their rights to accept or refuse care and to make advance directives (Ulrich, 1999), but this is not the case in the United Kingdom. Fourth, Manthorpe *et al.*'s (2009) participants noted concerns over the resources required to implement and monitor the act, and the risks associated with any deficiencies in its operation. Full assessment of capacity, including consultations with family, friends or independent mental capacity advocates, is time consuming and costly, and it is tempting to take shortcuts which could result in perverse decisions. In addition, surrogates and staff may not act in a person's best interests and the provisions for monitoring this are not well specified or resourced. Finally, there is no licensing or qualification system in the United Kingdom to guarantee that staff are knowledgeable and competent in implementing the act.

At a practical level, Myron *et al.* (2008) interviewed six carers and 20 service users in older adult and mental health services and identified several specific contextual elements that promoted involvement in decision making. These were being listened to, having a choice of communication mediums (oral or writing), being familiar with and trusting the staff involved and having conducive environments and positive, 'friendly' staff. Conversely, a number of factors were felt to militate against participation in decision making: circumstances that did not build up the confidence to make decisions, prejudice and stigma leading to assumptions that people with some health conditions were incapable of decision making, making decisions for someone in the knowledge that the person was different from their former self (carer specific) and feeling accountable for decisions made for others (carer specific).

Staff

The successful implementation mental capacity legislation depends crucially upon staff. However, research with staff prior to the implementation of the act in the United Kingdom revealed poor knowledge of mental capacity law (Jackson & Warner, 2002) and a lack of knowledge about policies for living wills (Schiff *et al.*, 2006). A similar state of affairs existed in the United States (Ganzini, Volicer, Nelson, Fox & Derse, 2004). Some have argued that medical practitioners generally lack the training and skills required for the manifold and nuanced nature of many capacity judgements (Silberfeld & Checkland, 1999). Deficiencies in staff knowledge of mental capacity legislations were also found in the questionnaire responses of 73 staff in UK mental health, older adult and learning disability services (Myron *et al.*, 2008). This sample exhibited different understandings of the nature of mental capacity and approaches to its assessment, and lacked confidence in their knowledge and skills in these areas. A key finding was that nearly all the staff in the study wished for more training and guidance on the operation of the act. Even more concerning, now that thrombolysis is used in the treatment of acute stroke, is a study (Evans, Warner & Jackson, 2007) that found emergency service workers in England have poor knowledge of the basic principles of the Mental Capacity Act 2005; that a competent person who refuses treatment should not be treated and that a relative's signature is not necessary to treat an incompetent person. In this study 33% of doctors, 90% of nurses and 100% of ambulance workers gave incorrect responses!

The problem of staff expertise is succinctly illustrated by the outcome of a large-scale postal vignette-based study of medical staff in the United States (Markson, Kern, Annas & Glantz, 1994). They found that medical staff were overly influenced by (erroneous) medical opinion and, despite knowing the standards for competence, many thought that competence depended on diagnosis rather than function. Finally, Gravel, Legare and Graham (2006) found that some key healthcare staff did not subscribe fully to the principles of shared decision making and patient autonomy, and felt that the approach lacks utility and is impracticable. As noted above, there is no requirement for staff to undertake training in the act or to reach any standard of proficiency. This contrasts with the Mental Health Act 1983 (England and Wales) where specific training is mandated for those who undertake the roles of Approved Mental Health Professional and Responsible Clinician. The lack of formal training opportunities is surprising in view of the expressed desire for training and guidance by staff (Myron *et al.*, 2008).

An empirical study of best interest's decision making for people with intellectual impairments (Dunn, Clare & Holland, 2008) demonstrated that staff operated on two levels. At one level, strategic life planning and healthcare decisions followed the formal model proposed for best interest's decisions, with full deliberation and consultation. But day-to-day decisions, such as choice of clothes or meals, were often accomplished spontaneously, and hinged upon the relationship between carer and recipient and the attainment of mutually beneficial outcomes. The stipulations of the act had little influence upon this kind of decision despite their pervasiveness and impact upon the person's life. Consequently, the authors proposed the integration of the National Minimum Standards for care with the provisions of the Mental Capacity Act 2005 in a manner that reflects the processes by which care is provided. In addition, they suggested that enhanced staff training, supervision and greater staff engagement with residents' care plans would increase the congruence between the care plans and the care received.

Conclusions

The involvement of service users in decision making is both beneficial and ethical, but that there are barriers to its realisation. Stroke is especially likely to impair decision making due to its effects on cognition, and this may result in the lack of capacity to make vital healthcare and welfare decisions. To address this developed countries have enacted laws to protect those who lack capacity and those who must make decisions on their behalf. There are similarities in the ways in which different jurisdictions endeavour to allow incapacitated people to participate in decisions, such as through advance directives and surrogate decision making. Despite the best intentions of legislators, all the approaches to addressing mental incapacity have shortcomings and flaws, and professionals and families are sometimes required to make difficult 'best interests' judgements with incomplete information. There are also major practical difficulties with fully implementing legislation and improving compliance with codes of practice. However, there are promising approaches to standardising and systematising the assessment of mental capacity, such as the Mac-CAT-T, and to increasing both the uptake of the provisions of legislation (Bisson *et al.*, 2009) and the participation of patients in decisions (Jeste *et al.*, 2009). Finally, decision making capacity becomes crucial when contemplating certain pivotal decisions such as end of life, deprivation of liberty and assisted dying. In these areas mental capacity assessment requires special safeguards, careful monitoring and well-developed psychological knowledge and skills.

Future research

Surprisingly, in view of the effect of stroke on cognition, and the high proportion of stroke patient admitted to hospital lacking capacity, there is a dearth of evidence about the impact of stroke on decision making, mental capacity and its assessment. This is a gap in knowledge that requires urgent attention. One particular question is the role and effectiveness of the various approaches to assisting decision making in this population.

The potential role of emotion in decision making, and its impact on mental capacity, has been noted by a number of authors (Akinsanya *et al.*, 2009; Breden & Vollmann, 2004; Owen *et al.*, 2009; Vellinga *et al.*, 2004). A sudden onset illness, such as stroke, occasions temporary psychological reactions of shock, numbness and anxiety, and it is important to understand the degree, nature and duration of the effects upon decision making and approaches to managing their impact. Despite this, there have been no empirical studies of the impact of emotional factors on the decision making of stroke patients.

Moye and Marson (2007) noted the paucity of data on ethnicity and decision making capacity, and the possible impact of incongruence between the value systems of healthcare professionals and members of some ethnic groups. Moreover, there has been little exploration of the reasons for the low uptake of advance decision making provisions in some ethnic groups, or of approaches to improving participation for these groups. These questions are especially important in view of the higher rates of stroke in black people than white people in the United Kingdom.

The implementation of mental capacity legislation throughout stroke care pathways, from the crucial decision about thrombolysis through to decisions about discharge and community care, is another fruitful area for investigation. The systematic approach to making advance decisions developed by Bisson *et al.* (2009) for progressive conditions might well be adapted for stroke, and investigations of its utility in stroke care would be informative. At the same time, it would be helpful to include the way in which capacity is assessed in the National Sentinel Audits of Stroke in the United Kingdom (Royal College of Physicians, 2008b) to obtain information about implementation of the legislation.

Finally, end-of-life decision making has received little attention in stroke patients, and if assisted dying should become legal in the United Kingdom, there will be important psychological research required to elucidate the nature of 'unbearable' suffering, and into the criteria for valid decisions.

Chapter 10

Neuropsychological Aspects of Rehabilitation

Introduction

The role of the neuropsychologist in stroke services should go well beyond the selection, administration and interpretation of cognitive tests. Within the complex intervention that is stroke rehabilitation, the neuropsychologist can contribute significantly to the work of the multidisciplinary team (MDT) on a number of levels. This is especially true if the neuropsychologist has a background in clinical psychology, and is therefore able to draw upon models of assessment and intervention from psychotherapy, neuropsychology and rehabilitation to develop holistic, person-centred formulations for each patient.

Neuropsychological rehabilitation can be defined as 'the amelioration of cognitive, emotional, psychosocial, and behavioural deficits caused by an insult to the brain' (Wilson, 2008). This broad definition, derived from McLellan (1991), highlights that neuropsychological rehabilitation should not be restricted to a narrow focus on the recovery of cognitive function alone. Furthermore, according to this approach, rehabilitation is not something that is 'done to' a patient. Rather, neuropsychological rehabilitation is a collaborative two-way process between the patient and the rehabilitation team. The goals of rehabilitation should be negotiated collaboratively by the patient and rehabilitation staff. Inevitably, this results in more functionally meaningful targets for the patient, who is often therefore more motivated to engage in the rehabilitation process (Gauggel & Fischer, 2001; Van den Broek, 2005).

Neuropsychological rehabilitation should be based on sound theoretical principles and models of intervention. The present chapter will attempt to link theories of neuropsychological rehabilitation to everyday clinical practice in busy stroke services. For example, Prigatano (2008) conceptualised neuropsychological rehabilitation as comprising of three interacting levels. The first involves

Psychological Management of Stroke, First Edition. Nadina B. Lincoln, Ian I. Kneebone, Jamie A.B. Macniven and Reg C. Morris.

interventions designed to facilitate recovery of damaged brain function (i.e. restitution of compromised cognition). The second level is said to involve the amelioration of disability associated with brain damage (i.e. compensation for permanent neuropsychological impairment in order to promote functional recovery). The evidence for the effectiveness of interventions primarily aimed at these levels of rehabilitation is discussed in the next chapter, 'Cognitive Rehabilitation'. The present chapter will primarily consider the third level of neuropsychological rehabilitation as described by Prigatano (2008): the patient's subjective experience of their brain damage and how the stroke rehabilitation multidisciplinary team can take account of the patient's experience in planning and implementing interventions.

The challenge within most stroke services is to undertake meaningful neuropsychological rehabilitation within typically very limited budgets. Resource constraints within most stroke services are such that the neuropsychologist will almost always rely heavily upon the multidisciplinary team to collaborate in assessment, formulation and in implementing clinical interventions. Effective team working is therefore essential for any stroke rehabilitation service. The present chapter will summarise key areas of interprofessional collaboration, such as goal planning, which are essential in enabling the multidisciplinary team to maximise a patient's rehabilitation potential.

Models of neuropsychological rehabilitation

Regardless of the specific service configuration in which the clinician is working, any neuropsychological rehabilitation approach should seek to apply sound theoretical principles to evidence-based practice. Clinical neuropsychology has a rich theoretical inheritance; the clinician has a broad range of theoretical cognitive models and theories upon which to base their own practice. Many early models of higher cognitive functions are still relevant today; for example, Luria's pioneering work with neurological patients emphasised cognitive rehabilitative strategies incorporating practice of 'higher cognitive functions' in order to restore or compensate for acquired neurological disability (Luria, 1962).

A detailed account of the many models of neuropsychological rehabilitation which can inform everyday practice in stroke services is beyond the scope of this chapter. Instead, the focus will be on the potential application of two influential approaches, those of Wilson (Wilson, 2002; Wilson, Gracey, Evans & Bateman, 2009) and Prigatano (2008). A third, closely related approach to neuropsychological rehabilitation, the biopsychosocial model, is also an important framework for practice within stroke rehabilitation (Williams & Evans, 2003). Clinicians working in stroke rehabilitation services should also be mindful of models of recovery from brain damage; Robertson and Murre's (1999) model will be briefly presented below.

Wilson's (2002) holistic model

Wilson's (Wilson, 2002; Wilson *et al.*, 2009) model (Figure 10.1) illustrates the importance of the need for neuropsychological rehabilitation to be based on a broad theoretical approach, acknowledging the many factors which influence a patient's experience after brain damage. The model describes the patient as central to the process of rehabilitation, with key contributing (e.g. family support), modulating (e.g. mood) and inhibitory factors (e.g. language impairment) incorporated into a framework. Such factors must be taken into account in rehabilitation services. Importantly, this model can inform the clinician as to the most appropriate clinical intervention for a patient. The

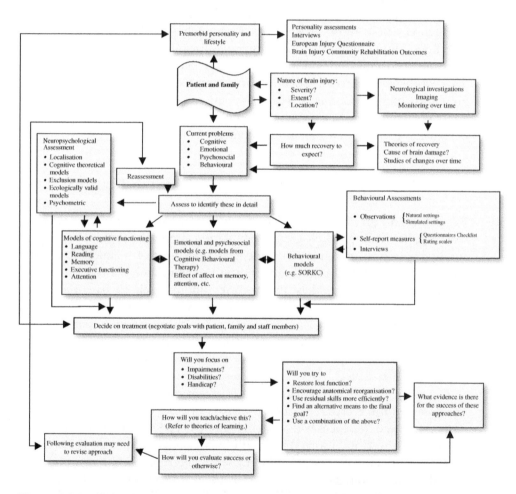

Figure 10.1 Wilson's provisional model of neuropsychological rehabilitation. Towards a comprehensive model of cognitive rehabilitation. (Reproduced with permission from Wilson, B.A., Gracey, F., Evans, J.J. & Bateman, A., 2009, *Neuropsychological Rehabilitation*, Cambridge University Press.)

overriding premise is that any intervention must be targeted at a patient's functional competence in everyday life. According to this model, for example, there is little point in encouraging a patient to focus on repetitive abstract cognitive exercises, as advocated by some cognitive remediation approaches, if this has little direct impact on that patient's everyday activities of daily living.

Wilson and colleagues' (2009) tentative holistic model emphasises five areas of particular importance: cognitive functioning, emotion, social interaction, behaviour and learning. Acknowledging cognitive models of Coltheart (1987), Baddeley and Hitch (1974), Norman and Shallice (1980), Wilson argued that an understanding of cognitive functioning is fundamental to the process of identifying appropriate interventions for people in neurorehabilitation. This understanding is fundamental, but on its own is insufficient. The clinician must also take account of the interaction between emotion and cognition (Harvey, Watkins, Mansell & Shafran, 2004) and the psychosocial impact of brain damage.

Wilson herself pointed out that this tentative model of neuropsychological rehabilitation omits some aspects of recovery and rehabilitation, such as motor functioning and physical recovery (Wilson, 2002), and these might be added in further revisions of the model to provide a fully comprehensive representation of the process of neuropsychological rehabilitation. However, the model as it stands is a very useful framework with which the clinician can design or benchmark their neurorehabilitation service.

Within any typical stroke rehabilitation service, the model is highly relevant. Even acute or hyper-acute stroke services should incorporate a similar framework in order to ensure that the service maximises every individual patient's rehabilitation potential.

Prigatano's (2008) third level of neuropsychological rehabilitation

Prigatano (2008) argued that the patient's subjective experience, the 'third level' of neuropsychological rehabilitation, is central to effective rehabilitation. According to this approach, in order to attempt to reduce the very common psychological symptoms associated with brain damage (e.g. frustration, confusion, anger, depression, anxiety, loneliness and shame), the psychologist must enter the patient's phenomenological field and attempt to experience rehabilitation from the patient's perspective (Prigatano, 2008). Prigatano suggested that attachment theory (Bowlby, 1973) and psychodynamic psychotherapy (Kohut, 1977) can provide insights into patients' behaviour that can transform their rehabilitation potential. Although research evidence for the effectiveness of such approaches had not yet been established, in clinical practice patients with apparently similar strokes and functional disability can often respond very differently to the rehabilitation process. Utilising a broad range of psychotherapeutic models can help the clinician collaboratively make sense of the patient's experience, develop a therapeutic alliance and through psychotherapy help the patient to engage in rehabilitation.

The presence of a therapeutic alliance has been shown to relate to neuropsychological rehabilitation outcome (Prigatano, Klonoff, O'Brien, Altman, Amin, Chiapello *et al.*, 1994), in that patients are more likely to be motivated and engaged in rehabilitation if they feel a collaborative bond with their therapist.

Prigatano (1999) presented 13 guiding principles for neuropsychological rehabilitation. Although not all are easily applicable in, or appropriate to, typical stroke rehabilitation services, the majority are useful in planning neuropsychological rehabilitation and are reproduced in Table 10.1.

The biopsychosocial model of neuropsychological rehabilitation (Williams & Evans, 2003)

Williams and Evans (2003) presented a special issue of the journal *Neuropsychological Rehabilitation*, in which they discussed the relevance of patients' emotional experiences to the process of neuropsychological rehabilitation. Psychological adjustment to acquired brain damage is seen as a central component of the patient's journey after stroke. Within stroke services, the biopsychosocial model reminds the clinician of the multiple factors which can influence the success or failure of a rehabilitation programme. Since Engel (1977) first argued for the medical profession to move away from a strict biomedical model, stroke rehabilitation has in many centres embraced the biopsychosocial approach, whereby the social and psychological consequences of a stroke are given as much attention as the biological and neurological sequelae. Modern neuropsychological rehabilitation holds the biopsychosocial approach as fundamental to effective patient-centred intervention.

Yeates, Gracey and McGrath (2008) presented a biopsychosocial framework within which the clinician can consider possible influences on a patient's apparent personality change following brain damage. This is illustrated in Figure 10.2. Within stroke services, family members of patients who have had a stroke may report that the patient is 'no longer the person they knew' pre-stroke. It is not uncommon for patients and their families to describe a change in personality after stroke. It is important to consider the neurobiological, psychological and psychosocial factors which can variously contribute to the perception of a changed personality after stroke. Yeates *et al.* (2008)'s framework, in this case describing factors influencing the perception of personality change, emphasises the utility of a biopsychosocial approach to neuropsychological rehabilitation. A similar framework can be applied to a multitude of clinical issues in stroke rehabilitation.

Models of recovery

Within neuropsychological rehabilitation, and especially within acute stroke rehabilitation services, it is important to take into account models of recovery of cognitive functioning when planning intervention. As Robertson (2005)

Table 10.1 Prigatano's Principles of Neuropsychological Rehabilitation. Reproduced with permission of Oxford University Press from *Principles of Neuropsychological Rehabilitation* by George Prigatano (1999): Table: Principles of Neuropsychological Rehabilitation (pp. 3–4) © 1999 by Oxford University Press, Inc.

Prigatano's Principles of Neuropsychological Rehabilitation	
Principle 1	The clinician must begin with patient's subjective or phenomenological experience to reduce their frustrations and confusion in order to engage them in the rehabilitation process.
Principle 2	The patient's symptom picture is a mixture of premorbid cognitive and personality characteristics as well as neuropsychological changes directly associated with brain pathology.
Principle 3	Neuropsychological rehabilitation focuses on both the remediation of higher cerebral disturbances and their management in interpersonal situations.
Principle 4	Neuropsychological rehabilitation helps patients observe their behaviour and thereby teaches them about the direct and indirect effects of brain injury. This may help patients avoid destructive choices and better manage their catastrophic reactions.
Principle 5	Failure to study the intimate interaction of cognition and personality leads to an inadequate understanding of many issues in cognitive (neuro)sciences and neuropsychological rehabilitation.
Principle 6	Little is known about how to retrain a brain dysfunctional patient cognitively, because the nature of higher cerebral functions is not fully understood. General guidelines for cognitive remediation, however, can be specified.
Principle 7	Psychotherapeutic interventions are often an important part of neuropsychological rehabilitation because they help patients (and families) deal with their personal losses. The process, however, is highly individualised.
Principle 8	Working with brain dysfunctional patients produces affective reactions in both the patient's family and the rehabilitation staff. Appropriate management of these reactions facilitates the rehabilitative and adaptive process.
Principle 9	Each neuropsychological rehabilitation programme is a dynamic entity. It is in a state of either development or decline. Ongoing scientific investigation helps the rehabilitation team learn from their successes and failures and is needed to maintain a dynamic, creative rehabilitation effort.
Principle 10	Failure to identify which patients can and cannot be helped by different (neuropsychological) rehabilitation approaches creates a lack of credibility for the field.
Principle 11	Disturbances in self-awareness after brain injury are often poorly understood and mismanaged.
Principle 12	Competent patient management and planning innovative rehabilitation programmes depend on understanding mechanisms of recovery and deterioration of direct and indirect symptoms after brain injury.
Principle 13	The rehabilitation of patients with higher cerebral deficits requires both scientific and phenomenological approaches. Both are necessary to maximise recovery and adaptation to the effects of brain injury.

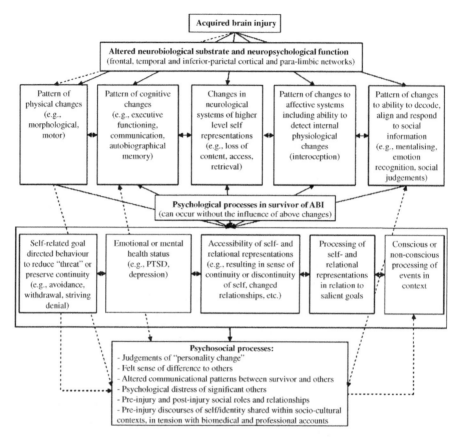

Figure 10.2 Biopsychosocial framework. (Yeates, G. N., Gracey, F., & McGrath, J. C., 2008, A biopsychosocial deconstruction of "personality change" following acquired brain injury, *Neuropsychological Rehabilitation*, p. 581. Reprinted with permission of Taylor & Francis Group LLC – Journals: http://www.informaworld.com)

discussed, when faced with a stroke patient who has hemiparesis, for example, the rehabilitation team has to decide whether to devote limited rehabilitation resources to facilitating the recovery of movement in the patient's arm, or alternatively to helping the patient develop compensatory strategies that will allow him or her to undertake activities of daily living and maximise quality of life. Robertson (2005) argued that this decision is especially significant as some attempts at compensation may have direct negative effects on a patient's brain function and outcome.

Robertson and Murre (1999) presented a neural network model of recovery from brain damage, based on empirical data. They concluded that, after brain damage, one subset of patients will spontaneously recover relatively normal function through neural self-repair processes. Other patients, usually with larger lesions, may not spontaneously recover significant function, and will instead rely on compensatory and functional reorganisation mechanisms in order to improve their functioning. According to Robertson and Murre's (1999) model, a third group of patients may have brain lesions that have the potential for restitution if a number of rehabilitative conditions are met. By this model, such conditions might include the availability of sufficient general stimulation (e.g. environ-mental enrichment), appropriately focused stimulation (e.g. stimulation of an affected hemiparetic limb in combination with the deactivation of the unaffected limb; Miltner, Bauder, Sommer, Dettmers & Taub, 1999), the absence of handicapping inhibition (i.e. nondamaged brain circuits inhibiting partially functioning circuits thus compounding the effects of the brain damage), adequate arousal levels and the capacity to unlearn faulty learning patterns. Crucially, this model implies that poorly designed rehabilitation has the potential to undermine a patient's potential for recovery.

Clinicians working in stroke rehabilitation should take into account devel-opments in our knowledge of the mechanics of recovery. Rehabilitation strat-egies must be appropriate for the individual patient. At present it is still a considerable challenge to 'triage' stroke patients into groups, as defined by Robertson and Murre (1999), but at the very least this model illustrates that one-size-fits-all stroke rehabilitation is flawed.

The impact of cognitive problems on daily life

Neuropsychologists can sometimes be accused of being more interested in psychometric data than in the practical 'real-life' problems associated with brain damage. However, this is unjustified. Genuine neuropsychological rehabilita-tion is entirely concerned with the patient's experience. Neuropsychological test data are used to help identify the causes of a patient's functional difficulties, and to develop focused, meaningful interventions. As highlighted by the models of Wilson *et al.* (2009), Prigatano (1999) and Williams and Evans (2003), cognitive problems must be identified in rehabilitation settings. Once identified, rehabil-itation interventions can focus on reducing the impact of cognitive impairment on the patient's activities of daily living and participation in the community.

'Pragmatic' neuropsychological rehabilitation in stroke services

Within many stroke services there are currently insufficient resources available for comprehensive neuropsychological rehabilitation to be undertaken. For example, in the United Kingdom, the National Health Service priorities are increasingly dominated by a focus on survival rates and reducing the length of stay in hospital. Some would argue that this service development ethos, while very welcome in undoubtedly increasing the proportion of patients surviving a stroke, has not simultaneously provided adequate resources to meet the increased rehabilitation needs associated with the ever-increasing number of stroke survivors. As discussed in chapter 2, there are signs that many stroke services are recognising this service development need, and rehabilitation services are beginning to receive more attention from commissioners. In the meantime, psychological services for people with stroke can be limited, and over-stretched psychologists working in such services often need to rely on very brief interventions. Rather than providing one-to-one formal psychotherapy and neuropsychological assessment and intervention, these psychologists often supervise other members of the team in implementing rehabilitation strategies.

Formal cognitive rehabilitation strategies supported by research evidence are described in chapter 11. Additional, less formal, psycho-education strategies can be recommended following a neuropsychological assessment, and often within stroke services can be discussed with the patient and their family as a set of interventions to begin in the acute rehabilitation setting and continue after discharge from hospital. Most members of the multidisciplinary team can contribute to this aspect of rehabilitation. Although the effectiveness of some of these strategies is yet to be established in robust research studies, clinical practice suggests that for many patients these strategies can be beneficial. Mateer and Sira (2008) provided excellent examples of some practical rehabilitation strategies which can be undertaken as part of the process of neuropsychological rehabilitation in stroke services. Caregiver and patient handouts were suggested, covering attention, memory, executive functioning and psychosocial strategies. Table 10.2 is an example of a caregiver handout describing some executive functioning strategies.

Table 10.2   Caregiver Handout: Executive Functioning Strategies (Copyright 2008 by Taylor & Francis Group LLC – Books. Reproduced with permission of Taylor & Francis Group LLC – Books in the format other book via Copyright Clearance Center; Mateer and Sira, 2008, p. 1005)

1. Set up a routine of daily activities and stick to it.
2. Try to set up the environment (or work or social role) so as to reduce novelty.
3. Try not to put time pressure on the person – allow extra time to complete tasks.
4. Employ environmental cues (audible alarms, signs, notes and calendars) to help remind and cue the person to do things.
5. Link behaviours that occur together naturally (e.g. always take medication at dinner).
6. Praise the person whenever they initiate, terminate or self-regulate appropriately.
7. If the person says or does inappropriate things, firmly correct them immediately after the behaviour. For example, say 'That statement was inappropriate' or 'You are not to touch me'.
8. If the person says and believes erroneous things, and is unable to give them up (delusional beliefs), gently redirect them and remind them of the true situation in a consistent manner.
9. When the person is learning something new, break down the problem into steps, and start with basic steps before moving to complex steps.
10. Employ a systematic and logical problem solving strategy – put the problem solving steps on a poster on the wall, or on a card the person can keep in their wallet until they memorise the strategy.
11. Rehearse and repeat strategies – practice makes perfect.
12. Make sure you and the person pace yourselves to minimise fatigue – don't take on too much.

As highlighted by the modern models of neuropsychological rehabilitation discussed earlier in the present chapter, it is important for any recommended strategies, such as those suggested in Table 10.2, to be agreed collaboratively with the patient. The patient may have a different perspective on the presenting problems, but may nevertheless recognise the importance of their family member's or caregiver's perspective, and agree to caregiver strategies such as those in Table 10.2.

Until stroke rehabilitation services are properly resourced, neuropsychological rehabilitation may remain over-reliant on psycho-education strategies, group interventions and the supervision of multidisciplinary interventions. Over time, increased prioritisation of neuropsychological rehabilitation by commissioners will allow comprehensive rehabilitation services to become more widespread. In addition to the enhanced quality of life arguments, the cost benefits of such services in terms of reduced readmission rates, reduced mental health service burden and enhanced return-to-work rates should more than justify the increased resourcing of stroke rehabilitation services.

Goal planning

There is a long history in healthcare rehabilitation of goal setting and goal planning being used as the basis for assessment and intervention (Kiresuk & Sherman, 1968; McMillan & Sparkes, 1999; Locke & Latham, 2002; Wade, 2009). In other settings, such as in education and industry, goal planning has been used for decades as a primary performance management technique. Several high-profile, high-quality neurorehabilitation centres in the United Kingdom rely on goal planning as fundamental to the success of their rehabilitation programmes. As Wilson *et al.* (2009) discussed, the advantages of goal planning include simplicity, relevance to everyday functioning and a natural focus on the individual. McMillan and Sparkes (1999) described some principles of effective goal planning, which include:

- The goals must be patient centred and agreed collaboratively with the patient.
- The goals must be challenging but also realistic and potentially attainable during the patient's time in the rehabilitation service.
- The goals must be clear and specific.
- The goals must have a definite time deadline.
- The goals must be measurable.
- The goals must be defined as long or short term.

Within stroke services, goal planning can be a useful method of coordinating multidisciplinary intervention, and it has the additional advantages of promoting team cohesion and efficient teamwork and facilitating good communication.

Additionally, McMillan and Sparkes (1999) suggested that further advantages may include:

- The clear documentation of rehabilitation aims
- An early focus on and consideration of discharge timing and destination
- The involvement of the patient and their family or carers in rehabilitation planning at the earliest possible stage
- Minimal staff training requirements

It can be challenging to introduce a goal-planning approach within acute stroke rehabilitation services. This is typically because of the focus on discharging patients from hospital as soon as possible, and because patients may have significant cognitive and communication problems. However, the above advantages of goal planning still apply. The initial longer-term focus for many patients is often, understandably, on recovery from physical disability, and in particular relearning to walk or to use an affected limb. However, even seemingly similar long-term goals can involve very different short-term goals requiring very different rehabilitative approaches. Goal planning can help patients and the multidisciplinary team to target specific barriers to longer term aims, and creates an environment in which such barriers may be more readily identifiable.

Patients may be reluctant to aim for challenging goals, or conversely may sometimes unrealistically be focused only on 'being exactly the same as I was before my stroke'. Setting and maintaining appropriate goals can therefore be challenging and require experienced leadership of the goal planning process. Goal planning can be a valuable approach to rehabilitation, and also provides an opportunity for service evaluation. Goal achievement (e.g. goals achieved, partially achieved or not achieved) is used by many rehabilitation services as the primary outcome measure (Bateman, 2009). Although this is very reasonable and appropriate, the multidisciplinary team must guard against the tendency to set only very easily achievable goals simply to provide encouragement for the patient or to demonstrate the effectiveness of the rehabilitation service. McMillan and Sparkes (1999) demonstrated that goal attainment can correlate well with objective measures of function or disability. However, not all goals are equal, and so this can be a simplistic and potentially misleading measure of outcome. More structured systems, such as goal attainment scaling, appear better proven than goal achievement (Hurn, Kneebone & Cropley, 2006), but may be too time intensive for routine use in clinical practice. The most balanced approach may be to use a combination of outcome measures (e.g. discharge destination, mobility, return to employment, independence in activities of daily living etc.), including goal achievement (Hurn *et al.*, 2006).

As yet, there is relatively little research evidence supporting the use of goal setting in neurorehabilitation (Levack, Taylor, Siegert, Dean, McPherson, & Weatherall, 2006). Holliday, Ballinger and Playford (2007) demonstrated that increased emphasis on the participation of patients in the goal setting process was preferred by patients, who subsequently perceived the rehabilitation process was more personally relevant to them. Unfortunately, there was no evidence in this study of any difference in patients' functional outcomes as compared with a standard goal setting process in which patients were not involved in goal planning. It should be noted that both of these interventions involved detailed, focused, multidisciplinary goal planning, which may be quite different to practice within some stroke rehabilitation services.

Examples of multidisciplinary intervention

In rehabilitation settings, collaborative multidisciplinary work enables patients to overcome their neuropsychological impairment by compensating for their acquired deficits. Some examples of collaborative multidisciplinary working are summarised in Table 10.3.

Working with families in neuropsychological rehabilitation

Oddy and Herbert (2003) examined the evidence base for family intervention in neuropsychological rehabilitation and concluded that, although there is a paucity of evidence concerning the effectiveness of family interventions, there is a significant literature highlighting the impact of brain damage on patients' families (see chapter 20). It makes intuitive sense to engage family members in the process of neuropsychological rehabilitation not only for the benefit of the patient, but also to ensure that the psychological needs of family members, who are often traumatised and struggling to adjust to the impact of brain damage on their loved one, are met. Within stroke services, there are practical reasons for engaging family members in the rehabilitation process, not least the fact that interventions initiated in stroke units can often only be maintained on discharge with the support of the patient's family.

Theoretical approaches to family intervention

As with neuropsychological rehabilitation more broadly, there are numerous psychological theories which can be used as the basis for family intervention in stroke services. Oddy and Herbert (2003) suggested that family intervention within neuropsychological rehabilitation can be informed by family systems, coping and cognitive-behavioural models. Theories of adjustment (e.g. Thompson, Sobolew-Shibin, Graham & Janigan, 1989), bereavement, grief and psycho-social transitions (e.g. Murray Parkes, 1971) also provide a framework within which to assess and formulate patients' and families' experiences. After stroke, themes of loss, adjustment and identity are highly relevant. In clinical practice,

Table 10.3 Case Examples of Multidisciplinary Working

Physiotherapy

Margaret, a 67-year-old woman on an inpatient stroke ward, was referred by her physiotherapist for becoming aggressive when practicing standing during treatment sessions. Margaret was reportedly friendly and cooperative when seated and in general conversation, but became hostile and abusive when physiotherapists attempted to help her stand. Psychological assessment revealed significant levels of anxiety, and neuropsychological assessment using visual screening (the CORVIST) and visuoperceptual assessment (the VOSP) highlighted some visuospatial impairment in the context of intact visual acuity and object perception. Observation of the physiotherapy sessions revealed a significant increase in anxiety precipitated by standing, which prompted Margaret's angry outbursts. Intervention, collaboratively agreed with Margaret, focused on anxiety management strategies (imagery and controlled breathing) and graded exposure, using positive reinforcement for small progress in each session (e.g. standing then immediately sitting down, then standing for a few seconds etc, then for a minute etc). Therapy progressed slowly, but crucially Margaret began to trust the physiotherapist, who consequently developed greater empathy with her. After several sessions, Margaret was engaging fully in her physiotherapy. Although the visuospatial impairment remained significant, she made functional progress and was able to continue to benefit from physiotherapy until her discharge from the inpatient unit.

Occupational therapy

Alfred, a 65-year-old man living at home, was referred by his community occupational therapist (OT). Alfred had been discharged from an inpatient stroke ward four months previously, three weeks after a partial anterior circulating artery stroke. The referral to the psychologist indicated that Alfred appeared to be unable to manage in the kitchen in his home, and his OT had some safety concerns. Although he presented as quite cognitively able in everyday conversation, Alfred became flustered and distressed when asked to show the OT how he made himself a cup of tea. A neuropsychological assessment was undertaken, which revealed largely intact language, visuo-perceptual and general intellectual functioning, but significant executive functioning impairment, with substantial qualitative evidence of distractibility and poor concentration. In particular, his performance on the Modified Six Elements task of the Behavioural Assessment of the Dysexecutive Syndrome highlighted very poor organisation and self-monitoring skills. Alfred's OT and the psychologist worked together with Alfred to introduce a number of rehabilitation strategies, including the use of clear labels on cupboards, and a series of laminated clear step-by-step logically sequenced instructions for the main kitchen tasks, such as making a cup of tea and making a sandwich. Over several sessions, the OT completed these tasks with Alfred, but gradually reduced her level of supervision and instruction. After several sessions, Alfred was able to undertake the key kitchen tasks safely and with minimal prompting, by relying on his instructions, ticking off the subtasks with a washable-ink pen as he undertook the tasks. Family members were included in the later sessions in order that in the future Alfred could increase the number of kitchen tasks without compromising safety. He remained dependent on the written instructions but was more confident and functionally able than prior to the neuropsychological assessment and intervention.

Table 10.3 (*Continued*)

Speech and language therapy

John, a 74-year-old man recently admitted to a stroke rehabilitation unit, was referred by his speech and language therapist due to concerns over his mood and apparent reluctance to engage in speech and language assessment for hesitant speech. An initial psychological assessment focused on mood, which revealed mild depressive symptoms, but also raised the suspicion of cognitive difficulties. A short battery of neuropsychological tests was administered, including the Raven's Progressive Matrices, National Adult Reading Test, Doors and People test, Brixton Test, Controlled Oral Word Association Test and Graded Naming Test. The results revealed severe memory and general intellectual impairment. Collateral history was obtained from the John's daughter, which revealed a history of possible memory difficulties for the past five years. CT imaging was inconclusive, suggesting moderate generalised cerebral atrophy probably consistent with his age in addition to the identified stroke lesion. A diagnosis of possible dementia was made by the consultant physician working within the MDT, subject to repeat neuropsychological assessment at six months, functional assessment and community rehabilitation team follow-up. Neuropsychological follow-up, with the potential for speech and language therapy and occupational therapy support, was arranged for six months after his stoke, in order to try to establish the potential for errorless learning strategies to help John maintain his knowledge of key people and places in his local village.

Nursing

Annie, a 62-year-old woman admitted several weeks previously to an inpatient stroke unit, was referred by nursing staff due to her reportedly being difficult to engage and hostile. Described as prone to lashing out at staff, Annie had developed a reputation for being a 'problem patient'. Initial assessment by brief interview with Annie and with several nurses, together with observation of her interactions with staff, suggested several possible hypotheses for the development and maintenance of the 'difficult behaviour'. Brief neuropsychological assessment utilising screening measures revealed significant expressive language impairment, impaired information processing speed and some right-sided visual inattention. The initial formulation was that Annie, a previously very independent and successful businesswoman, was struggling to communicate her needs to the nursing staff.

The staff felt too busy to spend the time needed to communicate effectively, and became more reluctant to engage with Annie due to her episodes of lashing out. These events were relatively infrequent, and appeared to have been precipitated by frustration and misunderstandings during care tasks, such as washing and dressing. Despite this, staff had begun to avoid working with Annie, which led to increased isolation and frustration, exacerbating her tendency to become frustrated with staff.

Intervention involved collaborative work between Annie, the speech and language therapist, nursing staff and the psychologist. A vertical picture board was developed to facilitate communication, and guidelines were established about interactions with Annie, emphasising the importance of patience and facilitating choice, while at the same time making sure that Annie and all staff working with her were safe. Staff training with the psychologist was also arranged to discuss working with patients with communication, cognitive and perceptual difficulties. One session focused on the importance of avoiding the understandable tendency for staff to sometimes label patients as 'difficult' or 'a problem patient'. Nursing staff reported that the sessions helped them to reappraise their interactions with patients and to cope with their own emotional responses to challenging behaviour. Annie made good progress in rehabilitation, and there were no further episodes of lashing out at staff.

some families can benefit significantly from the opportunity to discuss their feelings about the patient's stroke in a supportive group environment. Others simply need information about stroke, rehabilitation and community services. A minority of families require more substantial psychological intervention, and a key challenge within stroke services is in establishing which families require which level of input. Family intervention often provides the psychologist with an opportunity to work preventatively. The role of the psychologist within stroke services is not just to react to psychological distress, but also to try to prevent this wherever possible. Family intervention often allows the psychologist to facilitate the patient's adjustment to their stroke by engaging family members in rehabilitation strategies which can be continued by the family indefinitely.

Practical family engagement in stroke rehabilitation

Most stroke services have limited access to formal family therapy, and so the psychologist may have to rely on brief psycho-education or counselling intervention and support group work when working with families. The most useful first step is simply to meet with the patient and their family members in order to explain the patient's diagnosis and to discuss the process of rehabilitation. At this stage, ideally the patient and family should be engaged in the goal setting process so that the patient, rehabilitation team and the family are all invested in working towards the same end goal. As rehabilitation progresses, review meetings involving the patient and family should occur regularly, and especially whenever obstacles to rehabilitation are identified. In addition to family engagement in the rehabilitation process, some individual family members may benefit from counselling intervention at some point during the patient's rehabilitation. Although within many services there may be no scope to offer this level of support, this need can be met with support group interventions. Evidence for the effectiveness of such interventions is limited at present, although it is likely that early identification of and intervention for family members at risk of carer strain may help prevent significant psychological distress in patients and their family members (Blake & Lincoln, 2000).

Pitfalls of family engagement

As with any clinical intervention, there is always the potential for unforeseen problems to arise which can impede a patient's rehabilitation. There are various risks associated with family engagement in rehabilitation which should be anticipated, so that the impact of such problems can be minimised. Most of these problems can be avoided by careful assessment of the patient and their family at an early stage and patient and family engagement in goal planning. Effective communication is always vital, and is usually all that is needed to avert breakdown in collaborative working. It is important to manage the expectations of the patient and their family from the first meeting onwards. It is reasonable to adopt a stance of realistic optimism, in order to maintain the patient's motivation. However, unrealistic goals can simply set the patient up for failure, which can precipitate a major setback in rehabilitation. Equally, setting goals that are below the aspirations of the patient can undermine confidence and create frustration.

Occasionally, patients and their families will disagree with the philosophy of rehabilitation, particularly if the emphasis shifts from recovery to compensation. Conflict regarding individual therapy interventions, such as physiotherapy, is best avoided through patient and family involvement in goal setting and monitoring. If therapists believe that the patient has reached a plateau in recovery, this should be sensitively discussed with the patient and family. Patients and their family members can become frustrated with perceived slow progress, and occasionally this can lead to conflict between the patient and their family members. Counselling intervention exploring issues, such as role change, identity and relationships, can help to alleviate conflict and help the patient and family to refocus on maximising the patient's rehabilitation potential. A typology for the involvement of carers in treatment has been developed and may prove of use to the rehabilitation team (Dempster, Knapp & House, 1998).

Finally, it is worth recognising that some people who have a stroke and find themselves in rehabilitation do not necessarily feel motivated to engage in rehabilitation. This can be in the absence of any mood disorder, cognitive impairment or insight difficulties. In such circumstances, the patient's refusal to consent to therapy or rehabilitation should be respected, and the patient's family should be made aware, where possible, of the reasoning behind any decision not to persevere with rehabilitation.

Conclusions

Neuropsychological rehabilitation after stroke can maximise a patient's recovery from stroke, enhance their quality of life and facilitate the patient's re-engagement in their home, work and leisure activities. Several models of neuropsychological rehabilitation can inform the interventions provided within stroke services, all emphasising the importance of collaborative person-centred goal planning and the involvement of family members in the rehabilitative process. The psychologist's role within neuropsychological rehabilitation includes mood and neuropsychological assessment and the facilitation of cognitive rehabilitation strategies. However, given sufficient time and resources, neuropsychological rehabilitation can be much more than this, and can transform the stroke patient's rehabilitation potential across the patient pathway from the hyperacute stage to many years after community rehabilitation.

Chapter 11

Cognitive Rehabilitation

Introduction

Cognitive rehabilitation comprises the provision of therapeutic activities to reduce the severity of a cognitive deficit through either restitution of function or through the teaching of techniques to reduce the effects of cognitive impairment on functional abilities using compensatory strategies. The treatment of cognitive deficits is important because of the effect of cognitive impairment on functional abilities (Barker-Collo & Feigin, 2006) and quality of life (Kwa, Limburg, & De Haan, 1996; Mitchell Kemp, Benito-Leon & Reuber, 2010; Nys, van Zandvoort, van der Worp, de Haan, de Kort, Jansen et al., 2006). Patients with neglect following a stroke, for instance, progress less well with rehabilitation and it affects long-term outcome in independence in activities of daily living and quality of life (Jehkonen, Ahonen, Dastidar, Koivisto, Laippala, Vilkki et al., 2000; Jehkonen, Laihosalo & Kettunen, 2006b; Paolucci, Antonucci, Guariglia, Magnotti, Pizzamiglio & Zoccolotti, 1996; Paolucci, Antonucci, Pratesi, Traballesi, Lubich & Grasso, 1998). Those with memory and executive problems also progress less well in rehabilitation (Hanks, Rapport, Millis & Deshpande, 1999; Hoffman & McKenna, 2001). Attentional problems have been found to be associated with poor recovery (Hyndman & Ashburn., 2003; Robertson, Ridgeway, Greenfield & Parr, 1997; Stapleton, Ashburn & Slack, 2001; Hyndman, Pickering & Ashburn, 2008). Those with apraxia perform less well in activities of daily living than those without (Goldenberg, Daumuller & Hagman, 2001; Hanna-Pladdy, Heilman & Foundas, 2003; Sundet, Finsett & Reinvang, 1988; Walker, Sunderland, Sharma & Walker, 2004), and apraxia has a negative impact on functional abilities (Sunderland & Shinner, 2007). Variations between studies probably depend on the sensitivity

Psychological Management of Stroke, First Edition. Nadina B. Lincoln, Ian I. Kneebone, Jamie A.B. Macniven and Reg C. Morris.
© 2012 John Wiley & Sons, Ltd. Published 2012 by John Wiley & Sons, Ltd.

of the measures used to assess both cognitive abilities and outcomes, the timing of the outcome measurement and the criteria for selecting participants, but the general message emerging is that cognitive abilities are important predictors of functional outcome.

There are two main treatment strategies, restitution and compensation. The mechanism behind restitution is that the brain has plasticity of function, and that with appropriate timing, type and frequency of input, connections within the brain may be re-established (Robertson & Murre, 1999). By providing activities within a specific cognitive domain, the firing of cells will lead to increased connectivity (Robertson & Murre, 1999). The therapeutic activities need to be targeted so that they require the appropriate skills, and the more selective the activity the greater the chances of restoring the specific cognitive function. This requires a detailed neuropsychological assessment to identify the exact nature of the cognitive deficit. The effectiveness of treatment will depend on being able to provide a sufficient intensity of rehabilitation (Prigatano, 1999). In more severe lesions recovery of function does not occur, and but there is compensation by other brain areas taking over the lost functions (Robertson & Murre, 1999).

Compensatory strategies are designed to enable people to cope in daily life despite the cognitive impairment. The assessments to plan the treatment may be largely functional and not require the detailed identification of specific cognitive deficits. However, selecting the strategies likely to be effective does require a detailed knowledge of the pattern of impairment and the patients' specific strengths and weaknesses. As intact cognitive skills will be used in therapy to compensate for those that are impaired, it is important that those which are intact have been accurately identified. In some cases, compensatory strategies are used once attempts at restitution have been completed. In others, because these strategies tend to require less intensive treatment, they are used as the strategy of choice. Compensation is usually used once cognitive deficits are stable, but it may be appropriate to teach some strategies during the recovery phase so that they become well established early in rehabilitation. Also, some compensatory strategies require high levels of cognition in order for them to be used effectively, such as setting reminders on mobile phones, and therefore may need to be used when some recovery of cognitive abilities has occurred.

The delivery of cognitive rehabilitation in clinical practice is shared between psychologists, occupational therapists and speech and language therapists. The strategies used tend to be specific to the cognitive domains affected and therefore the speech and language therapists concentrate on language skills (see chapter 16), but because of the overlaps with memory, may also teach memory strategies. Occupational therapists and psychologists tend to provide rehabilitation for attention, memory and perceptual impairments, with the balance of provision varying between professions in different centres. Ideally any stroke service should have access to a neuropsychologist, to oversee the assessment and rehabilitation of cognitive deficits.

Evidence for effectiveness of cognitive rehabilitation after stroke

Techniques have been developed to deal with problems in all cognitive domains. Most of the evidence to support their effectiveness comes from single-case experimental design studies. Although these demonstrate that cognitive rehabilitation can improve functional outcomes, publication bias means that they give little indication of the overall effectiveness of the technique as used in clinical practice. In considering the effectiveness of cognitive rehabilitation, emphasis will be placed on results from randomised controlled trials where these are available.

Rehabilitation of visual neglect

Visual neglect is a common problem after right hemisphere stroke (see chapter 5). Like many cognitive impairments, it improves quickly over the first few weeks though many patients are left with residual problems (Jehkonen, Laihosalo, Koivisto, Dastidar & Ahonen, 2007; Kerkhoff & Rosetti, 2006). Strategies for the rehabilitation of visual neglect are probably the longest established and most comprehensively evaluated in cognitive rehabilitation. Treatments are classified into top-down approaches, in which patients are taught to compensate for their inattention, through increased scanning and the provision of external aids. Bottom-up approaches work on the principle that the underlying controlling factors that are responsible for the occurrence of spatial neglect, are modified (Parton, Malhotra & Husain, 2004; Pierce & Buxbaum, 2002). They include vestibular stimulation, optokinetic stimulation, neck vibration and alertness training. Some techniques involve both top-down and bottom-up strategies, such as limb activation training, while in clinical practice techniques are often combined so it is not clear which strategy is having an effect. Some suggest (Barrett, Buxbaum, Coslett, Edwards, Heilman, Hillis *et al.*, 2006) that top-down approaches on their own are unlikely to be sufficient to change a process which is due to 'a bottom-up stimulus driven deficit inaccessible to conscious, insight–oriented self-modification'. Several reviews have summarised the effectiveness of treatments for visual neglect (Barrett *et al.*, 2006; Bowen & Lincoln, 2007a, 2007b; Cappa, Benke, Clarke, Rossi, Stemmer & Heugten, 2005; Cicerone, Dahlberg, Malec, Langenbahn, Felicetti, Kneipp *et al.*, 2005; Lincoln & Bowen, 2006, Luaute, Halligan, Rode, Rossetti & Boisson, 2006; Manly, 2002).

A Cochrane review (Bowen & Lincoln, 2007b) found evidence that scanning training improved performance on standardised tests of neglect, but there was inadequate evidence to indicate whether or not there was an effect on functional abilities. Despite the lack of clear evidence to support its use, scanning training has become routine in some rehabilitation centres (Pizzamiglio, Fasotti,

Jehkonen, Antonucci, Magnotti, Boelen *et al.*, 2004; Schindler, Kerkhoff, Karnath, Keller & Goldenberg, 2002). Scanning training was first evaluated through a series of studies by Diller and colleagues from the Institute of Rehabilitation Medicine in New York (Diller & Weinberg, 1977, Weinberg, Diller, Gordon, Gertman, Liebermann, Lakin *et al.*, 1977). Patients were given regular practice on tasks which required them to scan the visual field. This included using a Diller board, in which there was an array of lights and patients were presented with one or more lights at a time and they were required to identify the light. Those with neglect tended to miss the lights on the left and had to be prompted to find them. The aim was to teach patients to be aware that they missed the left and to consciously scan the visual field. In addition scanning training usually involves practice on paper-and-pencil tasks which require people to work across the visual field, such as crossing out specific letters or words in page of text (Gordon, Hibbard, Egelko, Diller, Shaver, Lieberman *et al.*, 1985; Weinberg *et al.*, 1977; Weinberg, Diller, Gordon, Gerstman, Lieberman, Lakin *et al.*, 1979). The activities provide the therapist with opportunities to prompt patients to attend to the neglected side, with the aim that this behaviour will become more automatic, and for them to consciously use it as a strategy to compensate for their attentional failures. One problem in practice is that while patients improve during treatment sessions there is little generalisation to other activities. It has been observed that after actively reporting they must look to the left while doing treatment activities, patients bump into the door on their way out of the therapy room. Positive effects in scanning training studies have generally been found on measures that share characteristics with the training stimuli (Gordon *et al.*, 1985; Wagenaar, Van Wieringen, Netelenbos, Meijer & Kuik, 1992; Weinberg *et al.*, 1977). Many studies do not assess whether treatment effects generalise to daily life. Poor generalisation may be resolved by training patients on daily life tasks rather than relying on transfer effects from abstract tasks (Webster, McFarland, Rapport, Morrill, Roades & Abadee, 2001). However, despite the intuitive appeal of targeting real activities, this approach may be limited due to the range of activities requiring training (Manly, 2002). Scanning training is therefore most useful if the activities which patients require in daily life can be directly trained, such as reading and wheelchair navigation.

Limb activation training is based on the observation that left-sided inattention can be reduced by inducing patients to make movements with some part of their left side, such as arm or shoulder movements. The suggestion is that limb activation causes changes in lateral attention or spatial representation, whereas bilateral movements of both hands simultaneously abolish the beneficial effect of a single left movement by a left limb in the left hemisphere. Left-sided activation has been shown, using single-case experimental designs, to reduce neglect and improve functional abilities (Robertson, North & Geggie, 1992, Robertson & North, 1993, Robertson, Hogg & McMillan, 1998, Samuel, Louis-Dreyfus, Kaschel, Makiela, Troubat, Anselmi *et al.*, 2000). In a randomised controlled trial (Kalra, Perez, Gupta & Wittink, 1997), 50 stroke patients were randomly allocated to receive limb activation training or usual care. At 12 weeks after random allocation there were significant differences between the groups on some subtests of the Rivermead Perceptual Assessment Battery and the length of hospital stay was significantly shorter in the intervention group. Limb activation requires top-down processing in that patients need to initiate the movements in their left side, although automatic prompts may be provided. It has also been compared with scanning training in individual patients. For example, Worthington (1996) described a 60-year-old retired community nurse with visual inattention and neglect dyslexia after a right hemisphere stroke. An ABACA single-case experimental design was used, in which following baseline (phase A) treatment involved visuo-motor cueing to promote scanning (phase B) and, after reversal to baseline limb activation (phase C), a spatio-motor cueing strategy. The patient improved in reading ability with both treatments but the limb activation only produced an immediate effect on word reading, whereas scanning training produced benefits which were maintained 18 months after intervention. Limb activation has also been combined with scanning training in order to optimise the effects of both treatments (Brunila, Lincoln, Lindell, Tenovuo & Hämäläinen, 2002). ABA designs were used to evaluate treatment in four stroke patients. In the intervention phase patients were given four one-hour sessions a week for three weeks, and the effects were monitored on measures of visual inattention. Three patients showed improvement in article reading, and all showed some improvement on three cancellation tests. Unfortunately, the effects on daily life were not assessed in this study.

Other top-down approaches which manipulate visual input and thereby make patients more aware of their impairment are eye patching and hemi-spatial goggles (Arai, Ohi, Sasaki, Nobuto & Tanaka, 1997; Beis, Andre, Baumgarten & Challier, 1999; Rossi, Kheyfets & Reding, 1990; Zeloni, Farne & Baccinni, 2002). Patching the left eye can make patients aware of a reduced visual field and therefore they compensate for the loss by turning their head. Although patients have been demonstrated to benefit on measures of impairment, the effectiveness of the techniques seems to vary (Manly, 2002) and improvement in functional outcome has not been demonstrated. Similarly Fresnel prisms have been used to deflect the peripheral image from the left more centrally, thus reducing the extent of the neglected visual field. Although early versions of prisms were unsightly and cumbersome, stick on versions are available which can be attached to a patients ordinary glasses or a pair of reading glasses. The advantage of prism adaptation and hemi-spatial goggles are that they are non-invasive, require minimum supervision and do not require the voluntary orientation of attention to the neglected side. Prisms are also used as a bottom-up strategy to induce automatic adaptation. The basis is that people learn to compensate for wearing prisms but adjusting their internal spatial coordinates. This adaptation persists after removal of the prisms and can produce short-term reductions in neglect (Frassinetti, Angeli, Meneghello, Avanzi & Ladavas, 2002; Rossetti, Rode, Pisella, Farne, Li, Boisson *et al.*, 1998). However, longer term effects (Frasinetti *et al.*, 2002) have not been found. Only a few studies have examined the effect of prism adaptation on functional outcomes, though some (Keane, Turner, Sherrington & Beard, 2006) have found improvements in functional ability. Nys, de Haan, Kunneman, de Kort and Dijkerman (2008) compared prism adaptation, in which patients wore goggles inducing a 10^0 optical shift as compared with an attention placebo control in which they wore goggles with no field shift. Treatment was for four sessions, once a day for four days, while practising reaching tasks. Nys *et al.* (2008) found a beneficial effect of prisms on cancellation and line bisection but not copying or representational drawing. However, these effects did not persist a month after treatment. In a recent trial (Turton, O'Leary, Gabb, Woodward & Gilchrist, 2009), patients were randomly allocated to prism adaptation or sham treatment for 10 sessions in two weeks. The effects of intervention were highly variable and there was no evidence of any significant benefit on either a measure of visual inattention (Behavioural Inattention Test) or functional abilities (Catherine Bergego scale). One potential advantage of prisms is that they can be worn during functional activities rather than during artificial tasks, such a practising reaching, and can be worn for long periods of time. They would be providing a compensatory mechanism rather than remapping people's internal representation of space. However, apart from the early study by Rossi, Kheyfets and Reding (1990), they have not been applied in this way and have usually been used as a treatment delivered in specific sessions.

Bottom-up treatment strategies aim to remap the representation of space using sensory stimulation. These include caloric stimulation (Rode, Charles, Perenin, Vighetto, Trillet & Aimard, 1992) in which the patient's ear on the affected side is irrigated with cold water, and optokinetic stimulation (Pizzamiglio, Frasca, Guariglia, Inoccia & Antonucci, 1990; Pizzamiglio, Fasotti, Jehkonen, Antonucci, Magnotti, Boelen *et al.*, 2004; Thimm, Fink, Küst, Karbe, Wilmes & Sturm, 2009) in which a black and white pattern is moved across a computer screen from the ipsilesional to contralateral side to induce pursuit eye movements. Other sensory stimulation strategies include neck muscle vibration (Schindler *et al.*, 2002) and transcutaneous electrical stimulation (Polanowska, Seniow, Paprot, Lesniak & Czlonkowska, 2009; Rusconi, Meinecke, Sbrissa & Bernardini, 2002) in which an electrical stimulus is applied to the muscles of the neck, shoulder or hand on the affected side. Alertness training (Sturm, Thimm, Kuest, Karbe & Fink, 2006; Thimm, Fink, Kust, Karbe & Sturm, 2006) comprises practice on computerised attentional tasks, in some cases with the simultaneous presentation of a loud noise as an alerting stimulus. Evidence for the effectiveness of these treatments mainly comes from single-case experimental designs or examining patients with chronic visuospatial inattention, such that improvement would not be expected due to spontaneous recovery (Thimm *et al.*, 2006, 2009). Studies have shown improvements in measures of inattention, but few have evaluated the effects of treatment on measures of functional ability. A few studies have compared treatments. Kerkhoff, Keller, Ritter and Marquardt (2006) compared five patients who received optokinetic stimulation with five who received scanning training and found greater improvement on measures of inattention in those receiving optokinetic stimulation. A comparison of these approaches in a randomised controlled trial (Schröder, Wist & Hömberg, 2008) indicated that they can be combined with visual scanning training. Thirty patients with visual neglect following a first right hemisphere stroke were randomly allocated to receive 20 sessions over four weeks of either transcutaneous electrical stimulation and visual exploration therapy, optokinetic stimulation and visual exploration therapy or visual exploration therapy alone. Both stimulation methods produced significantly better performance on reading and writing tasks, but there were no significant differences on neglect tests. Follow-up only lasted one week so the long-term effects remain unknown. In a similar study, Polanowska *et al.* (2009) compared left-hand somatosensory stimulation combined with scanning training and sham stimulation with scanning training in 40 stroke patients. Following a month of treatment, patients in the electrostimulation group made significantly fewer errors on cancellation tasks but there were no significant differences in personal self-care, as assessed on the Barthel Index. However, the findings of these two studies support the suggestion (Barrett *et al.*, 2006) that bottom-up approaches may enhance the effects of top-down approaches, such as scanning training.

In clinical practice scanning and limb activation are most likely to be the initial therapy of choice. They do, however, require intensive treatment, as the effectiveness seems to be greater with intensive programmes and giving infrequent sessions is probably not worthwhile. Such sessions may be delivered as a specific training or incorporated into occupational therapy sessions (Edmans Webster & Lincoln, 2000). This approach may be supplemented by the use of Fresnel prisms or electrocutaneous stimulation, but any technique should be evaluated used single-case methodology, as patients seem to respond very differently. This may be due to different types of neglect or lesion locations (see chapter 4), but so far the relation between these factors and treatment effectiveness remains uncertain. The most practical application of top-down approaches is through transcutaneous electrical stimulation. However, it remains to be established whether any benefits persist long enough after the end of treatment to have an effect on daily life.

A case example is provided in Table 11.1.

Memory rehabilitation

Memory rehabilitation also uses both restitution and compensation approaches, although the latter is much more common in clinical practice. Restitution is concerned with improving memory ability though strategies such as rehearsal, chunking and attention retraining. Compensation approaches have focussed on teaching patients to use internal aids (such as mnemonics and mental imagery) and external memory aids (such as diaries, notice boards and lists) to help them remember and recall information.

Table 11.1 Case Example of Treatment of Visual Neglect

Angela was a 64-year-old woman who suffered right partial anterior circulation infarction, leaving her with left-sided weakness, sensory loss, homonymous hemianopia and inattention. Her progress with physiotherapy and occupational therapy had been limited, and she was referred by a social worker because of poor adjustment. As a result of the visual inattention, she was unable to engage in her previously enjoyed activity of reading and refused to join in Bingo. Baseline cognitive assessment showed average premorbid function based on the WTAR (predicted IQ 96–98). Her visual inattention was evident on the WASI Block Design and RBANS coding. On subtests of the BIT she identified 29% of targets on star cancellation, 31% on letter cancellation and 50% on line cancellation. Generally she appeared inattentive and often gazed round the room. An ABA design was used to evaluate the effects of scanning training. Each phase lasted two weeks, and the intervention comprised eight sessions of one-hour length. The tests showed relatively stable baselines and improvement following intervention, with improvement on three measures (Albert's test, Letter cancellation and Hair brushing) being maintained at follow-up two weeks after intervention. Results of the intervention are shown in Figures 11.1 and 11.2.

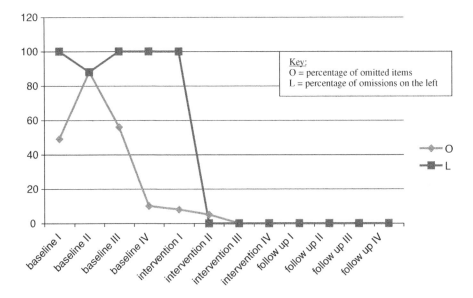

Figure 11.1 Results of Albert's test across sessions

There was a reduction in overall omissions from the second intervention session, and a reduction in omissions to the left of the right section, although these baselines showed some variability in performance prior to the intervention. Nevertheless, the gains were maintained at follow-up. The number of targets achieved to the left shows a very stable baseline followed by an improvement throughout the intervention and part way through the follow-up. However, there was no evidence of any effect of the treatment on reading,

(*Continued*)

Table 11.1 *(Continued)*

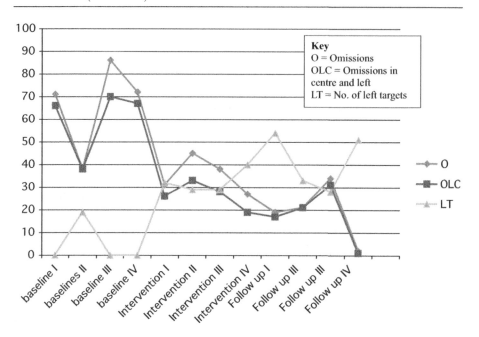

Figure 11.2 Results on letter cancellation across sessions

as assessed on the Indented Paragraph test. This may be due to the short duration of treatment, but as other measures showed improvement this seems unlikely. Functionally, it was noted at follow-up three months later that she was now engaging in Bingo at the care home, a previously enjoyed activity not engaged in since her stroke. Also, she was washing the whole of her body in the bath and brushing all of her hair, when previously she had only washed and brushed the right side.

Restitution approaches have been evaluated in stroke patients. Doornhein and De Haan (1998) compared memory strategy training on memory tasks that were practised during training (targeted memory tasks, forgetting names and remembering routes) and memory tasks that were not specifically practised (control memory tasks, auditory list learning and face recognition learning). They recruited 12 stroke patients who complained of memory problems and had evidence of memory impairment on neuropsychological testing. Treatment was two sessions a week for four weeks. Participants who received the training programme performed significantly better than those in the control group on the trained memory tasks but not on the control memory tasks; no differences were observed on subjective ratings of everyday memory functions.

Imagery training has also been evaluated in a mixed-aetiology group of patients. Kaschel, Della Sala, Cantagallo, Fahlböck, Laaksonen and Kazen (2002) compared a group of nine patients who received training in the use of visual imagery mnemonics with a group of 12 who received memory rehabilitation as part of their usual care. Participants were assessed at pre-baseline, at baseline, immediately post intervention and at three-month follow-up on general memory, domain-specific memory tests, and tests tapping other cognitive domains, such as attention. The results for the mixed-aetiology group as a whole suggested that the use of imagery mnemonics significantly improved performance on delayed recall of verbal material, such as stories and appointments, and observer-rated reports of memory failures. There was no significant improvement in scores on the Wechsler Memory Scale, Rivermead Behavioural Memory Test (RBMT) total score, or the self-report measure on the Memory Assessment Clinics (MAC) Rating Scale for the imagery group. However, while stroke-specific analyses were similar to these findings, they did not reach statistical significance (das Nair & Lincoln, 2007). Although the authors concluded that imagery mnemonics improved everyday memory performance for the group as a whole, this was not apparent from the stroke data.

Technological advances have facilitated the use of external aids, such as pagers (Wilson, Emslie & Evans, 2001), mobile phones (Wade & Troy, 2001), palmtops (Kim, 2000), voice organisers (Van den Broek, Downes, Johnson, Dayus & Hilton, 2000) and virtual environments (Rose, Attree, Parslow, Leadbetter & McNeil, 1999), to reduce patients' memory and planning problems. There is evidence to suggest that these improve everyday life functioning in studies with mixed-aetiology groups of patients including some patients with stroke (Cicerone *et al.*, 2005; Wilson, Emslie & Evans, 2001). However, there is evidence to suggest that those with stroke may respond less well to compensatory training than those with traumatic brain injury (Fish, Manly, Emslie, Evans & Wilson, 2008). Fish *et al.* (2008) analysed the results of a controlled trial (Wilson *et al.*, 2001) to evaluate training to use a pager. Stroke patients increased the percentage of target behaviours successfully completed and recorded in a diary following provision of a pager, but in contrast to patients with traumatic brain injury, gains were not maintained once the pager was taken away. Factors differentiating the stroke and traumatic brain injury groups were age, time since onset and the presence of executive deficits. Fish *et al.* (2008) examined the relation between these factors and maintenance of benefits of treatment, and found that in the traumatic brain injury group (n = 30), the score on the Six Elements test from the Behavioural Assessment of the Dysexecutive Syndrome, a measure of executive deficits, was associated with maintenance of benefit, but these factors were not significantly correlated with maintenance of benefit in the stroke group (n = 20). This may be due to differences in sample size. However, the findings do suggest that stroke patients may not benefit as much from external aids as those with traumatic brain injury.

In clinical practice, memory rehabilitation is often delivered in a group setting. This has the advantage of efficiency, but also it provides patients with an opportunity to learn from each other. Jennett and Lincoln (1991) compared a group for people with memory problems with a waiting list control in a cross-over study. There were no significant effects of treatment on the River-mead Behavioural Memory Test or the Everyday Memory Questionnaire, although there were significant reductions in the extent to which patients felt 'bothered' by their reported memory problems. There was a significant increase in the number of memory aids being used following treatment. Participants included those with both head injury and stroke, but there was no separate analysis for the stroke patients. Thickpenny-Davis and Barker-Collo (2007) also evaluated a memory group for people with traumatic brain injury or stroke. The results suggested that attending the group produced greater improvement on memory tests, relatives' ratings of the use of memory aids and strategies and knowledge about memory, than occurred in a waiting list control. However, there was no direct comparison of improvement with treatment to that while on the waiting list, so the specific effects of attending the group are unclear. Although it demonstrates that the intervention is appropriate for stroke patients, the efficacy for stroke patients remains unknown as there was only one patient with a stroke in each group. A similar problem arises in relation to an evaluation of a group intervention programme by Nair (Nair 2007; das Nair & Lincoln, submitted). Das Nair and Lincoln (submitted) compared restitution and compensation approaches, with a self-help group focussing on managing emotional problems as a control group. Patients were randomly allocated to the three types of group intervention and treated for ten sessions over three months. Comparison of the overall outcomes showed both treatment strategies improved patients on the use of internal memory aids but analysis of the 17 patients with stroke showed no significant benefits in this subgroup. However, this may be an effect of sample size and lack of evidence for effectiveness does not indicate the intervention was ineffective. The treatment was appropriate for those with stroke, and qualitative feedback from participants indicted that patients found it useful (Nair, 2007).

Although there have been trials to justify the provision of memory rehabil-itation for people with traumatic brain injury, the evidence for stoke is not as strong. Cicerone *et al.* (2000) suggested that the evidence for compensatory memory retraining with participants with mild memory problems was 'compelling enough to recommend it as a Practice Standard', and that there was no evidence to suggest that cognitive remediation aids in restoring memory function in participants with severe memory problems. However, in their updated review (Cicerone *et al.*, 2005), teaching patients to use external memory aids (including assistive devices) with direct application to functional activities was recommended as a 'practice guideline in subjects with moderate or severe memory impairment'. Similarly a report of a European Federation of Neuro-logical Societies task force (Cappa *et al.*, 2005) concluded that electronic external memory devices were probably effective but there was insufficient evidence to recommend other memory rehabilitation strategies. A Cochrane review (das Nair & Lincoln, 2007, 2008) found insufficient evidence to support or refute the effectiveness of memory rehabilitation in stroke patients.

A case example of memory rehabilitation is given in Table 11.2.

Table 11.2 Case Example of Treatment of Memory Problems

Brian was a 34-year-old man who had a left hemisphere stroke resulting in a right hemiplegia and mild aphasia. He was employed as a police officer before his stroke, and believed the stress of this contributed to the stroke happening. He made a good recovery from his hemiplegia and aphasia but reported persistent problems with memory. He had not resumed work at the time of starting treatment. He was referred for memory rehabilitation because he felt his memory difficulties were such that he would not be able to cope at work. At interview he reported problems in daily life with remembering to do things and forgetting peoples' names, including people he'd known for years. He also reported losing or forgetting things around the house. He used a diary to help cope with these difficulties and relied on his wife to remind him of things. His mood was within the normal range on the General Health Questionnaire 28. On formal cognitive testing he was of average premorbid ability on the NART. He obtained a maximum score on the Sheffield Screening test for Acquired Language Disorders. He was also within the average range on test of executive function, Trail Making and Stroop. On the RBMT-E he had a profile score of 2, which is average, but memory problems were identified on the Doors and People test with scores for visual memory, recall and recognition all lower than predicted from his premorbid level. On the Everyday Memory Questionnaire 28, he reported losing things round the house, forgetting when things happened, forgetting to take things with him, having a word on the tip of his tongue and forgetting where things were kept. His score of 29 was indicative of impairment of memory in daily life. He attended a memory rehabilitation group, which was run once a week for 10 weeks. In group sessions he was always well motivated, attending every week, and was open to ideas about what he was being asked to do, giving everything a go before deciding whether it was right for him or not. He seemed to be good at digit recall during chunking tasks but was less successful with lists of words. He found inventing a story to recall items on a shopping list very helpful and applied this to other lists of things to do. On reassessment three months later, all scores on the Doors and People test were within the average range and his EMQ score was 13 which is also within the average range. These improvements were maintained three months following the end of treatment. In terms of his daily life he was able to return to part-time employment with the police, cataloguing evidence.

Rehabilitation of attention and executive impairment

Attention is a prerequisite to many cognitive tasks and deficits in attention may underlie apparent problems with both memory and visual inattention. Attentional deficits recover over time (Hochstenbach, Den Otter & Mulder, 2003), but the detailed pattern of recovery has not been established. Attempts to retrain attention skills have relied on a restitution approach. Although there have been several well-designed studies of attention retraining in patients with traumatic brain injury (Niemann, Ruff & Baser 1990; Novack, Caldwell, Duke, Bergquist & Gage, 1996) and in mixed-aetiology groups (Gray, Robertson, Pentland & Anderson, 1992), there seem to be few studies specific to attentional deficits after stroke. A Cochrane review (Lincoln, Majid & Weyman, 2000) identified two studies of attention retraining after stroke (Schoettke, 1997; Sturm & Wilmes,

1991). Schoetke (1997) compared 16 stroke patients receiving attention train-ing with a control group of 13 patients who received standard rehabilitation. Training improved sustained attention, as measured on the Zahlen-Verbindungs-Test of concentration, but had no significant effect on functional abilities as assessed on the Barthel Index. Sturm and Wilmes (1991) evaluated training on computerised reaction training tasks. Comparison of early and late training in left hemisphere damaged stroke patients showed that attention training improved alertness and sustained attention, but there were no signif-icant effects on vigilance and no evidence of generalisation to verbal and nonverbal cognitive tests. A subsequent study (Sturm, Wilmes & Orgass, 1997) suggested this may be due to lack of consideration of all relevant aspects of attention. In a single-case series with 38 stroke patients, Sturm *et al.* (1997) found alertness and vigilance improved significantly more in response to specific training in alertness or vigilance, than to training on selective or divided attention. These results suggest that the effects of attention retraining are largely specific to the attentional skills being trained. In clinical practice this would require a clear classification of the nature of the attentional deficit. Training was also provided relatively intensively (14 hours in 3 weeks) and less intensive treatment may not be effective. The strongest evidence to support attention retraining comes from a randomised controlled trial of Attention Process Training (Barker-Collo, Feigin, Lawes, Parag, Senior & Rodgers, 2009). Barker-Collo *et al.* (2009) randomly allocated 78 stroke patients with impair-ments of attention to receive 30 hours of treatment or usual care control and found that attention training significantly improved outcomes on a measure of attention. There was a trend to suggest generalisation to everyday life as there was a difference between the groups on the Cognitive Failures Questionnaires, though this just failed to reach statistical significance ($p = 0.07$). It does, however, indicate that training of this type may be beneficial to stroke patients and should be investigated further.

Rehabilitation of executive problems has been less thoroughly investigated, even though executive problems are common after stroke (see chapter 4; Zinn, Bosworth, Hoenig & Swartzwelder, 2007). Although there are studies of the effects of cognitive rehabilitation for executive problems in traumatic brain injury (Cicerone, Levin, Malec, Stuss & Whyte, 2006) and in mixed-aetiology patients (Rath, Simon, Langenbahn, Sherr & Diller, 2003; Von Cramon, Matthes-von Cramon & Mai, 1991; Worthington, 2005) which indicate treat-ment can be effective, there is relatively little evidence specific to stroke patients. Problem solving training (von Cramon *et al.*, 1991) improved planning and behavioural measures in a group of 61 acquired brain injury patients, including 21 with stroke, who were identified on the basis of cognitive assessment as being poor problem solvers. Patients were alternately allocated to either problem solving training or memory training, which has the advantage of providing a realistic attention placebo control. The treatment was intensive (25 sessions in five weeks) and is also described in detail (von Cramon & Cramon, 1992). There were significant improvements in problem solving in the problem solving training group but not in the memory rehabilitation control group. Also, behavioural ratings showed significant improvement following problem solving training in contrast to memory rehabilitation. However, there was marked variability in the response to treatment and long-term functional outcomes were not assessed.

Levine, Robertson, Clare, Carter, Hong, Wilson *et al.* (2000) evaluated the effectiveness of goal management training, a problem solving intervention, on successful task completion. Participants received either one hour of goal management training or one hour of motor skills training. Goal management training was associated with improved performance on paper-and-pencil measures intended to simulate everyday activities. However, treatment was for only one hour, which may have limited its effectiveness, and the long-term benefits and effects on daily life were not assessed. However, a single-case report (Schweizer, Levine, Rewilak, O'Connor, Turner, Alexander *et al.*, 2008) with a patient with executive problems due to cerebellar damage suggested that seven two-hour sessions of goal management training enabled a patient to return to work as a result of increased awareness of situations in which he was likely to produce errors, realising the need to double check his work and staying focused on what he wanted to achieve. They attributed the gains to treatment rather than spontaneous recovery, as the patient was four months after stroke onset at the time that rehabilitation began. However, the data on recovery of executive problems after stroke are sparse, and it is not clear whether this interpretation is justified.

External cues have been used as prompts to regulate behavioural problems associated with executive impairments (Manly, Davison, Gaynord, Greenfield, Parr, Ridgeway *et al.*, 2004; Manly, Hawkins, Evans, Woldt & Robertson, 2002). Fish, Evans, Nimmo, Martin, Kersel, Bateman *et al.* (2007) evaluated the effect of linking a cue phrase 'STOP', an acronym for stop, think, organise and plan, with pausing current activity and reviewing goals. Patients with poor prospective memory following nonprogressive brain injury, including stroke, were included in the study. Patients were set the task of making a telephone call, at a specified time, to a voicemail service four times a day over three weeks. After a week baseline, patients were given one 30-minute training session, based on goal management training (Levine *et al.*, 2000), to teach them to use the executive review strategy. In the following two weeks, on five days (randomly allocated) the text message cue 'STOP' was provided and on five days it was not provided. The cues were sent eight times a day, determined at random with the constraint that they were not within an hour of a call time so that they did not directly prompt the target behaviour, they were also not within 15 minutes of each other or outside of working hours. There was a highly significant effect of cueing on the number of target calls made and the accuracy of timing of the calls. The study indicated that cues do not necessarily need to be task specific and can be content free. This is an advantage in terms of treating executive problems, in which the problem is in the way tasks are carried out in daily life rather than affecting discrete activities. However, the cue was closely linked to the task (i.e. a text message cue to use a 'phone'), so although content free in that they did not explicitly remind the patient to make a phone call, they were visually and spatially linked.

One of the clinical manifestations of executive impairment is lack of insight and lack of awareness of cognitive problems. This lack of awareness has been addressed in a group treatment programme (Ownsworth, McFarland & Young, 2000) with a group of 21 patients with acquired brain injury, three with stroke. The group treatment programme comprised a combination of cognitive-behavioural therapy, cognitive rehabilitation and social skills training. It included problem solving, guided self-reflection, relaxation, role play, developing compensatory strategies and practice of new behaviours. The group met once a week for 90 minutes over 16 weeks. The outcome assessment six months after baseline assessment indicated that patients improved in social interaction, alertness behaviour, emotional behaviour and communication skills. They also developed self-regulation skills, which Ownsworth *et al.* (2000) suggested was the main determinant of the maintenance of the gains achieved.

Thus although the evidence is not robust it does seem that executive problems are amenable to intervention. Given the negative impact they have on rehabilitation and long-term outcomes, attempts should be made to ameliorate these difficulties.

Rehabilitation of apraxia

Apraxia tends to improve over time (Smania, Girardi, Domenciali, Lora & Aglioti, 2000; Sunderland, 2000), but many patients are left with residual difficulties which do not recover (Basso, Capitani, Dellasala, Laiacona & Spinnler, 1987). Treatment is therefore designed to increase the speed of recovery and the level of ability reached.

Smania *et al.* (2000) conducted a partially randomised controlled trial to compare the effectiveness of training in using gestures and demonstrating object use with a control group, which received conventional aphasia therapy, in 13 patients with limb apraxia after left hemisphere stroke. The treatment involved practice on those activities which patients found to be difficult and therefore seemed to be based on the principles of restitution. There was no significant improvement on measures of apraxia in the group receiving conventional aphasia therapy, whereas those receiving treatment for apraxia improved on measures of both ideational and ideomotor apraxia. However, there was no direct comparison between the two groups. A subsequent study with 33 stroke patients (Smania, Aglioti, Girardi, Tinazzi, Fiaschi, Cosentino *et al.*, 2006) randomly allocated patients to strategy training or aphasia rehabilitation for 30 treatment sessions of 50 minutes. Outcomes were assessed blind to the intervention. Patients who received treatment improved significantly more on measures of ideomotor apraxia, gesture comprehension and importantly also increased their independence in activities of daily living.

In a larger trial with 113 stroke patients, Donkervoort, Dekker, Stehmann-Saris & Deellman (2001) compared strategy training integrated into occupational therapy with conventional occupational therapy. Strategy training involved teaching patients to verbalise while carrying out activities of daily living and they were assisted by writing down or showing pictures of the proper sequence of activities. The aim was to gradually teach the patient more efficient strategies. Subsequent comparison of trained and untrained tasks (Geusgens, van Heugten, Donkervoort, van den Ende, Jolles & van den Heuvel, 2006) showed that most improvement occurred on trained tasks, but that improvements in untrained tasks were greater following strategy training than in the control group, suggesting better generalisation following strategy training.

A review of the evidence for the rehabilitation of apraxia after stroke (Bowen West, Hesketh & Vail, 2009; West, Bowen, Heskethh & Vail, 2008) concluded that there was some evidence for an effect of intervention on functional performance at the end of the intervention period, but there was no lasting difference at six months after stroke. However, the number of studies was small, and the study by Geusgens *et al.* (2006) was not included in the review. Despite these positive results, it could be considered that providing a graded structured approach is in some ways inconsistent with the theoretical understanding of apraxia. Since the problem lies in carrying out behaviours under conscious control and automatic behaviours are well retained, it may be better to maximise opportunities for automatic behaviours. A case example is provided in Table 11.3.

Table 11.3   Case Example of Treatment of Apraxia

Joan was admitted to a stroke rehabilitation unit four weeks after stroke with major problems with apraxia. She had relatively good physical recovery and was able to walk but had limited movement in her right arm. She was not independent in many activities of daily living, such as making a hot drink and preparing a meal. She had great difficulty learning to dress herself, despite daily sessions with the occupational therapist. One morning the therapist was called to the telephone during dressing practice, and when she returned Joan had finished dressing herself. Joan could not describe how she had completed the task but reported she had 'just done it' It seemed that when the situation encouraged her to use automatic behaviours she was better able to dress than when being given instruction about the technique to use. The absence of the therapist seemed to facilitate the use of automatic behaviours, whereas when the therapist was present, she was putting in conscious effort to complete the task.

In a trial of rehabilitation of the ability to dress, Walker, Sunderland, Fletcher-Smith, Drummond, Logan, Edmans *et al.* (In Press) compared a neuropsychological approach, in which treatment strategies were based on the pattern of cognitive impairments, to dressing practice with the conventional approach commonly used by occupational therapists in the United Kingdom, in which practice is given in getting dressed. The results indicated that in patients with right hemisphere stroke, dressing practice which was informed by knowledge of cognitive deficits and included strategies, such scanning and alerting, produced greater improvements in dressing ability, than the conventional occupational therapy approach, though this difference just failed to reach statistical significance. However, in left hemisphere stroke patients there were no significant differences between the two approaches to dressing practice.

Visuospatial and visual agnosias

Damage to the occipital cortex of one hemisphere leads to hemianopia, whereas bilateral damage to the occipital cortex leads to cortical blindness. Patients with bilateral damage are functionally blind, although they may make automatic responses and avoid obstacles in their path. This ability to make responses to information which patients are not aware of seeing, blindsight, has been used as a basis for rehabilitation. Ro and Rafal (2006) reviewed the rehabilitation strategies used in the light of theoretical understanding of the phenomenon of blindsight. Schofield and Leff (2009) classified these strategies into three types, optical therapies, eye movement-based therapies and visual field restitution. Early rehabilitation studies attempted to restore vision through practice in pointing to targets on the border of the blind regions (Zihl, 2000). Eye movement therapies involve training patients to make saccadic eye movements in the blind hemi-field. For example Pambakian, Mannan, Hodgson and Kennard (2004) found search performance improved after 20 daily sessions of training over a month, and this was accompanied by improvement in activities of daily living. Visual restoration therapy (Sabel & Kasten, 2000, 2001; Sabel, Kenkel & Kasten, 2005) involves presenting a stimulus, changing in size, near the fovea in the sighted visual field. The stimulus is slowly moved across the midline until it disappears. This is signalled by the patient, at which point the stimulus is moved back into the sighted field, and the process repeated. By systematically working at the boundaries of the lost visual field, the field of vision can be expanded.

These therapies all rely on mass practice. 'Real-world' improvements have been achieved but the treatments require many hours of practice. A systematic review of the overall effectiveness of these techniques (Bouwmeester, Heutink & Lucas, 2007) has highlighted the methodological limitations of some of the studies. Most of the 14 studies identified used a repeated measures design and there were only two randomised controlled trials. Scanning training seemed to produce better results than visual restoration therapy, but there was limited evidence of effects on daily life functioning.

Visual agnosia is relatively rare and therefore treatment evaluations have exclusively relied on detailed study of individual patients (Riddoch & Humphreys, 1994; Wilson, 1999). These have shown that patients can relearn specific visual information but there is no generalization to untrained stimuli. Powell, Letson, Davidoff, Valentine and Greenwood (2008) obtained similar results in training patients with problems in face recognition. Patients trained using three face recognition techniques improved in their recognition of unfamiliar faces, and this improvement was significantly greater than achieved by control participants, who viewed all the faces under simple exposure conditions. However, this was a 'proof of concept' study and there was no evaluation of generalisation of face recognition skills in daily life.

Training of visuospatial abilities has relied mainly on practice on tasks which patients find difficult, a restitution approach. Evaluations of this approach (Edmans, Webster & Lincoln, 2000; Lincoln, Whiting, Cockburn & Bhavnani, 1985) have not shown training visuospatial abilities to improve either performance on perceptual tasks or increase independence in activities of daily living. Using a compensation approach by encouraging patients to use verbal cueing on spatial tasks has shown more promise (Young, Collins & Hren, 1983). For example, Davis and Coltheart (1999) treated patient KL who had difficulty acquiring new topographical information, which occurred as an isolated symptom following an episode of left hemiplegia. She was unable to construct mental maps. Treatment involved teaching the patient verbal mnemonics to recall the streets of her hometown. This led to a significant improvement in the names and locations of streets, which she was able to apply in daily life, but there was no generalisation to other locations. However, the studies are few, and lack of effective rehabilitation of visuospatial problems may be due to the lack of clear theoretical models for understanding these difficulties.

Conclusions

The evidence base for cognitive rehabilitation after stroke mainly supports the treatment of visual neglect, with limited evidence in other cognitive domains. In clinical practice, techniques can be used which have been demonstrated to be effective in other patients with acquired brain injury. Although the stroke population may differ in many characteristics from those of other acquired brain injuries, there are some stroke patients for whom these interventions will be useful. There are also ample single-case experimental design studies to support the provision of cognitive rehabilitation for individual stroke patients.

Chapter 12

Challenging Behaviour after Stroke

Introduction

As with many neurological conditions, stroke can affect an individual's emotional and cognitive status, level of consciousness and ability to communicate. It is not uncommon for people who have had a stroke to express high levels of distress, anger or anxiety, and therefore to be perceived by family members and carers as behaving very differently from before the stroke (Stone, Townend, Kwan, Haga, Dennis & Sharpe, 2004). Significant behavioural changes can present a challenge to services, to caregivers and to the individuals themselves. Psychologists can play a key role in helping the patient, professionals and family members understand the factors influencing behavioural change. Once an understanding is reached, everyone can work together to change, or adjust to, the behaviour.

Within stroke services, challenging behaviour is most likely to be evident in the hyper-acute, acute and early rehabilitation phases of recovery. Often the stroke patient who presents with challenging behaviour will be in an acute medical or rehabilitation setting. Behavioural challenges in these stages will be the main focus of the present chapter, although examples from the post-acute phase are also presented. In each of these settings, behavioural intervention and environmental modification offer the best means of resolving challenging behaviour. Behavioural difficulties in the post-acute phase of recovery are likely to relate to a mood disorder, or to severe cognitive impairment, especially executive dysfunction (Carota, Staub & Bogousslavsky, 2002). The principles of behavioural management remain relevant across all phases but, in the context of mood disorder as a causative factor for the development of challenging behaviour, the clinician is more likely to rely on cognitive-behavioural approaches to behaviour change, which are addressed in chapter 16.

Psychological Management of Stroke, First Edition. Nadina B. Lincoln, Ian I. Kneebone, Jamie A.B. Macniven and Reg C. Morris.
© 2012 John Wiley & Sons, Ltd. Published 2012 by John Wiley & Sons, Ltd.

The effect of challenging behaviour on carers and family members should be considered. Carers of people with challenging behaviour can experience significant emotional distress; there is some evidence that cognitive-behavioural interventions with formal and informal carers may enable them to minimise the impact of the challenging behaviour (Dagnan, Trower & Smith, 1998). It can also be helpful for staff and family members to learn that some challenging behaviour will resolve spontaneously, especially that which occurs during the hyper-acute and acute phases of recovery. The present chapter will describe challenging behaviour as it is commonly manifested after stroke. The causes and consequences of challenging behaviours will be illustrated with case examples. Management strategies will be reviewed, and the evidence to support their use summarised.

Defining challenging behaviour

The term 'challenging behaviour' was adopted in order to emphasise the interaction between the characteristics of an individual and the characteristics of their environment as the cause of a behavioural 'problem' (Allen, 2008). Emerson (1995) defined this as 'culturally abnormal behaviours of such frequency or duration that the physical safety of the person or others is likely to be placed in serious jeopardy, or behaviour which is likely to seriously limit or result in the person being denied access to ordinary community facilities'. Such behaviours include aggression, disinhibition, noncompliance, persistent screaming, disturbed behaviour and destructiveness. By emphasising the role of a person's environment and social context in the development and maintenance of challenging behaviour, the individual is less likely to be blamed for the behavioural problem. Solutions to the challenging behaviour do not therefore necessarily involve intervention directly targeting the individual. Although most often seen within traumatic brain injury and learning disability services, challenging behaviour is also occasionally evident in stroke services. Such behaviours include aggression, apathy, compulsive behaviours, disorders of emotional expression or control, loss of empathy, impulsivity and disinhibition (Carota *et al.*, 2002). The above definition of challenging behaviour remains relevant, as challenging behaviour in these settings is often the product of deficiencies within the service and the patient's environment, rather than solely the result of psychological changes within the patients themselves.

Emerson (1995) remains an excellent resource for clinical intervention in challenging behaviour. Any clinician struggling with a behavioural problem would do well to consult this text in the first instance. The present chapter summarises the principles of intervention in challenging behaviour as described by Emerson (1995) and others, such as Zarkowska and Clements (1994). Adherence to basic principles in the analysis of and intervention for challenging behaviours encountered in stroke services, as outlined below, may often be sufficient. For guidance regarding more entrenched behavioural difficulties, the reader is advised to refer to these original texts.

Aetiology of challenging behaviour

Within acute stroke settings, challenging behaviour is most likely to emerge in the context of communication problems, cognitive problems and associated disorientation arising from brain damage. Poor communication and disorienting environments are almost characteristic of some inpatient stroke wards. For example, in hyper-acute and acute settings there can be a large number of staff rushing around, substantial noise associated with medical equipment and numerous critically ill, unconscious patients. The confusion and disorientation caused by such environments will be substantially exacerbated by internal patient characteristics, such as dysphasia or transient delirium. Patients with relatively little acquired cognitive impairment can feel very disoriented in busy medical environments, and may have relatively little opportunity for social interaction or engagement in activity. In such circumstances, behaviours, such as verbal and physical aggression, may simply be attempts to communicate or elicit social contact. When acquired language impairment, other cognitive problems, such as memory and attentional impairment, and medical symptoms, such as fatigue, pain and nausea, are factored in, it is perhaps not surprising that some patients occasionally demonstrate challenging behaviour. It is essential that potential medical or physical causes of challenging behaviour are eliminated prior to undertaking an observational or psychological assessment. The resolution of medical factors, such as pain or constipation, can elicit a significant reduction in challenging behaviour.

Stroke patients may be particularly vulnerable to behavioural change if they have acquired executive functioning impairment. As with frontal traumatic brain injury, anterior focal strokes may affect an individual's behaviour. Such patients may be described by family members as having sustained a personality change. Typically, the patient exhibits disinhibition and impulsivity, or may express aggression or frustration more readily than was characteristic premorbidly. As with other mechanisms of challenging behaviour, it is often the interaction between changes in the patient's cognitive abilities and the frequently confusing hospital or rehabilitation environment which precipitates the challenging behaviour.

Assessment

Accurate and detailed assessment of challenging behaviour is usually essential if the stroke team hope to resolve a behavioural problem (Alderman, 2001).

Table 12.1 Case Example of Challenging Behaviour Due to Severe Communication Problems

Mary was a 34-year-old married woman with two young children, aged 5 and 7. While looking after the children during the school holidays, she collapsed on the living room floor and was found by a neighbour and was rushed to hospital. She had sustained a brainstem stroke which left her tetraplegic and unable to communicate. Her only movement was eye blinking. She was initially managed in acute hospital with no specialist services either for stroke or for people with severe physical disabilities. The general hospital staff reported major problems with her behaviour because she would make a wailing noise whenever they engaged her in washing and dressing or rehabilitation tasks. Her only communication at this time was one eye blink for 'yes' and two for 'no', a strategy which was identified by her husband rather than professional care staff.

After several weeks, Mary was transferred to a specialist rehabilitation unit. She was referred to psychology because of her wailing and her reluctance to engage in rehabilitation.

Assessment
Assessment by observation revealed that Mary was particularly prone to wailing during the hoisting procedure used in most washing, dressing and rehabilitation tasks. When the behaviour occurred in other circumstances, this always appeared to be an apparent attempt at communication.

Formulation
It became clear that communication difficulties were fundamental to the development and exacerbation of Mary's wailing behaviour. In particular, it was hypothesised that she was attempting to communicate her distress associated with washing, dressing and rehabilitation tasks.

Goal
To facilitate effective communication with Mary in order to establish the source of her distress and enable this to be addressed.

Intervention
As Mary was still communicating through eye blinks, the initial focus of rehabilitation was on providing a more effective means of communication. She was provided with a computer-based system in which she was able to control the cursor through eye movements detected with an infrared detector. This enabled her to communicate her basic needs, but it was slow and laborious to use and she was only able to use the system when in bed or in a chair beside her bed. However, it did enable the team to establish that her wails on transfers were because she was afraid and felt she was going to be dropped. She also indicated that her head 'flopped', which she found distressing, and that she found it very upsetting when her wails were ignored by staff.

A graded programme was developed in which initially three members of staff helped with transfers to ensure that Mary felt secure. She was told that if at any time she felt insecure to indicate with a noise and they would stop and make sure she was adequately supported.

(Continued)

Table 12.1 (*Continued*)

Outcome

Over several weeks, the number of staff assisting with transfers was gradually decreased until she was able to tolerate being transferred by one person. This was important as the aim was for her to return home, where only her husband would be available to transfer her. It was also important that she was given control of her transfers by ensuring that any noises indicating distress were responded to, as these noises were her only means of communication in this situation. Ultimately, her frequency of wailing reduced significantly, but still occurred, appropriately, whenever Mary became distressed.

However, occasionally it can be sufficient to provide staff with behavioural guidelines and principles. These can be used to facilitate a redefinition of the patient's behaviour, prompting a change in staff attitudes and behaviour towards the patient. Sometimes this is all that is required to precipitate a reduction in the challenging behaviour.

Quite often staff and family members describe challenging behaviour in general terms. The clinician must establish a detailed account of the 'how, what, where and when' of the behaviour as the first step in assessment. As Emerson (1998) described, assessment of challenging behaviour is likely to have four primary aims:

- Identification of the precise nature of the behaviour
- Identification of the impact of the behaviour upon the person's quality of life
- Understanding of the processes underlying the person's challenging behaviour
- Identification of possible alternatives to replace the challenging behaviour

Identifying the exact nature of the challenging behaviour may involve interviewing staff members and family or friends of the patient. Detail is important, as the challenging behaviour may be manifested differently across settings or with different staff members. Typically, the behaviour may be more evident in situations in which demands are placed on the patient, such as during washing and dressing tasks or in physiotherapy sessions. Once the behaviour is well described (i.e. the 'what' of the behaviour), it is important to determine the 'how, where and when' of the behaviour, and to examine the effect of the behaviour on the patient and others in detail. Doing so systematically is much more likely to yield useful information for the clinical formulation, and therefore inform effective intervention.

Information gathering

Within stroke services, especially busy inpatient settings, it can be very difficult to collect reliable observational information about the context and circumstances of a particular challenging behaviour. Staff, who are already very busy, will understandably feel reluctant to complete record forms of the behaviour, or may become very avoidant of the patient, affecting the opportunity for observational recording. Without staff cooperation in the assessment process, however, the chances for effective intervention are slim. Any intervention is likely to rely on staff cooperation, and in particular a consistent approach to the patient's behaviour by all staff members. The clinician has to rely on effective team working within stroke services, and where teams are dysfunctional, this can be the first target for intervention before any team interventions can be effective. Usually, staff training is successful in helping team members to understand the principles of behavioural intervention, the importance of consistency, information gathering and effective communication, and the benefits to the patients and staff of working together.

ABC Charts

A useful method of information gathering involves the completion of 'antecedent–behaviour–consequence' ('ABC') charts by observers, typically staff members (Pyles & Bailey, 1990). Assuming adequate staff training, such forms can elicit key information regarding the maintaining factors for a patient's challenging behaviour. Table 12.2 provides an example of the column headings for a simple ABC chart which can be given to staff to complete after each episode of challenging behaviour. Detailed information about the events leading up to the behaviour allow for sequential analysis, which can provide simple solutions, such as the elimination of a particular demand which always precipitates the behaviour. Staff should be encouraged to be as specific as possible about the antecedent events, the exact behaviour exhibited and the consequences to the patient, other people and the environment following the behaviour.

Table 12.2 ABC Chart Derived from Emerson (1995)

Name:

Each episode of challenging behaviour should be recorded and described below in as much detail as possible.

Date and time	Antecedent	Behaviour	Consequence
	What happened before the episode? Who was present, what was said, and what activities were being undertaken?	What happened? Be as detailed as possible. Think: where, when, what and how?	What happened immediately after the episode? What changed for the patient?

The results of ABC chart recording can be used to make preliminary hypotheses about the precipitating and maintaining factors for a challenging behaviour, but the data are often subjective and observer accounts of the same behaviour can differ significantly across observers (Robson, 1993).

Communication problems

Within stroke services, given the prevalence of acquired language difficulties, challenging behaviour often occurs as a result of communication problems. Patients can simply become frustrated by trying to communicate their needs, and this can precipitate verbal or physical aggression. Additionally, some acute medical settings may involve relatively little staff–patient or patient–patient social interaction, and so misunderstandings or mistrust can easily develop. Where a patient also has dysphasia, these problems can be magnified. It is always therefore useful to approach assessment with the question 'What might this person be trying to communicate?' Liaison and joint working with speech and language therapy colleagues are usually the most effective initial approaches in addressing challenging behaviour expressed by people with language difficulties.

Neuropsychological assessment

A cognitive screen, or more comprehensive neuropsychological assessment, can be a useful adjunct to behavioural rating scales or observational measures in patients with challenging behaviour. The results can be very revealing, especially in the case of patients with severe cognitive impairment but relatively intact social skills. Some patients on inpatient stroke wards will have a premorbid history of cognitive decline as part of a dementing process. Occasionally such patients can present with relatively intact social skills, answering basic social questions appropriately. However, they may elicit challenging behaviour at other times, for example during the night when they are more prone to disorientation. Neuropsychological assessment can reveal striking impairments in general intellectual functioning or memory and new learning, which will obviously influence the formulation and therefore the most appropriate choice of intervention. For example, a patient with challenging behaviour who has a significant general intellectual impairment may benefit from a behavioural intervention or environmental modification approach. A patient with circumscribed memory impairment associated with their challenging behaviour (e.g. persistently asking staff and family members the same question) may require a specific compensatory memory strategy (e.g. keeping written or pictorial reminders with them at all times) rather than a behavioural intervention *per se*.

Table 12.3 Case Example of Challenging Behaviour Reinforced by Staff Behaviour

Rita was a 70-year-old woman who was an inpatient in a stroke unit. She was referred for psychological assessment eight weeks after she sustained a major right hemisphere stroke. Rita was a retired council employee. For the five years prior to the stroke, she had been caring for her husband who was 10 years her senior and had Alzheimer's disease. The severity of Rita's stroke meant she was unable to mobilise with the assistance of a wheelchair, required assistance with washing and dressing and had an indwelling catheter. Her language appeared unaffected.

Rita was referred on account of two problems. The first of these was that she would empty her catheter bag on the floor of the ward in a public area, and secondly on some occasions she would undress herself in the corridor within public view.

Assessment
The rehabilitation staff kept an antecedents–behaviour–consequences (ABC) chart. The clinical psychologist completed a cognitive screen that included the Repeatable Battery for the Assessment of Neuropsychological Status (RBANS) and the Hayling and Brixton tests. At interview, Rita was neither able to recall the events of concern nor comment on why they had occurred. She admitted to frustration with her circumstances but did not report significant symptoms of depression or anxiety. This was supported by a self-report screening measure (the Hospital Anxiety and Depression Scale (HADS)).

The ABC chart revealed that one or other of Rita's behavioural difficulties occurred daily. It was further identified that the behaviours were more likely after her regular visitors left and that she received a great deal of staff attention in response to the target behaviour. That is, staff would complain to her about having to clean up the urine and ask her repeatedly about why she had emptied the bag where she had. Indeed, the clinical psychologist observed an episode where staff verbally expressed extreme frustration at what had occurred. Similarly, when Rita removed her upper clothing in public view, staff came from all directions to cover her up and spent some time trying to establish why she had taken off her clothing particularly any physical cause for this (e.g. that she was too hot, felt her skin was too sensitive, etc.). The cognitive test results revealed memory and executive functioning impairment. There was evidence of damage to the frontal lobes consistent with this on the MRI.

Formulation
On the basis of the assessment, it was hypothesised that Rita's behaviour developed in the context of her brain damage from her stroke and was being reinforced and thus maintained by staff attention.

Goal
The impact of the behaviours were such that that team set a goal for complete elimination of both behaviours.

Intervention
On the basis of the assessment, a behavioural intervention was planned. The intervention included providing a competing activity at times when the behaviours

(Continued)

Table 12.3   (*Continued*)

were more likely to occur, such as when visitors were leaving. This included staff spending some time with Rita, drawing her attention to puzzles and so forth, something it was known she enjoyed. Staff were also asked to limit their response to the behaviours of concern, that is provide minimal attention to the catheter bag being emptied and clean up quickly and go straight on to their other duties. With respect to the undressing in an appropriate location, a stimulus control approach was determined: staff would simply instruct Rita that the corridor area was an inappropriate place to undress and take her back to the privacy of her room where this was acceptable.

These interventions utilized learning principles. With respect to the emptying of the catheter bag, the intervention involved reducing reinforcement for the behaviour in order to aid extinction. In respect of the competing activity, a reward for more appropriate behaviour was the chosen principle. With respect to the undressing, a stimulus control intervention exploited a classical conditioning procedure; learning by association. Placing Rita in her room when she undressed strengthened the association between her room and undressing (i.e. the appropriate place for the behaviour).

Outcome
Over a four-week period, incidents of catheter bag emptying reduced significantly. Ultimately, this behaviour was eliminated. After three incidents of undressing in public, with staff responding as planned, Rita ceased the behaviour for approximately one week. At that time there was a further episode. Staff enacted the planned response on this further occasion, and subsequently there were none over the next four weeks at which time Rita was discharged.

This case example illustrates the capacity of interventions targeted at reducing challenging behaviour to enhance quality of life. Rita's personal circumstances and her disability were such that she had to move to residential care. Her options as to where she could go increased significantly when she no longer exhibited the behaviours for which she was referred to the psychologist.

Formulation

Once some clinically meaningful assessment of the challenging behaviour has been undertaken, the clinician can begin to develop a formulation of the factors influencing the expression of the target behaviour. Clinical psychological formulations, as practised across mental health settings, are entirely appropriate and the reader is referred to the Clinical Case Formulations textbook (Ingram, 2006) for a detailed account of the process of clinical formulation across several different therapeutic models, including behavioural and learning models. As with formulation within other settings, it is essential to view the process as ongoing and subject to feedback from the patient themselves regarding the appropriateness of the formulation in accounting for the factors influencing the behaviour. Although challenging behaviour within stroke services may be more likely to occur in the context of significant language or other cognitive impairment, which might restrict the opportunities for genuine collaborative working with the patient, it is still essential for the clinician to approach the clinical problem as a product of several factors. These factors almost always include the environment and other people, not simply the patient themselves.

Hypothesis generation and testing

The formulation will evolve as assessment and intervention proceed. Typically in challenging behaviour interventions, the clinician identifies the most likely contributing factors for a behaviour, and tests this hypothesis through intervention. Depending on the success or failure of the intervention, new hypotheses are generated and then tested. Ultimately, the formulation should be refined until it exists as a satisfactory account of the development and maintenance of the challenging behaviour, at least for a particular moment in time. As with all aspects of assessment and intervention, the formulation should be as collaborative as possible. Developing and sharing the formulation with the patient, where appropriate, is sometimes sufficient intervention in itself, as this can allow the patient to view their behaviour from another perspective.

Models of intervention

Behavioural intervention

The prevailing psychological model by which challenging behaviour is conceptualised and addressed is the operant behaviour model (Skinner, 1953). In this approach, challenging behaviour is viewed as a mechanism by which people can exercise control over their environment. Within this model, environmental consequences which maintain behaviour are referred to as reinforcers (Skinner, 1953). Positive reinforcement is the mechanism by which the rate of a behaviour is increased by the presentation of a (positively) reinforcing stimulus, for example care and contact in response to a patient shouting out without good reason. Negative reinforcement refers to the increase in a behaviour as a result of the withdrawal of an aversive stimulus (Skinner, 1953), for example a patient's inappropriate shouting will be reinforced as a result of them being removed from an occupational therapy session which they find aversive.

As Skinner (1953) described, the behavioural approach involves attempting to establish the functional relationships between events. Reinforcing events for a particular challenging behaviour may vary according to changes in the environmental or social context in which they occur. It is therefore important within stroke services to avoid making assumptions about the maintenance of a particular challenging behaviour. Accurate assessment is essential in order to determine which specific events, in which context, precipitate the challenging behaviour. Without this, staff may often report that there is no antecedent event, or that the behaviour occurs randomly. While this is possible, it is more common for there to be a precipitating event (which may be internal), which can be revealed by careful assessment.

Another key concept in behaviour intervention is the idea of contextual control (Emerson, 1998). Depending on the context, the same event may be reinforcing or punishing. For example, 1:1 social contact may be positively reinforcing while the patient is in a side room, but may become intolerable in the context of the patients' dining area in which there are numerous distractions and attentional demands. In the latter situation, a well-intentioned intervention (in this case, social contact) can elicit rather than diminish challenging behaviour. Interventions therefore need to be framed in terms of the place and time in which they are to be undertaken, in order to avoid inadvertent reinforcement of challenging behaviour.

Another central principle of behavioural intervention is the idea of behaviour as a dynamic system (Emerson, 1998). Each behaviour may be subject to several reinforcing and aversive influences, and so intervention might usefully aim to develop alternative behaviours that are incompatible with the target challenging behaviour, rather than directly aim for the elimination of the target behaviour. In this way, the patient experience might be more positive, in that reinforcement of other behaviours is the goal of the intervention.

Cognitive-behavioural intervention

Challenging behaviour is most likely to occur within the acute phase of post-stroke recovery. Interventions based on the cognitive-behavioural approach may be less appropriate in this stage, given the likelihood of significant cognitive impairment and medical symptoms, such as pain or fatigue. However, it is sometimes useful to conceptualise the challenging behaviour in terms of possible dysfunctional beliefs or negative automatic thoughts, which may be acting as contextual reinforcers or antecedent events to the challenging behaviour. Where this is identified, thought challenging may be an appropriate intervention, assuming that the patient has adequate memory and language functioning to be able to monitor thoughts, and to record and retain information between sessions. However, in practice, cognitive-behavioural therapy is rarely appropriate as an approach to challenging behaviour in the first few months after stroke.

Environmental modification

Aside from behavioural intervention, environmental modification perhaps offers the best option for intervention in challenging behaviour after stroke. Assuming the triggers for challenging behaviour can be identified with careful assessment, it may simply be sufficient, at least in the acute recovery phase, to target intervention at minimising the potential for triggers to occur. For example, a patient who screams when left in a side room alone might benefit from being moved onto the ward where opportunities for interaction and activity are greater. Environmental modification assumes a more preventative approach, acknowledging that the challenging behaviour is likely to be a product of the interaction between the patient and their immediate context (Carr, Robinson, Taylor & Carlson, 1990).

Environmental modification may involve enrichment of the environment, changing the nature of preceding activities and changing the context of activities which precipitate challenging behaviour (Carr *et al.*, 1990). It makes intuitive sense that, for most patients, challenging behaviour is more likely to occur in impoverished environments, where opportunities for enjoyable activity and interaction are absent. Preceding activities, which themselves do not act as obvious triggers, may nevertheless increase the likelihood of challenging behaviour occurring. For example, a demanding personal care routine may increase the likelihood of challenging behaviour in a physically demanding physiotherapy session if the physiotherapy immediately follows the care tasks. Rescheduling the physiotherapy for later in the day may be sufficient to reduce the chance of the challenging behaviour occurring.

Finally, tasks which have been identified as aversive for the patient and likely to elicit challenging behaviour can be modified to maximise opportunities for positive reinforcement, such as frequent breaks, patient input into session length or tasks undertaken, and opportunities for social interaction. Table 12.4 lists a

Table 12.4   Recommended Environmental Modifications to Minimise Challenging Behaviour in Inpatient Settings

Structure the environment carefully with clearly expressed rules and boundaries for appropriate behaviour.

Maintain consistency across all staff – be especially alert to the small minority of staff who may say they 'don't have time' or 'can't be bothered' to monitor or intervene with challenging behaviour.

Maintain adequate staffing levels; interventions cannot be effective if basic care needs are not being met.

Promote clear, frequent and effective communication between staff and patients.

Promote routine.

Personalise interventions so that they are appropriate for the individual patient.

Promote frequent opportunities for social interaction and engagement in activity; inpatient staff can naturally congregate around the nursing station or ward office but should instead be encouraged to interact with the patients at such times.

Provide staff training in behavioural management – it is common for patients to be labelled 'difficult', 'a nightmare', 'stubborn', 'a troublemaker' etc. by staff who have not adequately assessed the behaviour.

Minimise distractions when patients are engaging in therapy, self-care, or a rehabilitation activity.

Table 12.5   Case Example of Challenging Behaviour Due to Memory and Executive Dysfunction

Bradley was a 48-year-old building project manager and father of three. He had a stroke, due to a ruptured middle cerebral artery aneurysm, just after he had completed a challenging mountain climb. He was evacuated by helicopter to the closest acute hospital. A scan revealed continued bleeding and raised intracranial pressure; neurosurgical intervention, involving clipping of the aneurysm, was required. Bradley was referred to psychology three months after his event when he was an inpatient in a post-acute rehabilitation setting. Staff were concerned about inappropriate comments of a sexual nature and his giving them notes with a sexual content to them.

Assessment
The rehabilitation staff kept an antecedents–behaviour–consequences (ABC) chart. This revealed that the behaviours occurred around ten times a week. They appeared to be reinforced by the attention Bradley received for them. Interestingly, responses varied: some staff laughed off the comments, while others were extremely offended, sometimes expressing their shock and anger to Bradley. Neuropsychological assessment revealed executive deficits and impaired delayed recall. A team meeting considered the issue of whether the behaviours were a concern or not. It was agreed that they were and that, if they continued, they were likely have a significant impact on Bradley's social activities once he was discharged into the community.

Goal
To reduce episodes of the behaviour to one or less per week.

Formulation
It appeared likely that Bradley had less control over his response to thoughts of a sexual nature due to the effects of his brain damage. Delayed memory problems meant that learnt information might be lost some time later. As a result, despite being reminded that a behaviour was inappropriate, he was likely to forget this and repeat the behaviour in the future. The responses he received to his comments, even when negative, were likely to have reinforced the behaviour.

Intervention
As it was thought that Bradley may not realise or might forget what was inappropriate, it was determined that at the time of any behavioural episode he should be clearly informed that the behaviour was inappropriate (e.g., 'that's the wrong thing to say to someone involved in your care; please don't do it'). Staff were advised to avoid engaging in more interaction than this and to refrain from laughing or entering into arguments or discussion. The instruction was repeated once if the behaviour continued. When possible, some withdrawal from care was incorporated. For example, the staff member could go away and come back five minutes later to continue with the care task, or ask another staff member to complete the task.
It was also decided that staff would not read any written material handed them by Bradley. Any notes were passed on to the psychologist for use in one-to-one sessions in which Bradley received re-education regarding socially acceptable behaviour. As it was reasonable and desirable for Bradley to have positive interactions with staff, regular contact with Bradley was programmed to occur at times when the behaviours of concern were not evident.

Outcome
Incidents of the targeted behaviour became rare after the intervention commenced and decreased to an average of one per week from a baseline of ten.

number of commonsense strategies to minimise challenging behaviour in inpatient settings, utilising environmental modification.

Neurobiological intervention

It is not uncommon, or unreasonable, for medical staff to attempt short-term pharmacological interventions for challenging behaviour. Often the patient will present as highly distressed or agitated, and staff may wish to alleviate the patient's symptoms with sedative medication. However, although medication can sometimes legitimately form part of an intervention, for example by helping the patient to sleep at night, thus enabling them to remain more alert during the day, it is not appropriate for patients to receive antipsychotic, sedative, or antidepressant medication as a form of pharmacological restraint. A psychiatric opinion should be sought in situations in which medical or nursing staff are considering psychoactive medication to 'treat' a behavioural problem.

Conclusions

Challenging behaviour can occur after stroke, especially within the hyper-acute, acute and early rehabilitation phases of recovery. Careful assessment and analysis of challenging behaviour will allow a meaningful formulation, which will inform the most appropriate intervention. Within inpatient settings, such intervention will usually involve behavioural intervention and environmental modification. Practical strategies rely on adequate staffing levels and a consistent staff approach to the challenging behaviour.

Section 3

Emotional Effects of Stroke

Chapter 13

Emotional Problems after Stroke

Introduction

Stroke can be an extremely challenging event. It is a condition that can involve loss of control of movement, speech and continence. The onset of stroke can be extremely frightening with fear of death and disability, for both the patient and those close to them. In such a context, it is not surprising emotional problems occur in many. These emotional problems include some that would be expected, such as depression and anxiety, but others perhaps less expected, relating to the event onset (post-traumatic stress disorder) and disability (fear of falling), and those more likely to be directly influenced by the brain damage, such as emotional lability, catastrophic reaction, mania, anger or aggression. Comprehensive stroke rehabilitation requires attention to all these sequelae in order to achieve optimum patient outcomes, in terms of both functional ability and quality of life.

Depression

Major depression is by far the most investigated emotion and is characterised by low mood, loss of interest and pleasure in activity, changes in appetite and sleep, suicidal ideas or other morbid thoughts, feelings of guilt or worthlessness, decreased energy and difficulties in thinking and concentrating. In the presence of an identifiable psychosocial stressor, the stroke, and fewer symptoms, the condition can be classified as an adjustment disorder with depressed mood (American Psychiatric Association, 1994). When it is considered a direct physiological consequence of a general health condition, such as a stroke, it can be termed 'mood disorder due to stroke'. Depression occurs in approximately one third of people after stroke (Hackett, Yapa, Parag & Anderson,

Psychological Management of Stroke, First Edition. Nadina B. Lincoln, Ian I. Kneebone, Jamie A.B. Macniven and Reg C. Morris.
© 2012 John Wiley & Sons, Ltd. Published 2012 by John Wiley & Sons, Ltd.

2005). The proportion depressed remains at about 30–40% regardless of time since onset, but some people become depressed early on and then recover, whereas other people develop depression later on (De Wit, Putman, Baert, Lincoln, Angst, Beyens *et al.*, 2008). The risk of suicide after stroke doubles (Stenager, Madsen, Stenager & Boldsen, 1998), but those with pre-stroke depression are at greater risk than those with stroke but no previous depression (Caeiro, Ferro, Santos & Figueira, 2006). Depression after stroke is of significant concern because it is not only distressing for the individual but also associated with several negative outcomes. These include poorer functional outcome (Herrmann, Freyholdt, Fuchs & Wallesch, 1998; Morris, Raphael & Robinson, 1992; Parikh, Robinson, Lipsey, Starkstein, Fedoroff & Price, 1990; Pohjasvaara, Vataja, Leppävuori, Kaste & Erkinjuntti, 2001; Van de Weg, Kuik & Lankhorst, 1999), worse social outcome (Feibel & Springer, 1982; Hermann *et al.*, 1998; Labi, Phillips & Greshman, 1980) and lower quality of life (Bays, 2001b; Neau, Ingrand, Mouille-Brachet, Rosier, Couderq, Alvarez *et al.*, 1998). People also seem to respond less well to rehabilitation, in that those with depression show poor engagement with rehabilitation treatments (Gillen, Tennen, McKee, Gernert-Dott & Affleck, 2001), increased outpatient visits after discharge (Jia, Damush, Qin, Ried, Wang, Young & Williams, 2006), increased rate of rehospitalisation (Ghose, Williams & Swindle, 2005) and greater risk of institutionalisation (Kotila, Numminen, Waltimo & Kaste, 1999). The evidence for an effect on length of hospital stay is equivocal with some finding a trend to longer hospitalisation in those with depression (Saxena, Koh, Ng, Fong & Yong, 2007; Schubert, Burns, Paras & Sioson, 1992) and others not (Gillen *et al.*, 2001). Mortality is also higher in those with depression (House, Knapp, Bamford & Vail, 2001; Morris, Robinson, Andrzejewski, Samuels & Price, 1993; Townend, Whyte, Desborough, Crimmins, Markus, Levi *et al.*, 2007b). However, reviews have indicated that many of the studies do not adequately control for confounding variables (Hackett *et al.*, 2005; Hadidi, Treat-Jacobson & Lindquist, 2009) and also in some cases the direction of the relationship is not clear. For example, although depressed stroke patients have impaired cognition relative to nondepressed patients (Dam, 2001; Morris, Raphael & Robinson, 1992; Robinson, Bolla-Wilson, Lipsey & Price, 1986; Spalletta, Guida, De Angelis & Caltagirone, 2002; Verdelho, Henon, Lebert, Pasquier & Leys, 2004), there are also indications that those with cognitive impairment are more likely to develop depression (Nys, van Zandvoort, van der Worp, de Haan, de Kort, Jansen *et al.*, 2006).

Lesion location

Much research has been undertaken to establish whether depression after stroke is of organic origin or is primarily the result of the psychosocial adjustment required by a challenging disease. The conceptualisation of depression after stroke as directly related to lesion location led to the notion of post-stroke depression as a specific diagnostic category (Robinson, Starr, Kubos & Price, 1983), but recent studies of lesion location in relation to depression after stroke have not supported the original hypotheses (Carson, MacHale, Allen, Lawrie, Dennis *et al.*, 2000; Singh, Herrmann & Black, 1998). Carson *et al.* (2000) reviewed studies of lesion location in relation to depression after stroke and found the pooled relative risk of depression after a left hemisphere stroke, compared with a right hemisphere stroke, was 0·95 (95% CI 0·83–1·10). For depression after a left anterior lesion compared with all other brain areas, the pooled relative risk was 1·17 (0·87–1·62). They concluded that there was no support for the hypothesis that the risk of depression after stroke is affected by the location of the brain lesion. Subsequent reviews (Fang & Cheng, 2009; Santos, Kovari, Gold, Bozikas, Hof, Bouras & Giannakopoulos, 2009a) have highlighted that the variability in studies may mask important messages. Some (Dieguez, Staub, Bruggimann & Bogousslavsky, 2004; Santos, Gold, Kovari, Herrmann, Bozikas, Bouras *et al.*, 2009b) have suggested that biological factors may be important determinants of depression in the acute stage but later on psychological variables may become more important. In addition, Santos *et al.* (2009a) suggested that a shift of research focus from patients with large cortical lesions to those with small macrovascular and microvascular lesions may increase our understanding of the development of post-stroke depression. So it seems that biological factors may contribute to the occurrence of depression after stroke, but this relationship is not the sole determinant.

Psychological factors

A number of psychological factors appear to be associated with depression after stroke, including divorce, pre-stroke alcohol consumption (Burvill, Johnson, Jamrozik, Anderson & Stewart-Wynne, 1997), activities of daily living impairment (Landreville, Desrosiers, Vincent, Verreault & Boudreault, 2009; Robinson, Starr, Kobos & Price, 1983), perception of social support (Morris, Robinson, Raphael & Bishop, 1991; Robinson, Bolduc & Price, 1987) and locus of control (Morrison, Johnston & MacWalter, 2000; Thomas & Lincoln, 2006). In a systematic review of studies up to 1985, Hackett *et al.* (2005) found that physical disability, stroke severity and cognitive impairment were consistently associated with depression. However, they criticised the methodological quality of many of the studies and their small sample sizes. Similar concerns were raised by Snaphaan, Van der Werf, Kanselaar and de Leeuw (2009), who identified that a major problem with previous research was the failure of studies to control for potential confounders, such as pre-existing depression, white matter lesions and atrophy. They prospectively evaluated clinical and neuroimaging correlates occurring before and after stroke in relation to post-stroke depression. They found that functional limitations were the major determinants of depression after stroke, as opposed to stroke-specific factors, such as location or size of lesion on neuroimaging evidence. The evidence indicated that people

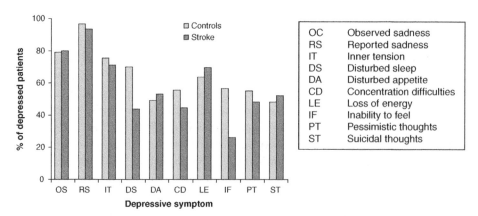

Figure 13.1 Comparison of symptoms of depression between stroke patients and healthy controls. From Cumming, T., Churilov, L., Skoog, I., Blomstrand, C., & Linden, T. (2010). Little evidence for different phenomenology in poststroke depression. *Acta Psychiatrica Scandinavica*, 121, 424–30. Reproduced by permission of John Wiley & Sons, Ltd.

with more severe disability after stroke were more likely to become depressed, but the accuracy of any prediction was insufficient for advising individuals or changing clinical management. Evidence to support the idea that post-stroke depression is not just dependent on biological factors is the fact that the symptoms of depression after stroke are very similar to those with depression but no other physical illness. Cumming, Churilov, Skoog, Blomstrand and Linden (2010) compared patients with depression after stroke and patients with depression with no known physical cause. They found depressed patients with no physical cause reported higher levels of anhedonia (the inability to experience pleasure from normally pleasurable activities) and more disturbed sleep, than depressed stroke patients, but otherwise they had a similar profile of symptoms. These are illustrated in Figure 13.1. There were no significant differences between the groups in the proportions of somatic and psychological symptoms. They concluded that clinicians should not necessarily dismiss somatic symptoms in stroke patients, as reflecting the direct physical consequences of stroke. Rather, they should evaluate these symptoms in relation to depression, as they would with depressed patients without stroke.

Cognitions

Further evaluation of the symptoms of stroke has indicated that even in the absence of depression, there may be negative cognitions. Hackett, Hill, Hewison, Anderson and House (2010) found that up to 28% of stroke patients who were not depressed according the General Health Questionnaire 28, nevertheless endorsed items indicating they had negative cognitions, such as hopelessness, worthlessness or suicidality. These were more frequent in stroke patients who were older, were more dependent in activities of daily living or did not have a partner. They raised the concern that the simple application of screening measures might lead these people to be missed, and yet such cognitions may be amenable to psychological interventions.

Other studies have focussed on examining correlates of depression to help understand the nature of distress in order to inform the development of appropriate treatment strategies. For example, Townend, Tinson, Kwan and Sharpe (2010) examined the role of acceptance of disability in depression after stroke. They assessed non-acceptance of disability, using a modified version of the Acceptance of Illness Questionnaire, and depression was independently assessed by psychiatric interview. They interviewed 60 stroke patients about their main concerns regarding their stroke and used qualitative analysis to identify participants' beliefs about their disabilities, related personal meanings and ways of coping with these. They then examined the relation between these concerns and depression status, as determined by psychiatric interview. This confirmed the relation between stroke severity, physical disability and depression, but additionally showed that non-acceptance of disability was significantly associated with depressive disorder after correcting for other variables. Qualitative analysis indicated that although many had negative feelings, these were 'stronger or darker' in those who were depressed. Many patients reported concerns about their ability to carry out activities of daily living, but those who were depressed tended to report these in terms of what they 'should' be doing rather than what they were able to do. Participants who were depressed were more negative about their reliance on other people and reported feeling 'useless', whereas there was greater acceptance of the changes in those who were not depressed. This study provides valuable insights into the nature of depression after stroke, and has direct implications for the potential for employing psychological treatments to address beliefs in the management of depression after stroke.

Self-esteem

Vickery *et al.* (Vickery, 2006; Vickery, Sepehri, Evans & Lee, 2008; Vickery, Evans, Sepehri, Jabeen & Gayden, 2009) conducted a series of studies to investigate the relation between self-esteem and depression after stroke. Self-esteem is a reflection of the extent to which people have a positive or negative evaluation of themselves. Patients' views of themselves have been shown to change following stroke (Ellis-Hill & Horn, 2000), and a negative self-concept has been found to be related to depression and anxiety (Vickery, 2006). In a consecutive sample of 79 inpatients with acute stroke, both the level of self-esteem and the stability of self-esteem over four days were found to be significantly related to depression, as assessed on the Geriatric Depression Scale (Vickery *et al.*, 2008). They highlighted that as stability of self-esteem is important, self-esteem should be assessed over time and not just at a single time point, especially in the acute stage. A subsequent study with 120 stroke patients in a rehabilitation setting (Vickery *et al.*, 2009) also found the level of self-esteem to be associated with depressive symptoms at discharge. Patients with high but unstable self-esteem were likely to report symptoms of depression at discharge from the rehabilitation unit, as were patients with low but stable self-esteem. Therefore, both the level and the stability of self-esteem seem to be associated with depression after stroke. Self-esteem may therefore be a potential target for psychological intervention.

Generally, the recognition of the importance of psychological factors as determinants of depression has important implications for the treatment of depression after stroke (see chapter 15) and the provision of psychological services.

Emotional lability

'Emotional lability' refers to inappropriate or uncontrollable crying or laughing which is out of proportion to the precipitating event. For example, Giacobbe and Flint (2008) described a patient who was referred for assessment and treatment of depression two weeks after a stroke. He had been crying 'for no reason' several times a day but reported no symptoms of depression. The episodes of crying occurred during an interview and seemed to be independent of the topics being discussed. Another example is Vic, a 54-year-old man with an extensive right middle cerebral artery stroke, who suffered from bouts of inappropriate laughter following his stroke. This caused him particular distress when he felt unable to attend a relative's funeral because he was so worried that he would laugh at an inappropriate time. This phenomenon has received a range of nomenclature in the literature. These include pathological laughing and crying (Parvizi, Arciniegas, Bernardini, Hoffmann, Mohr, Rapoport *et al.*, 2006; Robinson, Parikh, Lipsey, Starkstein & Price, 1993), emotionalism (House, Dennis, Molyneux, Warlow & Hawton, 1989a) emotional dyscontrol (Annoni, Staub, Bruggiman, Gragmina & Bogousslavsky, 2006), excessive crying (Nieuwenhuis-Mark, van Hoek & Vingerhoets, 2008), pseudo-bulbar affect and emotional incontinence (Chriki, Bullain & Stern, 2006). Recently there has been a call for standardisation of definition to 'involuntary emotional expression disorder' (Cummings, Arciniegas, Brooks, Herndon, Lauterbach, Pioro *et al.*, 2006). Basically these terms all refer to inappropriate or uncontrollable crying or laughing. The reactions can occur in response to an appropriate stimulus, for example sad news or relatives leaving after a visit, but are disproportionate to events. At other times they may occur in response to emotionally significant stimuli, such as relatives or pets, or without any apparent reason. There is also variation in the extent to which people have voluntary control over these reactions, with many reporting lack of control. However, it is important to note that there is also variation in the extent of control over normal crying (Nieuwenhuis-Mark *et al.*, 2008).

Estimates of the prevalence of emotional lability and related problems vary between studies according to the source of recruitment, timing of assessment and methods of evaluation. Generally estimates are between 10% and 40%. For example, House *et al.* (1989a) in a community sample of first-ever stroke patients found 15% demonstrated emotionalism at one month after stroke, 21% at six months and 11% at 12 months. Other studies have obtained slightly higher rates, such as 18% (Tang Chan, Chiu, Ungvari, Wong & Kwok, 2004), 21% (Calvert, Knapp & House, 1999), 29% (Eccles, House & Knapp, 1999) and 34% (Kim & Choi-Kwon, 2000). There is improvement in symptoms over time, though 10–15% of patients have problems persisting to a year after stroke (House *et al.*, 1989a; Giacobbe and Flint 2007).

The origins of emotional lability are suggested to lie in damage to various parts of the brain (Nieuwenhuis-Mark *et al.*, 2008) particularly the frontal lobes, brain stem, cerebellum (Parvizi et al., 2009) and thalamus (Tang, Chen, Lu, Mok, Xiang, Ungvari *et al.*, 2009a; Tang, Chen, Lam, Mok, Wong, Ungvari *et al.*, 2009b). Although the symptoms of emotional lability are often acute and short-lived, they can be distressing and embarrassing for those affected, and lead to avoidance of social situations (Calvert, Knapp & House, 1998; Chriki, Bullain & Stern, 2006). Emotional lability has also been found to be associated with depression after stroke (Carota, Berney Aybek, Iaria, Staub, Ghika-Schmid *et al.*, 2005), although it may also occur independently of depression. Parvisi *et al.* (2009) highlighted that it is a disorder of emotional expression, rather than one of emotional experience, as occurs in mood disorders. Despite this, previous research has shown that patients with emotionalism have more psychological distress than those without (Calvert *et al.*, 1998; House *et al.*, 1989a) and Eccles *et al.* (1999) found those with emotionalism had more intrusive thoughts and used more avoidant coping strategies. It is not possible to determine cause and effect from these studies, but it does suggest that emotionalism may require more consideration of the psychological effects and may not simply reflect the damage to specific neural networks.

A 'catastrophic reaction' is an intense reaction to an inability to perform tasks after neurological damage (Goldstein, 1942). Research suggests up to 20% of those who have had a stroke exhibit catastrophic reactions (Carota, Rosetti, Karapanayiotides & Bogousslavsky, 2001; Starkstein, Federoff, Price Leiguarda & Robinson, 1993), though the larger scale study by Carota *et al.* (2001) obtained a lower estimate of 4%. Occurrence has been found to be related to personal and family experience of psychiatric disorder, aphasia, greater subcortical damage and left middle cerebral artery lesions (Carota *et al.*, 2001; Starkstein *et al.*, 1993). Although Starkstein *et al.* (1993) found that catastrophic reactions were more frequent in those with depression, they concluded that depression was not sufficient to account for a catastrophic reaction and that some patients who were depressed did not display catastrophic reactions. Similarly Carota *et al.* (2001) found that that catastrophic reaction was not related to depression in the acute stage, but about two thirds of those with catastrophic reaction went on the develop depression later. Catastrophic reactions can occur when denial of disability is challenged by experience. Such denial, or anosognosia, is a neuropsychological impairment in the ability to be aware of or have insight into disability, and may contribute to this reaction (Chriki *et al.*, 2006).

Anxiety

Anxiety disorders are a range of conditions that include generalised anxiety disorder, panic attacks, obsessive-compulsive disorder and post-traumatic stress disorder. An associated condition is fear of falling. While anxiety has received less research attention in those who have experienced stroke than depression, generalised anxiety disorder, post-traumatic stress disorder and fear of falling have all been studied.

Generalised anxiety disorder

Generalised anxiety disorder is a condition that is characterised by excessive anxiety and worry, typically associated with a range of physical symptoms including restlessness, being easily fatigued, concentration difficulties, irritability, muscle tension and sleep disturbance (American Psychiatric Association, 1994). About one quarter of individuals seem to be affected be generalised anxiety disorder after stroke (Astrom, 1996; Castillo, Schultz & Robinson, 1995; De Wit *et al.*, 2008) and anxiety persists over time (Astrom, 1996; Bergersen, Frøslie, Sunnerhagen & Schanke, 2010; De Wit *et al.*, 2008; Morrison *et al.*, 2005). It can also co-exist with depression (Astrom, 1996; Bergersen *et al.*, 2010). Leppävuori, Pohjasvaara, Vataja, Kaste and Erkinjuntti (2003) differentiated two subgroups of generalised anxiety disorder: primary, which occurred in 11%, and secondary, which was generalised anxiety specifically due to stroke and occurred in 9%. They identified four factors that in combination were able to differentiate these two groups between three and four months later. These were the level of psychosocial functioning, a history of migraine, anterior circulation stroke localization and a history of insomnia. However, the reasons why these factors differentiated the two groups are not clear.

Lander (2009) conducted a qualitative study of patients' experience of anxiety after stroke and found that anxiety was associated with dependence, vulnerability and inability to meet expectations. Expectations appeared to be linked to pre-stroke beliefs and experiences of the self. Participants compared themselves with what they were like before the stroke and anxiety seemed to be associated with failure to meet pre-stroke expectations. For example, participants identified loss of autonomy, loss of roles and perceived negative appraisals by others to be contributing factors. Post-stroke anxiety seemed to relate to discrepancies between actual self and how stroke survivors thought that they 'ought' to be. This was suggested (Lander, 2009) to give rise to feelings of anxiety as a result of prolonged cognitive dissonance.

Anxiety early after stroke was found to be the best predictor of anxiety later on (Morrison *et al.*, 2005; Sagen, Finset, Moum, Morland, Vik, Nagy *et al.*, 2010), but some people who developed problems with anxiety did not have significant levels of anxiety early after stroke (Townend, Whyte, Desborough, Crimmins, Markus, Levi *et al.*, 2007b). Generalised anxiety after stroke does not appear to be consistently related to size or location of lesion (Bond, Gregson, Smith, Rousseau, Lecouturier & Rodgers, 1998; Kim, Kim, Choi, Kim, Moon & Chung, 2003). Evidence on the effects of age and gender on anxiety are conflicting (Barker-Collo, 2007). In addition anxiety is associated with the presence of cognitive impairments (Barker-Collo, 2007). As with depression, the presence of anxiety can affect outcomes. Its occurrence has been associated with reduced social contact, delayed recovery in activities of daily living (Astrom, 1996) and handicap (Sturm, Donnan, Dewey, Macdonell, Gilligan & Thrift, 2004b).

Few studies have examined anxiety disorders, other than generalised anxiety. Agoraphobia has been identified in 2–9%, of stroke patients (Burvill, Johnson, Jamrozik, Anderson, Stewart-Wynne & Chakera, 1995; House, Dennis, Mogridge, Warlow, Hawton & Jones, 1991; O'Rourke, MacHale, Signorini & Dennis, 1998) and panic disorder in 2% (Sharpe, Hawton, House, Molyneux, Sandercock, Bamford *et al.*, 1990). The prevalence rate for phobias has been reported as between 3% and 5% (House *et al.*, 1991; Sharpe *et al.*, 1990). In addition there are specific fears related to the stroke, such as the fear of recurrence of the stroke (see chapter 1) and the fear of falling. Townend, Tinson, Kwan and Sharpe (2006) investigated fear of recurrence from both a quantitative and qualitative perspective. Interviews with a sample of 89 patients indicated that about half the patients reported a fear of recurrence and in particular fear of further disability or communication problems. Patients were aware of the risk factors for further stroke, but many perceived that the prevention of a further stroke as out of their control. There were also concerns among several that overexertion could bring on another stroke. Although fear of recurrence reduced over time, there was only a slight increase in the perceptions of control over the recurrence. Fear of falling can be considered a lasting concern that leads an individual to avoid activities (Tinetti & Powell, 1993). Fear of falling is considered in further detail in chapter 17.

Post-traumatic stress disorder

Post-traumatic stress disorder (PTSD) can follow exposure to an extreme traumatic stressor. It involves the loss of the feeling of being in control of one's life and seeing the world as dangerous, with an associated autonomic reaction (American Psychiatric Association, 1994). In this condition, any memory of the traumatic experience is often so frightening that triggers to recall are avoided. There can be intrusive thoughts, nightmares and flashbacks to the traumatic event. This may lead to avoidance of reminders about the event. For example,

Scott and Barton (2010) reported that one patient used to avoid driving past the hospital where he was admitted following his stroke. The existence of PTSD may become apparent only during treatment for other emotional problems. Scott and Barton (2010) described a 52-year-old woman who had significant visual problems after stoke and was referred to the clinical psychologists because of anxiety. During treatment for anxieties about going out, it emerged that she also had post-traumatic symptoms relating to the stroke event. They were then able to address the PTSD in treatment as well as the anxiety.

The incidence of post-traumatic stress reaction after stroke appears to be between 5% and 30% (Bruggimann, Annoni, Staub, von Steinbuchel, Van der Linden & Bogousslavsky, 2006; Sampson, Kinderman, Watts & Sembi, 2003; Sembi, Tarrier, O'Neill, Burns & Faragher, 1998) with variation due to different methods of assessment and differences in sample selection criteria. These studies all used self-report screening measures of PTSD rather than diagnostic interviews and hence may have overestimated the prevalence of PTSD. Bruggimann *et al.* (2006), who obtained the highest estimate (31%), also had a poor return rate on questionnaires as only about half those invited returned them, so the sample may not be representative of the stroke population.

The stroke event, being sudden, potentially life threatening and uncontrollable, may be the source of symptoms of PTSD (Gangstad, Norman & Barton, 2009). However, this may not be specific to stroke but a reaction to any life-threatening health condition. For example Sampson *et al.* (2003) compared stroke patients with older patients on acute medical wards and showed a similar proportion (6%) of both groups showed signs of PTSD. PTSD after stroke has been found to be associated with both anxiety and depression (Bruggimann *et al.*, 2006; Sembi *et al.*, 1998). In particular intrusive images of illness seem to be related to depression (Sampson *et al.*, 2003). Negative cognitions about the self have been found to be associated with the severity of PTSD (Field, Norman & Barton, 2008; Merriman, Norman & Barton, 2007) suggesting that the way in which the traumatic event was processed and appraised may determine whether PTSD symptoms develop. Therefore it seems that PTSD may occur in a small proportion of patients after stroke in response to the traumatic health event. As suggested by Sampson *et al.* (2003), the implication is that stroke patients should be informed about vivid intrusive memories that may be experienced following a stroke, with the aim of reducing the negative appraisal of those events and the associated avoidance which may lead to PTSD.

The positive effects of trauma have also been investigated. Gangstad *et al.* (2009) evaluated post-traumatic growth in a sample of 60 stroke patients who had attended a rehabilitation centre. They found that some patients reported post-traumatic growth and that this was associated with positive cognitive restructuring, downward comparisons, resolution and denial, as assessed on the Cognitive Processing of Trauma Scale (Williams, Davis & Millsap, 2002). Positive cognitive restructuring involves being able to identify positive aspects to the situation. For example, one patient was able to take stock of his life, recognising his stroke as a second chance and an opportunity to do the things that he had not done before. He bought a dog and went walking every day, which improved his physical health and also improved his relationships with his family. He felt mentally stronger and reviewed what was important to him. Once he had tackled the stroke, he felt he could tackle anything (Barton, personal communication). Downward comparisons involve recognising that the situation could have been worse and that other people suffer more from a stroke. Resolution includes an acceptance of the situation and an ability to look to the future. Denial involves a rejection of the events, such as pretending the stroke never happened. Thus, although PTSD occurs, not all the consequences are negative. However, the proportion of people who experience post-traumatic growth is difficult to ascertain as those with positive experiences may be more likely to take part in research. PTSD can also be an issue for certain cohorts, such as those with stroke who are also concentration camp survivors (Pachalska, Grochmal-Bach, Duncan-MacQueen & Franczuk, 2006). The role of brain damage in post-traumatic stress disorder after stroke remains unclear. Independent from neurological trauma, PTSD has been linked to memory, attentional and executive problems (Horner & Hamnner, 2002; Kanagaratnam & Asbjornsen, 2007; Leskin & White, 2007), but this has not been investigated after stroke.

Anger

Anger can be a difficulty after stroke. This can range on a continuum from irritability to verbal and physical aggression and is surprisingly often directed towards carers and loved ones (see chapter 1). Diagnostically a number of terms might apply when this occurs after stroke, including 'intermittent explosive disorder' if serious assault or destruction of property are involved, 'personality change due to a general medical condition', 'aggressive type' or 'dementia with behavioural disturbance' (American Psychiatric Association 1994). In the acute phase after a stroke, 17–35% of individuals report significant aggressiveness (Aybek, Carotal, Ghika-Schmid, Berney, Van Melle, Guex *et al.*, 2005; Santos, Caeiro, Ferro, Albuquerque & Figueira, 2006). The variation is partly due to differences in the method of assessment. Aybek *et al.* (2005) used an observational scale, the Emotional Behavior Index (EBI), which comprises 38 items assessing emotional behaviours observed after stroke. These were grouped into seven categories; sadness, passivity, aggressiveness, indifference, disinhibition signs, adaptation and denial. Each item was rated according to the frequency of occurrence over four days. The frequency of problems identified on this scale varied between 82% displaying problems with adaptation and only 17% displaying aggressiveness. In contrast, Santos *et al.* (2006) used items from three psychiatric scales and recorded anger if the patient scored on at least one of the eight items and obtained a higher estimate of problems (35%). In the rehabilitation phase, Kim, Choi, Kwon and Seo (2002) found that 32% of patients had an inability to control anger or aggression.

The evidence is contradictory about an association between anger and damage to different areas of the brain. In the acute stage, Santos *et al.* (2006) found no significant relationship between anger and neuroimaging variables, but research in the rehabilitation phase suggested it was associated with lesions affecting cortical and subcortical areas in the territory of the middle cerebral artery, as well as the occipital lobe, the lenticulocapsular area and the pons (Kim *et al.*, 2002). There were no differences in the frequency of anger or aggression between those with anterior, middle or posterior cerebral artery strokes. Botez, Carrera, Maeder and Bogousslavsky (2007) examined aggressiveness in patients with posterior cerebral artery strokes. They described three patients (7%), from a series of 41 with posterior cerebral artery strokes who all presented with aggressiveness in the acute stage. This rapidly resolved over a period of about two weeks. Botez *et al.* (2007) concluded that the more extensive the lesions in territory of the posterior cerebral artery, the greater the risk of becoming confused, agitated or aggressive. In addition, demographic and clinical variables have been found to be related to anger. Aybek *et al.* (2005) found aggressiveness was correlated with a personal history of depression and the presence of haemorrhage. Kim *et al.* (2002) found inability to control anger or aggression was related to motor dysfunction, dysarthria and post-stroke emotional incontinence. The lack of consistency between studies may be due to small samples and differences in assessment methods, and suggests there may be some chance findings.

While 'personality changes' after a stroke are commonly reported by carers, what carers mean by this may be that patients display changes in emotional responding. There has been little investigation specifically of this; however, Stone *et al.* (2004) collected information suggesting major changes to be reduced patience, increased frustration, reduced confidence, increased dissatisfaction and 'a less easy going nature'. It may be that carers are describing low-level alterations in behavioural style, evident to someone who knows the patient well, that fail to reach the criteria for clinical concern but are indicators of changes of mood.

Apathy

Apathy has been noted as a feature of depression after stroke (Caiero, *et al.*, 2006) but may also be a feature of behaviour independent of depression. It is a state in which patients demonstrate a lack of emotion, interest or concern (Marin, 1990). Angelelli, Paolucci, Bivona, Piccardi, Ciurli, Cantagallo *et al.* (2004), in an evaluation of neuropsychiatric disorders after stroke, identified apathy in 27% of a sample of patients with a unilateral ischaemic stroke. The main features of behaviour observed were a decrease in activities (84%), lack of attention to usual interests (68%), loss of interest in plans of family members or other relevant people (62%), reluctance to start a conversation (50%) and being less frequently spontaneous or loving (15%). Apathy was more common six months or more after stroke, rather than in the acute stage. Mayo, Fellows, Scott, Cameron and Wood-Dauphinee (2009) examined factors related to apathy in a sample of 408 patients with first stroke who also had a carer to provide proxy ratings. They found that 33% had minor levels of apathy and only 3% had high levels of apathy, and the rates remained stable over the first year after stroke. Apathy was associated with cognitive impairment, high levels of disability and a high number of comorbidities. They reported that apathy had a negative effect on physical function, participation, health perception and physical health. Apathy seems to be independent of depression (Angelelli *et al.*, 2004), but it is not clear the extent to which it may be a manifestation of cognitive impairments, particularly impairment of executive function. It also seems to be associated with the presence of small vessel disease (Staekenborg, Su, van Straaten, Scheltens, Barkhof & van der Flier, 2010) which is present in many stroke patients.

Coping and adjustment

Coping

In addition to direct effects on mood, the emotional effects of stroke may be influenced by the ways people cope with a frightening and life threatening condition. Lazarus and Folkman (1984) defined coping as 'the constantly changing cognitive and behavioural efforts to manage the specific external or internal demands that are appraised as taxing or exceeding the resources of the person'.

People tend to use either problem solving strategies, which are active attempts to do something active to alleviate stressful circumstances, or emotion focused coping strategies, which are attempts to regulate the emotional consequences of stressful or potentially stressful events. Donnellan, Hevey, Hickey and O'Neill (2006) reviewed studies of coping after stroke and identified five studies which examined the relation between coping and various factors (emotionalism, nursing follow-up, depression, training of patient and anxiety) and two which investigated coping as a predictor of outcome. These studies produced conflicting findings on the use of active problem oriented coping in patients with stroke. In two studies (Finset & Andersson, 2000; Hermann, Freyholdt, Fuchs & Wallesch, 1997), stroke patients used more active problem oriented coping strategies, and in one (Herrmann, Curio, Petz, Synowitz, Wagner, Bartels & Wallesch, 2000) they used fewer. Similarly, there were inconsistent findings on the use of problem-focused as opposed to emotion-focused strategies (De Sepulveda & Chang, 1994; Rochette & Desrosiers, 2002). The coping strategies used did not change over time suggesting they were dispositional approaches. Donellan *et al.* (2006) found anxiety and depression were associated with more frequent use of avoidant coping strategies. These strategies include both behavioural avoidance (e.g. avoiding situations which are difficult, such as rehabilitation) and cognitive avoidance (e.g. trying to forget a bad experience) to avoid confronting problems occurring as a consequence of stroke. In addition, they reported that few studies showed significant correlations between coping and other psychological domains apart from one (Wahl, Martin, Minnemann, Martin & Oster, 2001) which showed that information seeking and search for affiliation were significantly correlated with subjective well-being and autonomy, suggesting they were adaptive strategies for coping. In addition, Darlington, Dippel, Ribbers, van Balen, Passchier and Busschbach (2009) have shown in a longitudinal study of 80 stroke patients discharged from hospital that the use of effective coping strategies was significantly related to quality of life a year after stroke. Qualitative evaluation of the process of coping (Rochette, Tribble, Desrosiers, Bravo & Bourget, 2006) has also shown that effective coping after stroke requires patients to realign their expectations to bring them more into line with the reality of their situation.

Adjustment

There have been suggestions that people gradually adjust to the effects of stroke over time. Adjustment is a process of adaptation to disability. Stroke patients progress through stages of emotional experience, which are very variable in their length but show consistency in the pattern of emotions experienced. These have been likened to the process of grieving. For example, Holbrook (1982) put forward a four-stage model of the process of adjustment after stroke. The initial phase was a crisis phase characterised by shock, confusion and anxiety. This was followed by a rehabilitation phase in which there were high expectations of recovery, denial that disability would be permanent and periods of grieving. The third phase was characterised by emotional reactions, including anger, rejection, despair, frustration and depression, as patients came to realise that they would not fully recover. The final phase then involved a gradual acceptance of the new reality as a disabled person. Alaszewski, Alaszewski and Potter (2004) examined the use of this bereavement model of adjustment after stroke by healthcare professionals. This confirmed the central concept of loss, not only for patients but also to enable healthcare professionals to understand the psychological effects of stroke.

In a qualitative evaluation, Kirkevold (2002) interviewed nine stroke patients in depth on several occasions over a year. Kirkevold (2002) also identified four phases of emotional adjustment; the first initial onset phase was characterised by surprise and shock at the occurrence of the stroke. This was followed by an active rehabilitation phase in which the focus is on regaining lost functions through hard work. After discharge from hospital, there was a phase of continued rehabilitation which included psychosocial and practical adjustment. In the fourth phase, the emphasis was on adapting to their changed lifestyle. Support for these phases mainly comes from qualitative studies. For example, Eilertsen, Kirkevold and Bjørk (2010) conducted in-depth qualitative interviews with six women after stroke and also identified four similar stages of readjustment after stroke; initially patients were concerned with understanding the nature of bodily changes that had occurred as a result of the stroke, and this was followed by an emphasis on achieving independence in activities of daily living. The later phases were characterised by dealing with the emotional effects of stroke. During the third phase, patients began to realise the permanence of their difficulties and had begun to process what had happened emotionally. At this stage, grief was linked

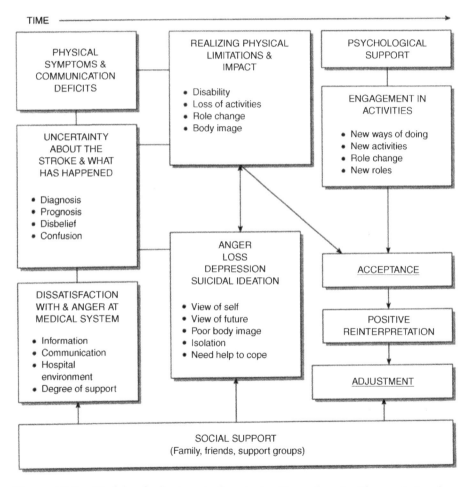

Figure 13.2 Models of adjustment after stroke. Reproduced with permission from Ch'Ng, A., French, D., & Mclean, N. (2008). Coping with the challenges of recovery from stroke: long term perspectives of Stroke Support Group members. *Journal of Health Psychology*, 13, 1136–46.

to a realisation of what they had lost. There followed a stage in which patients became more accepting of the changes that had occurred and there was greater emotional stability. Ch'Ng, French and Maclean (2008) held focus groups with 26 participants and also found patients progressed through stages of adjustment. Most emotional adjustment occurred after discharge from hospital, with problems arising from a sense of loss, despair and a loss of self-esteem. These led to depression in some while others managed to resolve their difficulties. Many highlighted a lack of attention to their emotional needs. Ch'Ng *et al.* (2008) presented a useful model summarising the challenges and ways of coping based on the reports of their participants, as shown in Figure 13.2.

Thus, there is consistency in the pattern of emotional changes which occur over time, and the implication is that when designing interventions to promote emotional adjustment and reduce distress, account should be taken of these stages of change. The emotional support needed will differ at each stage, and the challenge is to ensure that appropriate psychological interventions are available at each of the stages.

Conclusions

There are therefore many ways in which stroke has an effect on emotions. Although problems with depression are now widely recognised, there are other emotional reactions to stroke which are just as important. Clinical teams need to be aware of these problems, so that they can identify them when they occur and instigate appropriate management strategies. This requires appropriate screening of all stroke patients (chapter 14). Some reactions are important early after stroke, such as anger and emotional lability, whereas others may predominate later, such as apathy. The pattern is, however, very variable, and multiple factors determine the reactions that patients display. To discriminate between different emotional reactions and to determine whether the level of emotion experienced is appropriate or whether it signifies significant levels of distress, which need specialist intervention, require a comprehensive psychological assessment, as discussed further in chapter 14.

Chapter 14

Screening and Evaluation of Emotional Problems After Stroke

Introduction

The assessment of mood problems in stroke patients is complicated by the presence of concomitant neurological impairments, such as aphasia, memory problems, anosagnosia and visual neglect (Roger & Johnson-Greene, 2009; Salter, Bhogal, Foley, Jutai & Teasell, 2007; Spencer, Tompkins & Schulz, 1997). In addition, the symptoms of depression and anxiety may overlap with the direct consequences of stroke, such as fatigue, sleep and appetite changes. This has led some to suggest that somatic items should be removed from mood screening measures (Salter *et al.*, 2007; Thomas & Lincoln, 2008a) whereas there is other evidence to indicate that somatic items may be among the best discriminators between stroke patients with depression and those who are not depressed (de Coster, Leentjens, Lodder & Verhey, 2005; Spaletta, Ripa & Caltagirone, 2005). Therefore, it is necessary that any assessment methods used are appropriate for those with stroke and assessments developed in other contexts need to be independently validated for use with stroke patients. In addition, the characteristics of mood disorder may differ according to the patients' age (Palmer, Jeste & Sheikh, 1997), and some assessments may have an age bias (Jorm, 2000); therefore, the psychometric properties need to be checked in the different subgroups to ensure that the information obtained from the scales is valid.

Purpose of mood assessment

There are three main reasons for assessing mood in stroke patients, and for each of these, different measures may be needed. One purpose of mood assessment is to identify those with a potential problem with low mood so that they may be evaluated further. For this purpose, screening measures are needed that are short

Psychological Management of Stroke, First Edition. Nadina B. Lincoln, Ian I. Kneebone, Jamie A.B. Macniven and Reg C. Morris.
© 2012 John Wiley & Sons, Ltd. Published 2012 by John Wiley & Sons, Ltd.

and easy to administer by nonspecialist staff. They need to be practical to administer in a variety of settings, including acute hospital wards. They also need to be sensitive (i.e. to detect most of those people who do have a problem). For them to be efficiently used in clinical practice, they also need to be specific (i.e. to not classify those with no problem as having one). The positive predictive value is the proportion of patients scoring as having low mood on the test who have low mood, and the negative predictive value is the proportion of those scoring within the normal range who do not have low mood. The positive predictive value should be much higher than the probability of having mood disorder on the basis of population characteristics alone.

The second purpose of mood assessment is to gain an understanding of the nature of the mood problem in order to plan treatment. This needs to determine the severity of the problem, to differentiate between different types of mood disorder and to assess factors relevant to the choice of treatment strategy. The third reason for assessment is to monitor change in mood over time. Measures are needed which will be sensitive to change in individuals, in order that progress with therapy can be identified. Similarly they need to be reliable so that when no change is occurring scores do not change. These measures are also likely to be used as outcome measures in intervention trials, and so it must be feasible to administer the assessment with no prior knowledge of the patient, so that the outcome assessments can be conducted blind to the intervention.

Although there are many measures for assessing mood problems, only some have been validated for stroke patients. A consequence of this is there is great uncertainty about the frequency and severity of mood disorders after stoke. In this chapter, measures for mood problems will be reviewed and recommendations made for their use with stroke patients. Separate consideration will be given to measures for people with communication problems, as these present a particular difficulty in clinical practice.

Screening measures for people without communication problems

The main aim of screening measures is to detect those with common emotional problems after stroke: depression and anxiety. For people with other mood problems, such as anger, frustration and emotionalism, there are few screening measures available and therefore full assessment is needed.

Screening

Studies to assess the suitability of measures for screening purposes have administered a brief screening measure and compared the results with a gold standard measure. In most cases, this gold standard has been a structured clinical interview. Ideally, the gold standard measure should be conducted blind to the results of the screening assessment. Structured clinical interviews, such as the Present State Examination (PSE; Wing, Cooper & Sartorious, 1974), Schedules for Clinical Assessment in Neuropsychiatry (SCAN; World Health Organisation, 1992b) or Structured Clinical Interview for DSM-IV (SCID; Spitzer, Williams, Gibbon & First, 1992), provide a clinical diagnosis of anxiety and depression. In some studies, both major and minor depression have been considered separately. However, it has been questioned (Roger & Johnson-Greene, 2009; Salter *et al.*, 2007; Thomas & Lincoln, 2008a) whether some of the diagnostic criteria can be validly applied after a stroke. Most, but not all, studies have conducted the criterion measures blind to the screening measure scores.

Screening measures are usually administered by nonspecialist staff and need to be short; otherwise they will not be used. Clinical interviews are not usually practical for screening purposes as they take too long and require skilled interview techniques. Often the best option is to use standardised questionnaires, which can be either self-administered or administered by a healthcare professional. For ease of administration a standard response format is useful, so that patients can remember the categories of responses that they need to use. Measures which may be used for screening purposes to detect anxiety and depression are summarised below, and recommended cut-offs for stroke patients are shown in Table 14.1.

Screening questionnaires

Several questionnaires have been validated to identify depression and anxiety in stroke patients.

- The Beck Anxiety Inventory (BAI; Beck & Steer, 1993) is a 21-item scale assessing symptoms of anxiety. It may be appropriate for screening purposes as it is brief and has consistent response options. Schramke, Stowe, Ratcliff, Goldstein and Condray (1998) found the BAI was sensitive to anxiety as diagnosed on the SCID-R with patients who had had a stroke but the specificity was poor, although exact figures were not quoted. They suggested that in stroke patients the scale may measure general distress rather than specifically an anxiety disorder. However, it is one of the few measures of anxiety appropriate for stroke patients available.
- The Beck Depression Inventory II (BDI-II; Beck, Steer & Brown, 1996) and its forerunner the Beck Depression Inventory (BDI; Beck & Steer, 1987) are well-established measures of depressive symptoms which have been frequently used with stroke patients (Andersen, Vestergaard, Ingeman-Nielsen & Lauritzen, 1995; Dam, Pederson & Ahlgren, 1989; House, Dennis, Mogridge, Warlow, Hawton & Jones, 1991; Kotila, Numminen, Waltimo & Kaste, 1998; Pohjasvaara, Vataja, Leppävuori, Kaste & Erkinjuntti, 2001; Rochette & Desrosiers, 2002). The BDI-II comprises 21 items in two domains: cognitive and somatic. Concerns have been raised about the

Table 14.1 Recommended Cut-Offs for Screening Mood Problems in Stroke Patients

Screening measure	Study	Stroke sample	Criterion measure	Cut-off	Sens' %	Spec' %	PPV %	NPV %	Agree[t] kappa
Beck Anxiety Inventory	Schramke et al., 1998	n=44 Community patients > 12 mpo	SCID-R	15/16	high	low			
Beck Depression Inventory	House et al.,1989	n=76 Community patients 1 mpo	PSE						
	Aben et al., 2002	n=166 First stroke 1 mpo	Any depression	8/9	92				
			SCID major depression	9/10	80	61	22	96	
			SCID any depression	9/10	77	65	38	91	
	Lincoln et al., 2003	n=143 20 inpatients and 123 from CBT trial	SCAN depression	15/16	91	56	18	95	0.05
	Berg et al., 2009	n=100 2 weeks and 2, 6, 12 and 18 mpo	DSM-III-R, DSM-III-R2 major depression						
			2 weeks	9/10	80	93			
			12 months	9/10	63	92			
Beck Depression Inventory Fast Screen	Healey et al., 2008	n=49 patients in rehabilitation	SCID major depression	3/4	71	74	31	94	0.29
Brief Assessment Schedule Depression Cards	Healey et al., 2008	n=49 patients in rehabilitation	SCID any depression		62	78	50	85	
			SCID major depression	6/7	100	95	78	100	0.85
			SCID any depression	6/7	69	97	90	90	

Measure	Study	Sample	Criterion standard	Cutoff					
Center for Epidemiological Studies Depression Scale	Shinar et al., 1986	n =27	PSE any depression	15/16	73	100	100	84	
	Parikh et al., 1988	n=80 consecutive patients < 3 mpo Non-aphasic patients	Psychiatric interview	15/16	86	90	80	93	
	Agrell & Dehlin, 1989	n=40 Elderly Mean 14 mpo	Psychiatric interview	19/20	56	91	82	75	
	Rybarczyk et al., 1996	n=50	SADS	25/26	65	82	65		
	Schramke et al.,1998	n=44 Community patients > 12 mpo	SCID-R	16/17	high	low			
	Roger & Johnson-Greene, 2009	n=67 Inpatient rehabilitation	SCID-CV	14/15	66	68	34	35	
General Health Questionnaire 30	O'Rourke et al.,1998	n=133 Patients from a trial 6 mpo	Depression SADS any diagnosis	8/9	80	76			
General Health Questionnaire 28	Johnson et al., 1995	n=66 Consecutive community cohort 4 mpo	PAS						
	Lincoln et al.,2003	n=143 20 inpatients and 123 from CBT trial	Depression	5/6	78	81	50	94	
			Anxiety	4/5	71	56	30	88	
			SCAN depression	11/12	81	68	21	100	0.12
Geriatric Depression Scale	Agrell & Dehlin, 1989	n=40 Elderly Mean 14 mpo	DSM-III-R Depression Anxiety	9/10	88	64	58	88	

(continued)

Table 14.1 (Continued)

Screening measure	Study	Stroke sample	Criterion measure	Cut-off	Sens[y] %	Spec[y] %	PPV %	NPV %	Agree[t] kappa
	Johnson et al.,1995	n=120 Consecutive community cohort 4 mpo	PAS Depression	10/11	84	66	53	90	
Geriatric Depression Scale 15	Lee et al., 2008	n=253 First stroke 1 mpo	Anxiety	14/15	65	79	51	86	
			Depression with DSM-IV criteria	4/5	84	77	75	85	0.60
	Roger & Johnson-Greene, 2009	n=67 Inpatient rehabilitation	SCID-CV	2/3	67	73	31	32	
			Depression						
Hospital Anxiety and Depression Scale	Johnson et al., 1995	n=92 Consecutive community cohort 4 mpo	PAS Depression	4/5 (D)	83	44	26	92	
	O'Rourke et al.,1998	n=111	PAS Anxiety	5/6 (A)	80	46	31	89	
			SADS depression	6/7 (D)	80	79			
			SADS anxiety	6/7 (A)	83	68			
	Aben et al., 2002	n=171 1 mpo first stroke	SCID major depression	7/8 (D)	73	62	41	95	
			SCID any depression	11/12 (T)	92	66	30	98	
				6/7 (D)	73	79	51	91	
				11/12 (T)	87	70	45	95	
	Healey et al., 2008	n=49 Patients in rehabilitation	SCID major depression	7/8 (D)	86	69	32	97	0.32
			SCID any depression	7/8 (D)	62	69	42	83	

Scale	Study	Sample	Diagnostic standard	Cutoff					
	Sagan et al., 2009	n=101	DSM-IV any depression	4/5 (D)	84	73	42	95	0.42
		4 mpo	one anxiety	11/12 (T)	90	83	55	97	0.58
			disorder	4/5 (A)	83	65	41	93	0.36
				6/7 (T)	83	60	38	92	0.30
Montgomery-Åsberg Depression Rating Scale	Lightbody et al., 2007	n=24 Patients in hospital	Psychiatrist diagnosis of depression	6/7	100	65	54	100	0.60
	Sagan et al., 2009	n=103	DSM-IV any depression	6/7	90	66	39	97	0.38
		4 mpo		8/9	85	71	40	41	0.40
Patient Health Questionnaire 9	Williams et al., 2005	n=316	SCID major depression	10/11	91	89	80	95	
			SCID any depression		78	96	94	84	
Patient Health Questionnaire 2	Williams et al., 2005	n=316	SCID major depression	3/4	83	84	72	91	
			SCID any depression	3/4	78	95	93	85	
Stroke Inpatient Depression Inventory	Rybarczyk et al., 1996	n=50 inpatients on rehabilitation unit	SADS depression	16/17	71	94	86		
	Roger & Johnson-Greene, 2009	n=67 Inpatient rehabilitation	SCID-CV Depression	9/10	66	72	32	37	
Symptom Checklist 90 depression scale	Aben et al., 2002	n=176	SCID major depression	24/25	89	61	28	97	
Wakefield Depression Inventory	Lincoln et al., 2003	1 mpo first stroke n=143 20 inpatients and 123 from CBT trial	SCID any depression	24/25	88	66	44	95	
			SCAN diagnosis of depression	20/21	86	50	21	100	0.12

(*continued*)

Table 14.1 (*Continued*)

Screening measure	Study	Stroke sample	Criterion measure	Cut-off	Sens[y] %	Spec[y] %	PPV %	NPV %	Agree[t] kappa
Yale question	Watkins et al., 2001	n=79 acute stroke wards 2 weeks	MADRS	0/1	86	78	82	82	
	Watkins et al., 2007	n=122 acute stroke wards	MADRS						
		2 weeks		0/1	86	84	86	84	
		3 mpo		0/1	95	89	93	91	
	Lightbody 2007	n=74 acute stroke wardsds	SCID any depression	0/1	70	70	58	81	

SADS: Schedule for Affective Disorders and Schizophrenia; SCAN: Schedule for Comprehensive Assessment in Neuropsychiatry; SCID: Structured Clinical Interview; PAS: Psychiatric Assessment Schedule; HADS: Hospital Anxiety and Depression Scale; D depression subscale, A anxiety subscale, T total score; mpo: months post onset; Sens[y]: sensitivity; Spec[y]: specificity; PPV: positive predictive value; NPV: negative predictive value.

validity of the BDI and BDI-II, due to the inclusion of somatic items, such as questions about changes in sleep patterns and appetite and loss of libido. The scales are difficult to administer to stroke patients because of the long complex response categories. Despite this, the BDI has been found to be acceptable for detecting depression after stroke (Aben, Verhey, Lousberg, Lodder & Honig, 2002; Berg, Lonnqvist, Palomaki & Kaste, 2009; Lincoln, Nicholl, Flannaghan, Leonard & Van der Gucht, 2003) with a recommended cut-off of 9/10. The Beck Depression Inventory Fast Screen (BDI-FS; Beck, Steer & Brown, 2000) includes seven items from the Beck Depression Inventory-II (Beck *et al.*, 1996). It does not include somatic items in order to make it suitable for assessing medical patients. Healey, Kneebone, Carroll and Anderson (2008) found it was a useful measure for stroke patients, but it was not as sensitive or as specific as the Brief Assessment Schedule Depression Cards (BASDEC; Adshead, Cody & Pitt, 1992).

- The Brief Assessment Schedule Depression Cards (Adshead *et al.*, 1992) comprise 19 items developed for use with older people in a hospital ward environment. Each item is written on a separate card and respondents are asked to place the cards next to either a 'true' or 'false' card. Healey *et al.* (2008) reported that the BASDEC demonstrated excellent criterion validity in relation to the SCID in identifying stroke patients with major depression and was more accurate than either the BDI-FS or the HADS-D.

- The Center for Epidemiological Studies Depression Scale (CES-D; Radloff, 1977) is a 20-item scale to assess the frequency and severity depressive symptoms in older adults. Recommended cut-offs vary from 15/16 (Parikh, Lipsey, Robinson & Price, 1988) to 26/27 (Schramke *et al.*, 1998), but those evaluated by Parikh *et al.* (1988) included the same patients assessed on more than one occasion, which makes the results difficult to interpret. Salter *et al.* (2007) observed that in some studies, such as Toedter, Schall, Reese, Hyland, Berk and Dunn (1995), the CES-D was administered by interview rather than self-completion, which takes longer and may limit its applicability as a screening measure.

- The General Health Questionnaire (Goldberg & Williams, 1988) is a widely used self-report instrument for detecting psychiatric disorder (Burns, Lawlor & Craig, 1999). The 30-item (GHQ-30), 28-item (GHQ-28; Goldberg & Hillier, 1979) and 12-item (GHQ-12; Goldberg, 1992) versions are all derived from the original 60-item version (GHQ-60). Because it compares the patients' present state with the 'usual state', it is unlikely to detect chronic disturbance (Bowling, 1995), but this has the advantage that it excludes the persistent effects of stroke. There are recommended cut-offs for stroke patients for the GHQ-28 (Johnson, Burvill, Anderson, Jamrozik & Stewart-Wynne, 1995; Lincoln *et al.*, 2003) and GHQ-30 (O'Rourke, MacHale, Signorini & Dennis, 1998) in relation to depression and for the GHQ-28 in relation to anxiety (Johnson *et al.*, 1995) but not for the GHQ-12. It has generally been found to be sensitive, but specificity values are moderate.

- The Geriatric Depression Scale (GDS; Yesavage, Brink, Rose, Lum, Huang, Adey & Leirer, 1983) is a 30-item scale developed for use with elderly people. Cut-offs for stroke patients have been recommended as 10/11 for identifying depression (Agrell & Dehlin, 1989; Johnson *et al.*, 1995) and 14/15 (Gillen, Tennen, McKee, Gernert-Dott & Affleck, 2001; Johnson *et al.*, 1995) for anxiety. The GDS has a simple yes-no response format and does not include somatic items. However, items such as 'Do you feel full of energy?' may not be appropriate and statements such as 'Do you prefer to stay at home, rather than going out and doing new things?' are not applicable in hospital. It has been suggested that administering the GDS in the context of an interview enables a higher proportion of patients to be assessed on the GDS (Creed, Swanwick & O'Neill, 2004). Only half of those who obtain high scores do have depression, and so it leads to high follow-up rates. Short forms of the GDS with 15, 10 and 4 items (Sheikh & Yesavage, 1986) are available. The GDS-15 showed as good agreement with clinical diagnosis as the full GDS-30 in a large sample of acute stroke patients (Lee, Tang, Yu & Cheung, 2008). However, Roger and Johnson-Greene (2009) found very poor positive and negative predictive values in a rehabilitation sample.
- The Hospital Anxiety and Depression Scale (HADS; Zigmond & Snaith, 1983) was designed to assess both depression and anxiety, excluding the physical indicators of psychological distress. Even so, some items may occur as a direct result of the symptoms of stroke rather than reflecting low mood. For example, items such as 'I can enjoy a good book or radio or TV programme' may reflect language or cognitive impairments and 'I feel as if I am slowed down' may reflect motor, language or cognitive problems. A useful feature of the HADS is that there are separate anxiety and depression subscales. Recommended cut-off points for stroke patients range from 4/5 (Sagen *et al.*, 2009) to 7/8 (Aben *et al.*, 2002) for depression and from 4/5 (Sagan *et al.*, 2009) to 5/6 (Johnson *et al.*, 1995) for anxiety. The HADS total score has also been used as a measure of psychological distress (Aben *et al.*, 2002; Johnston, Pollard & Hennessey, 2000; Sagan *et al.*, 2009; Townend, 2004) for detecting both depression and anxiety. The HADS has been directly compared with other scales. It has been found to be comparable to the GHQ-30 (O'Rourke *et al.*, 1998), Beck Depression Inventory, Hamilton Depression Rating Scale and Symptom Check List 90 (Aben *et al.*, 2002) but less satisfactory than the GDS-30, GHQ-28 (Johnson *et al.*, 1995), BASDEC (Healey *et al.*, 2008) and Montgomery-Åsberg Depression Rating Scale (MADRS; Montgomery & Åsberg, 1979) (Sagan *et al.*, 2009). Sensitivity and specificity values were satisfactory but the positive predictive values were low, leading to many patients requiring further evaluation.
- The Montgomery-Åsberg Depression Rating Scale (Montgomery & Åsberg, 1979) is a clinician-rated scale for measuring the presence and severity of depressive symptoms. The MADRS comprises 10 items, which combine observation, self-report and information gathered from other informants, each

rated on a scale from 0 to 6. Sagan *et al.* (2009) compared the MADRS with the HADS using published cut-offs, rather than those specific to stroke, and found that the MADRS had higher sensitivity (MADRS, 70%; HADS-Depression, 58%), but otherwise the scales were comparable. One advantage of the MADRS is it can be used with people who have communication problems. It was found that 76% of aphasic acute stroke patients could be assessed with MADRS and 90% six months later (Laska, Martensson, Kahan, von Arbin & Murray, 2007). However, the subjective nature of the ratings and the multiple sources of information may make it difficult for inexperienced healthcare staff, who are often responsible for screening patients, to administer.

- The Patient Health Questionnaire (Spitzer, Kroenke & Williams, 1999) (PHQ-9) is a 9-item self-administered questionnaire for screening and diagnosis of depression. Each item is scored from 0 to 3, and the standard cut-off used is 10/11. Williams, Brizendine, Plue, Bakas, Tu, Hendrie and Kroenke (2005) found that it performed well as a screening for depression after stroke, but most participants were outpatients, so although there is some support for using the scale in community settings, there is no information on its suitability in acute stroke wards.

- The Stroke Inpatient Depression Inventory (Rybarczyk, Winemiller, Lazarus, Haut & Hartman, 1996) is a 30-item scale with yes-no responses. It includes items which are appropriate for stroke patients in hospital. The suggested cut-offs vary between 9/10 and 16/17, so there are wide discrepancies between studies.

- The Symptom Checklist 90 (Derogatis, Lipman & Covi, 1973) is a self-rated scale that consists of eight psychiatric symptom domains, including a 16-item depression subscale. The SCL-90 has been used as a measure of distress and to screen for depression in one study (Aben *et al.*, 2002), but there is no independent verification of the recommended cut-offs.

- The Wakefield Depression Inventory (Snaith, Ahmed, Mehta & Hamilton, 1971) is a 12-item scale which was designed to assess the severity of depression. It uses a consistent format of response categories which makes it simpler to administer to stroke patients than some scales. However, there are some items affected by the somatic symptoms of stroke, such as 'I find it easy to do the things I used to'.

- The Wimbledon Self Report Scale (Coughlan & Storey, 1988) is a 30-item scale which was developed to measure of mood in patients with neurological disorders, and is not specific to either symptoms of anxiety or depression. It is included in care assessment pathways in clinical services but there is no validation study of the scale in stroke patients. It was evaluated by Bunton (2008), as one component of the Mood Assessment Care Pathway (Field, Personal communication), but only eight patients were assessed on the scale. It was sensitive to major depression and minor depression, as assessed using a structured clinical interview, but the sample sizes were very small so confidence intervals were wide.

- The Yale question (Lachs, Feinstein & Cooney, Drickamer, Marottoli, Pannill & Tinetti, 1990; Mahoney, Drinka, Abler, Gunterhunt, Matthews, Gravenstein *et al.*, 1994) 'Do you often feel sad or depressed' has also been evaluated as a screening measure. Watkins *et al.* (Watkins, Daniels, Jack, Dickinson & van den Broek, 2001; Watkins, Lightbody, Sutton, Holcroft, Dickinson, van den Broek & Leathley, 2007) administered the MADRS and the Yale to 122 stroke patients in hospital two weeks and three months after stroke and found very close agreement between the two measures. Lightbody (2007) examined the relation between the Yale question completed by a research nurse and psychiatric interview completed blind to the Yale results in 74 of the 112 patients included in the study by Watkins *et al.* (2007). The Yale had moderate sensitivity and specificity (70%), but the sensitivity was higher for those with communication problems (79%) than those without (65%), suggesting it should only be used when other measures are not available. The main advantage is that it is very quick and simple to use.

The general message emerging is that for most measures, using the standard cut-off points may not be appropriate and stroke-specific cut-offs are required to detect stroke patients who need further evaluation, so that no patients with significant mood problems are missed. For many measures there is a trade off between sensitivity and specificity, such that low cut-offs may be used if it is important not to miss any patients who require further evaluation, but this will not necessarily be the most efficient, and in some circumstances it may be necessary to take greater account of specificity. Most of the screening measures are sensitive, but many lack specificity, so a large proportion of patients will require further evaluation. Although it might be expected that because some symptoms of depression overlap with those of stroke, the cut-offs might need to be higher for stroke patients, whereas in many cases lower cut-offs are recommended for stroke patients as compared with normative samples. The positive predictive values are very variable, but many of the scales are better at identifying those that do not have low mood (negative predictive values are high) than those that do (positive predictive values are low).

Screening measures for people with communication problems

In some studies (Hilari, Northcott, Roy, Marshall, Wiggins, Chataway *et al.*, 2010; Townend, Brady & McLaughlan, 2007c), mood measures have been modified in format to make them suitable for people with aphasia. However, interviews, verbal self-report and questionnaires may not be practical with many patients with communication problems, particularly in the acute stage after stroke. Even when questionnaires are presented in an adapted format, it has been suggested that the responses may not be meaningful or reliable (Price, Curless &

Rodgers, 1999; Turner-Stokes & MacWalter, 2005). Often it is the content of the question that is difficult for patients to understand, rather than the response categories, and therefore modifications to the scale will affect validity. Gordon and Hibbard (1997) advised that multiple sources of information are required to assess mood in stroke patients who are unable to complete a clinical interview or self-report measure. This includes using observational methods, which require a nurse, carer or relative to rate both behaviour, such as sadness or crying, and symptoms, such as sleep and appetite disturbances. For valid reports, the informant should have frequent contact with the patient (Carota & Bogous-slavsky, 2003). It is also important to take account of the fact that responses may also be affected by the observer's mood (Berg *et al.*, 2009; Klinedinst, Clark, Blanton & Wolf, 2007). Although the ideal is to use measures which have been standardised in relation to psychiatric interview, interviews may not be practical with a significant proportion of aphasic patients, and therefore cut-offs have been identified in stroke patients who can communicate, as they can complete interviews or questionnaires, and then results have been generalised to patients with aphasia.

Screening measures

Two types of measures have been used to screen for low mood in those who are unable to complete standardised questionnaire measures; one is observational scales based on observables behaviours, and the other is to use pictorial or visual analogue scales in which the items are presented nonverbally. The advantage of these measures is that they were all developed for people with communication problems rather than by adapting existing measures. The available scales are summarised below, and the recommended cut-offs for stroke patients are shown in Table 14.2.

- The Aphasic Depression Rating Scale (ADRS; Benaim, Cailly, Perennou, & Pelissier, 2004) is a nine-item observer-rated measure developed for aphasic patients. It was derived from behavioural items in existing depression scales which could be observed by another person, and the scale was validated in a group of aphasic patients. Some items are scored on a three-point scale and others on five- or six-point scales, which may be confusing for raters and effectively differentially weights items. The ADRS was validated against a rating from 0 to 100 made by a psychiatrist. This was then converted to depressed–not depressed categories, although the way this was achieved was not explained.
- The Depression Intensity Scale Circles (DISCS; Turner-Stokes, Kalmus, Hirani & Clegg, 2005) were developed as a simple, self-report screening measure, based on a criticism that the spatial relations of visual analogue scales can be difficult for stroke patients. The DISCS comprises six circles with an increasing proportion of grey shading. The DISCS was evaluated in

Table 14.2 Recommended Cut-Offs for Screening Mood Problems in Stroke Patients with Communication Problems

Screening measure	Study	Stroke sample	Criterion measure	Cut-off	Sens' %	Spec' %	PPV %	NPV %	Agree[t] kappa
Aphasic Depression Rating Scale	Benaim et al., 2004	n=50 Patients in neurorehabilitation unit	Psychiatrist rating of depression	8/9	83	71			
Depression Intensity Scale Circles	Turner-Stokes et al., 2005	n=114, 76 with stroke patients in neurorehabilitation unit	DSM-IV criteria for depression	1/2	60	87	75	77	
Signs of Depression Scale	Watkins et al., 2001	n=137 consecutively admitted acute patients	MADRS	1/2	70	56	65	62	
	Bennett et al., 2006	n=70	HADS-D	1/2	86	62	36	95	0.32
		patients in acute hospital wards	HADS-A	0/1	63	29	18	76	0.04
	Lightbody et al., 2007	n=71 acute patients in hospital	Psychiatrists diagnosis of depression	1/2	64	61	47	76	
Smiley faces	Lee et al., 2008	n=253 one month after first stroke	DSM-IV diagnosis of depression		76	77	74	79	0.53

Measure	Reference	Setting	Comparator	Cutoff					
Stroke Aphasic Depression Questionnaire 10	Leeds et al., 2004	n=65	GDS 15	14/15	70	77			
	Sackley et al., 2006	n=82 residents in care homes	HADS	14/15	77	78	40	95	
Stroke Aphasic Depression Questionnaire Hospital version 21	Bennett et al., 2006	n=69	HADS-D	17/18	100	81	62	100	0.67
		patients in acute hospital wards	HADS-A	9/10	75	40	27	84	0.09
Stroke Aphasic Depression Questionnaire Hospital version 10	Bennett et al., 2006	n=70	HADS-D	5/6	100	78	57	100	0.62
		patients in acute hospital wards	HADS-A	4/5	75	50	31	87	0.17
	Hacker et al., 2010	n=125 acute inpatients	BASDEC	6/7	68	79	58	85	
Visual Analog Mood Scales	Bennett et al., 2006	n=79	HADS-D	223/224	81	51	31	86	0.20
		patients in acute hospital wards	HADS-A	255/256	71	66	36	89	0.27

(continued)

Table 14.2 (*Continued*)

Screening measure	Study	Stroke sample	Criterion measure	Cut-off	Sens[y] %	Spec[y] %	PPV %	NPV %	Agree[t] kappa
Visual Analog Mood Scales sad item	Bennett et al., 2006	n=79 patients in acute hospital wards	HADS-D	22/23	88	62	37	95	0.33
	Berg et al., 2009	n=100	DSM-III-R2 major depression 2 months	49/50	20	84			
			12 months	49/50	0	93			
Visual Analogue Self-Esteem Scale	Bennett et al., 2006*	n=79 patients in acute hospital wards	HADS-D	32/31	19	95	50	82	0.06
			HADS-A	34/33	24	81	25	79	0.02

DSM: Diagnostic and Statistical Manual; BASDEC: Brief Assessment Schedule Depression Cards; MADRS: Montgomery-Åsberg Depression Rating Scale; Sens[y]: sensitivity; Spec[y]: specificity; PPV: positive predictive value; NPV: negative predictive value; HADS: Hospital Anxiety and Depression Scale D depression subscale, A anxiety subscale, T total score mpo: months post onset.

2, 6, 12 and 18 months after stroke.

*In the original paper, low scores were not reversed to indicate low mood.

younger adults with acquired brain injury in a neurorehabilitation unit, with the majority (67%) having had a stroke. A cut-off of 1/2 was recommended (sensitivity, 60%; specificity, 87%) for identifying depression as defined by DSM-IV criteria. Validation of the scale with older stroke patients would be useful.

- The Signs of Depression Scale (SODS; Hammond, O'Keefe & Barer, 2000) is a six-item scale of observable mood symptoms, which is a shortened version of a scale developed for elderly medical patients in hospital. It was validated early after stroke against the Montgomery-Åsberg Depression Rating Scale (Watkins, Leathley, Daniels, Dickinson, Lightbody, van den Broek *et al.*, 2001). It was able to detect depression in patients in hospital (Bennett, Thomas, Austen, Morris & Lincoln, 2006; Lightbody, Baldwin, Connolly, Gibbon, Jawaid, Leathley *et al.,* 2007; Watkins *et al.*, 2001) but not anxiety (Bennett *et al.*, 2006). Although the SODS is easily completed by staff on hospital wards, the efficiency is not high. It may be possible to increase this by requiring high scores on more than one occasion or from different observers.

- Smiley faces have been used as an alternative to visual analogue scales. These comprise diagrammatic faces with a smile, neutral or sad expression. Lee *et al.* (2008) evaluated smiley faces as a measure appropriate for those with low levels of literacy and from various cultural backgrounds. Stroke patients were asked to rate the frequency of having various facial expressions over the past week. Reporting having a sad face in the past week was more closely related to a diagnosis of depression using DSM-IV criteria than having a neutral face or a happy face. However, Lee *et al.* (2008) noted that the sensitivity of the faces was not very high and some patients with depression were missed. The Smiley Faces may, however, be useful when other methods are not practical.

- The Stroke Aphasic Depression Questionnaire (Sutcliffe & Lincoln, 1998) and Hospital Stroke Aphasic Depression Questionnaire (SADQ-H; Lincoln, Sutcliffe & Unsworth, 2000) were developed to assess mood in aphasic patients using observed behaviours. The 21 items were derived from those in standardised questionnaires which could be observed by another person, such as 'Did he/she initiate activities?' The four response options differ between the two scales. The original version (Sutcliffe & Lincoln, 1998) used 'often', 'sometimes', 'rarely' and 'never' as the response categories, and these were found to be acceptable in a community sample when ratings were being provided by carers. However, in hospital settings the reliability of nurses using these categories was low and therefore the hospital version has response categories based on the frequencies of the behaviours ('every day this week', '4–6 times a week', '2–4 times a week', and 'less than twice this week'). These frequencies were intended to be guide frequencies and recording behaviours on a daily basis is not required. There are ten-item short forms for each version (Sutcliffe & Lincoln, 1998; Lincoln *et al.*, 2000). Independent validation studies have identified cut-off points for various versions of the scale to identify depression (Bennett *et al.*, 2006;

Hacker, Stark & Thomas, 2010; Leeds, Meera & Hobson, 2004; Sackley, Hoppitt & Cardoso, 2006), but the SADQ-H was not found to be suitable for screening for anxiety (Bennett *et al.*, 2006). It is important to note that none of the versions of the SADQ has been validated in relation to psychiatric interview. In clinical practice the scale is administered weekly, and high scores are required on two consecutive weeks before patients are referred for further evaluation of their mood.

- The Visual Analog Mood Scales (VAMS; Stern, 1997) consist of eight visual analogue unipolar scales: afraid, confused, sad, angry, energetic, tired, happy and tense. Stern (1997) suggested a cut-off of 50 on the 'sad' item to identify possible depression or anxiety, but this has not been supported by other authors (Bennett *et al.* 2006). Berg *et al.* (2009) evaluated a happy-sad item, but noted that it had low sensitivity was no easier for aphasic patients to complete than questionnaire measures. They also found no significant correlation between the VAMS happy-sad item and the BDI a year after stroke. Similarly Benaim, Decavel, Bentabet, Froger, Pelissier and Perennou (2010) noted that 18% of their sample of stroke patients was unable to complete the VAMS sad item. One problem with the eight-item VAMS scale is that the neutral item is always presented at the bottom of the page and thus the positive items, energetic and happy, are not reversed relative to the negative items, such as sad, angry and tense. Kontou (2010) demonstrated that reversing the happy and energetic items produced less inconsistency of responding than the standard format. Thus, the revised version (Kontou, 2010) may be more accurate than the original, but this needs verification.
- The Visual Analogue Self-Esteem Scale (VASES; Brumfitt & Sheeran, 1999a, 1999b) is a 10-item scale designed to assess self-esteem in aphasic patients. Each item consists of a pair of pictures representing the following constructs: not being understood/understood, not confident/confident, cheerful/not cheerful, outgoing/not outgoing, mixed up/not mixed up, intelligent/not intelligent, angry/not angry, trapped/not trapped, not optimistic/optimistic and frustrated/not frustrated. Depressed/not depressed is used as the practice item. Bennett *et al.* (2006) evaluated the inclusion of depressed/not depressed as part of the scale, but this had very little effect on the overall screening ability of the measure. Although Bennett *et al.* (2006) found the VASES had good sensitivity for detecting both depression and anxiety, the specificity was so low that the authors concluded that the scale was not suitable for screening purposes.

In general, observational measures are the most practical for screening for low mood in people with communication problems and these can be followed up using visual analogue measures to verify the mood state. It has been recognised that collaboration between psychiatrists, psychologists and speech and language therapists is needed for a comprehensive evaluation of mood disorders in those with communication problems (Brumfitt & Barton, 2006; Creed *et al.*, 2003) and that standard criteria may need to be adapted (Townend *et al.*, 2007c). Further evaluation of many of the measures is needed in relation to comprehensive clinical evaluation.

Assessing mood to plan treatment

Once screening measures have been completed and potential problems with mood identified, patients should be assessed further in order to confirm the type of mood disorder and to plan treatment. In many cases this further assessment should comprise a structured clinical interview. Some of the measures reviewed above will also be useful for the further evaluation of stroke patients. The administration of additional measures will serve to confirm the presence of a mood disorder and to indicate particular features, which may be relevant to planning treatment. Some measures were designed to assess the severity of the mood disorder rather than just detecting its presence. For example the CES-D and WDI were both designed assess the frequency and severity depressive symptoms. The GHQ-30 or GHQ-28 will supplement information from the GHQ1-2 and, using a 0,1,2,3 scoring instead of a 0,0,1,1, scoring will indicate severity of distress. The GHQ-28 also has subscale scores. The BDI-II may sometimes be too long and complex to use as a screening measure, but will be appropriate for the more detailed evaluation prior to therapy. It will also differentiate cognitive and somatic components of depression. Berg *et al.* (2009) examined the cognitive and somatic subscales of the BDI-II in a follow–up study of 100 stroke patients taking part in a treatment study. Both subscales were significantly correlated with the total BDI score, with slight variations in the strength of the correlations at different times after stroke (cognitive subscale with total $r_s= 0.78$ to 0.91 and somatic subscale with total $r_s= 0.75$ to 0.89, $p<0.001$). The internal consistency of the cognitive subscale was acceptable (0.85 to 0.91), but that of the somatic subscale (0.37 to 0.56) was not. In addition, cognitive items (i.e. discouraged about the future, feeling like a failure, feeling guilty and looking unattractive) were found to be significant predictors of major depression in the acute phase. At 18 months, sadness, dissatisfaction, discouraged about the future, feeling disappointed, loss of interest in people and difficulty with decisions were the best predictors of major depression. This suggests that the cognitive subscale of the BDI may be particularly relevant when assessing the severity of depression after stroke.

Several studies have examined the symptoms of depression in order to obtain a diagnosis based on DSM criteria. The Hamilton Rating Scale has been the most commonly used for this purpose. However, it has been suggested (Gainotti, Azzoni, Razzano, Lanzillotta & Marra, 1997) that stroke-specific criteria should be used. The Post-Stroke Depression Rating Scale (PSDRS; Gainotti *et al.*, 1997) comprises ratings of the symptoms commonly seen in depressed stroke patients. It requires an interview by a 'professional examiner' who then rates the presence and severity of these symptoms in ten sections on a scale from 0 to 5. It was validated in relation to the Hamilton Rating Scale. Gainotti *et al.* (1997) identified differences in the profile of symptoms between stroke patients with major depression and psychiatric patients with endogenous depression, whereas patients with major and minor depression following stroke showed a similar profiles of symptoms. A validation study (Quaranta *et al.*, 2008) of the Hamilton Depression Rating Scale and the Post Stroke Depression Rating Scale in relation to psychiatric interview and diagnosis using DSM-IV criteria indicated that both scales were reliable diagnostic tools. The optimum cut-off for detecting major depression with the Hamilton Depression Rating Scale was 17/18 (sensitivity, 82%; specificity, 81%; PPV, 60%; NPV, 93%) and for the Post Stroke Depression Rating Scale 17/18 (sensitivity, 76%; specificity, 93%; PPV, 79%; NPV, 92%). However, the higher positive predictive value of the Post Stroke Depression Rating Scale, which was more marked in aphasic patients, led to its recommendation for use in clinical practice.

Since cognitions seem to be important determinants of mood, and cognitions may be particularly relevant for those who are being considered for cognitive behavioural therapy, further evaluation of cognitions may be needed. Hackett, Hill, Hewison, Anderson and House (2010) considered individual items on the depression section of the GHQ-28 in order to identify negative cognitions. However, the Stroke Cognitions Questionnaire Revised (SCQR; Thomas & Lincoln, 2008b) is a 21-item scale specifically designed to assess the frequency of positive and negative cognitions after stroke. The items were constructed from treatment notes and diaries of depressed stroke patients (Nicholl, Lincoln, Muncaster & Thomas, 2002). The SCQR was evaluated with 50 stroke patients in hospital. It had high internal consistency, interrater reliability and test–retest reliability and was significantly correlated with the BDI-II. There are no published cut-offs as the scale was not developed for screening purposes. However, the SCQR may be useful for identifying cognitions to be addressed in treatment and to monitor progress, but the sensitivity to treatment effects remains to be established.

Measures of self-esteem may also be useful in planning therapy. Bennett *et al.* (2006) examined the Visual Analogue Self-Esteem Scale (VASES; Brumfitt & Sheeran, 1999) and concluded that although not a good screening measure, the VASES could be used as part of a comprehensive assessment of mood. Support for this comes from Vickery (2006) who found that the VASES was highly correlated with measures of mood and was not significantly affected by demographic variables, such as age, education, gender and race, or stroke-related variables, such as visual acuity, language, abstract reasoning and visuo-perceptual impairment.

Anxiety is not well evaluated using standard screening assessments, and therefore additional assessment of anxiety may be required. Although the HADS anxiety subscale and Beck Anxiety Inventory will detect some patients with anxiety, their specificity is low and so there will be people with anxiety disorders who are missed using screening measures. Further evaluations might include the Speilberger State Trait Anxiety Inventory and the Symptom Checklist 90, but they require validation in patients with stroke.

Emotionalism is an additional problem which may need to be evaluated. There is one standardised measure developed in stroke patients, the Pathological Laughter and Crying Scale (PLACS; Robinson, Parikh, Lipsey, Starkstein & Price, 1993). The PLACS may be used to assess the severity of emotionalism and as a measure of change over time. It includes consideration of the duration, level of voluntary control, appropriateness to the context and feelings of well-being. For each item severity is rated on a scale from 0 to 3. Eight items assess pathological laughing, and eight pathological crying. It has been shown to be sensitive to the effects of drug treatment for emotionalism (Robinson *et al.*, 1993). As the PLACS was designed to be administered by a trained interviewer, it is best suited to being used as part of a comprehensive evaluation of mood state. A similar scale, the Center for Neurologic Study- Lability Scale (CNS-LS; Moore, Gresham, Bromberg, Kasarkis & Smith, 1997), was developed as a self-report measure of affective lability but was validated in people with multiple sclerosis. It has seven items, four measuring labile laughter and three measuring labile tearfulness. It may be appropriate for stroke patients, but validation studies are needed.

It has been recognised that post-traumatic stress disorder (PTSD) may occur following stroke (Sembi, Tarrier, O'Neill, Burns & Faragher, 1998) and may need to be evaluated. Several authors have used standardised scales to assess aspects of PTSD in stroke patients. Sembi *et al.* (1998) used the Impact of Events Scale (Horowitz, Wilner & Alvarez, 1979) and the Penn Inventory of PTSD (Hammarberg, 1992). The Impact of Events Scale is a self-report measure of current emotional distress related to a specific event, which has 15 items in two subscales, Intrusion and Avoidance. The Penn Inventory of PTSD is used as a measure of severity of PTSD. The cut-offs used were based on published data and not specific to stroke. However, these measures of PTSD were independent of physical disability suggesting they may not be significantly affected by the symptoms of stroke. Sampson, Kinderman, Watts and Sembi (2003) used the Post Traumatic Stress Disorder Checklist (Weathers, Litz, Herman, Huska & Keane, 1993), a 17-item self-report rating scale, and used a cut-off of 43/44 to indicate PTSD. Gangstad *et al.* (2009) used the Posttraumatic Growth Inventory (Tedeschi & Calhoun, 1996) and Cognitive Processing of Trauma Scale (Williams, Davis & Millsap, 2002). They adapted the Posttraumatic Growth Inventory by changing the words 'my crisis' to 'my stroke'. These scales seem to have been useful in research to evaluate PTSD in stroke patients and may be appropriate with individual patients in clinical practice.

Important aspects of the ways people deal with the emotional effects of stroke are the extent to which they cope and adjust emotionally. Donnellan, Hevey, Hickey and O'Neill (2006) reviewed measures of coping and adjustment after stoke. Although they identified ten measures, modified versions of the Ways of

Coping Questionnaire (Folkman & Lazarus, 1988) and the Coping Orientation for Problem Experiences (COPE; Carver, Scheier & Weintraub, 1989) were the most commonly used, with a few studies using scales to assess mental adjustment. There is also a short version of the COPE (Carver, 1997). However, the psychometric properties of these have not been established in stroke patients.

Sensitivity to change

Few measures have been demonstrated to be sensitive to the effects of psychological intervention after stroke. This may reflect problems with the sensitivity of the scales or lack of effectiveness of the interventions. However, there is some indication of measures which would be the most likely to be suitable for assessing change. The GHQ-28 has been shown to be sensitive to change over time and to the effects of interventions (e.g. House, 2003; Juby, Lincoln & Berman, 1996; Watkins, Auton, Deans, Dickinson, Jack, Lightbody *et al.*, 2007a). The BDI showed statistically significant change in the year after stroke (House *et al.*, 1991) and was sensitive to the effects of antidepressant treatment (Turner-Stokes, Hassan, Pierce & Clegg, 2002). It may be suitable as a measure of change, particularly in response to cognitive therapy, as in a treatment trial, Lincoln and Flannaghan (2003) showed significant change over time on both the BDI and GHQ-28. The Aphasic Depression Rating Scale has been shown to be sensitive to change over a month (Benaim *et al.*, 2010), but further validation is required to determine whether other observer measures, such as the Signs of Depression Scale and the Stroke Aphasic Depression Questionnaire are responsive to changes. In addition, although visual analogue measures have been used to evaluate progress with treatment (Cunningham & Ward, 2003; Ross, Winslow, Marchant & Brumfitt, 2006), they have not shown significant change. It is not clear whether this is due to lack of change in mood or lack of sensitivity of the measures, and therefore the responsiveness to change needs to be established. A measure of adjustment, the Cognitive and Instrumental Readjustment Scale (Ben Sira & Eliezer, 1990), has been shown to be sensitive to the effects of stroke unit rehabilitation (Juby *et al.*, 1996) and could be useful for monitoring progress with therapy.

It is clear from this review that many scales are available to assess mood in people with stroke. Many have cut-offs developed with stroke patients, such that they can be used to identify patients who need further evaluation of their mood. Different scales are suitable for different stroke patients, and not everyone can be assessed using the same measure. In addition different measures will be appropriate at different stages after stroke. The scales may be used as part of a comprehensive evaluation of mood within the context of an overall care pathway. These have been described in the literature (Turner Stokes & Hassan, 2002; Kneebone, Baker & O'Malley, 2010), and some examples are provided below.

Examples of mood assessment care pathways

In acute settings, time constraints may limit the use of questionnaire measures in the majority of patients and therefore observer measures are used as an initial criterion. They may then be followed up with questionnaires or interviews by specialist members of the team. For example, in Figure 14.1 a care pathway is shown which relies almost exclusively on the SADQH10 Dale, personal communication. Any patients with high scores are assessed by a psychologist.

In other settings, guidance is given to other members of the team to use a range of measures according to the patients' abilities. For example, Field (Personal communication) developed the Mood Assessment Care Pathway (MACP) in which the questionnaire measures were used according to patients' characteristics. The implementation is summarised in Figure 14.3.

The accuracy of this pathway was evaluated by Bunton (2008) in relation to clinical interview. They used the MACP to identify patients with depression and then compared the findings with a structured clinical interview, blind to the questionnaire results in an acute stroke setting. The individual screening measures were found to be sensitive to major and minor depression (71% to 100%), and most had adequate specificity (40% to 84%). The overall sensitivity of the pathway to major depression was 88% (specificity 65%) and to minor depression 74% (specificity 68%). However, kappa coefficients showed only slight agreement between the MACP and the structured clinical interview.

Mood assessment pathways may also be classified according to age (Kneebone *et al.*, 2010) as it is recognised that some measures have been validated in different age groups and the symptoms of low mood may vary according to age. Examples are shown in Figures 14.4 and 14.5.

Mood assessment pathways have also been classified according to the setting. Examples are shown in Figures 14.6 and 14.7.

These assessment pathways are mainly based on evidence for the individual scales included. Overall evaluation of the pathways in relation to comprehensive clinical evaluation has rarely been carried out, the notable exception being the evaluation of the MACP by Bunton (2008).

Adherence to guidelines for mood assessment

Although these mood assessment pathways are available in many stroke services, it is apparent that the assessment of mood does not occur in a way that is recommended. The first edition of the 'National Clinical Guidelines for Stroke' (Royal College of Physicians, 2000) included eight recommendations for mood disturbance. One was that 'patients should be screened for depression and anxiety within the first month after stroke and their mood kept under review' (p.46). The guidelines also recommended referral to an experienced clinical psychologist or psychiatrist when the mood disorder 'is causing

Mood pathway for acute stroke

Please ensure that the SADQ H10 is filled in for every person every week as a routine procedure. This is in order that we can monitor a person's mood and detect whether a person may be at risk of developing a mood disorder.

Please highlight at each case conference/MDT meeting each person's emotional well-being and identify any concerns regarding mood or psychological difficulties.

If you have any concerns about a person's mood as a first step please ensure the following:
- Use your listening skills.
- Be patient and empathic about their situation.
- Identify and encourage them to take part in activities that they may enjoy or find rewarding (ask them or their carers for ideas).
- Give positive feedback on achievements.
- Promote involvement in planning and decision making where possible.
- Ask if they would like more information about their condition and prognosis and in what form.
- Help them to problem solve difficulties.
- Involve carers in treatment if appropriate.

If the team would like further support in identifying and managing mood difficulties, refer onto Clinical Psychology or Psychiatry.

Refer to Clinical Psychology when:
- A patient scores 6 or above on the SAD QH 10 for two or more weeks. Depending on the circumstances, the psychology intervention may involve supporting the team or carers to manage the patient's mood, or direct contact with the patient. Techniques used include environmental changes, increasing social support, talking therapy (e.g. CBT, narrative and brief therapy), and behavioural therapy.

Refer to Psychiatry when:
- Advice is wanted on diagnosis or medication, for example diagnosis is uncertain, there is inadequate response to medication (allow at least two weeks to take effect), or there are unwanted or unpleasant side effects of medication.
- Or if you are worried about a person's suicidal intentions.

Please ensure on discharge that;
- Any concerns about mood and any recommendations including the clinical psychology discharge summary are passed on to the person's GP and relevant agencies, for example early supported discharge team or community stroke teams.

For any further information please contact Dr X, Clinical Psychologist, Stroke Services

Figure 14.1 Mood assessment on an acute stroke ward. From Dale (personal communication).

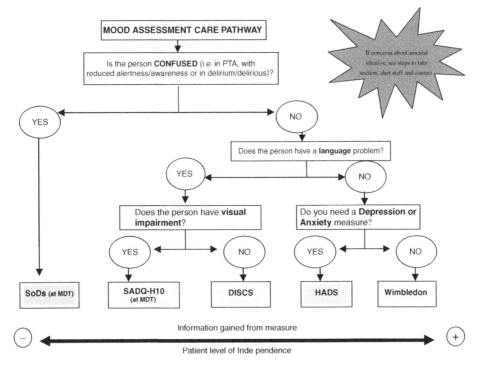

Figure 14.2   Mood Assessment Care Pathway. Reproduced with permission of Field (unpublished).

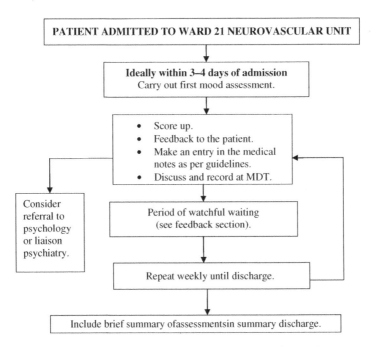

Figure 14.3   Implementation of Mood Assessment Care Pathway. *Source*: Reproduced with permission of Field (unpublished).

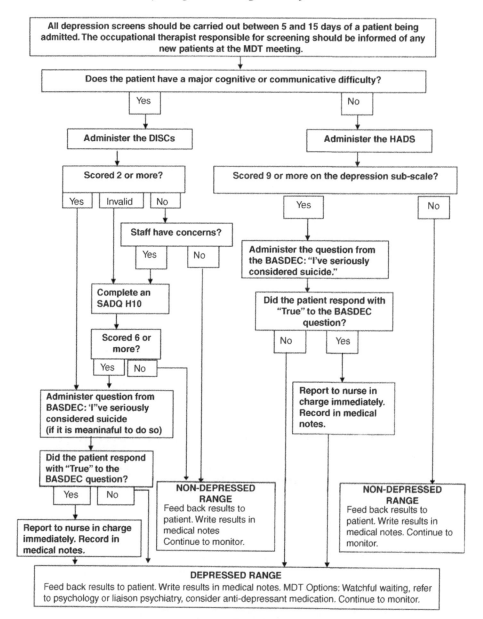

All depression screens should be carried out between 5 and 15 days of a patient being admitted. The occupational therapist responsible for screening should be informed of any new patients at the MDT meeting.

Does the patient have a major cognitive or communicative difficulty?

Yes — Administer the DISCs

No — Administer the HADS

Scored 2 or more?

Scored 9 or more on the depression sub-scale?

Yes | Invalid | No

Staff have concerns?

Yes | No

Complete an SADQ H10

Scored 6 or more?

Yes | No

Administer question from BASDEC: 'I''ve seriously considered suicide (if it is meaninaful to do so)

Did the patient respond with "True" to the BASDEC question?

Yes | No

Report to nurse in charge immediately. Record in medical notes.

Yes — Administer the question from the BASDEC: "I've seriously considered suicide."

Did the patient respond with "True" to the BASDEC question?

No | Yes

Report to nurse in charge immediately. Record in medical notes.

NON-DEPRESSED RANGE
Feed back results to patient. Write results in medical notes
Continue to monitor.

No — NON-DEPRESSED RANGE
Feed back results to patient. Write results in medical notes. Continue to monitor.

DEPRESSED RANGE
Feed back results to patient. Write results in medical notes. MDT Options: Watchful waiting, refer to psychology or liaison psychiatry, consider anti-depressant medication. Continue to monitor.

Figure 14.4 Flow chart for people younger than 65 years. Reproduced with permission from Kneebone *et al.* (2010).
BASDEC = Brief Assessment Schedule Depression Cards; DISCs = Depression Intensity Scale Circles; MDT = Multidisciplinary Team; SADQ-H10 = Stroke Aphasic Depression Questionnaire-Hospital, ten-item version.

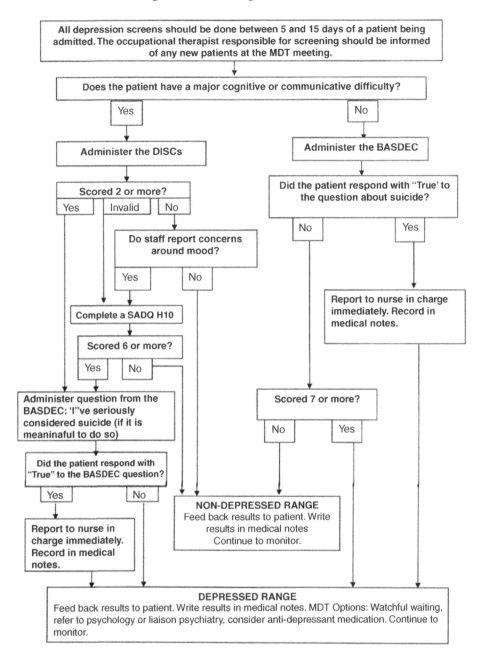

Figure 14.5 Flow chart for people aged 65 years and older. Reproduced with permission from Kneebone *et al.* (2010).
BASDEC = Brief Assessment Schedule Depression Cards; DISCs = Depression Intensity Scale Circles; MDT = Multidisciplinary Team; SADQ-H10 = Stroke Aphasic Depression Questionnaire-Hospital, ten-item version.

Mood assessment care pathway

In Hospital

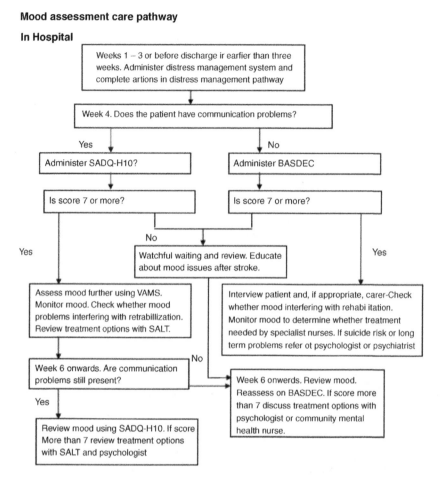

Weeks 1 – 3 or before discharge ir earfier than three weeks. Administer distress management system and complete artions in distress management pathway

Week 4. Does the patient have communication problems?

Yes — Administer SADQ-H10?

No — Administer BASDEC

Is score 7 or more?

Is score 7 or more?

No

Watchful waiting and review. Educate about mood issues after stroke.

Yes

Yes

Assess mood further using VAMS. Monitor mood. Check whether mood problems interfering with retrabillization. Review treatment options with SALT.

Interview patient and, if appropriate, carer-Check whether mood interfering with rehabi itation. Monitor mood to determine whether treatment needed by specialist nurses. If suicide risk or long term problems refer ot psychologist or psychiatrist

No

Week 6 onwards. Are communication problems still present?

Yes

Week 6 onwerds. Review mood. Reassess on BASDEC. If score more than 7 discuss treatment options with psychologist or community mental health nurse.

Review mood using SADQ-H10. If score More than 7 review treatment options with SALT and psychologist

Figure 14.6 Mood screening pathway for acute hospital stroke wards.

persistent distress or worsening disability' (p.46). A national audit of the RCP guidelines for assessing mood (Bowen, Knapp, Hoffman & Lowe, 2005) showed that compliance with the guideline was low. In an audit of hospital notes carried out in the UK in 2001–2002, there was a median compliance rate of 50% for hospitals following the guidelines for mood screening, by 2008 (Royal College of Physicians, 2008c) this had improved to 65% of patients being screened for low mood after stroke. In the 2001–2002 audit comparison of the 31 hospitals with psychologist input with the 80 hospitals without showed no significant difference (60% vs. 50%) in the rate of compliance with mood screening, but this was not available for the 2008 audit. After discharge from hospital, there was evidence of mood being reviewed in only 54% of patients in the 2001–2002 audit. Thus, although there were mood screening measures available, they were not being used in clinical practice at that time. Field *et al.* (in preparation) conducted an audit before and after implementation

Mood assesment care pathway

After discharge from Hospital

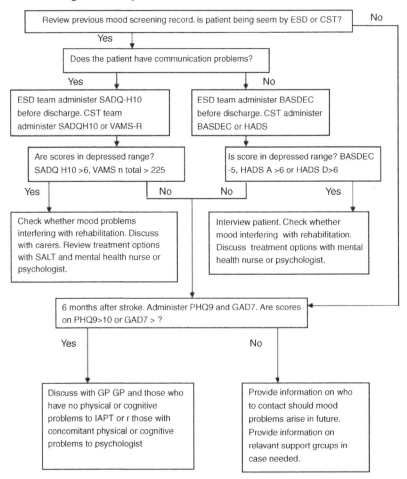

Figure 14.7   Mood screening pathway after discharge from hospital.
CST: community stroke team; ESD: early suported discharge team.

of their Mood Assessment Care Pathway and found that the rate of screening increased from 13% of patients to 44%, but despite training doctors to use the care pathway over half the patients were not assessed for mood problems. In addition, despite providing six measures suitable for different types of patients, in the sample studied only two of the measures were used in practice. It may be that the allocation of responsibility for screening should be spread across more professions, according to the setting and the timing of assessment in the stroke pathway. It will also depend on the availability of clinical psychologists to support the process, provide consultation for complex cases and to monitor for drift.

Staff training

There are various reasons why low rates of screening may occur. One reason is that staff on wards do not have the skills to identify the symptoms of mood disorder and therefore they do not carry out the required assessments. Several authors have commented that nurses may require greater training to identify the symptoms of depression (Berg *et al.*, 2009; House *et al.*, 1989b; Lightbody *et al.*, 2007). The implication is either that nurses need training in eliciting symptoms of depression or that greater use is made of self-report measures which are less dependent on the interpretation of symptoms. Hart and Morris (2008) developed a questionnaire to explore the reasons that screening for mood disorders was not carried out in compliance with guidelines. They evaluated the responses of 75 staff participants using the theory of planned behaviour to understand compliance behaviours. They found that the barriers to mood screening were lack of time, feeling uncomfortable using available question-naires and a concern that screening might trigger depression. They suggested that staff training could be provided to increase knowledge and skills, to identify treatment options and the benefits of screening, and to 'demystify' post-stroke depression. They also identified that lack of consensus about appropriate screening measures for stroke patients contributed to the failure to screen patients in practice.

Conclusions

There are several measures available to screen for low mood after stroke. Although there is variation between studies, the overall ability of the measures to identify patients with low mood is satisfactory and there are recommended cut-offs available. The measures suitable for those with communication pro-blems are less robust but provide an option when standardised questionnaires are either not possible or not practical. There are far more measures available to identify depression than other mood states. In most cases, a high score on a screening measure will need to be followed up by further assessment of mood. A variety of measures will be needed according to the patients' abilities and the setting, as is reflected in care pathways used in clinical practice. The advantage of such care pathways is that they help to ensure that the effects of stroke on mood are considered. Few of the mood measures have been used as outcome measures and so the sensitivity to change has not been well documented, though many are used clinically for this purpose. However, although standardised measures have their place, mood assessment requires more than administering a questionnaire and those with problems with low mood should always be assessed more comprehensively in order to identify the most appropriate treatment strategy.

Chapter 15

Managing Emotional Problems after Stroke

Emotional problems after stroke are common and have a negative impact on rehabilitation outcome and quality of life. Therefore, they require treatment. Treatments provided include both pharmacological and psychological interventions.

Treating emotional problems after stroke

Depression and associated disorders

A review by Hackett, Anderson, House and Xia (2009) identified a small but significant effect of medication on depressive symptoms and on treating depression in stroke samples. Medications that have been trialled include the selective serotonin re-uptake inhibitors (SSRIs; Citalopram, Fluoxetine and Paroxetine), Nortriptyline, Amitriptyline, Deanxit, Aniracetam, Reboxetine and Trazodone. Unfortunately, a major problem in the research is the short length of the trials completed. This has meant that the reviewers were unable to make statements as to whether one medication was more effective than another. The reviewers also raised concerns about the downside of medication for depression after stroke. It is associated with an increase in adverse events, most particularly nervous system and gastrointestinal effects (Hackett *et al.*, 2009). A trial of electroconvulsive therapy (ECT) for depression after stroke supported its use (Currier, Murray & Welch, 1992); however, randomised evidence on the efficacy and safety of ECT in depressed people with concomitant cerebrovascular is lacking (Van der Wurff, Stek, Hoogendijk & Beekman, 2003).

Hackett *et al.* (2009) considered the effect of psychotherapy on depression and depressive symptoms. They found no evidence of benefit in the small

Psychological Management of Stroke, First Edition. Nadina B. Lincoln, Ian I. Kneebone, Jamie A.B. Macniven and Reg C. Morris.
© 2012 John Wiley & Sons, Ltd. Published 2012 by John Wiley & Sons, Ltd.

number of randomised controlled trials completed. While there is a literature on a range of therapies for depression after stroke, including hypnotherapy (Crasilneck & Hall, 1979), problem-focussed family therapy (Watzlawick & Coyne, 1980), counselling (Forster & Young, 1996), differential reinforcement (Jain, 1982), human givens (Tapper, 2006) and cognitive-behavioural therapy (CBT; Lincoln, Flannagan, Sutcliffe & Rother, 1997) much more is required to establish the effectiveness of these approaches. CBT is the most researched of all therapies and appeared to offer promise (Kneebone & Dunmore, 2000) but is as yet unproven in a randomised controlled trial (Lincoln & Flannaghan, 2003).

A number of studies have considered pharmacological intervention for emotionalism after stroke. In a review of these, Hackett, Yang, Anderson, Horrocks and House (2010) considered studies that included tricyclic anti-depressants (TCA), SSRIs, and monoamine oxidase inhibitors (MAOIs), among others. They concluded that antidepressants can reduce post-stroke crying, in terms of both intensity and frequency, but were guarded in identifying any one class of medication as more effective than another. Further trials of improved quality are required for solid conclusions to be drawn on the medication of choice for emotionalism.

Information on what psychological approaches are useful for emotionalism after stroke is restricted to one case series. Sacco, Sara, Pistoia, Conson, Albertini and Carolei (2008) used a psychological intervention in four individuals with locked-in syndrome after stroke, when emotionalism had proved unresponsive to medication. The treatment trial was a competing response and exposure paradigm. A psychologist, with the assistance of a physiotherapist, instructed patients to tense facial respiratory muscles they were able to control and presented with trigger stimuli. After 6–8 weeks of treatment (30 minutes, five times weekly), some degree of control was achieved for the four participants. While not available within the literature, some clinicians (personal communication) report that relaxation training (once again, as a competing response) and finger tapping (as a distraction) are useful for emotionalism after stroke. No consideration has yet been given specifically to treatment of 'catastrophic reactions' after stroke.

A case study is given in Table 15.1.

Treating anxiety and related disorders after stroke

Information on what is effective treatment for anxiety after stroke is highly limited, with only one trial of pharmacotherapy. Ohtomo, Hirai Terashi Hasegawa and Araki (1991) trialled Aniracetamand and found some benefits in anxiety reduction. First-line pharmacotherapy, such as SSRIs and noradrenergic and serotonin re-uptake inhibitors (SNRIs), are the preferred options in treatment of anxiety in the nonstroke population (Bandelow, Zohar, Hollander, Kasper & Moller, 2002). Acupuncture has been suggested as an alternative to medication in the treatment of anxiety after stroke. It performed as well as alprazolam in a comparison trial (Ping & Songhai, 2008). In another Chinese

Table 15.1   A Case Example of Psychological Treatment of Emotionality after Stroke

Jim was an 80-year-old retired civil engineer who experienced a right hemisphere stroke with left hemiparesis when gardening on a cold winter's day. He clearly recalled the event, his assessment and transport to hospital by the paramedics and his stabilisation there. He further recalled becoming 'easily moved' a week or so after his stroke. Some cousins, to whom he was very close, had travelled some hundreds of miles to the acute hospital to see him. He found himself weeping 'uncontrollably' when they left. He found this embarrassing and completely out of character. This reaction continued over the following three weeks. He was referred to a psychologist because of concerns by the therapists at the post-acute stroke unit that he was depressed. At assessment he indicated that visits from family, sad items on the evening news and praise from therapists about success all provoked tearfulness and even, on occasion, wailing that he found impossible to control. He was concerned not only about the loss of control itself, but also because he felt he was being weak by 'not coping' better and that he was upsetting those close to him, most particularly his wife of 56 years, Jean, who he felt he had put though enough.

Assessment by the clinical psychologist failed to find any evidence of frank depression. Apart from the episodes of tearfulness and his concerns relating to them, Jim was coping reasonably well. He had some fatigue that he put down to his stroke, but he was eating and sleeping well, and enjoyed reading, TV shows and regular banter with the nursing and therapy staff. He had no significant personal or family psychiatric history.

Formulation

It appeared Jim was exhibiting post-stroke emotionality. The origins of this were likely to be a direct consequence of his stroke-related brain damage. Possible additional contributors to his difficulty were considered to be his own self-deprecation for the emotionality as well as embarrassment and concern as to its effect on others, particularly his wife.

Intervention

The psychologist provided both Jim and his wife with education, including written information, on emotionality after stroke. Jim accepted a prescription of citalopram from the stroke physician and agreed to a cognitive-behavioural programme to assist his affect management. This consisted of training in a brief yoga breathing exercise, for use when the emotionality arose, and considering the view he took of his emotionalism. Over the course of the three-session psychological intervention, he went from self-criticism for the emotionality to a view of 'While I don't like it, it is part of the stroke, just like my difficulty in using my left arm and I can cope with it'. He addressed his concerns about the reaction of others as follows: 'The staff here are used to this and are not concerned when I am tearful. Jean has told my friends and reassured them it is a part of the stroke and it doesn't mean I am deeply distressed'.

Outcome

Over the course of the intervention, Jim's emotionality was assessed on the Post Stroke Crying Scale (Robinson, Parikh, Lipsey, Starkstein & Price, 1993). On this instrument, he improved from 19 to 7 on the crying dimension of the scale. He also became much more accepting of his reaction, a combination of his changed view and the reduced frequency of his emotionality. Jean was very pleased and relieved to receive the education about emotionality after stroke. She had been very concerned that her husband was not coping. She became able to accept his reassurances that he was generally feeling and managing well.

study, slow-stroke back massage reduced anxiety relative to controls, though the follow-up period was only three days (Mok & Woo, 2004).

Psychological therapy that is considered highly effective for anxiety in older and working-age people, such as CBT (Ayers Sorrell, Thorp & Wetherell, 2007; Butler, Chapman, Forman & Beck, 2005), remains to be evaluated in this population, as do supportive and psychodynamic approaches (Hunot, Churchill, Silva de Lima & Teixeira, 2007). Evidence of the positive effects of treatment of generalised anxiety, combined with neurorehabilitation for those with traumatic brain injury, suggests that CBT may be effective for anxiety after stroke (Soo & Tate, 2007).

To date there are no reports of pharmacological interventions that are successful in treating post-traumatic stress disorder or post-traumatic stress symptoms after stroke. Pharmacologically, the antidepressants, particularly the SSRIs do appear to have some effect in people with post-traumatic stress disorder (Stein, Ipser, & Seedat, 2006). In terms of psychological treatment, there is considerable evidence that trauma-focused CBT is effective for post-traumatic stress in the general population (Bisson & Andrew, 2007). That this might be successful after stroke is suggested from evidence that it is useful in those with head injury, including those with cognitive dysfunction (McMillan, Williams & Bryant, 2003; Soo & Tate, 2007), and in those with other neurological conditions, such as hydrocephalus (Kneebone & Hull, 2009).

A case example of psychological treatment for post-traumatic stress disorder after stroke is shown in Table 15.2.

There is, as yet, no outcome research supporting any particular approach to reducing fear of falling solely among people with stroke. A CBT (Tennstedt, Howland, Lachman, Peterson, Kasten & Jette, 1998b) approach has been considered useful, though there is also support for tai chi, exercise and the use of hip protectors (Zijlstra, van Haastregt, van Rossum, van Eijk, Yardley & Kempen, 2007).

Treatment of anger after stroke

As with anxiety, the treatment of anger after stroke largely remains to be investigated. The first issue for the clinician, however, is whether or not anger is the primary concern. Anger, for instance, can be one aspect of depression (Busch, 2009). Further, anger can be salient in PTSD, can emerge in psychosis and is an attribute of some personality disorders (Novaco, 2010). It follows that differential diagnosis is important in clinical decision making. Anger itself is rarely considered a diagnosis itself.

Glancy and Knott (2003) provided an algorithm for pharmacological treatment of aggression that considers the origin of the disorder. Should investigations reveal the possibility of temporal lobe epilepsy or EEG abnormalities, anticonvulsive medications, such as Carbamazepine or Valporate, are recommended. For first-line treatments when there is dementia caused by a general medical condition, such as stroke, they recommended a mood stabiliser, such as

Table 15.2 Case Example of Psychological Treatment of a Stroke Patient with Post-Traumatic Stress Disorder

Arthur was a 57-year-old divorced civil servant. He was about to go away on holiday abroad when he had a major left hemisphere stroke. At onset of his stroke, he presented with a significant expressive aphasia and was unable to transfer from bed to chair unassisted. He was unable to walk at all. Because he lived alone and he was expected to be away, he was not found for two days. He had additional nerve damage because he had lain on a stone floor over this time. He spent nine weeks at the acute hospital before he was considered medically stable enough for transfer to a rehabilitation ward.

Arthur was referred to a clinical psychologist because he complained of being unable to sleep, appeared to be fearful of mobility tasks in therapy and was not engaging with therapists on this account. He would also withdraw to his room at any opportunity. He refused to discuss return home, consistently saying he wished to go to his parents' home after his discharge.

Assessment by the psychologist identified Arthur was experiencing nightmares in which he saw himself as lying on the floor of his kitchen incapacitated and unable to cry out. He tried not to think of his experience but felt it was constantly popping into his head. He also described feeling consistently 'on edge' and unable to concentrate in therapy for fear of falling to the ground. Additional worrying thoughts mainly concerned his future, such as whether he would be able to work again or play golf, his main leisure and social pursuit.

Formulation

Arthur's reaction appeared to have developed as a response to an extremely painful frightening event that had caused him to fear for his life. It included troubling nightmares, anxiety and avoidance (not wishing to go home, and avoiding therapy where physically he felt less stable). It appeared to be maintained by this avoidance. Arthur felt better when he didn't have to undertake tasks or consider going home.

Intervention

The nature of post-traumatic stress was discussed with Arthur. The effectiveness of exposure-based treatments was also considered. With some hesitance, as Arthur was unable to write or read following his stroke, he used a dictation machine to record in detail what he recalled of the event and his thoughts and feelings at the time. He was then asked to revise his recording several times, adding anything he had missed. With the help of the psychologist, he then produced a fully inclusive tape that was used for exposure sessions. His main thoughts were concerns about the extreme pain in his side, that he would not be found, that was going to die and that he would not see his friends or family again.

Attendance and engaging in therapy were considered in sessions with the psychologist. A decisional balance was used for Arthur to consider the pros and cons of therapy avoidance. This quickly established that despite the small risk of a fall, he had more to gain than to lose from therapy attendance.

Arthur was asked to listen to his tape at least three times a week, four to five times on each occasion. He did this over a five-week period. Additional sessions with the psychologist considered his losses, as regards his vocation and leisure activity, and problem solving, in terms of what he might pursue as alternatives, was undertaken.

(*Continued*)

Table 15.2 (*Continued*)

Outcome

Arthur began to report sleeping better about three weeks into his exposure programme. About the same time, therapists noted better attendance, enthusiasm and compliance with physical therapy. Scores for both intrusions and avoidance on the Impact of Events Schedule reduced substantially over the period of the exposure, as did anxiety scores on the Hospital Anxiety and Depression Scale. Depression on the HADS remained unchanged in the borderline range. Arthur agreed to a home visit, provided the psychologist accompanied him. While there was significant anticipatory anxiety about this, once at home Arthur coped well.

Arthur considered the intervention had been very successful. He felt he had put the event behind him and was working towards his future. He accepted he was close to retirement and that leaving his work would not leave him financially insecure. He had started to play Wii golf but identified this was no replacement for his usual round. He planned to continue as a social member of his golf club. He considered his borderline depression score was highly valid; while he was coping, he had lost much and was looking at a substantially changed life as a result of his stroke.

Lithium, be considered. When aggression appears anxiety related, as a second-line treatment they recommend beta blockers, such as Trazodone, Buspirone and atypical antipsychotics. Where major depression is identified, they considered SSRIs are indicated with adjunctive Buspirone and beta blockers. When an underlying psychiatric condition is not thought to be present, SSRIs are the first choice with appreciation that different SSRIs suit different individuals. Second-line treatments in this circumstance include beta blockers, commencing at low dosage. Glancy and Knott (2003) admitted that a mood stabiliser, such as lithium, along with Buspirone and Trazodone, might also prove useful.

No trial has yet addressed psychological treatment for anger occurring after stroke. A number of meta-analyses however have supported the use of psychological interventions to treat anger in adults. DiGiuseppe and Tafrate's (2002) review concluded that psychological interventions reduce aggression and increase positive behaviours. One review concluded that CBT for driving anger, anger suppression and trait anger, and relaxation therapy for state anger, were supported (Devecchio & O'Leary, 2004). Other reviewers, however, consider evidence to guide clinical recommendations as to the most useful treatment including combined psychological and pharmacological ones, is awaited (Saini, 2009).

Conclusions

To date, evidence as to the usefulness of both pharmacological and psychological therapies, or indeed their combination, for emotional changes after stroke requires further investigation. Even where there does seem to be a body of work supporting a therapy, such as antidepressants for depression, there are troubling findings about side effect profiles. Cognitive-behavioural therapies are supported in the general population for most psychological disorders that are common after stroke, so there is an expectation they may prove useful, though modification to suit the stroke population may be required (Kneebone & Dunmore, 2000). Due to the heterogeneous nature of stroke, including variations in cognitive and communication ability, it remains that different psychological treatments may be useful for different groups. It may also be that while psychological distress after stroke is relatively constant in its frequency over time, treatments may be differentially useful according to the length of time since the stroke. For instance, strategies useful in the acute phase may be different from those used post acute and in the long term, given the different challenges that may be occurring for individuals at these different times.

Chapter 16

Behavioural and Cognitive-Behavioural Therapy for Depression after Stroke

Behavioural therapy and cognitive-behavioural therapy

A multitude of psychological therapies have evolved over the past 50 years to treat depression in the general population. Among the most prominent of these are behavioural therapy (BT) and cognitive-behavioural therapy (CBT). Behavioural models of depression (Ferster, 1973; Kazdin, 1977) provide the basis of behavioural therapy. Essentially, these models consider depressed behaviour as a result of reinforcement for this behaviour in combination with a lack of reinforcement of nondepressed behaviour. The potential for deterioration with depression is acknowledged, in that aversive social consequences may occur over time as individuals lose social responsiveness as a consequence of their presentation (Coyne, 1976). On this basis, behavioural therapy for depression emphasises the gaining of access to pleasant experiences alongside attempts to reduce aversive experiences (Lewinsohn & Graf, 1973). The core component of treatment under this approach is behavioural activation: daily monitoring of pleasant and unpleasant events alongside monitoring of mood, in concert with behavioural strategies, such as activity scheduling to increase access to positive events (Brown & Lewinsohn, 1984). Social skills training, problem solving training and even time management approaches are also used.

CBT, as its name suggests, adds consideration of cognition (thoughts, attitudes and beliefs) to BT. In addition to the strategies described above, it involves clients directly considering the role their thinking plays in the development and maintenance of their depression. 'True CBT' is more than this, however. The approach is seen as requiring specific agenda setting for sessions, a collaborative joint effort between therapist and client, alongside a Socratic questioning style and the regular integration of homework to support change (White, 2001). Agenda setting involves ensuring sessions are structured and

Psychological Management of Stroke, First Edition. Nadina B. Lincoln, Ian I. Kneebone, Jamie A.B. Macniven and Reg C. Morris.
© 2012 John Wiley & Sons, Ltd. Published 2012 by John Wiley & Sons, Ltd.

planned. Routinely an agenda will include a summary and consideration of any prior session, a review of homework and a review of recent experience and circumstances with respect to mood. At the end of a session summarising, setting further homework and review of the session's content occurs. Collaboration in CBT refers to the way in which the other content of sessions is determined by negotiation between the therapist and the patient; they work as a team to support the resolution of difficulties. Socratic questioning involves guided discovery. The therapist aims to facilitate the patient's own discovery of alternative, more useful ways of considering their experience. Active involvement in CBT is usually achieved by the patient completing homework tasks between treatment sessions. Commonly these will involve challenging the assumptions patients are making that contribute to emotional disorder. For instance Jeffrey, hemiplegic after a stroke, who was convinced he would be rejected because of his physical appearance, visited his old workplace to find the opposite. His colleagues were warm and welcoming.

Behavioural therapy and cognitive-behavioural therapy: the evidence base

There is evidence that both BT (behavioural activation, problem solving) and CBT are effective treatments for mild to moderate depression in the general population (Cuijpers, van-Straten, Andersson & van Oppen, 2008). They also appear to offer benefits to those with neurological conditions, including those with depression with multiple sclerosis (Mohr & Goodkin, 1999), to those encountering emotional distress after brain injury (Bradbury, Christensen, Lau, Ruttan, Arundine & Green, 2008) and in the context of other physical disorders, such as diabetes (Lustman, Griffith, Freedland, Kissel & Clouse, 1998). Among older people, who make up the majority of those who have experienced stroke, BT and CBT are both effective and as effective as medication in the treatment of depression (Fraser, Christensen & Griffiths, 2005; Pinquart, Duberstein & Lyness, 2006; Scogin, Welsh, Hanson, Stump & Coates, 2005). Further, in older people these therapies have been demonstrated as useful for depression in those with medical conditions, such as elevated cardiovascular risk (Strachowski, Khaylis, Conrad, Neri, Spiegel & Taylor, 2008) and illness precipitating attending primary care (Arean, Hegel, Vannoy, Fan & Unutzer, 2008) and, in the case of BT, of possible benefit in nursing home settings (Hussian & Lawrence, 1981).

No psychological therapy can currently be judged empirically efficacious in treating depression after stroke (Hackett, Anderson, House & Xia, 2008b). However, evidence from a variety of sources suggests BT and CBT hold promise. Two studies have investigated CBT within mixed sample of older people with disability, some of whom had strokes (numbers unspecified). Kemp, Corgiat and Gill (1991/1992) used a group approach to treat depression, comparing the responses between two groups, one with and the other without disability. They concluded the intervention was equally effective initially, in terms of change from baseline, but suggested longer treatment or booster sessions for those in the disability group as, unlike those in the nondisabled group, these participants did not appear to continue to improve at six- and 12-month follow-ups. Lopez and Mermelstein (1995) compared, among other measures, the Center for Epidemiological Studies Depression Scale (CES-D) scores (Radloff, 1977), between those who received individual CBT who had presented as distressed at the outset of an older person community based rehabilitation programme (n=21) with a group (n=52) who did not present as distressed and received care as usual. Depression significantly reduced in the group that received CBT, to a level comparable to the nondistressed group.

The evaluation of the use of BT and CBT in depression occurring specifically post stroke is limited to date. A randomised controlled trial of behavioural activation is currently underway (Thomas, Lincoln, Walker, Macniven & Haworth, 2010). The possibility that the results for this might be positive comes from studies by occupational therapists into leisure rehabilitation. Drummond and Walker (1996) found that providing advice and equipment to enable leisure pursuits, combined with liaison with specialist agencies, resulted in fewer intervention participants with diagnosable depression after intervention. Unfortunately a subsequent multicentre trial failed to replicate these findings (Parker *et al.*, 2001). Disappointing results were also obtained for an intervention by stroke family care workers that incorporated a problem solving (BT) approach alongside counselling, goal setting and specific stroke advice (Dennis, O'Rourke, Slattery, Staniforth & Warlow, 1997). With a large sample (n=417), they found no benefit of their treatment group over controls. In contrast, House (2003) in a randomised trial found patients visited by a community mental health nurse, who provided training in problem solving, to benefit in terms of their scores on a measure of general psychological distress, the General Health Questionnaire (Goldberg & Hillier, 1979), that includes items sensitive to depression.

The earliest reference to CBT for depression after stroke appears in a case study in the mid-1980s. Hatcher, Durham and Richey (1985) described CBT as one part of a multidisciplinary approach that also included a rationalisation of medication and moving accommodation to a non-institutional setting. The CBT components of this included attention to negative thinking, assertion training and the development of a supervised activity programme. Unfortunately conclusions as to efficacy were based on subjective descriptions of improved mood and self-esteem. In 1992, Hibbard, Grober, Stein and Gordon (1992) also reported a case study. They used CBT, modified to be sympathetic to stroke, over 52 sessions to treat depression in an individual after stroke. Multiple assessments of response to treatment included therapist and spousal ratings on psychometric scales and formal diagnostic interviews. These established the patient as 'not depressed' following treatment (over six months) and at a 12-month follow-up.

Two papers have reported AB experimental design case series evaluations of CBT for depression after stroke. Lincoln, Flannaghan, Sutcliffe and Rother (1997) recruited 19 participants who received and average of 8.4 sessions of CBT for depression after stroke. They assessed the outcome predominantly by considering symptom change on the Beck Depression Inventory (Beck, Ward, Mendelson, Mock & Erbaugh, 1961) on the basis of visual inspection, comparison of pretreatment results with those post treatment and consideration of the proportion of scores below the lowest baselines achieved. Overall a statistically significant decrease in BDI pre- to post intervention was evident, but based on all their criteria it was considered that four patients showed evidence of consistent benefit, six patients some benefit and nine patients no benefit from the treatment. Sampling issues, reservations about the therapists' training and experience and limited treatment dosage have been put forward to explain this case series outcome (Kneebone & Dunmore, 2000). More recently, a further case series considered the utility and feasibility of CBT for people with post-stroke depression. Rasquin, Van De Sande, Praamstra and Van Heugten (2008) used a single-case AB design that incorporated three-month follow-up, with five participants experiencing significant depressive symptoms attending an outpatient rehabilitation clinic after a first stroke. Four patients reported improved mood and at three-month follow-up, three patients had reduced depressive symptoms. Both therapists and patients considered the intervention feasible. To date, only one randomised controlled trial has evaluated CBT for depression after stroke. Lincoln and Flanagan (2003) randomly allocated those with significant depressive symptoms (n=39) to receive individual CBT or an attention placebo intervention (n=43) or usual care (n=41). They found no significant difference between groups on any of the depression measures. The authors considered a range of reasons for their findings including the brevity of the CBT relative to other studies, therapist training, sample size, recruitment strategy, and selection criteria. It may be CBT is more appropriate to a post-acute than an acute setting, as retrospective analysis of data indicated that those recruited later improved substantially more relative to controls, though a lack of power prevented this difference proving statistically significant. In addition, evidence of substantial improvement in the control group suggested a period of watchful waiting maybe appropriate before therapy is commenced. As post hoc analysis also revealed those who benefited least had greater communication problems (Thomas & Lincoln, 2006), this trial has influenced the development of the investigation of behavioural therapy referred to above. The presence of cognitive deficits and subtle communication changes may mean BT is more suited to the majority of those with depression after stroke.

Taken together, the empirical evidence for the effectiveness of BT and CBT for depression after stroke is lacking. More work is required to establish whether it works and, if it does, for whom and at what time after stroke. However, in clinical practice BT and CBT are widely used and some patients seem to benefit, so they are worth considering as treatment strategies for those who are depressed.

Modifying behavioural therapy and cognitive-behavioural therapy for those with stroke

Assessment

A number of instruments are now available that have been determined, valid and reliable to screen for depression after stroke (Healey, Kneebone, Carroll & Anderson, 2008; Bennett & Lincoln, 2006). Protocols also exist for screening in specific environments, such as stroke units (Kneebone, Baker & O'Malley, 2010). While questions on these screens offer some insight into the views that can be addressed by cognitive therapy, for example 'I feel life is hardly worth living' is a question on the Brief Assessment Schedule Depression Cards (BASDEC; Adshead, Cody & Pitt, 1992), clinical interview and observation are required to identify adequately the full range of behavioural changes and cognitive distortions that may play a role in depression after stroke. Despite this the clinician may be helped in assessment by a questionnaire, the Stroke Cognitions Questionnaire–Revised (Thomas & Lincoln, 2008b). The questionnaire is made up of 21 items that represent common positive and negative thoughts people often have following a stroke. It attempts to assess the frequency with which these occur.

Cognitive deficits may also produce lack of insight into changes after stroke. This is not limited to physical and cognitive changes, but may extend to personality and mood. In such cases it has been recommended that carers be involved in assessing the presence of depression (Gordon & Hibbard, 1997; Hibbard *et al.*, 1992), though this is not without its problems (Berg, Lönnqvist, Palomäki & Kaste, 2009).

Treatment

In a narrative review of psychological treatments for depression, Kneebone and Dunmore (2000) proposed that both BT and CBT interventions for depression after stroke should be considered as one. Implicit in this is an integrated approach, where the balance between cognitive and behavioural strategies depends on the presentation of the client. As cognitive deficits and communication disorder increase, the balance between cognitive and behavioural interventions should be adjusted by the therapist. With increasing deficits, behavioural strategies predominate and the role of carers in instructing and supporting therapy increases. Allowing behavioural therapy as the basis of any treatment has some support. While BT and CBT appear equally effective in treating depression, the most active elements of the treatments are considered by many to be behavioural (Hopko, Lejuez, Ruggiero & Eifert, 2003).

As noted, a role for carers in the treatment of depression has been identified (Kneebone & Dunmore, 2000). This acknowledges that initiating behavioural activities can be limited in those with communication or cognitive difficulties after stroke. Due consideration of this is required and the nature of the pre-stroke relationship, among other things, should be taken into account. Kneebone and Dunmore (2000) suggested using a typology developed by Dempster, Knapp and House (1998) to help determine whether, how and when to include carers in treatment. Carer types to which Dempster *et al.* (1998) referred include generally supportive carers, such as the 'collaborative carer' who joins in actively and takes naturally to participation in therapy, to the generally unsupportive carer, such as the 'antagonistic carer' who will participate yet with seemingly their only purpose to disrupt or prove the procedure pointless. In the former case the implication is to include them in treatment, in the latter, not to include them or to consider their discontinuation if they have been involved.

Adding motivational interviewing techniques to the more traditional CBT approach to depression after stroke has been suggested (Broomfield, Laidlaw, Hickabottom, Murray, Pendrey, Whittick & Gillespie, 2010). Motivational interviewing is a patient-centred counselling technique that addresses perceived barriers to patients achieving individual goals. This has intuitive appeal for use particularly when patients are in active rehabilitation. It also has support (independent of CBT) in a randomised controlled trial in this population (Watkins *et al.*, 2007).

More specific modifications have been offered for treating depression after stroke using cognitive and behavioural approaches. Hibbard, Grober, Gordon and Aletta (1990a) indicated cognitive deficits should be taken into account and maintained that cognitive rehabilitation can be important to ameliorate depression after stroke. A straightforward example of how this might occur is the case of Pat, an individual on an inpatient stroke unit, who had memory loss that contributed to depression. Pat reported feeling lonely, isolated and unsupported. Assessment identified a major contributor to this was that she was forgetting those who had visited. The simple treatment for the depression then was the provision of a visitors' book complete with pictures of the main family members. Using this booklet and drawing the client's attention to it, meant she fully recovered from her affective disorder. From a BT and CBT point of view this can be considered as increasing pleasant events, by bringing to mind the support the patient was experiencing, and changing negative appraisals about their circumstances. Cognitive deficits also mean that every opportunity should be taken by practitioners to reinforce the work completed in sessions. Strategies that support memory, that are already recommended for successful CBT with older people, should be incorporated wherever possible. For instance some therapists will write down, or indeed have the patients write down, disputes of irrational ideas within sessions, so they are readily available for the individual when the thoughts recur (Granholm, McQuaid, McClure, Pedrelli & Jeste, 2002). Others use recordings of sessions, so that key messages can be reinforced and rehearsed in the time between sessions (Hibbard, Grober, Gordon & Aletta, 1990a; Zeiss & Lewinsohn, 1986). Mnemonic strategies, such as SLEEPS (**S**elect a regular bedtime and wake time, **L**imit use of the bedroom, **E**xit the bedroom if you are not asleep in 10 to 15 minutes, **E**liminate naps and **P**ut your feet on the floor at the same time every morning) may help with insomnia (Stanley, Diefenbach & Hopko, 2004). The 3 Cs 'catch it, check it and change it' with respect to unhelpful thoughts can also be useful (Granholm *et al.*, 2002). Changes in concentration and speed of information processing can occur after stroke, as occurs in older people (Zeiss & Lewinsohn, 1986). It may be appropriate that sessions are shorter and at a slower pace. Use of more concrete, less abstract, cognitive intervention may also be more appropriate after stroke, as it is for older people (Church, 1986). For instance, the therapist might specifically consider a patient's distress due to it being unfair that they have had a stroke, without attempting to dispute an underlying demand that things must be 'the way they want them to be'. As Ellis (1991) noted, therapists may need to develop coping self-statements for those who are rigid, less sharp or very upset. For example, 'when next you find yourself upset about how awful your stroke is, take out the card we have prepared with the re-assurance on it', 'yes it is tough, having had this stroke and the rehabilitation is hard work, but things are improving'. Multimodal presentations that support retention are also recommended for older people (Zeiss & Lewinsohn, 1986) and are appropriate for those with stroke.

Hibbard, Grober, Gordon, Aletta and Freeman (1990b) emphasised the importance of acknowledging the mourning of losses after stroke when providing CBT for depression. Beck's (1979) cognitive model emphasises consideration of the 'depressogenic triad', the negative view of the self, the world and the future. The inexperienced therapist will threaten rapport if they do not join with their client in recognising their understandable emotional reaction and acknowledge what could in reality be a substantially changed self and future. In this context it is important to also consider second-order distress, that is, the client's discomfort at the experience of depression. Acceptance and normalising the reaction are important prior to addressing any attitudinal distortions that might be augmenting their adjustment reaction. Time must be allocated for this. Indeed the initial sessions may be devoted to this prior to education in the CBT model.

Those with depression after stroke are a highly heterogeneous group; for some a substantial physical recovery might be possible, while for others this is less likely. It follows that the goals of psychological therapy might need to be modified. For instance, generally it will not be appropriate to aim for a patient to 'feel happy' when they think of their stroke-related disability, but it would be more reasonable to aim for affects, such as sad, regretful and disappointed, at least initially. Activity planning should be sympathetic to premorbid preferences and lifestyle (Hibbard, Grober, Gordon & Aletta, 1990a). Pleasant event scheduling, as part of behavioural activation, should be considered in light of the levels of disability (Laidlaw, 2008; Zeiss & Lewinsohn, 1986), and modified versions of formal pleasant events schedules used whenever possible. Occupational therapists may be invaluable in developing an appropriate behavioural activation programme. They can determine what a patient may be able to do despite their stroke, that will give them pleasure and a sense of mastery, thereby helping to ameliorate the depression. The frequent contact with other members of the multidisciplinary team means that the use of cognitive-behavioural principles to both prevent and manage depression after stroke needs not be confined to the CBT therapist (Kneebone, 1999). A milieu in which team members all cooperate has great potential to support emotional health in any rehabilitation setting.

The provision of homework is an important element in CBT. In those with disability, inability to write or communication problems may mean the opportunities for this are limited. Whenever possible homework, even if it is in a simplified form, should be utilised. Its completion has been identified as an important contributor to change in CBT interventions with older people (Wetherell, Hopko, Diefenbach, Averill, Beck, Craske *et al.*, 2005)

With any intervention, clarifying what has happened, the prognosis and treatment processes, including medication and secondary prevention measures, can be very important. Particular types of cognitions can contribute to distress and depression after stroke. Some patients for instance are understandably fearful of a further stroke, and this should be addressed. One common counter of this concern includes a self–statement along the lines of 'yes having had a stroke means I'm at risk, but I am on a preventative medicine now and looking after myself, so I'm doing what I can. Worry doesn't help the process – what can I do instead?'

Unrealistic expectations can be common after a stroke. It is important that these are also addressed. Patients can find themselves tyrannised by what they consider they 'should' be able to do and this may well be unrealistic if they have not factored in their stroke. For instance, 'I should be able to dress myself easily' can be countered with 'Hold on, I'm hemiplegic since the stroke that's why I need help. It's frustrating but I do cope with it every day'.

Recognising and attending to discrepancies between actual and perceived losses are important issues for both patients and families and have indeed been seen as crucial within CBT treatment post stroke (Hibbard, Grober, Gordon & Aletta, 1990a). After a stroke, individuals may misrepresent their disability. It is not unusual to find a patient with depression and mobility problems stating 'I can't walk' when the truth of the situation is they just can't walk *like they used to*. Families may both exaggerate and minimise the person with the stroke's disability. If a family member undertakes things for a patient that they can do themselves, they can inadvertently reinforce disability and dependence, thus augmenting mood disorder. Conversely if the family have expectations of the patient that exceed their ability, this can set a patient up to fail, thereby also contributing to low mood. Table 16.1 sets out the negative cognitions from the Thomas and Lincoln (2008b) Stroke Cognition Questionnaire–Revised, and considers some counter-arguments that may prove useful in cognitive therapy after stroke when these ideas present.

Some case examples are provided in Tables 16.2–16.3 and 16.4 to illustrate the application of CBT with stroke patients.'

Table 16.1 Common Negative Stroke-Related Cognitions and Useful Responses Negative cognitions in stroke based on Stroke Cognitions Questionnaire–Revised (Thomas, S. & Lincoln, N.B., 2006, Factors relating to depresssion after stroke. Reproduced with permission from the British Journal of Clinical Psychology © The British Psychological Society)

Cognition
1 **I feel inadequate and helpless.** My stroke does mean I need help from others and that's disappointing, but I can still do many things and take control of my life despite the limitations.
2 **I get irritated easily.** That's to be expected, it's really stressful having a stroke but if I relax like I've been shown and accept things aren't how I want them I can reduce my frustration and it will be less of a problem.
3 **I feel a burden to others.** Yes things have changed and the family have to make time to support me, but isn't that OK? I'd do it for them. After all family isn't just for the good times. I've helped them in the past, its OK for them to give something back?
4 **I'm frustrated about not being able to do the things that I want to.** Yes it is frustrating and sad that I can't do what I want, but the therapists are showing me how to do more things. If I can't do the things I used to enjoy, I'll find other things and do them instead.
5 **I wonder what the point of living like this is.** Things have changed, I've lost a lot, but aren't there still good things in my life?
6 **There is no point in doing things if I can't do them as well as before.** Hold on, do I have to do things perfectly to enjoy them? When I think about it, I was a never a Michelin-starred chef but I did enjoy getting a meal together.
7 **I am no good at anything.** Hold on, where's the evidence to support that I'm no good at anything? Where's it written that I have to be good at things? Just getting by is an achievement after the stroke.
8 **I feel alone and unwanted.** It's true I see people less since the stroke and indeed some friends have dropped away, but some good friends still visit and my family have been supportive; I've actually grown closer to my granddaughter.
9 **I feel like a failure.** OK, I've failed to return to work but that doesn't mean I'm a failure as a person? After all I really tried my best. Come to think of it, people who don't walk can still do remarkable things.
10 **I've lost confidence in myself.** Well, that's to be expected. I suppose when you can't do what you're used to doing. Perhaps if I set some goals, achieved things therapists say I'm capable of, that will help.
11 **I dwell on what I'm unable to achieve.** Well there are lots of things I can't do now and from time to time I'll be sad about that, however thinking about them all the time doesn't get me anywhere. I'll look at what I can do, concentrate on those things. If I make the whole 'me' about my stroke, that's not going to help.

Table 16.1   (*Continued*)

Cognition

---

12 **I can't be bothered to do anything.**
Well hello! That's no surprise, so many things take much more effort now. But where will not doing things get me? More physical problems? Unhappier? Perhaps if I just get back to some things – I'll start that book even if it's just for five minutes to be getting on with.

Table 16.2   Case Example of Cognitive-Behavioural Therapy

John, age 64, experienced a stroke while on holiday in Malaysia. The stroke resulted in mild cognitive changes, an altered gait pattern and fatigability.

Formulation
John became depressed a year after the stroke, following the realisation he was not likely to make a complete recovery. He had expected a full recovery as he'd been given this re-assurance by a doctor in Malaysia when he first presented. One year later he realised he was unable to return to work and on this basis considered his 'life was over', there was 'nothing good in it' and he was a 'failure' for not having recovered as the doctor had said he could. It was very clear that this thinking maintained his depressive disorder.

Intervention
Through monitoring of daily activities, John realised that he was in fact doing many things he enjoyed. For instance he had learned to use the Internet and was participating in an audit of butterfly prevalence by watching in his back yard and reporting online. He noted he had regular visits from friends and outings that he enjoyed, all things he had previously discounted. His view that he had failed in rehabilitation was disputed in therapy by having him consider whether the original prognosis of a full recovery by an accident and emergency physician was credible and re-assurance from John's therapists and indeed himself that he had done all that had been asked of him in his rehabilitation and had in fact made a very good, though not a full, recovery.

Outcome
John recognised the good things in his life and thus changed his review of his recovery as a success story rather than one of failure. Significant changes on the Hospital Anxiety and Depression Scale (Zigmond & Snaith, 1983) supported the gains noted by the therapist. Scores on the Depression Scale went from 16 to 7, the latter below the cut-off for significant disorder.

Table 16.3   Case Example of Cognitive-Behavioural Therapy

Catherine was 55 years old, a divorcee and a high school geography teacher, when she suffered a major left hemisphere stroke leading to expressive dysphasia and mobility changes. Catherine was able to produce only single words reliably, including 'yes' and 'no', but unable to understand simple sentences delivered on a one-to-one basis. Her mobility was impaired by right-sided weakness to the extent that she was initially unable to walk at all. Sleep, appetite and mood were all significantly impaired.

(*continued*)

Table 16.3   (*Continued*)

Formulation

Catherine had become considerably depressed four weeks after the stroke. The main context that had contributed appeared to be her reduced communication and limited mobility. It was observed she would get agitated if she could not get her message across, and became frustrated when assisted with activities of daily living.

Intervention

Five one-to-one sessions were conducted used using simple communication aids. As a result of discussion with family members, a chess board was obtained so that Catherine could participate in something for which she had a flair and that was largely nonverbal. Catherine's family also brought in videos of dog shows in which she had judged and taken part, which she had collected over the years. This had been her main leisure pursuit prior to her stroke. Catherine was also taught a brief relaxation strategy to enable her to manage her agitation and support her communication. Further, a goal list indicating what her rehabilitation goals had been and what she had achieved was placed in Catherine's room. A key worker (physiotherapist) went through this list regularly with Catherine so that she would be aware of what she was achieving. The therapist used physical demonstrations to assist Catherine's understanding of her progress.

Outcome

Catherine became more relaxed, her communication improved and she did well in physiotherapy, progressing to walking independently with a quad stick. On the Depression Intensity Scale Circles (DISCS; Turner-Stokes, Kalmus, Hirani & Clegg, 2005) over a six-week period, her score went from 5, the maximum score on this instrument and well above the cut-off for depression (2) to 0, which is 'nondepressed'.

Table 16.4   Case Example of Cognitive-Behavioural Therapy

Keith, an 84-year-old man, was seen in a day hospital setting six weeks after he had a second stroke. His first stroke had been three years previous, and he had made a full recovery from it. Keith had a supportive family and regularly saw his daughter and a female friend with whom, though they did not co-reside, he had had an intimate relationship for ten years. His wife had deceased 15 years previously. Keith had experienced cognitive changes following the second stroke. Essentially his thinking was more concrete. He was also unsteady on his feet, though he could walk unaided with concentration. The second stroke itself had been extremely traumatic in that he had been at home for several days before being found, as the family had been away on holiday, and he had been close to death. Keith felt extremely low and reported intrusive recollections of the event, feeling extremely uncomfortable when left alone, and avoided bathrooms. He would only bathe weekly with assistance as opposed to every second day, as he had before the second stroke. Keith was feeling extremely despondent about his future, thinking it would consist only of a further stroke and greater disability. He also felt he was becoming a burden on his daughter by living with her, whereas but for his anxiety, he would have been able to live on his own with occasional care assistance. He was aware he found it hard to take information in and sort out problems he encountered. In addition to the depression, there was

Table 16.4 *(Continued)*

evidence of significant post-traumatic stress symptoms. Keith had experienced a life threatening event, as when he collapsed he had not been found for two days. His anxiety was augmented by frequent recollection of this event and avoidance.

Formulation
Keith had become depressed and suffered post–traumatic stress symptoms in the context of a second stroke. His depression was principally maintained by his fear of a further stroke, concerns that he was a burden and was less intellectually astute than he had been. Anxiety was also high, in the context of dramatic recollection of the event. His feeling better when someone was with him or when he managed to keep away from a bathroom, reinforced avoidance.

Intervention
Keith being a burden to his family was considered in therapy. He was able to reflect that he himself had looked after his elderly parents when they had needed assistance and acknowledged that while not a physical disability his anxiety was understandable and valid particularly in the context of how it had developed. His concerns about another stroke were considered. He discussed with the physician the likelihood of this occurring and then was able to set this in the context of his whole life. He was able to make a decision that he did not wish to spend his remaining time full of worry about having another stroke rather than 'enjoying the moment'. Keith set a goal to return to his own home. Concerns about traumatic stress symptoms were addressed by exposure. Keith tape-recorded his version of the events of his second stroke. He checked and revised these regularly with the assistance of family. The pros and cons of treatment, essentially reassurance but dependence if he stayed at his daughter's versus independence but having to confront his anxiety if he went home, were considered with Keith. He agreed to attempt to overcome his anxiety. To support Keith, a coping self-statement list was drawn up, alongside a hierarchy of goals that would lead Keith to assuming more independence. The hierarchy of goals ranged from Keith's daughter standing outside the bathroom rather than being within the room when he was bathing, to him bathing every second day in his own home. Exposures to the traumatic event recording were daily over a period of five weeks. A trainee clinical psychologist helped Keith slowly advance through the anxiety hierarchy.

Outcome
Keith's score on the Hospital Anxiety and Depression Scale (Zigmond & Snaith, 1983) went from Anxiety 27 and Depression 14 to Anxiety 9 and Depression 6. On the Impact of Events Schedule (IES; Horowitz, Wilner & Alvarez, 1979), his overall combined intrusion and avoidance scores went from 40 to 14, the latter being below the cut-off considered of clinical significance (DeVilly, 2005). Eventually Keith was able to move back to his own home. Unfortunately he did not achieve full independence as, prior to going home, an occupational therapy assessment recommended care assistance for showering because of stroke-related mobility changes.

Conclusions

Successful treatment for depression after stroke is highly desirable not only because of the distress of the emotional disorder itself for those who experience it, but also because of its effects on rehabilitation outcome. To date, no one psychological therapy has demonstrated convincing efficacy in the treatment of diagnosed major affective disorder or depressive symptoms after stroke (Hackett *et al.*, 2008). BT appears promising (Drummond & Walker, 1996) and remains under investigation (Thomas *et al.*, 2010). Despite the findings of one RCT (Lincoln & Flannaghan, 2003) CBT shows promise at the clinical level (Kemp *et al.*, 1991/1992; Lincoln *et al.*, 1997; Lopez & Mermelstein, 1995; Rasquin *et al.*, 2008), its efficacy may yet be proved. It may well be that the most important consideration is what therapy for what patient at what point after stroke.

Chapter 17

Stroke and Fear of Falling

Stroke and falls

Unsurprisingly, given the reduced physical function that commonly occurs with a stroke, falls are common in this population. In inpatient rehabilitation settings, the incidence can be as high as 39% (Nyberg & Gustafson, 1995) and patients an average of 10 years after stroke fall more than twice as often as age and sex matched controls (Jorgensen, Engstad & Jacobsen, 2002). Most stroke patients within inpatient rehabilitation settings fall indoors from their bed or chair, often when attempting transfers (Czernuszenko & Czlonkowska, 2009). In contrast, after discharge from hospital those with stroke who fall usually do so while walking (Jorgensen *et al.*, 2002). A large number of factors have been identified to predict falls after stroke. In the first six months after stroke, these include a history of falls, reduced physical function, greater medication usage and hemi-neglect (Mackintosh, Hill, Dodd, Goldie & Culham, 2006). In the longer term, a history of near falls in hospital and reduced upper limb function, meaning one is unable to save oneself from a fall, were found to be the best predictors of falls (Ashburn, Hyndman, Pickering, Yardley & Harris, 2008). From a psychological perspective, what is most intriguing is research indicating that depressive symptoms increase the relative risk of falling after stroke (Jorgensen *et al.*, 2002; Takatori, Okada, Shomoto & Shimada, 2009). Finally, reduced executive function has also been implicated in falls risk after stroke (Liu-Ambrose, Pang & Eng, 2007). Falling after stroke is associated with subsequently being less socially active, lower mood and greater stress for carers (Forster & Young, 1995). The consequences can be serious for a minority, as 4% experience a fracture in the two years after stroke, 1% of which is hip fracture (Dennis, Lo, McDowall & West, 2002).

Psychological Management of Stroke, First Edition. Nadina B. Lincoln, Ian I. Kneebone, Jamie A.B. Macniven and Reg C. Morris.
© 2012 John Wiley & Sons, Ltd. Published 2012 by John Wiley & Sons, Ltd.

Fear of falling

Historically, the theoretical and clinical considerations of fear of falling have been hampered by lack of an agreed definition. It has been variously defined as a loss of confidence in one's ability to keep one's balance (Maki, Holliday & Topper, 1991), a concern about falling sufficient that it limits the performance of an activity (Tinetti & Powell, 1993) and low efficacy (confidence) in terms of one's ability to avoid falls (Cumming, Salkeld & Szonyi, 2000). Consistent with a recent consensus (Lamb, Becker, Jørstad-Stein & Hauer, 2005), we accept the fear of falling definition as that utilised by Tinetti and Powell (1993), that is 'a lasting concern about falling that leads to an individual avoiding activities'.

Numerous attempts have been made to investigate the factors that contribute to fear of falling, particularly as it is both a consequence of falls as well as a risk factor for future falls. Drawing upon research and clinical experience, Hull and Kneebone (2007) developed a model that attempted to cover the majority of relevant variables. As can be seen in Figure 17.1, the model takes a predominantly cognitive behavioural approach in order to explain fear of falling and its ability to increase the risk of future falls. In terms of predisposing and precipitating factors, those considered in the literature to be independently related to fear of falling include being aged over 80 years (Murphy, Dubin & Gill, 2003), having visual impairment, being female (Arfken, Lach, Birge & Miller, 1994) and adopting a sedentary lifestyle (Bruce, Devine & Prince, 2002). Interestingly, while a previous history of falls is associated with an increased risk of the fear (Arfken et al., 1994), it is not a necessary precursor (Legters, 2002). Depression may also play a role (Arfken et al., 1994), possibly as a consequence of the reduced activity that can arise when people are afraid of falling. The identification of a concern (i.e. of perceived threat) is seen as the first in a range of cognitive factors that may be involved in the fear of falling. In the stress and coping literature, the identification of threat is seen as the first step in a stress response (Lazarus & Folkman, 1984). Self-efficacy beliefs, one's confidence in the performance of activities of daily living without falling, have long been recognised as a factor in fear of falling, indeed having previously been considered as a definition of the fear itself (Tinetti, Richman & Powell, 1990). There is strong evidence that falls self-efficacy is related to poorer health and function in older people (Scheffer, Schuurmanns, van Dijk, van der Hooft & Rooij, 2008). The importance of outcome expectations has only recently been acknowledged as a potential factor in increasing the risk of fear of falling and falls (Lach, 2006). This is consistent with self-efficacy theory: what an individual considers will be the outcome of their behaviour has a significant influence upon it (Bandura, 1997). In the case of deactivation, certain behaviours may be avoided because of expectations that a fall could lead to an injury, even if that 'injury' might be damage to identity (hurt pride) in terms of one being seen as frail. All these

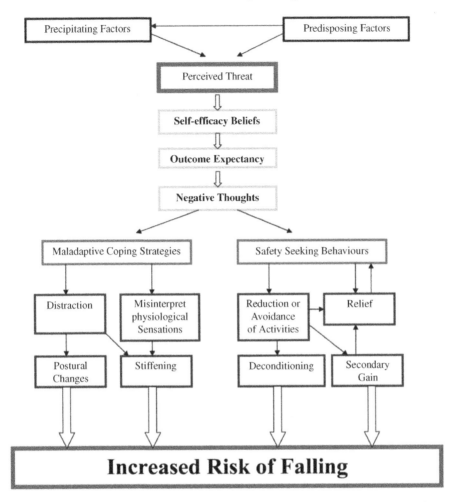

Figure 17.1 Revised cognitive-behavioural model for fear of falling (Hull & Kneebone, 2007).

viewpoints can combine into a sequence of negative thinking in relation to action that provokes safety-seeking behaviour: behaviours that reduce anxiety in the short term but prevent more adaptive beliefs developing in the longer term (Salkovskis, 1989). In the case of fear of falling this may mean the unnecessary use of an aid, such as a walking stick, or activity avoidance without the presence of a trusted other. Also consistent with an anxiety model, is the relief achieved by activity avoidance, which itself reinforces the avoidance. Of course, the presence of a trusted other can be a social reinforcer further supporting the avoidance, so-called secondary gain (Delbaere, Crombez, Vanderstraeten, Willems & Cambier, 2004). Activity avoidance over the longer term can result in physical deconditioning (Howland, Lachman, Peterson, Cote, Kasten & Jette, 1998), thereby increasing the risk of a fall. The association of coping with physical and psychological health outcomes is well established (Penley, Tomaka & Wiebe, 2002); however, while consistent with Lazarus and Folkman's (1984) model of stress and coping, coping strategies are considered important in understanding fear of falling (Filiatrault & Desrosiers, 2010). It remains for any mediational role between the fear and actual falls to be established.

Negative thoughts about falling can be destructive in the short term. If an individual is vulnerable to a fall, such as someone with balance problems, the cognitive and physiological aspects of the fear can distract them from concentrating on what is required to succeed at a physical task to the detriment of performance, ultimately increasing the risk of a fall (Yardley, 2004). The physical changes associated with anxiety can also directly reduce performance (Jacob, Furman, Clark & Durrant, 1992), while balance and gait changes can predict the development of the fear (Kressig, Wolf, Sattin, O'Grady, Greenspan, Curns *et al.*, 2001; Vellas, Wayne, Romero, Baumgartner & Gary, 1997). In the presence of fear of falling, a stiffening strategy (being "scared rigid") may be adopted, which is also counter-productive with respect to performance (Carpenter, Adkin, Brawley & Frank, 2006).

Fear of falling after stroke

Research considering fear of falling in those with stroke is limited. Watanabe (2005) found 29 of 33 (88%) of stroke patients developed a fear of falling to some extent following a fall in the 12 months after discharge from hospital. Of the patients that were found to have a fear of falling, 16 (48%) indicated that they were afraid of falling 'almost all the time'. Unfortunately Watanabe's study restricted questions about fear of falling to only those who had actually had a fall. As noted in the older population generally, fear of falling is not necessarily only evident in those who have fallen. Consistent with this, Andersson, Kamwendo and Appelros (2008) found 20% of stroke patients who reported low fall-related self-efficacy had not experienced a fall and 11% of those who had a history of falls reported high fall related self-efficacy. Nonetheless in general terms in this study, and as in other research (Belgen, Bininato, Sullivan & Narielwalla, 2006), fear of falling after stroke was associated with poor physical function and a history of falls. Impaired balance self-efficacy has been identified in those living in the community after stroke and to explain significant variance in perceived health status in these individuals (Salbach, Mayo, Robichaud-Ekstrand, Hanley, Richards & Wood-Dauphinee, 2006). Interestingly, there is also a disparity between actual and perceived ability; falls efficacy and objective assessment of balance were only associated to a low or moderate degree in two samples of stroke unit patients assessed on the Berg Balance Scale and the Falls Efficacy Scale (Engberg, Lind, Linder, Nilsson & Sernert, 2008). Pang and Eng (2008) identified that falls-related self-efficacy, and not balance or mobility performance, was related to accidental falls in stroke patients with low bone density, a group at enhanced risk of fracture (Marsden, Gibson, Lightbody, Sharma, Siddigi & Watkins, 2008). This reinforces the view that confidence and fear play major roles in the risk of future falls. Qualitative research has suggested that fear of falling after stroke often commences with a fall that occurred as part of the initial stroke event, which is then augmented by a loss of trust in one's body in terms of balance, strength and stability (Schmid & Rittman, 2007).

Assessment of fear of falling in those with stroke

As noted, the avoidance of activities one is capable of doing is a key component of fear of falling. On this account, multidisciplinary assessment is required to establish an individual's likely physical ability. Such assessments should take into account cognitive contributors to falls risk. Further, it is important to establish the specific details of the avoidance to aid goal setting, including what makes a difference to the presence and intensity of the fear, such as others being present or the use of an aid. Taking a history of any falls, including their outcome, places the experience of the client in context and facilitates the development of rapport. It is important not to overlook the experience of pre-stroke falls and the possibility that a client's difficulty may have arisen after observing another person fall. While depression and generalised anxiety commonly co-occur with fear of falling and may need review, particular attention should be given to excluding the presence a of a post-traumatic stress disorder. Even following less severe stroke, PTSD may be present in up to 31% of survivors (Bruggimann, Annoni, Staub, von Steinbüchel, Van der Linden & Bogousslavsky, 2006). Care should be taken to establish that avoidance of activities is not accompanied by persistent re-experiencing of the fall event, through for example intrusive re-collections or nightmares, in the presence of pervasive hyperarousal and numbing of respon-siveness. These are the hallmarks of PTSD (American Psychiatric Association, 1994). PTSD from a fall after stroke requires a different treatment approach.

A recent systematic review identified ten instruments considered to be in use for measuring fear of falling (Scheffer *et al.*, 2008). The majority of these were variations of the original Falls Efficacy Scale (FES) developed by Tinetti *et al.* (1990) and the Activities Specific Balance and Confidence Scale (ABC; Powell & Myers, 1995). In addition, single-item questions, such as 'At the present time are you very fearful, somewhat fearful or not fearful that you may fall?' (Arfken et al., 1994), were used in several studies. In terms of clinical use, the versions best suited for screening and assessing response to treatment are the Falls Efficacy Scale International (FES-I; Yardley, Beyer, Hauer, Kempen, Piot-Ziegler & Todd, 2005) and the original ABC.

The FES-I asks those completing it to rate, on a scale from 1 to 4 (from 1 = 'not at all concerned' to 4 = 'very concerned'), their concern about falling when undertaking 16 particular activities of daily living. Total scores are a summation, giving a range from 16 to 64. The higher the score, the greater is the concern about falling. The FES-I has content validity derived using an expert panel and demonstrates good internal and test–retest reliability (Yardley *et al.*, 2005). The Swedish modification of the FES (FES-S) has acceptable test–retest reliability in stroke survivors (Hellstrom & Lindmark, 1999). The Activity-specific Balance Confidence Scale (ABC; Powell & Myers, 1995) is also a 16-item measure. It requests information on balance confidence (from 0% = 'no confidence' to 100% = 'complete confidence') with respect to indoor and outdoor activities. The total score for the questionnaire is obtained by adding the scores from each question and then dividing by 16 (score range 0–100). The ABC's content validity was also derived by an expert panel and the views of a sample of older people. It is internally consistent and demonstrates good test retest reliability, including in stroke survivor samples (Botner, Miller & Eng, 2005; Salbach *et al.*, 2006; Scheffer *et al.*, 2008). Most clinicians also screen and assess for fear of falling using Likert type scales. Even though reliability or validity data are largely unavailable for these (Scheffer *et al.*, 2008), the time efficiency of administration makes them attractive.

A new area considered to be important in fear of falling is outcome expectancy (Lach, 2006). When working one to one, information on this might be obtained by clinical interview. However, there may be some advantages in using a specific scale to assess outcome expectancy more thoroughly. Some individuals may not have thought through their fear in these terms and the use of a questionnaire might facilitate this process. The Consequences of Falling Scale (CoF; Yardley & Smith, 2002) measures outcome expectancy with respect to falls. Those completing the questionnaire rate 12 items in terms of their level of agreement or disagreement about the consequence(s) of a fall. A statement such as 'I will feel foolish' is rated on a four-point Likert response in which 1 = 'disagree strongly', 2 = 'disagree', 3 = 'agree' and 4 = 'strongly agree'. Two subscales can be calculated from the CoF. These reflect items related to Loss of Functional Independence (CoF-LFI) and Damage to Identity (CoF-DI). There are six items for each subscale, which are summed to obtain the subscale scores (range 4–24). A total score, the sum of all 12 items, is also calculated (range 8–48). The higher the score, the greater levels of concern identified. The CoF subscales are internally reliable and demonstrate adequate test–retest reliability (Yardley & Smith, 2002). The scale's psychometric properties remain to be established with stroke survivors.

While questionnaires may be useful for the detection and evaluation of progress, in clinical practice the main concern is improvement relative to individual goals; that is achieving goals in terms of behavioural activity within physical capability, not evident prior to intervention. For instance, if a client has been unable to walk upstairs and becomes able to do so, this is a substantial outcome. In addition, the use of questionnaires needs to be considered in the context of a stroke population. Those with significant cognitive or communication impairment may not be able to complete even the simplest instruments. Cognitive or communication disorder aside, some people without these difficulties will have a fear of falling that is evident to an observer, but to into which they themselves do not have insight. In addition, fear of falling may not be expressed or observable, as those with fear of falling may have ceased undertaking activities such that the fear is never evident. Unfortunately, family and formal carers can support this avoidance by interpreting that it is due to stroke-related disability rather than due to fear. They may then take over tasks that a patient is capable of doing. It is a challenge for the physiotherapist to identify such individuals and to set appropriate goals with those referred for rehabilitation on the basis of their physical potential.

Interventions for fear of falling

Although there is currently no outcome research supporting a particular approach to reducing fear of falling among people with stroke, a number of studies have considered this in older people, some of whom have experienced a stroke. From the earliest randomised controlled trial (Tennstedt, Howland, Lachman, Peterson, Kasten & Jette, 1998), a cognitive-behavioural therapy (CBT) approach has been considered the most appropriate to deal with fear of falling. Interventions for fear of falling include: cognitive therapy to change attitudes about the risk of falling, education about the fear of falling and recognition that it is controllable, goal setting to increase relative activity levels of participants and to provide a graduated exposure to fearful situations, environmental modification to reduce the risk of falling, increasing physical exercise and maximising strength and balance. A manualised approach is available, which is particularly useful for nonpsychologically trained therapists (Tennstedt, Peterson, Howland & Lachman, 1998).

Zijlstra, van Haastregt, van Rossum, van Eijk, Yardley and Kempen (2007) completed a systematic review of interventions to reduce fear of falling in community living older people. Their review considered any intervention that assessed fear of falling, rather than those that specifically targeted this within their intervention. They concluded that interventions that showed an effect on fear of falling were five multifactorial programmes (such as that described above), three tai chi interventions, two exercise interventions and one hip protector intervention. The multifactorial interventions all included a CBT approach as described above.

Psychological management of falls and fear of falling

Childs and Kneebone (2002) considered psychological management of fear of falling in a clinical setting. They emphasised the importance of setting realistic goals in the context of fear of falling. Their view was that any falls programme, whether it addresses fear of falling specifically or not, should consider an approach that emphasises 'falls reduction' rather than 'falls prevention'.

This is in order to reassure a client who may be pessimistic about preventing falls that the programme has value and allow open discussion of a client's fears in this context. This also allows the client to admit to falls over the course of intervention without concern that they will be personally blamed for an incident. This approach is also seen as helpful to staff. As preventing all falls is unrealistic, if staff can judge their interventions on the basis of falls reduction, they too are less likely to see themselves as having failed.

Childs and Kneebone (2002) also accepted that in the clinical setting a major opportunity to manage a fear of falling is in falls groups, in which only some of the participants may be fearful of falls. Some patients may fall every day and wish to minimise this for safety's sake but may not be fearful. On this basis, it is recommended that group interventions for falls incorporate steps and advice appropriate for people who may not admit to fear of falling, those who avoid activities which may precipitate the fear, and indeed those in whom abstract thinking skills, such as those required to understand the cognitive model, may not be present. The most important components of such an intervention should be to increase patients' self efficacy in relation to reducing falls risks, how to manage situations that may present a risk of falling and how to manage if one does fall. Programme components that can support confidence without fear being specifically acknowledged, include normalising falls across the population, considering factors to increase or reduce falls risk, conducting exercises which manipulate extrinsic and intrinsic factors to reduce the risk of falls, relaxation approaches and attentional strategies. The aim is to direct participants to develop specific approaches to enable them to mobilise well. Training in how to get up once one has fallen and in means of accessing help can also serve to allay fear. Currently research to support the use of such strategies within general falls groups remains to be undertaken.

When psychological therapists see individuals who acknowledge a fear of falling, intervention can be more explicit. Childs and Kneebone (2002) considered the importance of beginning by acknowledging the validity of the fear. In the context of stroke, where balance and other aspects of mobility are compromised, this is essential. For many after a stroke, the fear of falling is not phobic but a reality-based concern. They may well have fallen or seen others fall over during the course of rehabilitation. The fear can be protective, and some wariness and caution in the context of mobilisation when one is frail are entirely appropriate; the difficulty arises when this is out of proportion to the risk and leads to immobility and paradoxically greater risk. It can be helpful to explain to patients that staying seated and avoiding risk is understandable though counter-productive in the long term. The role of therapists is to educate their patients as to how this understandable reaction is counter-productive. This includes the identification of obtainable physical goals that will not be achieved, the likelihood of deconditioning and other consequences of immobility, such as constipation and pressure sores. In inpatient settings, the fear may lead to inability to return to one's home. In some cases a decisional balance can be considered for a

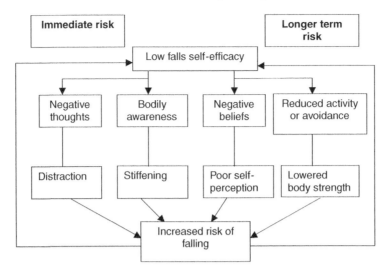

Figure 17.2 Fear of falling as a risk factor for future falls. Based on Childs, L., & Kneebone, I. I. (2002). Falls, fear of falling and psychological management. *International Journal of Therapy and Rehabilitation*, 9, 225–31.

client that leads to a decision to pursue mobilisation goals 'despite the risk of a fall'. While the model proposed earlier (Figure 17.1) is complicated, a more straightforward version, similar to that proposed by Childs and Kneebone (2002) as seen in Figure 17.2, can be useful to educate patients. More advanced intervention, such as motivational interviewing, can be used if required. This approach directly addresses barriers to mobilisation and problem solving to address these barriers. Motivational interviewing has been shown to have great potential in healthcare settings (Rollnick, Miller & Butler, 2007) and has already proved successful in improving mood after stroke (Watkins *et al.*, 2007).

Once patients are educated and agree their goals, they are trained in physical and cognitive techniques to manage their fear. Physically this can include a variety of relaxation and breathing exercises. Three–part breathing for instance (Winkler, James, Fatovich & Underwood, 1982), can be used 'on the spot' by patients. Pre-prepared self-statements, in the manner of stress inoculation therapy (Meichenbaum, 1985), provide the cognitive support to the behaviour. This might include self-statements that acknowledge the risk of a fall, alongside reassurance that if they 'relax and concentrate' on what they need to do to perform the activity, this risk is reduced (Childs and Kneebone, 2002). A reminder list, prepared in conjunction with a physical therapist, of what they need to do is the final cognitive element. Essentially while interventions can be individually tailored, the process is brief relaxation, cognitive coping statements and a shift in attention to the task at hand. Additional components to support successful intervention include collaborative negotiation of a hierarchy of goals and giving control to the client over when new goals are to be attempted.

With the cognitive and communication disorder evident in some stroke survivors, the ability to engage in cognitive behavioural therapy can be reduced. Essentially intervention for fear of falling with such patients emphasizes the behavioural components over the cognitive (i.e. relaxation and attention diversion become more prominent). Some case studies that illustrate interventions for fear of falling after stroke are shown in Tables 17.1, 17.2 and 17.3.

Table 17.1   Case Example of Fear of Falling

Dorothy, aged 82, was seen when an inpatient in a post acute rehabilitation service (stroke unit) six weeks after a stroke. She had a history of falls with a fractured neck of femur as a result of one of these, three years prior to her stroke. Her Mini Mental State Examination score was 24/30. She had no other significant medical conditions. The stroke had left Dorothy with left sided weakness and poor sitting balance. She was continent, independent in feeding and all aspects of grooming. The physiotherapist referred Dorothy as she was refusing to attempt to mobilise from her bed. On assessment, Dorothy was found to be 100% convinced that she would fall and that she would be badly injured if she attedmpted to stand unassisted.

Formulation
The difficulty with fear of falling appeared to have arisen in someone prone to anxiety, in the context of stroke-related mobility difficulties and following a past fall that had lead to a painful injury, surgery and hospitalisation. The difficulty was maintained by the belief that she would be certain to fall and injure herself. A further contributor appeared to be the adversarial interaction that had developed with her physical therapists; they were unable to accept that she would not cooperate with therapy and kept attempting to persuade her to undertake her exercises.

Intervention
On the basis of a consultation with the unit clinical psychologist, it was decided to:

1. Make it clear to Dorothy that it was her decision as to whether she participated in rehabilitation or not and that it was our role to inform her of our best opinions, not only as to what would be useful but also the consequences of nonparticipation. These consequences included immobility and discharge to a nursing home rather than to her own home.
2. Provide daily communication sessions with the physiotherapist in which the above was reiterated and during which the stages and process the physical therapy were explained in terms of the stepping stones that could build up to Dorothy walking again.

Once the pressure from therapists had ceased and following the detailed explanations by therapists that reinforced that participation was under Dorothy's control, Dorothy achieved the first goal of treatment: sitting at the side of her bed with a table in front of her. Subsequent to this, her therapy proceeded within normal expectations. She quickly progressed to standing with a table in front of her. She was easily able to walk more than 20 metres when discharged to her own home.

Table 17.2   Case Example of Fear of Falling

Yvonne aged 55, was an inpatient in a rehabilitation unit for younger people with neurological disability. She had a history of one fall prior to her stroke, from the top of the stairs in her own home. This was considered an accident not related to any medical condition. She was reviewed two months after a stroke that had led to right-sided weakness, mild language problems and concentration difficulties. Rehabilitation was proceeding well to the extent that Yvonne was independent in transferring with supervision, walking on flat ground and up stairs, with one person for standby assistance. While her performance was affected by fatigue and she had reduced standing tolerance and safety awareness in the kitchen, she was fully independent in feeding and all personal self-care apart from washing her feet. The strength in her right, dominant arm had returned to 80% of that of her left. Unfortunately, Yvonne became fearful of going downstairs when this goal was addressed in therapy. It was most important that she do this, not only for general community access but also for access to the upper floor of her home.

Formulation

The fear of falling difficulty had arisen after a stroke in someone who was generally coping well. It was brought on when she first stood at the top of the stairs and looked down, a position she had not been in for some time. Although prior to this the previous fall had not been a concern, in the context of disability and being stood for the first time at the top of stairs, a fear was precipitated. The fear appeared to be maintained by the view that a fall was likely and would result an injury that would probably lengthen hospitalisation and her ability to be discharged on her target date. Avoidance also played a role; Yvonne felt relieved when she was taken away from the stairs.

Intervention

The patient's goals were clarified with her, that is, that she wished to be discharged home and to be able to use the upper floor of her home, which would require her coming down the stairs. A decisional balance was then used, empathy was shown for the patient's concerns about falls and the risk of a fall was not denied but was placed in perspective. As there would initially be a therapist behind and a therapist in front of her as well as handrails on either side, she agreed a fall was unlikely.

Training included a brief relaxation strategy to allow the physical components of fearfulness to be contained. A list of coping self-statements was drawn up, and a goal hierarchy was established. Two trials then took place in pursuit of the agreed goals. In contrast to earlier physical therapy sessions, this included a lower flight of stairs made of a material considered less harmful in the event of a fall, than the stairs used on previous attempts. Therapists made sure that the client was agreeing to each goal and that these were pursued when she was ready. An occupational therapist, a physiotherapist and a psychologist were present to prompt the use of coping responses and to manage concerns about falls.

The patient became able to independently go up and down stairs in the hospital, then in her own home, through a trial on weekend leave. Yvonne was discharged home successfully.

Table 17.3 Case Example of Fear of Falling

Petros was a 76-year-old man living with a female companion. He had had a stroke five years prior to the referral. He had made an almost complete recovery from his stroke with the exception of mild balance problems that he managed with the support of a stick. Twelve months prior to his referral to an older peoples' day hospital, Petros had declined to mobilise without standby assistance and supervision. Nor would he go out unaccompanied. He only went out once a week, when his daughter took him shopping.

Formulation

The problem for Petros had arisen when he had attended an open air theatre in the previous summer. Despite having made a good recovery from his stroke, his balance was still mildly affected. He came close to falling when, after the intermission, he was bumped by the 'throng of the crowd', returning to see the second half of the performance. He fell over on the grass without injury. Following this event Petros became nervous, restricted his activities and avoided mobilising when not in the presence of others. At the time of the initial review, Petros was able to walk anywhere within the hospital and its grounds with standby supervision. He even did this holding his stick in front of him as he proceeded, which meant it offered him no support. It was evident that the difficulty was maintained by concerns about having a fall, this being embarrassing and possibly dangerous. It also seemed likely that the care provided by his partner and his daughter was a further maintaining factor.

Intervention

The initial component of intervention was education about fear of falling and how fear of falling could precipitate future falls. This included the handout in Figure 17.2. The risk of falls was considered relative to Petros' disability. The need to mobilise was considered in terms of potential physical health gains, and independence benefits, such as the ability to go to the toilet without standby assistance during the day (Petros' partner worked).

Petro's risk of falling was considered alongside the health and independence benefits of increasing his mobility. He was keen to be able to toilet without standby assistance during the day when his partner was out at work. The intervention included goal setting, relaxation, developing appropriate coping self-statements and attention management. Petros became independently mobile within his home but remained unwilling to mobilise independently out of doors. It was considered the dedicated weekly visits of Petros' daughter were such that he would not pursue outdoor mobility because of the possibility that these visits might end. Petros acknowledged this possibility, but was reluctant to set a goal to overcome this.

Conclusions

People fall when they have a stroke and are also at risk of a fall subsequently on account of disability. Regardless of an actual fall after stroke, individuals can develop a fear of falling that can impact, through avoidance, their physical and emotional state. There are approaches to understand fear of falling after stroke and instruments that may prove useful in assessing and screening for it. While there is no randomised controlled trial evidence to indicate the effectiveness of treatment for this condition within this specific population, cognitive-behavioural approaches trialled with older people appear promising. These should be subject to further investigation in a stroke population. There also remains the opportunity for further investigation of the factors that contribute to the development of fear of falling after stroke. Further information on this could inform both prevention and treatment.

Chapter 18

Prevention of Psychological Distress after Stroke

Introduction

The problem of low mood after stroke has been considered and interventions to improve mood are available. The evidence reviewed so far has focussed on responding to those who develop problems with their mood. However, a better approach is to prevent the development of mood disorders after stroke. Some strategies have been employed specifically to prevent people becoming depressed; but most aim to reduce the likelihood of general psychological distress and therefore serve also to prevent anxiety and other emotional difficulties.

Ward-based prevention strategies

Rehabilitation

While patients are in hospital, there is evidence to suggest that psychological distress is less likely if patients are treated on a specialist stroke unit and have an active rehabilitation programme. Most trials of the effectiveness of stroke units have concentrated on death and disability as the main outcomes. However, some studies have considered psychological outcome measures. For example, Juby, Lincoln and Berman (1996) included the GHQ028 as a measure of psychological distress in their randomised trial of stroke unit care as compared with rehabilitation on conventional general medical and healthcare of the elderly wards. Patients treated on the stroke unit had significantly lower scores at 12 months after randomisation than those on conventional wards. They were also better adjusted at six months, and this adjustment process may in part explain the better outcome in mood. At the time, this was one of the few stroke

Psychological Management of Stroke, First Edition. Nadina B. Lincoln, Ian I. Kneebone, Jamie A.B. Macniven and Reg C. Morris.
© 2012 John Wiley & Sons, Ltd. Published 2012 by John Wiley & Sons, Ltd.

rehabilitation units to have a clinical psychologist as a member of the multidisciplinary team, and few of the other stroke units evaluated in the early randomised trials had a significant level of psychological input.

Observational studies have indicated that there are variations in the level of
activity of patients in different ward settings. An important difference between
stroke units and general medical wards is that rehabilitation is provided more
intensively on stroke units. For example, Lincoln, Willis, Philips, Juby and
Berman (1996) observed patients in the above-mentioned randomised trial of a
stroke unit (Juby *et al.*, 1996) and showed that those on the stroke unit spent
significantly more time actively engaged in rehabilitation. Patients on the stroke
unit spent 31 minutes in an eight-hour day in interactions with nurses and
36 minutes with therapists, in contrast to those on conventional wards, who
spent 18 minutes in an eight-hour day with nurses and 21 minutes with
therapists. On the basis that inactivity tends to be associated with low mood,
one reason for less psychological distress on the stroke unit may be that there was
more interaction with rehabilitation staff. However, an observational study
comparing four stroke rehabilitation units (De Wit, Putman, Dejaeger, Baert,
Berman, Bogaerts *et al.*, 2005) did not support the view that more active
rehabilitation improves mood, as there were no significant differences between
the units in the levels of anxiety and depression assessed on the Hospital Anxiety
and Depression Scale scores, despite very different intensities of rehabilitation. It
is possible that this was partly due to the use of a screening measure to assess
mood rather than a measure of the severity of the mood disorders.

Occupational therapy

A similar conclusion may be reached on the basis of the evidence for the
effectiveness of occupational therapy. A meta-analysis of trials of occupational
therapy (Legg, Drummond & Langhorne, 2006; Legg, Drummond, Leonardi-Bee,
Gladman, Corr, Donkervoort *et al.* 2007) showed no significant benefit in
mood or distress scores in patients receiving occupational therapy as compared
with those not. However, these results were based on the four occupational
therapy trials which provided results of mood as an outcome and therefore the
analysis may not be powered to detect differences in mood. An individual patient
data meta-analysis of trials of occupational therapy examined the effects of
occupational therapy on mood assessed using the General Health Questionnaire
(Walker, Leonardi-Bee, Bath, Langhorne, Dewey, Corr *et al.*, 2004). Although
there were no significant effects on GHQ scores, only three trials were included
(Logan, Ahern, Gladman & Lincoln, 1997; Parker, Gladman, Dewey, Lincoln,
Barer, Logan *et al.*, 2001; Walker, Gladman, Lincoln, Siemonsma, & Whitely,
1999), and the forest plot indicates the trends were in the predicted direction.
The results for the pooled analysis at the end of the treatment phase, were OR
0.76 (95% CI 0.54 to 1.07), so quite close to being a significant reduction in
GHQ scores (good outcome), but at the end of the trial phase the OR was 1.10

(95% CI 0.74 to 1.63) showing no significant effect at 12-month follow-up. It is possible that there was an effect at the end of treatment phase, but there might not have been enough power to detect it. One specific study (Drummond & Walker, 1996) indicated that introducing patients to leisure activities may improve mood. Patients were randomly allocated to receive leisure rehabilitation, additional occupational therapy for personal self-care activities or usual care. Those who received treatment focussing on leisure activities had significantly lower scores on the Nottingham Health Profile three months after discharge from hospital than those allocated to either extra occupational therapy or usual care and the proportion with scores in the definitely depressed range of the Wakefield Depression Inventory was also less. The reason that this form of occupational therapy had more beneficial effects than other trials of occupational therapy may be because the focus was on identifying activities which people enjoyed doing, whereas many of the others were designed simply to promote independence in activities of daily living. However, the beneficial effect of leisure rehabilitation was not supported in a multicentre trial (Parker *et al.*, 2001), so the findings obtained by Drummond and Walker (1996) may have been due to chance. Subsequent analysis of results on the Nottingham Leisure questionnaire (Walker *et al.*, 2004) suggested leisure rehabilitation did improve leisure outcomes, but the effects on mood were not ascertained.

Music therapy

Music therapy has been investigated in acute hospital settings and found to reduce distress. Nayak, Wheeler, Shiflet and Agostinelli (2000) recruited 18 patients with low mood who had suffered a traumatic brain injury or a stroke, and assigned them to either a music therapy group or a usual care control group. The music therapy group engaged in various activities including singing, composing, playing instruments and listening to music. The patients in this group met two to three times a week for a maximum of ten treatments. Outcome measures included a self-report measure of mood, a family rating and therapist ratings. The results showed that the music therapy group exhibited a greater improvement in mood and social interaction compared with control group. However, the results were only preliminary and the groups were not randomly allocated.

Sarkamo, Tervaniemi, Laitinen, Forsblom, Soinila, Mikkonen *et al.* (2008) conducted a randomised controlled trial of daily listening to music as compared with daily listening to audio books or no intervention. Outcomes were assessed three and six months after stroke on a shortened Finnish version of the Profile of Mood States (McNair, Lorr & Droppleman, 1981). This contains 38 items assessing tension, depression, irritability, vigour, fatigue, inertia, confusion and forgetfulness. At three months there was a significant difference between the groups in depression and confusion, as assessed on the Profile of Mood States. Post hoc tests indicated that the depression score was significantly lower in the music group than in the control group. These differences were maintained at six

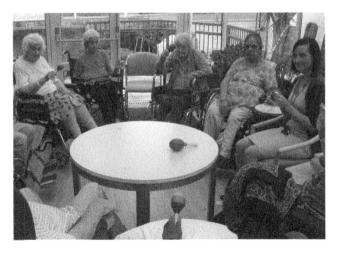

Figure 18.1   A music therapy group.

months in favour of the music group, although the difference was no longer statistically significant. However, the mechanism by which these changes were achieved is not clear. Although other studies have indicated music has a beneficial effect on motor function (Altenmüller, Marco-Pallares, Műnte & Schneider, 2009) and mood (Forsblom Laitinen, Sarkamo & Tervaniemi, 2009; Koelsch, 2009), music listening may be a form of activity. The differences between music listening and listening to audio books were minimal on the mood measure and so the results could be due to increased activity. However, as suggested by Sarkamo *et al.* (2008), music may have a specific effect on arousal and attention and produce structural changes within the brain, which could equally account for the effects observed. Regardless of the mechanism, it does suggest that listening to music may be a strategy to improve mood in the acute stage in hospital and thus reduce the likelihood of psychological distress. An example is shown in Figure 18.1.

Individual psychological interventions

The prevention of mood disorders may require more specific interventions than simply increasing the level of activity.

Distress Management System

A Distress Management System originally developed for use within an oncology service has been adapted for use in rehabilitation stroke wards with the intention to develop it further within acute and community settings (Williams, personal communication). The system encompasses a training programme to develop multidisciplinary staff knowledge and to provide the skills to identify and alleviate distress.

Part of the Distress Management System is the Distress thermometer (adapted from the National Comprehensive Cancer Network's 'Clinical Practice Guidelines in Oncology', 2004). The distress thermometer (see Figures 18.2 and 18.3) is used to inform a discussion between patients, carers and staff about

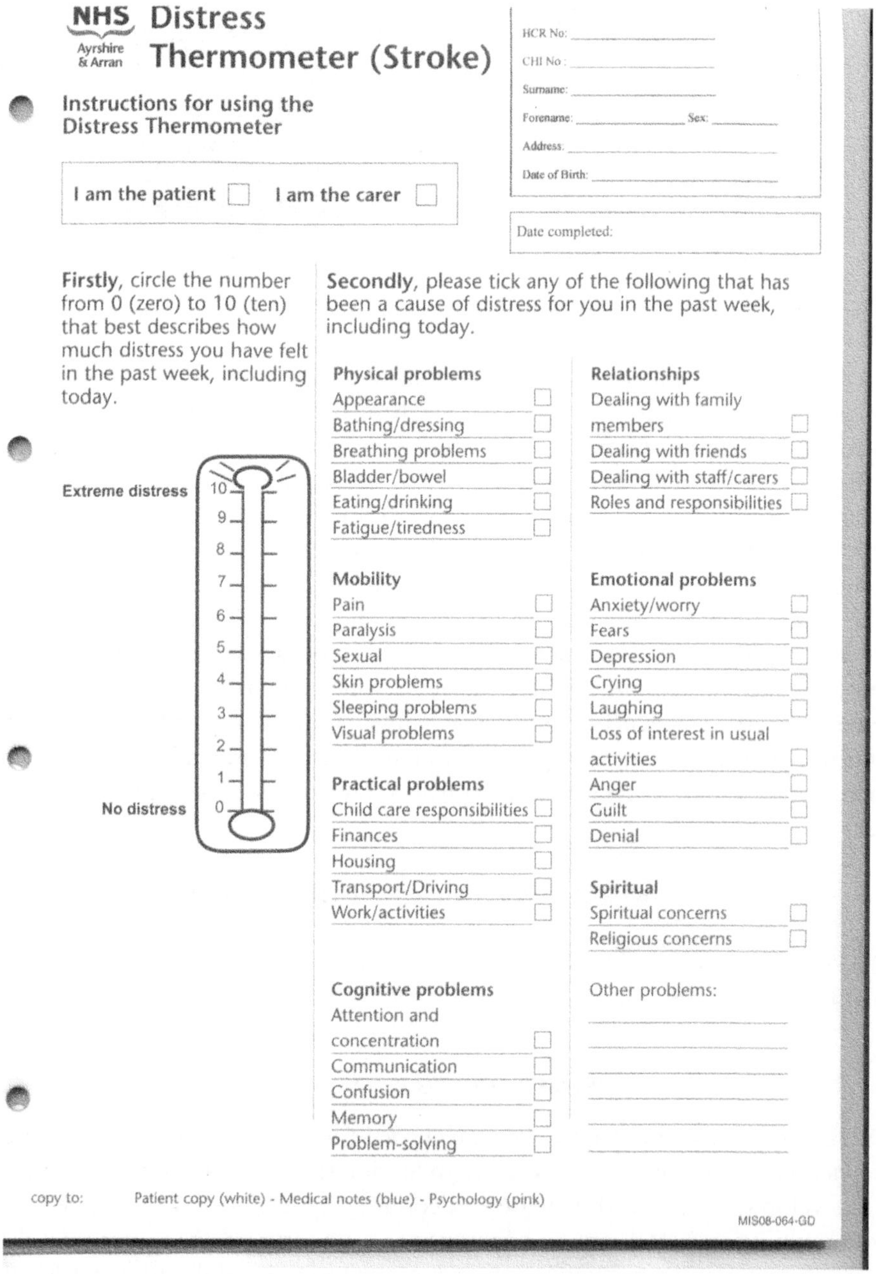

NHS Ayrshire & Arran

Distress Thermometer (Stroke)

HCR No:

CHI No:

Surname:

Forename: Sex:

Address:

Date of Birth:

Instructions for using the Distress Thermometer

I am the patient ☐ I am the carer ☐

Date completed:

Firstly, circle the number from 0 (zero) to 10 (ten) that best describes how much distress you have felt in the past week, including today.

Extreme distress 10 9 8 7 6 5 4 3 2 1 0 No distress

Secondly, please tick any of the following that has been a cause of distress for you in the past week, including today.

Physical problems
Appearance ☐
Bathing/dressing ☐
Breathing problems ☐
Bladder/bowel ☐
Eating/drinking ☐
Fatigue/tiredness ☐

Mobility
Pain ☐
Paralysis ☐
Sexual ☐
Skin problems ☐
Sleeping problems ☐
Visual problems ☐

Practical problems
Child care responsibilities ☐
Finances ☐
Housing ☐
Transport/Driving ☐
Work/activities ☐

Cognitive problems
Attention and concentration ☐
Communication ☐
Confusion ☐
Memory ☐
Problem-solving ☐

Relationships
Dealing with family members ☐
Dealing with friends ☐
Dealing with staff/carers ☐
Roles and responsibilities ☐

Emotional problems
Anxiety/worry ☐
Fears ☐
Depression ☐
Crying ☐
Laughing ☐
Loss of interest in usual activities ☐
Anger ☐
Guilt ☐
Denial ☐

Spiritual
Spiritual concerns ☐
Religious concerns ☐

Other problems:

copy to: Patient copy (white) - Medical notes (blue) - Psychology (pink)

MIS08-064-GD

Figure 18.2 Distress thermometer.

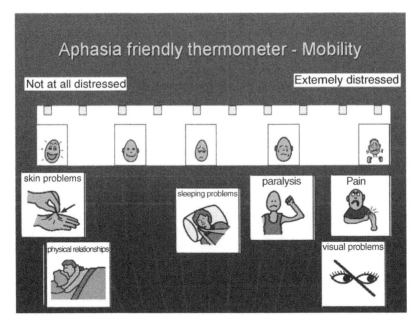

Figure 18.3 Aphasia-friendly distress thermometer. Reproduced with permission of Talking Mats, www.talkingmats.com, and DynaVox Mayer-Johnson for the use of The Picture Communication Symbols © 1981–2010.

patients' individual needs and causes of distress. This discussion in itself reduces distress by helping patients identify and prioritise their own distress, and by setting a shared agenda. Having identified the nature of distress this is managed by appropriate information provision, key clinical skills, monitoring, consultation or referral to a specialist. The system ensures the members of the multidisciplinary team communicate with patients about their concerns on a regular basis and provides staff with a range of actions when faced with a patient in distress. It has been recognised that information provision improves mood (Smith, Forster, House, Knapp, Wright & Young, 2008; Smith, Forster & Young, 2009) and so a key element of the Distress Management System may be that it provides a structure to ensure patients are provided with appropriate information at a time when they need it.

An audit of the Distress Management System (Williams, personal communication) showed that the system was used with 94% of stroke patients and that 59% of patients' distress was managed by patients themselves or nonpsychology staff. Qualitative feedback from the team, through content analysis of evaluation questionnaires, was positive. The benefits were an improved provision of psychological care through increasing staff skills and access to psychological therapy, and also the benefits this brings to overall rehabilitation. The training and experience of using the Distress Management System improved staff confidence in managing patients who were distressed. Staff members were using consultation to help support and to advise patients on managing distress and

Table 18.1   Case Example of the Distress Management System

Case Example

Malcolm was described by staff as agitated, anxious and aggressive. He was refusing to take his medication, not engaging well with the therapists, lacked insight into his condition and staff perceived that he was having difficulty accepting his diagnosis. A physiotherapist carried out the distress thermometer with him and three main areas were identified. He was extremely worried about financial issues, but did not want to worry his family and did not think it was anything to do with hospital staff; he decided that he just needed to get home so he played down what was wrong with him. Information was provided on benefits available, and he contacted social work services to arrange a meeting. He stated that he was a heavy smoker and was really agitated because of not being able to smoke; a referral was made to the smoke cessation team. He also reported that the medication was making him tired, and so he had decided to stop taking it but perceived that staff were trying to force him to take it and this led to thoughts that they were trying to keep him sedated. The consultant was made aware of this, and he took time to explain to Malcolm and his wife each of the medications prescribed and the physical impact of stroke in terms of fatigue. They were also given written information on fatigue. A short time later Malcolm, who was making poor progress initially, had established good engagement with the therapists and was making progress towards discharge earlier than expected.

recognising when it was appropriate to refer to specialist services. However, one major aspect highlighted was that the team only felt confident to use the Distress Management System knowing that they had access to a clinical psychologist for support when the levels of distress were beyond their capability to manage. An example patient is given in Table 18.1.

This intervention included the provision of information and there is evidence from a Cochrane review of information provision that this has a beneficial effect on mood. Smith *et al.* (2008) reviewed studies of information provision, seven of which included mood as an outcome. In addition to improving knowledge, there was a small statistically significant difference on depression questionnaires scores (WMD 0.52, 95% CI 0.93 to 0.10) but no evidence of any difference on anxiety questionnaire scores (WMD 0.34, 95% CI 1.17 to 0.50). Results are shown in Figure 18.4.

Problem solving

Problem solving interventions have been evaluated in community settings. Forster and Young (1996) randomly allocated community patients to receive support from a specialist nurse or usual care. The role of the specialist nurses was to provide visits as needed over the course of a year to offer information, advice and support. The intervention was based on a counselling and enabling model, intended to address psychological factors. It included training in problem solving, goal setting, advice on specific issues and the provision of information

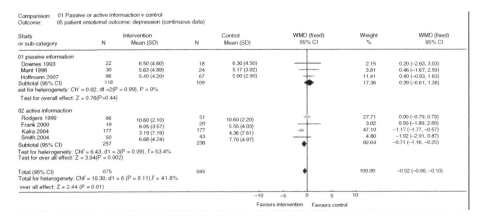

Figure 18.4   Forest plot of the effect of information on patient depression. Smith, J., Forster, A., House, A., Knapp, P., Wright, J. J., & Young, J., Information provision for stroke patients and their caregivers, *Cochrane Database of Systematic Reviews 2*, 2008. © Cochrane Collaboration, reproduced with permission.

booklets. There were no significant differences between the groups in the level of well-being as assessed on the Nottingham Health Profile (excluding the physical function section). However, qualitative studies (Dowswell, Lawler, Young, Forster & Hearn, 1997; Dowswell, Lawler, Dowswell, Young, Forster & Hearn, 2000; Lawler, Dowswell, Hearn, Forster & Young, 1999) suggested that patients and carers had found the intervention useful and some felt that the intervention had facilitated emotional adjustment. Goldberg, Segal, Berk and Gershkoff (1997) conducted a randomised trial in which the treatment comprised weekly phone contact, monthly home visits and a home-based therapeutic team to attend to psychosocial stressors and prevent significant psychosocial problems from accelerating. The treatment was delivered by a multidisciplinary team, which included a psychiatrist, psychologist, recreational therapist, research program case manager and social worker, and continued for a year after stroke. Although the Center for Epidemiological Studies Depression Scale was administered at outcome, the groups were not compared on this measure. Qualitative feedback was positive, including the emotional support provided. These two interventions showed limited effectiveness, but problem solving was only one component of a package of care. Other studies have provided more structured and intensive problem solving training.

House (2000, 2003) evaluated problem solving training in an acute stroke setting, but few details are available. Stroke patients were randomly allocated to problem solving training, an attention placebo control or usual care. Problem solving training was delivered by specialist mental health nurses for one to ten (median five) fortnightly sessions. The attention placebo was delivered by trained volunteers for one to 42 (median six) fortnightly contacts. Patients who received training in problem solving had significantly lower scores on the GHQ-28, a measure of psychological distress, at the end of treatment. There is also more recent evidence to support the use of problem solving training in acute stroke (Robinson, Jorge, Moser, Acion, Solodkin, Small *et al.*, 2008). Robinson *et al.* (2008) randomly allocated 176 nondepressed stroke patients within three months of a stroke. Patients were randomly allocated to the anti-depressant, escitalopram, placebo or problem solving therapy. The structure of the problem solving therapy programme was based on a treatment manual (Mynors-Wallis, Gath, Lloyd-Thomas & Tomlinson, 1995) and comprised six treatment sessions in the first 12 weeks and six reinforcement sessions in the following period up to a year after randomisation. The treatment was delivered by therapists who were trained through supervised practice of five cases prior to the study. The likelihood of developing depression was lower in both the escitalopram and problem solving groups, as compared to placebo. There was also an interesting observation that five patients recruited to the study were assigned to problem solving therapy because they refused pharmacological therapy. Although they were not included in the analysis, the observation does support the need for psychological interventions to be available in addition to pharmacological. Although Robinson *et al.* (2008) found support for the use of a drug treatment in the prevention of depression, an earlier meta-analysis (Hackett, Anderson, House & Halteh, 2008) which included 11 trials did not find any evidence of benefit. Patients treated with antidepressants were no less likely to develop depression than those who received a placebo. In addition, many patients do not meet the inclusion criteria for these trials, and some people also prefer not to take medication as a preventative strategy.

Motivational interviewing

Another psychological intervention for improving emotional outcomes in the acute stages after stroke is motivational interviewing. Watkins, Auton, Deans, Dickinson, Jack, Lightbody *et al.* (2007) evaluated motivational interviewing with patients on acute stroke wards in comparison with a usual care control. Patients were invited to take part in a study of problems adjusting to life after a stroke. They were informed that a type of counselling, called motivational interviewing, has been used previously to help people resolve adjustment problems in other disorders and they were invited to take part in a study to find out whether it was helpful after stroke. They were randomly allocated to receive motivational inter- viewing or usual care. Motivational interviewing is a specific talk-based therapy which is used to improve motivation to make changes in health behaviours. The aim was to provide early intervention to support and build patients' motivation to adjust and adapt to having had a stroke. Patients were encouraged to make psychological adjustments and to identify realistic personal goals for their recovery. The treatment was provided by nurses and psychologists, who were trained and supervised by an experienced clinical psychologist. Patients were treated for up to four half-hour sessions delivered on a weekly basis. The content of a sample of sessions was recorded to check that the therapists complied with the principles of motivational interviewing. The clinical psychologist reviewed the content of 20 therapist utterances from each session and classified them into utterances which were motivational interviewing-consistent and those which were not. The motivational interviewing-consistent utterances included open questions, reflections, advise with permission, affirm, emphasize control, reflect, reframe and support. Utterances which were rated as motivational interviewing-nconsistent, included advise without permission, confront, direct, raise concern without permission and warn. The percentage of motivational interviewing-consistent utterances was determined, and results showed that the delivery of intervention was of high quality and on average 98.1% of utterances were motivational interviewing consistent. The outcomes were assessed three months and a year after stroke. At three months, there was a significant benefit of motivational interviewing over usual care on the dichotomised GHQ-28 scores (normal <5 or low >5). The odds ratio was significant (p 0.03; OR [normal mood]: 1.60, 95% CI: 1.04 to 2.46). Normal mood was found in 70 (41.9%) of those receiving usual care and 94 (54.7%) of those who received motivational interviewing. There was also a protective effect of motivational interviewing against depression on the Yale question (Lachs, Feinstein & Cooney, 1990) as a screening question (p 0.03; OR: 1.65, 95% CI: 1.06 to 2.58). Scores in the intervention group decreased from a median of six to a median of 3 at both three months and a year, which is within the normal range, whereas the median of the control remained at 6 at three months, having also been 6 at baseline, though there was a reduction to a median of 5 at the one-year follow-up. This suggests that the benefits of the intervention persisted over a year. An example patient is illustrated in Table 18.2.

Motivational interviewing is a brief directive cognitive therapy that worked well with stroke patients in the acute stage. Although the participants in the treatment trial (Watkins *et al.*, 2007) were not referred for mood treatment or presenting with a salient psychological issue, the motivational interviewing approach helped them to use their inner resources to develop self-efficacy, by affirming their own skills and attributes, rather than focussing on behavioural rehabilitation strategies. Further verification of the effective elements of motivational interviewing is required, but it seems to be a promising strategy to reduce distress after stroke.

Overall effectiveness

The overall evidence to support the provision of psychological interventions in the prevention of psychological distress after stroke comes from a Cochrane review (Hackett *et al.*, 2008a) involving 902 participants from two studies (House, 2000; Watkins *et al.*, 2007). There was a small significant benefit of psychological therapy in the proportion of participants meeting the study criteria for depression at the end of treatment (OR 0.64; 95% CI 0.42 to 0.98) in comparison with usual care controls. There was also a reduction in psychological distress scores on the GHQ-28 scale (mean difference − 1.37; 95% CI − 2.33 to − 0.40). This provides evidence to support the use of psychological therapies in the prevention of depression after stroke. Results are shown in Figure 18.5.

Table 18.2   Case Example of Motivational Interviewing

Case example

Freda was a 37-year-old female who was in work. She suffered a stroke that left her with a right-sided weakness in her arm and leg, as well as slight speech and swallowing problems. She also had lack of sensation in her right arm, and could not differentiate between hot and cold. She lived with her partner who worked in the same place.

The motivational interviewing programme was delivered over four weekly sessions of up to one hour duration. Because of the brief nature of the programme and the focus of the intervention, the therapists were sensitive to the areas in which they could engage the patients. The main approach is to encourage conversation, express empathy, develop discrepancy, roll with resistance and support self-efficacy. This is facilitated with the main tools: open questions, affirmations, reflections and summaries.

Formulation

Psychometric measures suggested that Freda was depressed. She exhibited high levels of frustration at the lack of control over her situation, which was underpinning her depression. All of the sessions were conducted after discharge from hospital, and she consistently stated that she felt she was ready to drive her car and return to work as soon as possible and could not understand why she was prevented from doing this. Freda claimed that she would bring this about by her own motivation and efforts. In the early session she exhibited frustration and anger at her lack of control over her life and could not understand why 'people' were not giving her the information or answers she wanted.

Treatment

Freda rated importance in regaining control over her life as 10 out of 10, and she rated her confidence in her ability to achieve that as 9 out of 10. These ratings were at odds with her depression score. By encouraging her to engage using open questions, reflecting what she stated and affirming where appropriate, it soon became clear that the lack of control went much deeper than the residual stroke problems. Issues in the relationship with her partner became evident early on in the sessions. The therapist used summaries as sophisticated reflection techniques, and Freda, though still very anxious and frustrated in sessions 1 and 2, became more composed and calm in session 3. This was achieved by supporting her self-efficacy. For example she had developed strategies for coping with two sources of strain in her job, and dealt with this better than her colleagues. Though stressful, she expressed an affection for her job, reflecting this back over a number of sessions. It became clear that she felt a high level of self-esteem and personal control in relation to work. However, in her relationship with her partner she had low levels of control and she felt that her partner used strategies to lower her self-esteem as often as an opportunity arose.

Outcome

By the final session she was very calm and previous anxieties and frustrations had subsided. She indicated that on reflection, she felt out of control with her illness and her relationship; her job presented her only place of control and safety. She also realised that she was not ready to return to work and her earlier urge to do so was almost a denial of her condition. She came to realise that the issue of control in relation by her partner may have been borne out of consideration or affection, but it was still not welcome. Latterly, she felt strong enough to put strategies in place to cope with this situation. In the final session, when asked to quantify importance and confidence in the final session, she admitted that her original 10 and 9 were over-optimistic but felt that such scores were now realistic. She also expressed how helpful the sessions had been to enable her to focus on her strengths and to develop approaches to build on them.

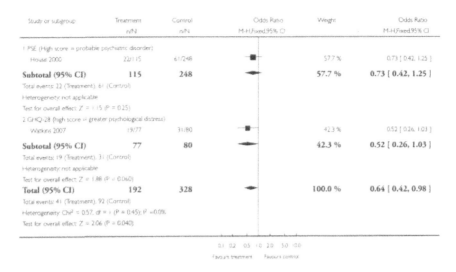

Study or subgroup	Treatment	Control	Odds Ratio	Weight	Odds Ratio
	n/N	n/N	M-H,Fixed,95% CI		M-H,Fixed,95% CI
1 PSE (High score = probable psychiatric disorder)					
House 2000	22/115	61/248		57.7 %	0.73 [0.42, 1.25]
Subtotal (95% CI)	**115**	**248**		**57.7 %**	**0.73 [0.42, 1.25]**
Total events: 22 (Treatment), 61 (Control)					
Heterogeneity: not applicable					
Test for overall effect: Z = 1.15 (P = 0.25)					
2 GHQ-28 (high score = greater psychological distress)					
Watkins 2007	19/77	31/80		42.3 %	0.52 [0.26, 1.03]
Subtotal (95% CI)	**77**	**80**		**42.3 %**	**0.52 [0.26, 1.03]**
Total events: 19 (Treatment), 31 (Control)					
Heterogeneity: not applicable					
Test for overall effect: Z = 1.88 (P = 0.060)					
Total (95% CI)	**192**	**328**		**100.0 %**	**0.64 [0.42, 0.98]**
Total events: 41 (Treatment), 92 (Control)					
Heterogeneity: Chi² = 0.57, df = 1 (P = 0.45); I² =0.0%					
Test for overall effect: Z = 2.06 (P = 0.040)					

0.1 0.2 0.5 1.0 2.0 5.0 10.0
Favours treatment   Favours control

Figure 18.5   Effect of psychological interventions for the prevention of depression after stroke. (Hackett, M. L., Anderson, C. S., House, A., & Halteh, C. 2008. Interventions for preventing depression after stroke. Vol. 3, p. 200. Copyright Cochrane Collaboration, reproduced with permission.)

Group psychological treatments

There have been a few studies of group interventions to prevent psychological distress. These have been used both in the community after discharge from hospital and more recently in the acute stages in hospital.

Community groups

Barton, Miller and Chantor (2002) described a seven session group psychological intervention designed for patients who were approximately six months after stroke in the community. The aim of the group was to help patients to cope psychologically, to develop an understanding of their experiences of the stroke, to learn to accept their disabilities and changed health circumstances, and to give patients an opportunity to share experiences with each other. In addition, the aim was to increase individual control and self-esteem, and encourage patients to develop a positive attitude. The topics covered include feelings associated with loss, understanding the grieving process, the balance between hope and despair, the potentially dysfunctional nature of unrealistic hope, redefining self and identity, individual goal planning and ways of coping. Initial qualitative feedback was positive. In the later groups, participants were ask to give ratings of feelings about how they were coping, and these also showed positive change. Scott and Barton (2010) described case studies of patients who received this psychological support. The benefits seemed to stem from identifying ways of coping. For example, Scott and Barton (2010) identified that the group setting provided an opportunity for people to speak about their concerns, to problem solve, for humour and to plan for the future. In addition people said it made them feel human again and increased confidence (Barton, personal communication). Two examples of patients are a 78-year-old man, who was reluctant to attend the group, but did. Before the group he was not progressing well in rehabilitation and was physically able to do more than he was doing. For example he was capable of going to collect his pension, but was not going. When he first attended the group, he talked about thinking of going into long-term care and had been to visit a couple of places. By the end of group he had decided to stay in his own home, and to have a telephone installed. He was also going out daily to do tasks, such as his shopping, and to collect his pension. A young 34-year-old woman with speech difficulties reported that attending the group increased her self-confidence. During group programme, she investigated going to get a job, had a job interview and got a job. She reported that it was the group that had been essential in enabling her to do this.

Regaining confidence after stroke course

A similar programme was developed by Townsend (2003). Regaining Confidence after Stroke is a course provided to stroke patients after discharge from rehabilitation. The objective of the course is to promote psychological recovery and adjustment. The aims are regaining confidence, promoting coping skills, improving mood and the ability to manage difficult times through increased self-efficacy. The course provides an opportunity for participants to share experiences with other stroke survivors and their carers and gain support from each other. This is intended to provide emotional support, in the context of a group of peers, each confronting the same challenges. The aim of the course is to bridge the gap between reliance on professional rehabilitation staff and having the independence and confidence to lead their own lives again. It provides people with the opportunity to understand themselves and to provide them with the skills and knowledge to continue the process of recovery on their own. It is suitable for stroke patients who are able to communicate with others, not necessarily through speech, and to participate in group discussion. However, those with very severe communication, cognitive or physical problems may not derive as much benefit as those without.

It is run as 11 weekly sessions, each lasting about two hours. Supporters are invited to attend three of the sessions. The initial session involves setting the ground rules for all sessions: that everyone must have a chance to speak, it is everybody's job to make sure that each person gets this opportunity and what is said within the sessions is confidential. Each session includes the presentation of a topic, such as tips and tricks for solving problems, setting realistic targets, emotional ups and downs, other people in your life and coping with change. The sessions include discussion on the topic and structured activities. The materials for each session are provided on a CD, with all the required handouts and materials for activities. This is accompanied by a DVD of videos giving patients' stories, which are used as the basis for discussion.

The course recognises that the process of psychological recovery and adjustment may take many months or even years. People have to deal with many changes, such as changes in mood, lower levels of energy, lack of self-confidence, loss of ability and changes in family roles and relationships. Having the stroke may also have been a traumatic experience. Feedback from group participants suggested that attending the course increased optimism, improved mood, increased social support and produced a more positive personal identity. Feedback has been obtained though audits of groups run in several centres. For example, Ford and Foley (2009) reported that in a small sample of 12 patients who completed the course, scores on the Hospital Anxiety and Depression Scale decreased showing improvement in mood, and confidence increased as assessed on the Stroke Self Efficacy Questionnaire (Jones, Partridge & Reid, 2008). Townsend and Lincoln (unpublished data) found that there was a significant improvement ($p < 0.05$) on a measure of confidence in a small group of 12 participants who attended the RCAS course.

Group interventions provided in hospital have included a modified version of the Regaining Confidence after Stroke course. Vohora and Ogi (2008) described an adapted in-patient version of the course, which comprised five sessions over two and a half weeks. Each session lasted about an hour and was facilitated by a clinical psychologist and assistant psychologist. A manual was created to produce a standard format for the operational rules of the group, as well as the content of each session. Results from six patients were presented which indicated that most patients liked the sessions, and overall most of the feedback was positive.

Inpatient groups

Gurr 2009a, 2009b) described two types of intervention group for stroke patients in hospital. The Share Your Story Group (Gurr, 2009a) was run for two consecutive weeks and open to anyone who wished to attend. In the first sessions participants were encouraged to share their experiences of having had a stroke, and the second session focused on exploration of participants' thoughts and feelings about rehabilitation, and hopes for the future. A before and after evaluation was conducted using the Hospital Anxiety and Depression Scale and a rating the helpfulness of the group for participants' recovery process. Outcome data from 34 of the 80 patients invited to take part in the group showed no significant difference in scores on the Hospital Anxiety and Depression Scale. The average rating for the usefulness of the group was 7, on a 1 to 10 scale, suggesting they found it useful. Qualitative comments also showed positive feedback. The author commented that one reason for lack of significant change was the short duration of intervention, which was due to patients being discharged before sessions had been completed. Gurr (2009b) also described a well-being group which was designed to promote the adjustment experiences gained in the Share Your Story group. This group was provided as a rolling programme so patients were able to join at any stage. It was run once a week for one and a half hours and included both cognitive behavioural techniques and relaxation practice. Evaluation of the progress of 16 patients out of the 26 who attended the group showed a significant decrease in scores on the anxiety scale of Hospital Anxiety and Depression Scale and an improved ability to relax. In addition qualitative feedback was positive.

In addition some groups have included both stroke patients and carers. Hull, Hartigan and Kneebone (2007) described a group comprising six sessions each lasting about 90 minutes. Each session had a stand-alone format so that participants could join the group at any stage. The main feedback was that the group provided enjoyable activities and group members reported feeling better after the group. However, no formal evaluation was carried out.

Effectiveness of group interventions

Thus, although there are some well-developed group interventions to address psychological adjustment at various stages after stroke, the evidence of their effectiveness is lacking. The feedback is generally positive and trends on questionnaire outcomes are in the right direction, but the studies do not have the power to detect statistically significant change. The measures used may not be appropriate to detect the changes being achieved and there is no consideration of long-term outcomes. Further evaluation is required. However, in the meantime provision of such psychological support seems to be appropriate and may help to reduce levels of distress and thus prevent further psychological problems. The need for such groups is supported by views derived from focus groups with both stroke patients and their carers (Hull *et al.*, 2007). In addition, patient examples provide an indication that some patients appear to benefit.

It may also be necessary to provide psychological support in other parts of the stroke care pathway. For example, psychological input into TIA clinics is variable, and often absent. There may be a case for preventative psychological intervention into these clinics in order to support lifestyle adjustment and to address anxiety and low mood. In addition, patients who are discharged from hospital after a few days are rarely referred though to psychological services, but they too may experience significant levels of distress and might benefit from discussion of emotional adjustment coping strategies.

One key feature of those studies which have provided most evidence of effectiveness is the level of training and supervision of the therapists. In both randomised trials which individually showed evidence of effectiveness (House, 2000; Watkins *et al.*, 2007) treatment was delivered by trained therapists who received regular supervision in the delivery of the intervention. Therefore, even though the interventions can be provided by nurses and assistant psychologists, to deliver effective psychological intervention requires training and supervision from an appropriately qualified healthcare professional, most likely a specialist mental health nurse or clinical psychologist. The availability of clinical psychologists within stroke services may therefore be crucial to the successful delivery of these types of interventions. None of the trials of psychological interventions to prevent depression has included a cost-effectiveness analysis, and this is urgently needed. In addition, other psychological interventions (Barton *et al.*, 2002, Townsend, 2003; Vohora & Ogi, 2008; Williams, unpublished) which qualitatively seem useful, even though there are as yet no randomised trials, also require supervision from clinical psychologists.

Conclusions

Several strategies have been used in clinical stroke services to prevent the development of psychological distress. Meta-analysis (Hackett, Anderson, House & Halteh, 2008) has shown that psychological interventions prevent the development of depression. However, while it is clearly important to prevent depression, it is also important to prevent anxiety and reduce general levels of distress. Many of the psychological interventions aim to improve confidence and self-efficacy and these may have an important effect on overall quality of life. However, these have rarely been formally assessed within randomised trials and so evidence for their effectiveness is limited. The feedback from patients and carers is positive suggesting that strategies to prevent psychological distress should be provided in clinical stroke services.

Chapter 19

Pain and Fatigue

Introduction

Aside from mood and cognitive problems, stroke produces a range of other impairments. Some, such as pain and fatigue, may be amenable to psychological interventions. This chapter therefore reviews psychological interventions for pain and fatigue and briefly summarises the evidence base to support their provision.

Pain

Pain has been subject to multiple definitions. For our consideration of pain after stroke we accept the perspective taken by the UK Department of Health (Department of Health, 2009c, p.12) that it is 'an unpleasant sensory and emotional experience associated with actual or potential tissue damage or described in terms of such damage' (Merskey & Dogbuk, 1994) and that it is also 'whatever the person experiencing the pain says it is, existing whenever the person communicates or demonstrates it does' (McCafferey, 1968). An agreed classification of post-stroke pain subtypes is currently not available. Research is clouded by an overlap in definitions and the fact that mixed aetiologies are common and current classifications form no foundation for treatment choice (Roosink, Renzenbrink, Van Dongen, Buitenweg, Geurts & IJzerman, 2008). Clinically speaking, however, there appear to be three main types of pain that occur after a stroke. These are central post-stroke pain, pain considered of neurological origin and viewed as related to lesions affecting the spinothalamic pathways in the brain; nocioceptive pain, often affecting the shoulder and considered mainly related to the effects of weakness in the limb affected by the stroke; and tension-type headaches, related to muscle tension in the head (Widar, Samuelsson, Karlsson-Tivenius & Ahlstrom, 2002).

Psychological Management of Stroke, First Edition. Nadina B. Lincoln, Ian I. Kneebone, Jamie A.B. Macniven and Reg C. Morris.
© 2012 John Wiley & Sons, Ltd. Published 2012 by John Wiley & Sons, Ltd.

The prevalence of pain after a stroke appears to vary, dependent on how the pain is measured and the time period since the stroke. Jonsson, Londgren, Hallstrom, Norvving and Lindgren (2006) identified moderate to severe pain in 32% of survivors four months after stroke. Twelve months later fewer had pain (21%) but the intensity was more severe. In respect of shoulder pain, Lindgren, Jonsson, Norrving and Lindgren (2007) recruited 416 first-ever stroke patients and followed them up at four months and 12 months after stroke. Close to a third of patients developed shoulder pain, the majority at moderate to severe intensities. Widar *et al.* (2002) reviewed pain after stroke in a Swedish sample. Fifteen patients (35%) reported central post-stroke pain, 18 (35%) nocioceptive pain, principally shoulder pain, and 10 (23%) tension-type headache. Four months after stroke, Jonsson *et al.* (2006) found predictors of pain were age (younger patients were more likely to have pain), gender (female) and overall recovery (less recovery). Twelve months later, predictors were gender (female), higher Geriatric Depression Scale–20 (Swedish version) score (Gottfries, Noltorp, Norgaard, 1997), better Mini-Mental State Examination (MMSE) scores and raised glycosylated haemoglobin. The finding for depression was not surprising given the established link between pain and depression, though despite a longitudinal study, the researchers presented no information on the direction of the relationship. They suggested the findings with respect to cognitive impairment may be due to reduced activity levels in those who are cognitively impaired, leading to less opportunity for provocation of pain, though this would seem to go against accepted evidence that reduced activity can do the reverse (White, 2001). Lindgren *et al.* (2007) found impaired arm function and reduced overall recovery (NIH Stroke Scale score) predicted shoulder pain principally, as measured by a visual analogue scale (range 0–100). Widar *et al.* (2002) also identified that 16 (37%) of their sample considered stress and anxiety increased their pain, 13 (30%) considered peace and quiet reduced their pain and 18 (42%) that rest helped them.

For patients with pain after stroke, 58% reported that it disturbs sleep and 40% required rest for relief (Jonsson *et al.*, 2006). Widar, Ahlstrom and Ek (2004) also found pain after stroke affected health and quality of life, as measured by qualitative interview, the Hospital Anxiety and Depression Scale and the Short Form health survey (SF36) scale.

Fatigue

So-called normal fatigue is considered to be tiredness as a consequence of over-exerting oneself that can be assisted by rest (de Groot, Phillips & Eskes, 2003). Conversely, clinical fatigue is often considered to be independent of exertion and much less amenable to rest (Piper, 1989). It is 'a feeling of physical tiredness and lack of energy' described as pathological, abnormal, excessive, chronic, persistent or problematic (de Groot *et al.*, 2003, p.1715). De Groot *et al.* (2003) reviewed

Table 19.1   Proposed Criteria for Post-Stroke Fatigue. Preprinted from *Archives of Physical Medicine and Rehabilitation*, 11, M. H. De Groot, S. J. Phillips, G. A. Eskes, Fatigue associated with stroke and other neurologic conditions, 1714–20. Copyright (2003), with permission from Elsevier.

The following symptoms should be present every day during a two-week period in the past month:
- Significant fatigue (defined as overwhelming feelings of exhaustion or tiredness), diminished energy or increased need to rest, disproportionate to any recent exhaustion levels, plus any three of the following:
  - Experience of sleep or rest as unrefreshing or nonrestorative
  - Disrupted balance between motivation (preserved) and effectiveness (decreased)
  - Perceived need to struggle to overcome inactivity
  - Difficulty completing or sustaining daily tasks attributed to feeling fatigued
  - Post-exertional malaise lasting several hours
  - Marked concern about feeling fatigued

over 1000 relevant research articles considering neurological patients and identified fatigue as a common complaint. On the basis of their review, they recommended a set of criteria for post-stroke fatigue (Table 19.1). These criteria highlight the level of subjectivity involved in ascertaining the presence of the condition. Despite such criteria, research continues to define fatigue in a variety of ways, often viewing it as on a continuum. On this account, as with pain, estimates of the prevalence of "pathological" fatigue after stroke appear to vary depending on measurement strategies used and the time since stroke.

Ingles, Eskes and Phillips (1999) considered the frequency and outcome of fatigue in 88 stroke patients in a community setting, comparing them to 56 older people also living in the community. Self-report of fatigue, as measured on the Fatigue Impact Scale, was significantly greater in those who had experienced a stroke (68%) than in healthy older people (36%). Of note, 40% of those reporting fatigue in the stroke group considered it one of their worst symptoms. Interestingly, while fatigue was independent of depressive symptoms in this study, depression significantly influenced the reports of the impact of fatigue on functional ability. Glader, Stegmayr and Asplund (2002) excluded stroke patients with depression when they considered fatigue in 3667 patients two years after their stroke. Ten percent of their patients considered they 'always felt tired', and an additional 29.2% 'often tired'. Naess, Nyland, Thomassen, Aarseth and Myhr (2005) considered fatigue an average of six years after ischaemic stroke in 192 younger patients using the Fatigue Impact Scale. Compared with 212 controls, fatigue was much more common at this point after stroke. Winward, Sackley, Metha and Rothwell (2009) found that fatigue was a problem even in those with mild stroke and transient ischaemic attack (TIA). They found that 41 (56%) of a sample of 76 with minor stroke and 22 (29%) of 73 with TIA reported significant levels of fatigue, as assessed on the Chalder scale. Naess *et al.* (2005) found fatigue after stroke was associated with less good functional outcome and depression. Further, in terms of the impact of fatigue, when they controlled for age Glader *et al.* (2002) found fatigue was an independent predictor of having to make a move to institutional care, dependency in primary activities of daily living, and, three years after stroke, a higher mortality rate.

The pathogenesis of post-stroke fatigue remains unclear. Research considering an association with brain stem lesions is contradictory (Ingles *et al.*, 1999; Naess *et al.*, 2005; Staub & Bogousslavsky, 2001) and the proposition that fatigue after stroke may be related to cortisol dysregulation remains to be investigated (McGeough, Pollock, Smith, Dennis, Sharpe, Lewis *et al.*, 2009). Fatigue is common in depression that is also prevalent after stroke (Hackett, Yapa, Parag & Anderson, 2005), and there is support that this is a contributing factor to fatigue after stroke in many, but not all, studies (Ingles *et al.*, 1999; Naess *et al.*, 2005). Clinically, one certainly comes across patients who experience substantial fatigue without depression.

Assessment and treatment of post-stroke pain

Assessment of post-stroke pain

Depression and anxiety are common in those with chronic pain (Gormsen, Rosenberg, Bach & Jensen, 2009). It follows that any assessment of pain should include screening for these disorders, with consideration given to whether treatment for these should be initiated prior to, or contiguous with, treatment for pain. Screening by physicians for medically treatable causes of pain is also warranted, though most patients will be referred to a psychological therapist when medical treatments have not been not successful or cannot be tolerated.

Ideally, any attempt to assess pain after stroke should involve the patient completing a pain diary. This almost always includes information on pain intensity, activity levels and medication intake. Cognitive records detailing attitudes to activity and pain are also useful for those for whom cognitive-behavioural therapy is being considered. Academic studies of pain after stroke have tended to use straightforward visual analogue scales to measure pain intensity, for example 0 to 10 on a 10 cm horizontal line. The 0 anchor point is assigned 'no pain', and the end of the line is 10 equalling 'the worst imaginable pain' (Jonsson *et al.*, 2006; Widar *et al.*, 2002). Other studies have used similar visual analogue scales but with multiple numerical points (Kim, 2003). Clinically, such scales can be useful for outcome evaluation of psychological interventions. More comprehensive measures of pain provide more detail of the pain experience. The McGill Melzack Pain Questionnaire (MMPQ; Melzack, 1975), for instance, is one of the most comprehensive pain assessments. The questionnaire includes adjectival pain descriptors covering sensory, affective and evaluative elements, an assessment of pain variation over time and what relieves or exacerbates the pain, as well as a single measure of pain intensity. The MMPQ is useful for pre- and post treatment, rather than continuous assessment. The short form of the MMPQ (Melzack, 1987), that contains only the adjectival pain descriptors, has been used to assess sensory sequelae of medullary infarction in men (Kim and Choi-Kwon, 1999) and central post-stroke pain in those who have had lenticulo-capsular haemorrhages (Kim, 2003).

For those with significant cognitive deficits and receptive aphasia, a pain intensity scale has recently developed which can be administered with the minimum of verbal production by the stroke patient (Turner-Stokes, Disler, Shaw & Williams, 2008). The Scale of Pain Intensity (SPIN) instrument presents the patient with a sequence of six red circles in a vertical alignment, each with an increasing proportion of shading, from the bottom to the top. The lower anchor point is labelled 'no pain', the upper point 'pain as bad as it could be'. The concurrent validity of the SPIN, with respect to a numeric graphic rating scale, has been considered in a neurorehabilitation setting. Seventy percent of participants preferred the SPIN. Test–retest reliability and responsivity also appeared promising for the scale (Turner-Stokes *et al.*, 2008).

For those with more severe cognitive or communication problems after stroke, using pain measurement systems developed for those with dementia has been suggested (Helfand & Freeman, 2009). The two instruments which appear to have the best support in the dementia population (Herr, Bkoro & Decker, 2006; van Herk, van Dijk, Baar, Tibboel & de Wit, 2007; Zwakhalen, Hamers, Abu-Saad & Berger, 2006a) are the Pain Assessment Checklist for Seniors with Limited Ability to Communicate (PACSLAC; Fuchs-Lacelle & Hadjistavropoulos, 2004) and the Pain Assessment in Advanced Dementia (PAINAD; Warden, Hurley & Volicer, 2003). The PACSLAC is made up of four subscales: the first considers social, personality and mood indicators, such as appearing 'upset'; the second, facial expressions, such as grimacing; the third, activity and body movement, such as guarding a sore area; and the fourth, physiological and other factors, including eating, sleep changes and vocalisations. Sixty items are marked by an observer as present or absent. At this time, there is no recommended cut-off for significant pain on this instrument. The PAINAD assesses pain using five items: breathing independent of vocalisation, negative vocalisation, facial expression, body language and consolability. Each item is scored from 0 to 2. The PAINAD gives a score range from 0 for 'no pain' to 10 for 'severe pain'. The PAINAD's brevity is a considerable advantage in an applied setting, though nurses rated the clinical utility of the PACSLAC slightly higher than that of the PAINAD (Zwakhalen, Hamers & Berger, 2006b). Studies confirming the reliability of and validity of both the PACSLAC and PAINAD for patients with stroke are awaited.

A number of other scales may be useful in the assessment and management of pain after stroke. The Patient Stages of Change Questionnaire (PSCQ; Kerns, Rosenberg, Jamison Caudhill & Haythornthwaite, 1997) asks patients to rate their agreement or disagreement, on a five-point scale, with respect to statements that assess readiness to adopt a self-management approach to their pain. The PSCQ can form the basis for motivational interviewing (Rollnick, Miller & Butler, 2008) to assist a patient's determination to use strategies that will be likely to reduce pain. The Beliefs about Pain Control Questionnaire (BAPCQ; Brown & Nicassio, 1987) uses a similar rating system to the PSCQ to assess the degree to which patients consider their pain is under the control of internal versus external factors. Unfortunately, there is a dearth of evidence on the validity and reliability of both the PSCQ and BAPCQ specific to stroke patients.

Psychological treatment of pain after stroke

The rationale for psychological intervention for chronic pain comes from a number of sources. The most influential of these is the integrative 'gate control' model of pain first proposed by Melzack and Wall (1965). The most important aspect of this theory is that pain is no longer considered a direct response to a stimulus or lesion. It is proposed that neural mechanisms involved in pain perception are affected by psychological factors, including thoughts and emotions, and these augment or reduce the pain.

Treatment of pain by psychological means has a long history (Morley, Eccleston & Williams, 1999). There is good evidence for the benefit of behavioural therapy and cognitive-behavioural therapy (CBT) in most chronic pain disorders (Eccleston, Williams & Morley, 2009), including headache (Andrasik, 2007). Further, it has been recognised that biopsychosocial and cognitive-behavioural therapy approaches typically seen as applicable to nociceptive pain, such as pain caused by tissue injury in the joints, bones, muscles and various internal organs, may be relevant for understanding and treating pain of neuropathic origin (Daniel & van der Merwe, 2006). Unfortunately, there is little empirical support for psychological intervention for pain after stroke. In studies investigating CBT for chronic pain, there may well have been people with stroke, but unfortunately most authors have failed to describe the likely origins of pain experienced by the participants. The research on psychological treatments for nociceptive pain and headache supports the view that psychological interventions are likely to be useful if pain occurs in the context of stroke. Currently there is little support for behaviour therapy or CBT for neuropathic pain of any origin. That said, a single-case study (Edwards, Sudhakar, Scales, Applegate, Webster & Dunn, 2000) described the treatment of a 70-year-old female who experienced central post-stroke pain and ataxic movement of her right arm and hand following a left posterior cerebral artery infarction. Seven years after her stroke, she was treated successfully with a combination of interventions, including progressive muscle relaxation, behavioural pain coping skills training, CBT, forced use therapy and electromyographic biofeedback. Other support for the potential utility of CBT comes from evidence that it is applicable in other neuropathic pain conditions, such as peripheral neuropathic pain in people who have HIV (Evans, Fishman, Spielman & Haley, 2003).

Cognitive-behavioural therapy and behavioural therapy for chronic pain

Behaviour therapy and cognitive-behavioural therapy interventions dominate the literature in terms of the empirical validation of psychological interventions for chronic pain (Morley *et al.*, 2009). These therapies are protocol driven and are often combined with multidisciplinary programmes that consider physical and occupational elements (Eccleston *et al.*, 2009). CBT for chronic pain considers the thoughts and beliefs around the pain, and the consequences of these. Behaviour therapy, separate or within the context of CBT, considers the operant factors involved in pain, that is, what provides pain relief and particularly what might perpetuate the pain. For instance, having tasks done for one might 'reward' pain, as could medication contingent upon pain complaint. Typically CBT for pain, depending on the results of individual initial assessment, focuses on reducing catastrophisation and helplessness about the pain, improving perceptions of controllability and considering the view the patient takes of the impact of the pain on their activity level (White, 2001). The CBT therapist may use activity monitoring to consider the 'boom and bust cycle' that can add to the chronic pain experience. Patients with variable pain will typically use periods in which they experience less pain to maximise their activity levels while avoiding activity when the pain levels are greater for fear of exacerbation. Some patients also may be resigned to the pain, particularly if it has been longstanding. It may be necessary to promote the opportunity for management and control of pain, by providing education about how psychological factors might be exploited to reduce pain. CBT for chronic pain will initially commence with such education. The principal vehicle for this is often the gate control theory of pain. As noted, this presents a model of pain in which pain is not purely determined by physical pathology, but as an experience augmented by fear, anxiety and tension, and conversely reduced by distraction, activity and relaxation: the opening and closing of the 'pain gate'. The patient is also involved in setting realistic goals for the management rather than the eradication of pain. Goals for increasing activity levels despite the pain need to be informed by the physiotherapist and occupational therapist members of the team. They can consider the disability and baseline fitness levels to help design a remedial programme. Typically a gradual build-up in activity levels, avoiding a 'bust' and balanced with regular planned rest breaks, will be enacted until an optimum level of functioning is achieved (McCracken, 2005; White, 2001).

A case example is shown in Table 19.2.

Table 19.2 Case Example of a Patient with Pain

Nigel was an active 63-year-old who sustained a right hemiplegia after a stroke. He initially recovered well, regaining mobility with the use of a stick and only very occasionally using a wheelchair for longer social outings. He was independent in all washing and dressing and other personal activities of daily living. As an inpatient three weeks after his stroke, in the context of high levels of frustration, he received training in an autogenic relaxation strategy and had a brief cognitive therapy intervention from a psychologist, with significant benefit. He was discharged home after a six-week stay on a stroke unit. Three months after his stroke, Nigel was able returned to work in his computer cable supply company, albeit on reduced hours. This was his own business that he ran with his wife. Two weeks after his return to part-time work, Nigel started to experience frequent intense bouts of pain. A stroke physician diagnosed central post-stroke pain. The pain descriptors endorsed on the on the McGill Pain Questionnaire, in respect of this pain included 'searing', 'shooting', 'penetrating' and 'agonizing'. He scored 40 for the 'number of words chosen'. On the Hospital Anxiety and Depression Scale, he scored 4 for depression, below the cut-off for clinical concern, and borderline for anxiety (9). A pain diary identified that the pain was most common in the afternoon between 2 p.m. and 4 p.m. At these times, on a 0–100 scale, Nigel most often recorded the pain intensity as 90, requiring that he cease work. Recording also established that the pain was more likely on a Monday to Friday than at weekends, though it was evident on some Sundays. When he was in pain, Nigel's wife would encourage him to lie down at the back of their workplace, make him a cup of tea and provide analgesia. A number of drugs, the last of which was Gabapentin, had been trialled in an attempt to reduce Nigel's pain. Unfortunately, none of these had been well tolerated. The Gabapentin, for instance, while reducing the pain had made Nigel extremely nauseous.

Nigel was at first sceptical about the involvement of a psychologist for pain control, but having been assisted with frustration reduction on the stroke unit before his discharge, agreed to the consultation. His familiarity with the concept of considering relationship between events, thoughts and affect from his previous contact with a psychologist allowed the assessment to proceed smoothly. Nigel's thoughts when the pain struck included 'here we go again', 'this bloody stroke', 'it's happening again', and 'it's with me for life'. The therapist was able to clarify that 'it's happening again' related to an image Nigel had of the blood vessels in his head blocking and his view this was the origin of his pain. Nigel's activity diaries indicated that while working part-time he was taking few breaks in order that he would get as much as possible done before the 'pain hit'.

Formulation

The physician's diagnosis of central post-stroke pain was supported by the items Nigel endorsed on the MPQ. The activity records identified Nigel's part-time work was 10 a.m. to 4 p.m. with him often losing the last two hours to rest because of the pain. It was clear that he worked 'flat out' from 10 a.m. to 2 p.m. without a break in order to get orders filled before the 'pain time'. He readily admitted this was demanding, with the stress to complete orders added to by the anticipation of the pain to come. Nigel's wife was vigilant to the pain time, responding to his grimaces with urges for him to cease work and lie down. This was followed by a comforting cup of tea and medication (paracetemol). On this basis of the assessment, it appeared that possible augmentors to the pain were time urgency, failure to rest, and that the expression of pain was rewarded by a break, sympathetic reassurance from his wife, a cup of tea and medication.

(Continued)

Table 19.2   (*Continued*)

Intervention

Following sharing of the formulation with Nigel and his wife, the following was determined.

1. Nigel would take a break for lunch from 12.30 to 1.15 p.m., during which he would use the autogenic relaxation exercises in which he had been trained on the stroke unit, but had not practised since.
2. Nigel's expectation of his work output should be revised in light of his stroke. A significant reduction of work was negotiated that was still fiscally viable to the business.
3. Nigel would take responsibility for his own pain management, rather than act in response to prompts from his wife.
4. As part of step 3, Nigel was to reconsider the view he took of his pain, both in anticipation of the pain and when it was present. The cognitive intervention included the following. The view of the pain as 'inevitable and uncontrollable' was changed to 'OK, I do get some pain. That is challenging, but there are some things I can do about it, and I know it eventually passes'.
5. The image of the pain as being the stroke still happening, was countered by 'that's not so, the pain has its origins in my stroke but the stroke is over, the pain is intermittent not an extending stroke. If I relax it will pass more quickly'.

Outcome

Nigel gradually began to apply the strategies. As a consequence, his pain improved markedly. The number of pain descriptors on the McGill Pain Questionnaire reduced from 40 to six, and his pain intensity in the afternoon to a maximum of 50/100. At this point, he could continue with work and completed the hours he had set as his original goal. His score on the HADS anxiety scale reduced from 9 to 5 (below the cut-off for clinical concern). Nigel admitted he used his relaxation at times but found it hard to do this consistently every lunch-time.

Nigel's spouse initially found it hard to allow her husband to take responsibility for his own pain management. Agreeing that the couple have tea together at the start of Nigel's day rather than her ministering him later in response to his pain helped her to consider that she was not 'ignoring him'. Nigel's benefit from pacing and self-talk meant his pain was reduced, making it easier for him to manage. An afternoon break was also negotiated as Nigel extended his work hours. Over time, Nigel became able to work the 10 a.m.–4 p.m. day that was set as his goal. At his 12-month follow-up, Nigel and his wife had had to retire from their business but assured the team this was due to low demand at a time of economic recession, and not on account of his pain.

Assessment and treatment of post-stroke fatigue

Assessing fatigue

As with pain, when patients are referred with fatigue, the psychological therapist will need to ensure that the possible physical contributors that are amenable to change have been considered by a physician. In the case of fatigue, this includes nutritional imbalances (e.g., those related to hydration or electrolytes), systemic disorders (e.g., infection or hypothyroidism) and medication influences (de Groot *et al.*, 2003). Psychological assessment needs to consider not only the fatigue itself but also the primacy of any contributing or concurrent mood disorder. As with pain, treatment of these may take precedence over direct intervention for fatigue. Sleep disturbance likewise may need to be the initial focus of treatment. This includes conditions amenable to medical intervention, such as sleep apnoea that is common after stroke (Parra, Arboix, Bechich, Garcia-Eroles, Montserrat, Lopez *et al.*, 2000), as well as those which might benefit from psychological therapy, such as insomnia (Leppävuori, Pohjasvaara, Vataja, Kaste & Erkinjuntti 2002). Cognitive assessment is also useful for patients complaining of substantial fatigue. Clinical experience is that those with cognitive impairment often complain that their cognition is affected by fatigue (Krupp, Alvarez, La Rocca & Scheinberg, 1988). Fatigue may well affect cognition and vice versa. Cognitive rehabilitation by easing cognitive load might therefore be one component of an intervention for fatigue after stroke.

Lynch, Mead, Greig, Young, Lewis and Sharpe (2007) developed a brief interview system to identify the presence of clinically significant fatigue. Among other things, this system determines whether the fatigue is considered to be a problem or not, how often a patient is fatigued and how long the fatigue lasts. No scale has yet been developed specifically to assess post-stroke fatigue (Glader *et al.*, 2002). Mead, Lynch, Greig, Young, Lewis and Sharpe (2007) considered 52 fatigue scales with respect to face validity, selecting five for closer scrutiny. They found four scales valid and feasible to administer to patients after stroke: the Short Form-36 item Health Survey (SF36v2) vitality component, the Profile of Mood States fatigue subscale, the Multidimensional Fatigue Symptom Inventory general subscale and the Fatigue Assessment Scale (FAS). Of these, the FAS had the poorest internal consistency, though this was not considered a weakness but rather a reflection that it assessed more aspects of fatigue than the other instruments. The FAS (Michielsen, De Vries & Van Heck, 2003) requires patients to rate ten statements, such as 'I get tired quickly', on a one to five scale in terms of how they usually feel, where 1 represents 'never' and 5 'always'. Test–retest reliability, internal reliability and convergent validity for the FAS were acceptable. However, no cut-off for 'significant' fatigue is currently available for this measure.

The Fatigue Severity Scale (FSS) (Krupp, Larocca, Muirnash & Steinberg, 1989) assesses the severity of the fatigue experienced in nine situations with respect to the respondent's last week. Items such as 'fatigue causes frequent problems for me' are rated on a one to seven scale where '1' indicates 'strong disagreement' and '7' 'strong agreement'. Mead *et al.* (2007) rejected the FSS for use with stroke patients on account of a concern that they did not think patients could not separate the effect of their fatigue from their neurological deficit. However, many consider this scale is clinically useful, and it has demonstrated (as a German version) discriminant validity and excellent internal reliability in a sample of 852 neurological patients, including 135 with recent ischemic stroke (Valko, Bassetti, Bloch, Held & Baumann, 2008). A score of 36 or more is considered high on this instrument.

Visual analogue scales (VAS) are also often used to measure fatigue after stroke. A VAS 0–10, for instance, can be used with $0 =$ very alert and $10 =$ extremely fatigued. As is required with assessment of other variables after stroke, any visual analogue scale should probably be presented in a vertical orientation to minimise the impact of any visual neglect. Those with severe cognitive problems or dysphasia may only be able to be assessed with observational measures. Unfortunately, to date there are no observational scales available to assess fatigue in this population.

Treating fatigue after stroke

A recent systematic review (McGeough, Pollock, Smith, Dennis, Sharpe, Lewis *et al.*, 2009) identified three clinical trials that have evaluated interventions for fatigue after stroke. Two of the interventions were drug treatments (Choi-Kwon, Choi, Kwon, Kang & Kim, 2007; Ogden, Mee & Utley, 1998), and one was a multidisciplinary self management programme (Lorig, Ritter, Stewart, Sobel, Brown, Bandura *et al.*, 2001). The self-management trial involved 1140 community dwelling participants and investigated the effect of a chronic disease self-management programme on health status, healthcare utilisation and self-efficacy outcomes. The programme was administered over seven weekly sessions according to a manual and included teaching about exercise, nutrition, use of medication, fatigue and sleep management, communication, managing emotions and decision making. The intervention group performed significantly better than the controls six months post treatment, in terms of measures of health status and hospitalisation. McGeough *et al.* (2009) accessed the data for the 125 participants in the study who had had a stroke. Unfortunately, no significant differences were evident for this subsample. Based on their review, McGeough *et al.* (2009) called for more research to determine the effectiveness of treatments for fatigue after stroke and suggested cognitive interventions may be one way forward. Below is presented a brief overview of this approach and a case study illustration. Clinicians are already administering such interventions, although empirical support is awaited.

Cognitive-behavioural therapy for fatigue after stroke

Cognitive-behavioural therapy for fatigue management after stroke has its origins in the view that excessive avoidance and resting behaviour and all-or-nothing behaviour contribute to fatigue. Fatigue is added to by a patient's inactivity. When people have 'a good day', they work to excess to take advantage

Table 19.3 Case Example of a Patient with Fatigue

Harold was a 72-year-old man with mild cognitive problems, including executive deficits, after a stroke. He also had mild dysphasia and a right hemiplegia. At the time of the referral, he was an inpatient on a stroke unit and had progressed to walking with a frame with stand-by assistance. Physiotherapy staff referred him to the psychologist because they considered he had the potential to eventually walk with a stick, but his progress was being hampered by verbal aggression, irritability and occasional refusal of treatment. Staff monitoring identified that the aggression and irritability mainly occurred in the afternoons. Harold was usually cooperative in the morning even though there was concern within the session that he was valuing speed of performance over quality. The second physiotherapy session of the day was the one that he intermittently declined, on occasions quite rudely. Harold was screened for depression with the Brief Assessment Schedule Depression Cards (BASDEC) and scored well below the cut-off for depression. It was noted, however, that he endorsed the item 'I am not sleeping well', and enquiry confirmed frequent night waking and difficulty returning to sleep because Harold found it 'difficult to get comfortable'. The rapid responding in therapy appeared consistent with executive deficits, though Harold's premorbid hard-driving personality might also have contributed. The interview also established that following the morning session of therapy, Harold would continue to exercise in his room, despite being advised against this because of the absence of supervision and concerns about fatigue. Harold admitted to being washed out, tired and irritable in the afternoon and expressed some regret as to the way he had responded to staff on these occasions. On the Fatigue Severity Scale, Harold scored 51, well above the cut-off for significant fatigue.

Formulation

It appeared that fatigue was a major issue for Harold, contributing to his inability to progress in rehabilitation as well as he might. The fatigue had arisen following his stroke but was added to by a number of other influences. Harold had mild impairment of executive abilities on account of his stroke. Perseveration, aggression and disinhibition were all suggestive of executive function disorder (Wilson *et al.*, 1996). In the context of his hard-driven personality, these had probably contributed to his rapid responding in physiotherapy and his persisting in exercises after sessions, despite directions not to do this by staff. In addition Harold's not sleeping well added to his vulnerability to fatigue. It was also apparent that Harold's literal interpretation of the '24-hour approach to rehabilitation' proffered by the unit meant he was not taking rest as advised.

Intervention

The formulation was fed back to Harold verbally and in written form, to support his understanding. A treatment plan was agreed that included relaxation to aid return to sleep at night along with rest breaks during the morning and afternoon. These involved resting in a chair; day sleep was discouraged. Harold's acceptance of the plan required some work by the psychologist. Harold considered he must 'constantly' keep working to get optimum recovery from his stroke. This view was disputed by considering with him the advice of experienced therapists that he should include rest breaks. While this was partially useful, it was Harold himself recognising that his approach was not working, to the extent that at times he could not attend afternoon therapy sessions, which saw his acceptance of the plans.

(Continued)

Table 19.3   (*Continued*)

Outcome

With the aid of agreed prompts from staff, Harold took regular rest breaks. He also improved his sleep by using a brief relaxation exercise when he woke. Over the course of the intervention, this same technique was applied in therapy to allow him to slow his responses and to focus on quality over speed. Monitoring by staff indicated a reduction in the number of physiotherapy sessions declined by Harold and in the number of instances of verbal disinhibition in the afternoons. After two weeks, a repeat FSS identified a significant decline in fatigue, from a score 51 to 30. After four weeks, Harold was discharged home with support from the stroke team for early discharge. Handover on fatigue management was provided to the team. He had some significant problems with fatigue in the first ten days of being home, but with the help of community staff, strategies which were found useful at the hospital were applied and fatigue was again reduced.

---

of this with severe consequences. This matches the 'boom and bust cycle' briefly described earlier for chronic pain. A patient who has fatigue after stroke may not attempt to improve their activity for fear that it will exacerbate the fatigue. A prolonged period of inactivity can lead to concerns that they are not recovering. On such a basis, a burst of activity can result in an excessive response in terms of fatigue. CBT for chronic fatigue after stroke borrows heavily from treatments developed and found successful in the treatment of chronic fatigue syndrome. It focuses on patterns of inactivity that maintain fatigue and the thinking that contributes to these. A planned programme of graded activity and rest is developed, usually in collaboration with physical and occupational therapists. Based on a team assessment, realistic goals are established with an emphasis on achieving these gradually and consistently (Burgess & Chalder, 2005). A case example is shown in Table 19.3.

Conclusions

Pain and fatigue are common after stroke and can have a significant effect on recovery and quality of life. The opportunity to intervene psychologically for these problems has only recently been realised. The challenge for the future is to improve the evidence base to support the work being undertaken by psychologists and also to ensure the work undertaken by other therapists is psychologically informed.

Section 4

Social Dimensions of Stroke

Chapter 20

Carers of Stroke Survivors

Why consider stroke carers separately?

Over the past five decades, much attention has been devoted to understanding caring in a range of health conditions: physical, neurological and psychological. Every illness presents its own unique and specific challenges for carers. Some conditions, such as dementias, Parkinson's disease and motor neurone disease, all share neurological features with stroke. But these conditions do not have a sudden and unexpected onset, and have a declining course rather than an improving one. Other cardiovascular conditions, such as heart attack, may have sudden onset and an improving course in many cases, but do not generally have extensive neurological consequences. Sudden onset is important, in that carers do not have opportunity to prepare for their roles, and neurological impairments have psychological consequences that impact on cognition, adjustment, personality, relationships and family functioning in a more direct way than physical illnesses. Traumatic brain injury shares many features with stroke, but shows different demographic patterns, requires different medical treatments, and does not carry the same increased risk of further similar events. For these reasons, it is important to study stroke carers as a group (Low, Payne & Roderick, 1999).

It would be informative to compare the experiences and outcomes of carers from different conditions, if only to identify the importance of the factors discussed above. However, many studies are condition specific, and those that include carers of more than one condition normally do so to boost numbers, and are rarely designed specifically to make comparisons across conditions. There have been exceptions, but results often highlight global, high-order factors that are common across conditions, such as cognition, and do not identify significant concerns of carers for people with specific conditions (Thommessen, Aarsland, Braekhus, Oksengaard, Engedal & Laake, 2002).

Psychological Management of Stroke, First Edition. Nadina B. Lincoln, Ian I. Kneebone, Jamie A.B. Macniven and Reg C. Morris.
© 2012 John Wiley & Sons, Ltd. Published 2012 by John Wiley & Sons, Ltd.

Definitions

The UK government defines a 'carer' as 'someone who looks after and supports a friend, relative or neighbour who could not manage without their help. This could be due to age, physical or mental illness or disability' (Directgov, 2009). People, professionals and others, who provide care as part of their employment or for payment, are specifically excluded. The terms 'informal carers' and 'family carers' have also been used to describe this group of people, but in this chapter the term 'carer' is preferred for its simplicity, to avoid the additional connotations carried by the term 'informal' and to recognise that some carers are not family members. Caring activities and caring behaviour are less well defined than 'carer', and a plethora of definitions are found in the literature (McCance, McKenna & Boore, 1999). A common definition of caring as 'an activity that a carer carries out for, or on behalf of, someone who is not themselves able to perform the activity' begs the question of whether the caring activity actually benefits the recipient, and allows for a wide range of interpretations. For example, how should we account for time spent with the survivor providing companionship, being 'on call' but not actively caring, and time sharing a confining and life-limiting existence? Should caring include mutually beneficial activities, such as cooking a shared meal or going out together to see a film? There will inevitably be important subjective differences in what is considered as a caring activity, and surveys that allow the carer to decide what constitutes caring may lead to widely differing findings. A pragmatic strategy is to list a number of common caring activities, and then to allow carers to specify the number of hours spent on each. At the same time carers can be given space to describe other activities that they construe as caring, and these can subsequently be considered for inclusion.

Demographic factors

Over 80% of previously independent stroke survivors are discharged home (Royal College of Physicians, 2007; Rudd, Hoffman, Irwin, Lowe & Pearson, 2005) and between 40% and 50% require the assistance of unpaid carers, usually family members, to live independently in the community (Wilkinson, Wolfe, Warburton, Rudd, Howard, Ross-Russell et al., 1997). The England and Wales census in 2001, for the first time asked whether people provided unpaid care for a family member or friend and for how many hours. The census did not ask the reason that the person needed care, so unfortunately there are no data specific to stroke. However, the results include stroke carers and are relevant to their situation. There were 5.2 million carers in England and Wales (one in ten of the population), including over 3.9 million of working age; 3.56 million (68%) of carers provided care for up to 19 hours a week, 0.57 million (11%) for 20 to 49 hours and 1.09 million (21%) for 50 or more hours per week. Many of those providing care also did paid work, and 1.6 million carers held full-time jobs.

British carers were estimated to have saved the UK exchequer £87 billion each year at 2009 values (Buckner & Yeandle, 2007), and their economic value was recognised by the Department of Health (2006). An equivalent estimate for the United States (Arno, Levine & Memmott, 1999) set the saving at $196 billion for 1996. The 2001 UK census data (Office for National Statistics, 2009) demonstrated that, of those identifying themselves as carers, 58% were women and 42% were men. However, the gender ratio varied for specific caring roles so that, for physical care and taking the person out, the proportions of men and women were about equal, whereas women provided more personal care, supervision and company than men. Population studies of carers across a range of health conditions indicated that around 55% were spouses and around 20% were offspring (Hirst, 2002), leaving the other 25% to be filled by friends and other relatives. There are few reliable population statistics specifically for stroke carers, but one study in Australia examined primary carers from a systematically compiled database and found that 42% were spouses and 40% offspring, with friends and other relatives making up the remainder (Dewey, Thrift, Mihalopoulos, Carter, Macdonell, McNeil *et al.*, 2002). Anderson, Linto and Stewart-Wynne (1995), also in Australia, found that 59% of carers were spouses, 32% offspring and 9% other relatives; females carers greatly outnumbered males (wives 49%, husbands 10%, daughters 26% and sons 6%). It is not uncommon for young children to provide care. The 2001 Census indicated there were 175,000 children and young people under 18 in the United Kingdom providing care to family, friends or neighbours. The majority provided care for up to 19 hours per week, but in England 22,000 (16%) of young carers were caring for between 20 and 50 or more hours per week. Young carers have been studied by Dearden and Becker 1998; 2004) across a range of conditions in the United Kingdom and by van de Port, Visser-Meily, Post and Lindeman (2007) for stroke in the Netherlands. Ethnicity is an important factor in childhood caring (see chapter 21), but there are no demographic data that provide precise estimates of rates of child carers of stroke survivors. Patterns of caring are likely to be culture and age dependent.

Studies of stroke carers across all age groups have included mainly spouses, about 70% on average (Low *et al.*, 1999; Wade, Legh-Smith & Hewer, 1986). The proportion of spouses in research studies is greater than expected based on the estimates produced by Dewey *et al.* (2002) and Anderson *et al.* (1995), and there may be inclusion bias due to the greater accessibility of spousal carers than offspring carers, because the latter are more likely to have employment or childcare responsibilities that preclude participation in research.

> Our son helps lift her on the bed and will change her and all sorts. I guess it was a big adjustment for him . . . . I feel like he hasn't had a life as such . . . and my other son comes up almost every night. And I do feel a bit guilty about that. (Husband of survivor)

Legal and policy framework

In the United Kingdom, the Carers (Recognition of Services) Act 1995 (Her Majesty's Government, 1995) and the Carers and Disabled Children Act 2000 (Her Majesty's Government, 2000), stipulate that carers aged 16 or over who provide a regular and substantial amount of care for a disabled person have the legal right to an assessment of their needs as a carer. The legal rights of carers were further strengthened by the Carers' (Equal Opportunities) Act 2004 (Her Majesty's Government, 2004) which extended and amended existing legislation by:

- placing a duty on local authorities to ensure that all carers know that they are entitled to an assessment of their needs,
- placing a duty on councils to consider a carers' outside interests (work, study or leisure) when carrying out an assessment,
- promoting better joint working between councils and the health service to ensure support for carers is delivered in a coherent manner.

Over the past decades, the UK government has developed successive policy guidelines for the support and involvement of carers. For example, 'Caring about Carers' (Department of Health, 1999) provided for better information resources, better carer support, enhanced care for carers and improved financial support. This policy was reviewed in 2007 as part of the 'New Deal for Carers' (Hansard, 2007), and a new policy was produced, 'Carers at the Heart of 21st-Century Families and Communities' (Department of Health, 2008). This set out a ten-year plan to provide individualised, tailored support for carers that will enable them to balance caring with their own needs and lives. The new plan allocated an additional £255 million in total with more funding (£150 million) for respite care, and promised 1. improved support and services for carers through telephone help-lines, 2. expert carer programmes with training and instruction, 3. help in maintaining employment alongside caring and 4. special provision to protect children and young people who provide care from unreasonable burden (see chapter 21, 'Strokes in Young People'). Greenwood, Mackenzie and Harris (2008a) considered this package of proposals in the light of carers' actual wishes and needs revealed through surveys (Carers UK, 2008). They concluded that emergency respite care and individualised information that matched carers' diverse needs and preferences were priorities for carers. With regard to the recommendation of the Department of Health (2008), they noted the lack of conclusive evidence for the effectiveness of help-lines and expert carer schemes, and pointed out that these provisions did not clearly address stroke carers' priorities, and may attract limited uptake. A further barrier to effective support for carers is that carer assessment is not universally applied; the 2008 Sentinel Stroke Audit revealed that 24% of carers did not receive a separate needs assessment (Royal College of Physicians, 2009), and it has also been reported that 40–60% of carers' benefits were unclaimed (Carers UK, 2006). Despite the advent of new approaches to carers' assessment across England, Wales and Scotland between 2001 and 2002, there remain obstacles to full and effective implementation, such as insufficient staff awareness and training, a lack of effective partnership working and the inefficient sharing of information. Even when assessments are completed, their quality is variable (Seddon, Robinson, Reeves, Tommis, Woods & Russell, 2007; Seddon, Robinson & Perry, 2010).

Since April 2007 working-aged people in the United Kingdom caring for an adult who is a relative, or who lives at the same address, also have a statutory right to ask employers for flexible working under the Work and Families Act, 2006 (Her Majesty's Government, 2006). They also have the right to take (unpaid) time off work for dependants in cases of emergency. Carers may also receive financial benefits; carers' allowance and direct payments to support their caring role, and, if they are unable to work, pension protection and a carer premium are added to their income support. In some cases community support grants may also be available, and carers can also benefit from financial assistance provided to the stroke survivor, such as disability living allowance and attendance allowance. However, many of these financial benefits are income related, and serve only as a safety net for those with very low incomes rather than benefiting the majority.

> There is nothing in xxxshire for people like John . . . . And that made it very, very hard. We've got an elderly person's home down the road that takes respite, but they are so ill that there would be no communication at all. (Wife of survivor)

The Mental Capacity Acts for the United Kingdom home countries have further strengthened the role of carers and others concerned with the welfare of survivors. They require health and social care providers to consult with carers (under most circumstances) if the survivor is unable to make decisions for themselves. There is also a new 'lasting power of attorney' in England and Wales that gives an individual, or individuals, chosen in advance by the survivor, the power to act as a surrogate decision maker if they should lose the capacity to make a decision for themselves.

Most national clinical guidelines for stroke, including those for the United Kingdom (Royal College of Physicians, 2008a), make stipulations as to the assessment and support of carers, but Van Heugten, Visser-Meily, Post and Lindeman (2006) noted that the focus of guidelines is primarily upon care of the patient. Consequently this Dutch group conducted a systematic literature search for evidence relevant to stroke carers and convened a panel of experts who used the Delphi technique to agree upon 13 areas and 29 guidelines that form the basis of a comprehensive set of carer guidelines. Since these are the only guidelines available for stroke carers, they are reprinted in Table 20.1. Notable aspects of the recommendations are early assessment of carers at risk, formal

Table 20.1   Dutch Clinical Practice Guidelines for Care of Carers. (Reproduced with permission from van Heugten C., Visser-Meily A., Post M., & Lindeman E. 2006. Care for carers of stroke patients: evidence-based clinical practice guidelines. *Journal of Rehabilitation Medicine*, 38, 153–8.)

LEVELS OF EVIDENCE

Level 1 (strong evidence) supported by at least two independent studies, such as meta-analyses or high-quality randomized controlled trials.

Level 2 (moderate evidence) supported by at least two independent studies, such as randomized controlled trials or other studies comparing groups of patients.

Level 3 (limited evidence) supported by research other than level 1 or 2 (i.e. cohort studies, descriptive studies, control groups unknown, no blinded outcome assessment).

Level 4 (consensus), supported by expert opinion.

CLINICAL PRACTICE GUIDELINES

1.1. Partners at risk
Psychosocial burden in the long term can be predicted early in the rehabilitation process. Carers at risk of burden in the long term should be detected as early as possible and supported accordingly. At the start of the rehabilitation, carers at risk of high perceived burden are those with a depressed mood, a passive coping style and living with a stroke patient with severe physical and/or cognitive impairments (level 3).

1.2. Assessment of carer burden
A consultation should always be offered to patient and carer after discharge home. During this contact, carer strain should be measured with a standardized instrument. The instrument can be sent to the carer beforehand (level 4).

Carer strain can be measured adequately with a burden scale. The Caregiver Strain Index (CSI) is most often used and preferable in terms of time and effort. In addition, the CSI has a cut-off point (level 2).

1.3. Interventions for carers
Counselling, aimed at active problem-solving behaviour and support seeking behaviour of the carer, has a positive effect on the mood and emotional well-being of the carer and on his or her capacity to maintain social support (level 2). This effect can be found in all phases after stroke.

Carers with high levels of burden (on the basis of a standardized measure) or with a higher risk of developing burden (on the basis of predictors) should receive adequate professional care, such as counselling, or partner support groups (level 4).

After discharge there should be contact with the carer at predetermined moments, such as 1, 4, 6 and 12 months post-discharge. During these contacts the problems and needs of the carer should be discussed. Professionals should define who will initiate this contact (level 4).

1.4. Information provision and education
Carers of stroke patients should be given information about the stroke in combination with individual education. In this way carers gain more knowledge about the nature of the disease and the related problems (level 2).

Several years after the stroke carers may still have questions, which can change during the process from information on the stroke itself to information on cognitive and behavioural consequences. Information should be unequivocal, should be repeated more than once, and should be tuned to the demands of the individual carers (level 3).

Table 20.1 (*Continued*)

Current written information materials on stroke and its consequences are being read and rated positively by the carers. These materials should therefore be distributed or recommended in all phases after the stroke; websites can also be recommended as sources of information (level 3).

During the rehabilitation and chronic phase, information should be given about expected changes, such as financial changes and changes in family roles (level 4).

1.5. Differences in complaints between patients and carers
Patients and carers often do not agree about the consequences of the stroke when asked separately. This concerns mainly the less visible consequences, such as cognitive or emotional and behavioural problems. Healthcare professionals should be alert to these differences, especially during the chronic phase after stroke, because these differences can lead to family problems. When professionals are asked to intervene, it is important to assess the complaints of the patients and their carers separately (level 3).

1.6. Depression
Carers of stroke patients can become depressed and healthcare professionals should be alert to these problems during rehabilitation but also in the long term. Depression of carers is related to the degree of disabilities of the patient and the burden of the carer. Severe depression should be treated with education or information provision about the symptoms, time course and self management techniques, medication and support by the general practitioner (level 3).

1.7. Primary care
Professionals in primary care should keep in contact with the carers in all phases after stroke, because there is evidence that carers have specific needs (level 3).

Professionals should be alert to increase in burden in the chronic phase after stroke because the support from the environment can decrease and the health status of both patient and carer can decrease as well (level 4).

1.8. Involvement of carers in the rehabilitation process
Carers should be involved actively in the rehabilitation process because there is evidence that through active involvement satisfaction with care will increase. Active involvement can be realized by carers attending therapy sessions or organizing carer support groups (level 3). When stroke patients visit their own home at the weekends, these visits should be evaluated with both the patient and the carer; the carer may have questions or problems of his or her own (level 4).

During inpatient rehabilitation, a carer support group should be organized (level 3).

During inpatient rehabilitation, the multidisciplinary team should discuss which team members will support the family of the patient with stroke (level 3).

1.9. Long-term consequences
Even after 1 year post-stroke, carer strain should be reassessed regularly, because the strength and the supporting power of the carer can diminish, despite a stable status of the patient. Cognitive consequences can become more pronounced in daily life in the long term, which increases burden. In addition, disappointment about lack of recovery and lasting disabilities can influence the level of burden (level 3).

(*Continued*)

Table 20.1   (*Continued*)

1.10. Fellow sufferers
Carers in need of extra support should be recommended to join carer support groups of
fellow sufferers because there is evidence that these carers are more satisfied and
experience higher feelings of support (level 3).

1.11. Young children of stroke patients
The development of young children can be influenced negatively by the possible changes
in the family situation after stroke. Children should therefore be supported actively in
order to live with the lasting consequences of the stroke of the parent (level 3).

   Supporting children of stroke patients should be elaborated in a protocol and should
be offered with the consent of the parents. In the protocol should be written who, when
and how support to the children will be offered (level 4).

   Both the patient and the healthy parent should be supported in the changes within the
family and the role as parent. This should be a regular theme in the support of the
individual carer and can be a topic of the carer support group (level 3).

1.12. Sexuality and intimacy
Patients and spouses are often not satisfied with their sexual functioning after stroke;
sexuality and intimacy should therefore be discussed with (married) couples (level 3).

   Changes in sexual functioning should be discussed with patients and spouses at different
moments during the rehabilitation process, such as at discharge and at follow up.
Professional support should be offered when necessary. The multidisciplinary team should
discuss explicitly which members of the team will support the (married) couple (level 4).

   Sexuality and intimacy should be discussed during carer support groups. Information
should be given about the nature and causes of these changes (level 4).

1.13. Societal involvement
Respite care should be offered to relieve the carer and to create opportunities for societal
involvement of the carer (level 4).

---

assessment of carer strain and burden, regular monitoring of carers after
discharge, long-term assessment and support, involvement of carers in rehabilitation, encouragement to network with other carers and support for young
children of stroke patients.

   In addition to health services and local authorities, there are also third sector
charitable organisations which focus on carers. supporting research and development, campaigning for carers and acting as information exchanges (Carers UK
and The Princess Royal Trust for Carers). The influence of surveys carried out by
such groups upon the development of the recent carers' policy attests to their
importance.

Models and processes of caring

Survivors are affected by the care offered by carers, and carers themselves are in
turn affected by support from other family members, professionals and services.
The models discussed below are often applied separately to explain the outcomes
for survivors or carers. But there is much overlap, and, for example, Lazarus and

Folkman's (1984) transactional model of stress, which is commonly applied to carers, is equally applicable to survivors. The importance of having a conceptual framework to underpin knowledge and inform the development of complex interventions has been underlined in Medical Research Council guidance (Medical Research Council, 2008). However, caring is complex and multifaceted, and consequently several kinds of models may be relevant.

Social contact and social support

Caring inevitably entails social contact and elements of social support, and some of the benefits of caring may stem from these sources. There is ample evidence that social contact is beneficial. House, Landis and Umberson (1988) reviewed six large prospective studies and concluded that mortality is higher in more socially isolated people. Uchino (2006) reviewed studies of the relationship between social support and physiological functions and concluded that it is beneficial for cardiovascular, neuroendocrine and immune functions. The suggestion that biological functions may be affected by social contact is bolstered by animal studies. For example, Karelina, Norman, Zhang, Morris, Peng and DeVries (2009) studied male mice with surgically induced strokes and found that socially isolated male mice had shorter survival and more neuronal damage than those housed with a female. Two studies (Glass, Matchar, Belyea & Feussner, 1993; Tsouna-Hadjis, Vemmos, Zakopoulos & Stamatelopoulos, 2000) have demonstrated the benefits of social support in people with stroke. Glass *et al.* (1993) conducted a prospective study with measurements at one, three and six months after stroke and found that survivors with greater social support had better functional outcomes in terms of activities of daily living. The effect of social support was most pronounced for survivors with more severe strokes, and this group scored 65% higher on a scale of activities of daily living than those with the least social support. Tsouna-Hadjis *et al.* (2000) undertook a similar study using the same measurement periods, but included measures of depression and social involvement as well as functioning, and also ensured that measurements were made 'blind' to level of social support. They found that patients with more social support were less depressed, were more socially involved, and had better functioning than those with less social support. As in the study by Glass *et al.* (1993), more severely affected survivors showed greater benefit than those with milder strokes, but only with regard to functioning.

Social support implies much more than merely the provision of practical or instrument caregiving, and Wills and Shinar (2000) suggested the following may be implicated:

- Emotional support (esteem, confidant, intimacy)
- Instrumental support (practical care)
- Informational support (advice, guidance)
- Companionship (socialising, belonging)
- Validation (feedback, social comparison)

The social contact provided by supporters may have a *direct* effect on the health and well-being of the recipient. Specific pathways for this direct action include social influence and information that promote health-enhancing behaviours, such as a healthy diet and treatment adherence, as well as practical care. Information may also reduce uncertainty and anxiety and protect from psychological dysfunction. The direct effects of care benefit all recipients, but there may also be *indirect* effects that benefit only those experiencing stress. The buffering or moderator-mediator model holds that supporters influence health and well-being by limiting or removing the impact of stressors, such as by influencing the recipient's susceptibility or reactivity. This may occur through promoting a 'benign' appraisal of stressors (i.e. the appraisal that there are sufficient resources to meet demands), or through perceived or received social support that ameliorates the emotional responses or negative cognitions occurring as a consequence of stress (Thoits, 1986). This buffering effect of support is entirely commensurate with Lazarus and Folkman's (1984) transactional model of coping (described below), in which support and available resources affect secondary appraisal and this in turn affects coping and outcome. Cohen and Willis (1985) reviewed the literature on health maintenance and well-being and concluded that both buffering and direct effects occur, and that a person's perception of the availability of social support is crucial in buffering. These findings may not, however, hold for all conditions. Stroebe, Zech, Stroebe and Abakoumkin (2005) found evidence for a direct effect of social support, but no evidence for buffering effects in a large-scale study of depression in bereaved women. There is evidence that perceived, as well as actual, social support is linked to coping effectiveness in patients and in carers (Bennett, 1993; Hartke & King, 2003). It is important to distinguish between perceived and received support: perceived support has been shown to be linked with better functioning across a range of conditions, but paradoxically received, or practical, support is sometimes associated with greater impairment (Wills & Shinar, 2000). An obvious explanation for this finding is that more impaired people need and receive greater amounts of practical support. However, this may not be the only factor; Palmer and Glass (2003) proposed that too much practical support may be related to over-protection and an over-investment in caring by the carer that inhibits and restricts the independent functioning of the survivor.

Lazarus' and Folkman's transactional model

Caring is often understood in terms of stress coping theory, most commonly the theory of Lazarus and Folkman (1984). The majority of studies of interventions for carers reviewed by Brereton, Carroll and Barnston (2007) drew upon this theory, and it is also described in Morrison's (1999) review. A primary tenet of the model is that challenging events, such as the demands of caring, are the occasion for appraisal. The outcome of such appraisal may be the experience of stress which may in turn engender attempts to reduce or manage the stress which are referred to as 'coping'. This theory is transactional; the person and the environment are viewed as being in a dynamic, mutually reciprocal, bidirectional relationship. Coping is defined as a 'person's cognitive and behavioural efforts to manage (reduce, minimize, master, or tolerate) the internal and external demands of the person-environment transaction that is appraised as taxing or exceeding the person's resources' (Folkman, Lazarus, Gruen & De Longis, 1986). Coping stems from a dynamic interaction of the context, the person and the stressor itself. Some general aspects of coping may be dispositional traits, such as a tendency to investigate threats and obtain information, versus the tendency to avoid such potentially disturbing information by denial or distraction. These distinct styles have been referred to as 'monitoring versus blunting' by Miller (1987). However, most approaches to coping see it as primarily determined by particular contexts, events and the available resources, rather than by individual traits.

Figure 20.1 depicts the general framework of coping theory based on the work of Lazarus and Folkman (1984) and Pearlin, Mullan, Semple and Skaff (1990). The stressor, which may arise from any aspect of the carers' situation, including the demands and needs of the survivor, is evaluated by appraisal processes. The processes by which this occurs have been articulated by Lazarus (1993) and Smith and Lazarus (1993). The 'primary cognitive appraisal' process determines the stressor's potential psychological impact by assessing its relevance to the person and their goals, sense of self and self-esteem. A 'secondary appraisal' subsequently considers what, if anything, can be done to prevent negative outcomes or to increase well-being. Consideration of available resources and assets enter into the secondary appraisal, and several assessments are made; there is an assessment of whether the circumstances were caused by the person themselves or by an external agent; the potential for changing the situation by practical action is determined, and also the person's capacity to deal with the emotions aroused; then there is an assessment of the extent to which the situation is amenable to change. Following secondary appraisal,

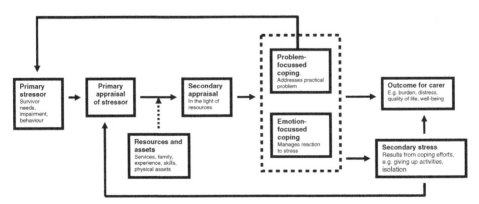

Figure 20.1   A model of stress and coping. Based on Lazarus and Folkman (1984).

coping efforts of two kinds may be initiated. The first kind of coping, 'problem-focussed coping', is aimed at addressing practical problems and could encompass actions for meeting the survivor's needs, obtaining information about how to access services or finding ways to minimise difficult behaviour. The second kind of coping, 'emotion-focussed coping', is used to manage the carers' own reactions to stressors and usually involves self-care activities such as taking time out, seeking support for one's self and religious worship. Finally, 'secondary stressors' may emerge from engagement in coping efforts and could, for example, stem from loss of activities and social contact and the resulting changes to self-image and self-esteem.

This model is a useful heuristic for developing supportive and therapeutic interventions since it identifies significant, distinct processes that may occur as a consequence of the caring role, and, above all, it highlights the importance of individual appraisal in determining the psychological outcome for the carer. It helps those working with carers to appreciate the pathways by which a carer arrived at their current situation and the kinds of influences that may shape their experience and behaviour. It can enable healthcare professionals to plan and implement individual, *ad hoc*, interventions, as well as informing service planners about what to consider when developing standardised, systematic interventions to support carers. But its recursive, dynamic nature renders measurement of key processes and outcomes complex. Moreover, Lazarus's model is by no means comprehensive, it has primarily spawned research focused on 'dis-ease', the negative, stressful, aspects of caring, and has been characterised as 'patho-logising' caring (Brereton *et al.*, 2007). There has been little attention to the positive effects of mild stress, and the positive benefits of caring have been largely ignored. While the model is useful as a means of understanding why and how carers react to challenges, it does not address the fundamental psychological processes that motivate people to adopt and to sustain caring roles in the first place. A model that provides a comprehensive account of caring behaviour, embracing motivation as well as adaptation to adverse circumstances, is needed.

The theory of planned behaviour

Ajzen's (1985) theory of planned behaviour was originally designed to explain the health-related behaviours of individuals, for example in terms of avoiding risks and adopting healthy habits. It has more recently been applied to the helping behaviour of professional care staff, including those in stroke services (Hart & Morris, 2008). According to the theory of planned behaviour (Figure 20.2), behaviour is determined by intention, which is itself determined by attitudes (positive or negative evaluations) towards the behaviour, subjective norm (percep-tions of others' views about the behaviour) and perceived behavioural control (beliefs about personal control over the behaviour). Each of these components is in turn determined. Attitudes stem from beliefs about outcomes of the behaviour and

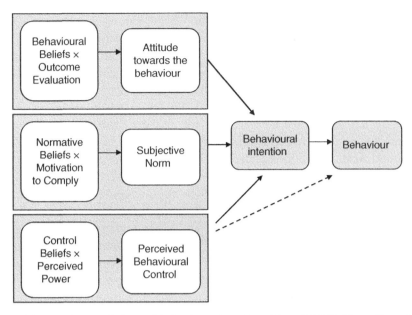

Figure 20.2 Theory of planned behaviour. Based on Ajzen (1985). From Hart, S., & Morris, R. (2008). Screening for depression after stroke: an exploration of professionals' compliance with guidelines. *Clinical Rehabilitation*, 22(1), 60–70.

evaluations of these outcomes. Subjective norm depends on perception of others' views of the behaviour and strength of the desire to comply with others. Perceived behavioural control is determined by the evaluation of factors that facilitate or hinder the behaviour and perceptions of the power of these factors. There is good empirical support for the theory as a predictor of intention and behaviour, and for the predictive power its major constructs, although there have been some modifications to the theory, one of which is the inclusion of moral norms as well as subjective norms (Armitage & Conner, 2001). Applied to caring, the theory of planned behaviour highlights particular aspects of individuals' belief systems that influence the decision about whether to become a carer. It may help to explain why some people readily adopt caring roles, while others eschew any involvement in caring. For example, caring is likely to occur when people possess a combination of attitudes and beliefs incorporating; a positive attitude to caring, based on the belief that carers can improve the well-being of a survivor; the perception that respected family members, or society in general, expect people to become carers, and a belief in their ability, given appropriate resources and support, to provide the necessary care. This analysis received some support from research into carer motivation which demonstrated that intrinsic motivation, typified by positive attitudes to providing care, resistance to other modes of care such as placement, a principled belief in caring and a belief in one's self as a carer, were all associated with greater satisfaction with caring (Lyonette & Yardley, 2003). However, this study also showed that some aspects of subjective norm, notably others' expectations and sense of duty, were negatively associated with satisfaction and positively related to stress.

The strength of the theory of planned behaviour is that its three major components (attitude, subjective norm and perceived behaviour control) identify possible targets for interventions that may facilitate positive change in intention and behaviour. This has the potential to inform the development of interventions to support carers and enhance and sustain the commitment to caring. Interventions based on the theory of planned behaviour are particularly applicable to individuals who are not intrinsically motivated at the outset (Hardeman, Johnston, Johnston, Bonetti, Wareham & Kinmonth, 2002). Elliott and Armitage (2009) identified 34 studies in which the components of the theory of planned behaviour were targeted in interventions designed to promote behaviour change. Eighteen of the studies reported changes in intention, and 15 found significant change in behaviour. Many of these studies had methodological limitations, but Elliott and Armitage's rigorously controlled study of driving behaviour found good evidence for change in reported behaviour. However, not all the model's components showed change, and the translation of the model's components into effective interventions is not straightforward, so the approach will require refinement and adaptation if it is to be applied to carers (Morrison & Bennett, 2009, pp.139–47).

Benefits of family care for survivors

In an extensive review of the evidence, Kwakkel, Wagenaar, Kollen and Lankhorst (1996) concluded that social and family support is one of the most prominent and reliable factors contributing to positive functional recovery after stroke. Palmer and Glass (2003) reviewed the evidence for the beneficial effects of families and carers of stroke survivors across a number of domains and found several studies demonstrating benefits; both the functioning and the psychological state of survivors were improved by the availability of support from family members (Glass *et al.*, 1993; Kriegsman, VanEijk, Penninx, Deeg & Boeke, 1997; Morris, Robinson, Raphael & Bishop, 1991). They also noted that the likelihood of rehospitalisation and institutionalization decreased, and treatment adherence increased, if effective social and family support were available. Similarly, Meijer, van Limbeek, Kriek, Ihnenfeldt, Vermeulen and de Haan (2004) found that marital status and social support were important predictors of discharge to home or placement. The involvement of family carers in treatment and rehabilitation is also a characteristic of effective stroke services, impacting on a number of performance and outcome measures (Stroke Unit Trialists' Collaboration, 1997).

Factors affecting the outcome of care for survivors

Palmer and Glass (2003) concluded that, while the availability of care by itself is beneficial, the quality and nature of care are also important. They identified the perception of the availability of emotional support as a crucial element that was frequently associated with improved progress in rehabilitation and better recovery. They found studies demonstrating that survivors' functional recovery and psychosocial state (including mood and cognitive functioning) were related to the quality of family functioning; particularly in the domains of communication, emotional support and empathy, absence of over-protection and effective problem solving.

It is salutary to note that the psychological state of the carer also impacts the survivor; Carnwath and Johnson (1987) found survivors with depressed carers exhibited elevated depression scores themselves, and depression in the caregiver was associated with poorer social rehabilitation for the survivor. Grant, Weaver, Elliott, Bartolucci and Giger, (2004) noted that depressed carers provided a poorer standard of care and were less able to meet the survivor's needs. Carers' attitude to care, particularly an over-protective stance, was reported to reduce the stroke survivors' motivation, and potentially their recovery (Maclean, Pound, Wolfe & Rudd, 2000). As expected, when the burden for the carer became too great, it was found to affect their ability to support the stroke survivor at home (Anderson, Linto & Stewart-Wynne, 1995). However, carer factors may also have a positive effect on survivors; Molloy, Johnston, Johnston, Pollard, Morrison, Bonetti *et al.* (2008), in a prospective study, demonstrated that spousal caregivers' confidence that there would be improvement in mobility predicted actual improvement in mobility and greater survivor self-efficacy for recovery.

Negative impact of family care for survivors

It is natural to assume that the caring activities involved in 'looking after' someone are invariably beneficial for the recipient, and the evidence reviewed above suggests this is generally the case, but it is not always so. It has already been noted that over-protection may lead to over-provision of care. Palmer and Glass (2003) cited evidence that over-protection is a relatively common occurrence, and that too much practical support may engender worse functional outcomes and encourage dependence. It may also result in under-stimulation and hamper the adjustment of both the survivor and the carer. In addition, Robinson, Francis, James, Tindle, Greenwell and Rodgers (2005) described how a 'fear orientation' may develop from anxiety about the survivor having another stroke and engender over-protection that hampers recovery.

> I was terrified really, because I was worried I didn't want him falling over, hurting himself, so I was maybe too mothering I suppose, but I just wanted to make sure that he was safe. (Wife of survivor)

Morrison's (1999) review concluded that caring activities are most beneficial when they are matched to specific stressors, and that over-helping may lead to survivor depression. She also reviewed evidence showing that survivor depression affected their perceptions of care: depressed survivors viewed caring activities less positively. Newsom and Schulz (1998) found that 40% of survivors had negative reactions to care, and these were associated with their attitudes to care, self-esteem and perceived control. Such negative reactions predicted depression one year later. Under-helping when help was needed produced distress, but surprisingly over-helping did not produce any negative effects.

Negative effects of caring upon carers

> My main and only role basically now, is a carer to Dawn. I feel I haven't got a life as such anymore. Not an individual life . . . . I can't do anything on the spur of the moment. I have no real individuality anymore. (Husband of survivor)

As described earlier, recent advances in social policy provision for carers have fostered a large research effort into carers in general, and the recent international focus on stroke as a major cause of morbidity (see chapter 2) has ensured that a good proportion of these studies have included stroke carers. As a result of this increased research effort, there have been several recent reviews of studies of the impact of caring for stroke carers (Greenwood, Mackenzie, Cloud and Wilson, 2008b; Greenwood, Mackenzie, Cloud & Wilson, 2009a; Han & Haley, 1999; Low *et al.*, 1999; McKevitt *et al.*, 2004; Morrison, 1999; Murray, Young, Forster & Ashworth, 2003; White, Lauzon, Yaffe & Wood-Dauphinee, 2004). A number of themes emerged in these reviews and are considered below.

A diverse range of carer outcomes have been studied; emotional well-being burden, quality of life, life satisfaction, stress, strain and psychological health. There is abundant evidence that carers have elevated rates of stress-related psychological problems across a broad spectrum: feelings of burden, concerns about competence, fatigue, depression, impaired social and family relationships and reduced sexual fulfilment (Anderson *et al.*, 1995; Berg, Palomaki, Loonnqvist, Lehtihalmes & Kast, 2005; Carnwath & Johnson 1987; Draper & Brocklehurst, 2007; Han & Haley, 1999; Low *et al.*, 1999; McCullagh, Brigstocke, Donaldson & Kalra, 2005; McKevitt, Redfern, Mold & Wolfe, 2004; Palmer & Glass, 2003).

> Oh for somebody to phone up and say 'oh, what are you doing, fancy coming down town?' Oh yes, I'd love to say 'yes' for once instead of saying 'oh no I can't'. But now nobody don't phone me up, because they know the situation. (Wife of survivor)

Carers also experience pervasive lifestyle changes (Periard & Ames, 1993; McKevitt *et al.*, 2004). They may feel under-valued, trapped by the need to be constantly with the survivor and burdened by the need to take on new and unfamiliar roles and by having to deal with altered relationships because of changes in the survivor's personality or dependency (Greenwood *et al.*, 2009a). In a review of 19 studies of quality of life after stroke, White *et al.* (2004) concluded that stroke carers' vitality and mental health at six months after stroke were lower than in the general population, but that levels recovered by 12 months. Thus there was no evidence for a consistent, long-term reduction in health-related quality of life. Several studies included in this review found quality of life and enjoyment declined after stroke, but there were no comparisons with healthy samples. The reviewed studies also provided evidence that life satisfaction declined following stroke to a lower level than in matched noncarers (White *et al.*, 2004). Buschenfeld, Morris and Lockwood (2009) found that isolation was an important negative experience in stroke carers, and this was echoed in the results of Brereton and Nolan (2002) who also found that carers felt their own needs were not considered. Other specific effects included feeling unprepared for the caring role (Brereton & Nolan, 2000).

Murray *et al.* (2003) reviewed 23 qualitative studies of carers and patients and found much overlap between the difficulties identified by these two groups. Over 25% of the problem areas identified in the reviewed studies related to carers and caregiving. Social and emotional consequences of stroke were the most frequently reported (39%) and included problems relating to mood, social changes, attitudes about recovery, self-perception and relationships. The second most frequently cited source of problems for carers was service deficiency (29%). Finally, there is emerging evidence that carers, as well as survivors, may experience severe and enduring effects of the trauma of the stroke event (Buschenfeld *et al.*, 2009; Robinson *et al.*, 2005).

> I don't talk about those first few days so much any more. They still have the same intensity . . . when I think back to that time it's the shock of seeing him as he was. And you never forget that. Somebody his age, and all the emotions come back. You'd think that after nearly five years, you'd be OK. (Wife of survivor)

Benefits for carers

> Whilst he relies on me, I rely on him, works both ways, I think the bond has got stronger, it definitely has got stronger. (Wife of survivor) It was a desperate thing to happen, but it did make us focus on what is really important in life . . . looking after your family, going out to experience different things in life, to use what you have to the best resource for your loved ones. (Wife of survivor)

Studies of stroke carers are generally designed to produce evidence of morbidity, and therefore use measurement scales designed to tap psychological problems in the form of strain, burden, depression and lifestyle change, or else they assess precipitating factors such as stress and disability. While the evidence clearly demonstrates that many carers experience major losses combined with increased vulnerability and burden, the picture is not entirely bleak, and many reviews make reference to positive outcomes of caring (Morrison, 1999; White *et al.*, 2004). In their review of qualitative studies, Greenwood *et al.* (2009a) noted findings demonstrating improved relationships between survivor and family, satisfaction and fulfilment through the caring role, the development of spiritual awareness and reappraisal of priorities. Greenwood, Mackenzie, Wilson and Cloud (2009b) found that positive experiences of caring and stroke increased in the first few months after discharge from hospital. Palmer and Glass (2003) reviewed studies that echoed this finding and concluded that some families demonstrate positive gains as a result of stroke or other serious illness. The benefits were similar to those reported by Greenwood *et al.* (2009b) and extended to spiritual growth, increased appreciation of life, a greater sense of the purpose of life and a reappraisal of values, as well as improved interpersonal relationships and increased self-confidence. Buschenfeld *et al.* (2009) also identified the theme of 'growth' in their study of long-term carers. This theme encompassed strengthening of relationships and new life opportunities, such as new employment. Haley, Allen, Grant, Clay, Perkins and Roth (2009), using a questionnaire-based interview, found that most carers positively endorsed all 11 questions in a 'positive aspects of care-giving' questionnaire, such as appreciating life more, feeling more needed and strengthening relationship. In the case of these three questions, over 86% of their sample of 75 gave positive responses. Finally, Mackenzie and Greenwood (2009) reported preliminary results of a review of ten studies that found positive outcome for stroke caregivers. The positive benefits reported in these studies stemmed from survivors' responses to their care and the carers' own appraisals of their situation. They identified six clusters of positive outcomes characterised as: feeling appreciated; demonstrated love through closer family ties; observing recovery and improvement of the survivor; mastery of the caring role, satisfaction in meeting needs and increased self-esteem; a sense of duty and reciprocity and a closer relationship with the survivor.

The perception of positive and negative aspects of caring, and their relative importance for individual carers, are not well understood, but the primary and secondary appraisal mechanisms identified in Lazarus and Folkman's model may be key factors. Similarly, factors highlighted by the theory of planned behaviour – attitudes to caring, the perception of others' expectations and values and perceived personal control and mastery – may be influential. Further research is needed in this important domain.

Factors affecting the impact of caring upon carers

Methodological issues

There have been numerous studies of factors affecting the psychological and physical response of carers and their capacity to continue caring. The results are illuminating, but studies in the area suffer from several problems. Quantitative studies of factors associated with carer outcomes use predetermined categories and produce, averaged, typical results which do not capture the range and diversity of reactions. None to date have used approaches such as structural equation modelling, to explore complex relationships between variables and pathways of influence including financial resources, skills and experience, family configuration and level of disability. Qualitative studies can highlight individualised and diverse reactions, but cannot be generalised to provide estimates of the prevalence of such reactions. There are also pervasive methodological issues that impede interpretation. Greenwood *et al.* (2009a) noted that the diversity of carers included in studies, the lack of consistent, comparable measures of outcome and differences in the timing of the studies after the stroke all limit the generality of the conclusions that can be drawn. Another important consideration is that *change* in circumstances after stroke, for example in income, lifestyle and social relationships, may be as important a determinant of outcome as the absolute level of these variables (Morrison, 1999). Despite this, most quantitative studies are cross-sectional with no opportunity to measure change, and change is not commonly used as a variable, even in longitudinal studies.

Attributes of the survivor

There is ample evidence that carer outcomes are related to stroke severity, physical disability, dependency and cognitive impairment; but other factors, including behavioural problems, mood and age, have also been shown to be influential (Greenwood *et al.*, 2008b; Haley *et al.*, 2009; Low *et al.*, 1999; McCullagh *et al.*, 2005). Most studies of carers of stroke survivors with aphasia have reported greater burden than for carers of non-aphasic survivors (Draper, Bowring, Thompson, Van Heyst, Conroy & Thompson, 2007), but evidence for the importance of aphasia has not been universally found (McClenahan & Weinman, 1998). The sheer number of caregiving tasks required affects outcome for carers, and has been shown to exacerbate stress through the curtailment of activities and to increase vulnerability to depression (Nieboer, Schulz, Matthews, Scheier, Ormel & Lindenberg, 1998).

Attributes of the carer

Caregiver attributes, such as physical health, level of optimism, psychological adjustment, emotional status and appraisal of coping capacity, have all been shown to be potent determinants of carers' well-being (Forsberg-Wärleby, Moller & Blomstrand, 2001; Greenwood *et al.*, 2009a; Low *et al.*, 1999; Scholte op Reimer *et al.*, 1998). Carers' age and gender (McCullagh, *et al.*, 2005) and coping style (Visser-Meily, Post, van de Port, Maas, Forstberg-Warleby & Lindeman, 2009) have also been reported to determine outcomes for carers. Ethnicity is a potentially important factor which unfortunately has been only sparsely explored. Having an African ethnic background may protect from depression to some extent (Greenwood *et al.*, 2008b), but Mackenzie, Perry, Lockhart, Cottee, Cloud and Mann (2007) found higher levels of burden in black and Asian carers than in white carers. For African-Caribbean carers in the United Kingdom, religious faith, close family ties and previous experiences of 'battling' with racism may help to bolster resilience, and a strong distaste for institutional placement may strengthen determination to cope (Strudwick & Morris, 2010). Financial resources also impact positively on quality of life, and financial problems impact negatively (White *et al.*, 2004).

Age determines carers' experiences and outcomes (McCullagh *et al.*, 2005). Unfortunately, there is a lack of consistency in how 'young' is defined in the literature (see chapter 21, 'Strokes in Young People'). The situation is further complicated by differences in the relationship between the survivor and the carer, which may lead to large age differences when the latter is an offspring or a parent. Younger spousal carers are more likely to become very long term carers due to the longer life span of survivor and carer, and the role of long-term adjustment is therefore particularly important (Buschenfeld *et al.*, 2009; Visser-Meily *et al.*, 2009). Few studies, with the notable exceptions of Periard and Ames (1994) and Mackenzie *et al.* (2007), have compared different age cohorts within a single design, but there exist many studies that have recruited spousal carers in different age bands, from 20 years old upwards. The comparison of these studies may also provide insights into the importance of age differences. For example, Banks and Pearson (2004) included carers aged 29–49, Buschenfeld *et al.* (2009) carers under 60 and Forsberg-Warleby *et al.* (2004) carers under 75. A principal source of difference between younger and older carers is that young carers are more likely to have dependent children, and will generally be of working age. Younger carers experienced more lifestyle change and caregiver strain (Mackenzie *et al.*, 2007), engaged in more coping activities and were less accepting of formal care than older carers (Periard & Ames, 1994). Younger female carers were less satisfied with care and communication with staff than their older counterparts, and younger carers of both genders experienced greater difficulty in talking things over with staff (Mackenzie *et al.*, 2007). Banks and Pearson (2004) and Buschenfeld *et al.* (2009) both highlighted changes in roles, responsibilities and the young carers' active efforts to adjust and cope with the changes and demands of caring. They also found evidence of major lifestyle changes and enduring effects on the self-image of the young carers.

Family and relationship factors

There is evidence that family factors and family dynamics influence outcomes for carers as well as for survivors. Studies and reviews have concluded that family support is associated with improved carer functioning (McCullagh *et al.*, 2005; Scholte op Reimer *et al.*, 1998) and improved quality of life (White *et al.*, 2004). One study investigated the level of agreement between patients' and carers' assessments of the patient's level of disability in the first few months after a stroke. It reported that agreement was usually rated lower by the patient than the carer (Knapp & Hewison, 1999), and the extent of the disagreement predicted carer strain. With the exception of the studies cited above, family factors have not been widely reported as determinants of carer outcome (Greenwood *et al.*, 2008b). Most of the 39 studies included in Greenwood *et al.'s* review recruited mainly spouses, and the authors noted the lack of information about different experiences and outcomes for other family members who provide care. There is, however, evidence that younger carers in particular, as well as those with multiple roles within the family, such as responsibility for children and wage earning, find their situation especially difficult (Banks & Pearson, 2004; Mackenzie *et al.*, 2007). Moreover, high levels of responsibility and multiple roles may lead to a decrease in satisfaction with responsibilities and roles (Enterlante & Kern, 1995).

Time since stroke

The comparison of cross-sectional studies of caring at different times after stroke suggest that some difficulties are enduring, such as the challenge of providing physical care and need for information; whereas others, such as initial shock, specific stressors and the quality of the relationship with the survivor, change over the course of time since the stroke. Studies conducted in the first few months after the stroke have shown that stress focussed on the confining nature of caregiving and the accompanying changes to personal and family life (DeLaune & Brown, 2001). Moreover, the level of stress in this period was related to the carers' previous physical health and amount of time required for caring (Forsberg-Wärleby *et al.*, 2001). Even when patients were still in hospital having rehabilitation, carers experienced 'role reversal' as they picked up roles that were formerly occupied by the survivor, such as childcare or managing finances; and this engendered strain and exhaustion (Hunt & Smith, 2004). At one year after, the stroke carers were still coming to terms with the dramatic changes in their lifestyles, and the caregiver role had become a central commitment (Kerr & Smith 2001; Smith, Lawrence, Kerr, Langhorne & Lees, 2004). Several studies of carers reviewed by Greenwood *et al.* (2009a) reported that carers needed time to themselves at this stage. Psychosocial difficulties persisted so that at three years after the stroke, significant burden was still experienced and was determined by the amount of care provided (Scholte op Reimer *et al.*, 1998). Carers continued to experience greater difficulty with emotional reactions, lack of sleep and social isolation than matched noncarers (Greveson, Gray, French & James, 1991). Even two to seven years after the stroke, carers reported that their lifestyle had changed significantly across several domains: home, employment and social life. Their self-identity also changed as a result of the experiences they lived through, their new caring roles and their increased social isolation (Buschenfeld *et al.*, 2009). The review by Greenwood *et al.* (2009a) included 17 qualitative studies of carers, all using carer interviews. Most of the studies focussed on the first year after stroke, but the range extended to 14 years after the stroke. Pervasive difficulties that persisted across all time points were the challenge of providing physical care, need for more information and need for more support.

Longitudinal studies of change in carers' experience and outcome have generally focussed on the first year after stroke (Forsberg-Warleby *et al.*, 2004; McCullagh *et al.*, 2005), and have produced mixed results for burden, emotional state and quality of life, variously showing improvements, stability and even deterioration (Visser-Meily *et al.*, 2009). In part, the inconsistent results of studies may have been due to the use of different measures and samples (Ilse, Feys, de Wit, Putman & de Weerdt, 2008). Fewer studies have looked at longer term adjustment, beyond one year after stroke, and the results show little evidence for change in carers' burden, depression or quality of life (Visser-Meily *et al.*, 2009). Visser-Meily *et al.* (2009) followed a group longitudinally across four measurement points from shortly after the stroke to three years, and this study did produce some evidence of change, but it was both positive and negative; burden and depression decreased in the years after stroke, but the quality of the relationship between carers and care recipient and their wider social relationships also decreased.

Coping by carers

> I think at the time the emotions don't come into it really, you just do what you have to do. I think for a long time I just ignored what I was going through and what I was feeling. (Husband of survivor)

Coping is a major feature of Lazarus and Folkman's model, intervening between the demands of caring and the outcome. It is therefore not surprising that research has identified coping as a major factor for carers. Buschenfeld *et al.* (2009) identified coping as a theme for their young (under 60) carers, and coping has been shown to be associated with psychological functioning and outcome (McClenahan & Weinman, 1998; Visser-Meily *et al.*, 2009). Active problem-focussed coping was considered more effective than passive coping by spouses (Buschenfeld *et al.*, 2009) and was associated with more positive outcomes (Visser-Meily *et al.*, 2009). Greenwood *et al.* (2009a) found that taking things one day at a time, establishing routines, asking for and accepting help, asking for information and being patient were all commonly reported methods of coping with caregiving stress.

Planning and evaluating interventions to support carers

A number of interventions for carers have been designed to meet their identified needs and to improve service provision.

Carers' needs

A reasonable first step in the development of interventions for carers is to enumerate their needs, and several studies have addressed this important topic. Bakas, Austin, Okonkwo, Lewis and Chadwick (2002) interviewed stroke caregivers and identified five major areas of need in the first six months after stroke: information about stroke, support with physical care, help with other practical difficulties, such as benefits, services, employment, managing the carers' own reactions and responses to caring. The need for information, and also for the accessibility of staff to answer questions, was corroborated in a questionnaire study of carers during the initial period of hospital treatment (van der Smagt-Duijnstee, Hamers, Abu-Saad & Zuidhof, 2001). This study also found that carers felt a need for supportive counselling, and this echoed two studies reviewed by Greenwood *et al.* (2009a), where carers identified emotional support as an important need. Greenwood *et al.* (2009a) also confirmed the prominence of informational needs, which were identified in six of the reviewed studies. Information needs encompassed general information about stroke and services, such as the likelihood of further strokes, financial benefits and available services, and also information tailored to individual survivors. The need for information about stroke, its treatment and services was also reported by MacKenzie *et al.* (2007) and McLean *et al.* (1991). These studies also identified a need for training to develop skills. A qualitative study by Greenwood *et al.* (2009b) highlighted uncertainty as a prominent concern for carers after discharge. Murray *et al.* (2003) reviewed studies of long-term survivors. Their analysis revealed that three of the 19 problem areas identified in the studies were expressions of carer need: for more social support, a break and more independence. Scholte op Reimer *et al.* (1998) found evidence for unmet psychosocial needs and unmet demands for practical assistance with daily activities.

On the basis of these studies, it would appear that carers require interventions and service enhancements that provide fuller information about stroke, its treatment and stroke services and benefits. The need is specifically for information tailored to their individual situation. Carers also require strategies for managing uncertainty, psychosocial and emotional support through counselling and respite from, and assistance with, practical tasks.

Carers' satisfaction and experience with services

Carers' satisfaction and experience of services are closely linked to their perception of their needs having been met. Hence, their views about services provide another route to identifying needs. Carers usually express overall satisfaction with hospital care (MacKenzie *et al.*, 2007; Morris, Payne & Lambert, 2007; Pound, Gompertz, & Ebrahim, 1993; Wellwood, Dennis & Warlow, 1995). Visser-Meily, Post, Meijer, Maas, Ketelaar and Lindeman (2005a) found that while 44% of their sample of 194 spouses of stroke patients was very satisfied with in-patient care, 23% felt that care was below standard. Participation in a group, attending the hospital and support from staff were all positively associated with satisfaction. Satisfaction with care after discharge from hospital is generally lower and a National Audit Office survey of 760 carers and patients in England (National Audit Office, 2010) found that less than half of the respondents rated services for carers as 'very good' or 'good' across the domains of information about stroke, a separate social care needs assessment, emotional support (such as counselling), access to respite care and training in how to support patients at home. For the last three areas, less than one third rated services as good.

Even carers who express overall satisfaction with a service may have significant unmet needs. This was illustrated by the results of Morris *et al.* (2007) who found that carers' satisfaction with hospital provision was complex and multi-dimensional; positive views about staff co-existed with negative evaluations of aspects of service provision. Factors that carers regarded as important included good information and availability of care and treatment, staff attitudes, considering the whole person and their context, accommodating patients' individual needs and the burden of care placed on the carer. In community settings, carers have identified inadequate consultation and consideration by professionals as areas of concern (Simon & Kumar, 2002). The adequacy of preparation for discharge is another major determinant of satisfaction, as are the availability and organisation of service provision after discharge (Kelson *et al.*, 1998; Kerr & Smith, 2001; MacKenzie *et al.*, 2007; Pound *et al.*, 1993; Wellwood *et al.*, 1995).

In addition to the interventions and enhancements indicated by studies of needs, these studies of service provision suggest that interventions should address the availability of services, staff attitudes, the consideration of the 'whole' person and their individuality, preparation for discharge and support after discharge.

Difficulties with research into efficacy of interventions

The economic and social importance of carers, coupled with government initiatives to support family carers, has stimulated the development of supportive interventions and services. It will become clear that the evidence for the efficacy of many of the approaches is inconclusive, but research in the area is complex and ideally should involve randomised controlled trials. The reasons for the difficulties with researching the area overlap with those identified by Greenwood *et al.* (2008b) as affecting studies of the impact of caring. First, interventions tend to deliver more or less standardised package of care, but, as described above, carers are diverse in terms of needs, expectations, background and ethnicity; the benefits that are appreciated by one carer may not suit others. Moreover, the characteristics and experience of those delivering the interventions are potent uncontrolled influences that may affect outcome, for example by their ability to develop a therapeutic partnership working with carers and their families (Sandberg & Eriksson, 2009). Added to this is that carers' needs change over the course of time since the stroke; an intervention that is acceptable in the period immediately after stroke may not be appropriate later (Cameron & Gignac, 2008). Many interventions for carers are delivered in the community after discharge from hospital; in this setting, carers experience a rich and diverse range of other influences and events affecting their functioning and well-being. Any beneficial effects of the intervention have to be detected against this backcloth, and large samples are required to produce the necessary statistical power. More importantly, carers are not passive recipients of care, and the community setting is not one in which researchers have control over participants' help seeking behaviour: those assigned to control or comparison conditions, and denied the particular intervention being evaluated, may benefit from developing their own strategies (McKevitt *et al.*, 2004), or from accessing alternative sources of support that meet their needs. The benefit derived from such alternative strategies could mask the beneficial effects of the intervention. Finally, there is poor agreement between researchers about primary outcomes. There are many facets that are potentially significant: mental health including anxiety and depression, quality of life, burden, stressors, strain, benefits of being a carer, satisfaction with care, social engagement, family functioning and relationships, self-efficacy, self-esteem and specific experiences in services. Even when the same conceptual outcome is addressed, for example quality of life or mood, the measures used are many and varied, and this complicates comparison between studies and the pooling of results. Individual carers may show improvements in different areas, and there may be subtle and difficult-to-capture effects where specific measures do not change, but the intervention fosters higher order change, such as acceptance of burden without any actual change in the level of burden itself, or increased resilience to stress without any change in the stressors encountered. A final complicating factor is that many interventions are complex and multifaceted and, for example, can involve education combined with counselling and/or support (Brereton *et al.*, 2007; Visser-Meily, Post, Meijer, van de Port, Maas and Lindeman, 2005b). Attributing positive outcomes to specific interventions is therefore not straightforward.

Reviews of the evidence for the efficacy of interventions

Despite the many problems of researching this area, there have been a large number of studies of interventions for stroke carers, and the evidence below relies on a number of systematic reviews of these studies. Visser-Meily *et al.* (2005b) reviewed 22 studies of interventions for stroke carers. The review used broad inclusion criteria encompassing randomized controlled trials, clinical trials and uncontrolled trials with measures taken before and after the intervention. Brereton *et al.* (2007) used more restrictive inclusion criteria; including only randomised controlled trials and excluding studies that used only educational or information-giving interventions. Five of the studies in Brereton *et al.* (2007), all published before 2003, overlapped with those in the review by Visser-Meily *et al.* (2005b). But there were also three additional, more recent, studies. Smith *et al.* (2008) furnished another systematic review of 17 randomised trials with a specific focus on information provision and educational interventions, and included 13 studies not covered by Visser-Meily *et al.* (2005b) or Brereton *et al.* (2007). Finally, a review of studies investigating family support liaison worker for stroke carers has been completed (Ellis, Mant, Langhorne, Dennis & Winner, 2010). The interventions reviewed included support after discharge, family liaison workers, education, counselling and peer support.

Support after discharge

Interventions that provide support after discharge are highly variable in both content and delivery mode. Content may include training in problem solving, problem solving partnerships, individual counselling and/or education about stroke and stroke care. Delivery may be initiated in hospital and followed up at home, or may be all home based. It may include groups (support, educational or training), individual home visits, telephone conferences, or individual telephone support.

The review by Visser-Meily *et al.* (2005b) included 11 studies of interventions after discharge. Only four studies reported benefits for carers, and there was no consistency in the particular outcomes that improved across these four studies. A review *by* Brereton *et al.* (2007) included three studies published since Visser-Meily *et al.* (2005b). These studies all had interventions with an element of support after discharge, and the results were more positive than those of Visser-Meily *et al.* (2005b). Most of the interventions reviewed took place in the period up to six months after discharge. Support groups and home visits led by nurses improved carers' coping skills, self-efficacy, efforts to obtain social support and confidence in knowledge about the survivor's care, but did not improve carers' well-being. A study of telephone support for individuals (Grant, 1999; Grant, Elliott, Weaver,

Bartolucci & Giger, 2002) did show benefits, compared with a control group, for measures of depression, problem solving and preparedness. But an intervention using group telephone conferences (Hartke & King, 2003) did not show gains compared with a control group. Brereton *et al.*'s conclusions were circumspect about the overall effectiveness of support interventions, and they pointed to a number of factors that prevented firm conclusions being drawn. The interventions were highly varied and did not allow results to be pooled for statistical meta-analysis; crucially some of the studies did not demonstrate improvements relative to control groups. There were sometimes before-after gains on some measures for carers in the intervention condition, but these might simply have reflected natural changes over time. The measures and measurement methods varied across studies, improvements were not consistent across studies and the methodological rigor of the studies was poor, especially with regard to matching of control groups.

Stroke liaison workers

A stroke liaison worker is a healthcare worker whose aim is to help return patients and their carers to normal functioning. They often provide emotional and social support and information for stroke carers and/or their family members, and liaise with services with the aim of improving their quality of life (Lilley, Lincoln & Francis, 2003). Ellis *et al.* (2010) conducted a meta-analysis of caregiver's outcomes from 15 intervention trials of stroke liaison workers that included data from 1775 carers. The review concluded that there was no evidence of benefit with respect to caregiver strain and subjective health, activities of daily living or mental health. In fact, the difference favoured the non-intervention conditions for two of the measures: caregiver subjective health status and caregiver extended activities of daily living. However, carers' responses to questions addressing information provision and satisfaction did demonstrate statistically significant benefits of the liaison worker in a meta-analysis, and in several individual trials. These questions were:

* 'I received all the information I needed about the nature and causes of the patient's illness' (three trials).
* 'I have received enough information about recovery and rehabilitation' (three trials).
* 'Someone has really listened' (two trials).
* 'I have not felt neglected' (two trials).

The lack of statistically significant benefit for many measures of caregiver outcome in the aggregated results of the trials included in Ellis *et al.* (2010) does mask heterogeneity in individual studies. Burton and Gibbon (2005), for example, found that follow-up after discharge by a stroke nurse reduced carer strain at three months as well as deterioration in the survivors' physical dependence between three and twelve months. However, both these effects in this trial only just reached statistical significance, and a detailed analysis by Ellis *et al.* (2010), in which trials were classified and grouped according to the emphasis of the intervention (social support, education or simply liaison), failed to reveal any consistent benefits for particular types of intervention.

Information, educational and training programmes

This encompasses a variety of methods: leaflets, small-group teaching sessions, seminars, individual feedback on assessment and telephone sessions. Content may include material on general knowledge about stroke and secondary prevention, information about services, development of problem solving skills, and coaching in exercise and care skills. Visser-Meily *et al.* (2005b) included six studies of educational programmes in their review and four showed improvements; as expected, knowledge about stroke was the outcome that most often improved. Brereton *et al.* (2007) concluded that the only training intervention which improved carers' well-being and quality of life by reducing psychological symptoms, such as depression, anxiety and burden, was the training of carers in nursing and personal care techniques. However, Lee, Soeken and Picot (2007) conducted a statistical meta-analysis of four studies of interventions designed to improve the mental health of stroke carers. These included two studies of educational interventions (Grant *et al.*, 2002; Rodgers, Atkinson, Bond, Suddes, Dobson & Curless, 1999). Lee *et al.* (2007) found evidence for a statistically significant positive effect on mental health outcome measures, such as depression and burden, across all four studies.

Perhaps the most conclusive evidence for the impact of information and education in stroke care comes from the Cochrane review completed by Smith, Forster, House, Knapp, Wright and Young (2008). The 17 trials in this review included 1773 patients and 1058 carers. Meta-analyses showed that information produced a significant improvement for carers' knowledge, but not for carers' mood or satisfaction. Qualitative analyses found no strong evidence of an effect for any other outcomes. A large-scale randomised trail from Sweden exploring the benefits of group support and education meetings prior to discharge for spouses of stroke survivors echoed these conclusions (Franzen-Dahlin, Larson, Murray, Wredling & Billing, 2008); there was no overall effect on psychological health, but knowledge of stroke did improve. It seems, therefore, that despite the ubiquitous finding of stroke carers' and survivors' desire for information, the benefits of information provision by itself are limited to improved knowledge. This is not to say that information is not beneficial, but that it may be effective only in combination with other interventions or support measures.

Counselling

Interventions employing counselling typically involve individual, one-to-one sessions of formal counselling or problem solving training. Visser-Meily *et al.* (2005b) found three out of four studies that provided carers with counselling showed positive benefits across a range of outcomes; coping, social support, emotional state, quality of life, activities and family functioning. Brereton *et al.* (2007) also found studies demonstrating the efficacy of counselling, and concluded that counselling combined with education was effective in improving knowledge and in reducing deterioration in family functioning.

Peer support

Peer support, usually through groups, is by no means new, and has for many years been the mainstay of support provided by third sector organisations such as the Stroke Association and Different Strokes. However, it has recently been included in the National Stroke Strategy for England (Department of Health, 2007a), both within its ten-point service improvement plan (point 7) and in four of the quality markers. Peer support has not been prominent in recent reviews of interventions for stroke carers, so it will be considered in some detail here.

Peer support is a social intervention, with the 'peer' being a person who shares similarities with the person requiring support, such as age, ethnicity, health concerns or situation. Peers also possess specific knowledge derived from personal experience rather than formal training. It is this personal experience that enables a peer supporter to understand and empathise with a person's situation. Peer supporters can impart experiential knowledge, and this differs from professional knowledge, in that it is pragmatically based rather than theoretical, here-and-now rather than long-term and holistic rather than segmental. Peer support groups enable the pooling of large amounts of such knowledge (Borkman, 1976). Peer support may be provided on an individual basis, face-to-face, by telephone or by computer. However, it is commonly delivered in group settings. Although there is some evidence for the efficacy of peer support across a range of conditions (Dennis, 2003; Doull, O'Connor, Welch, Tugwell & Wells, 2005), there have been few studies of peer support in stroke. One such study of the efficacy of peer support with stroke carers, (Stewart, Doble, Hart, Langille & MacPherson, 1998), investigated the impact of home visits by professionals (initial visit) and subsequent biweekly one-to-one visits for 12 weeks over 18 months by peer supporters. There were 20 carers of stroke survivors in the study, but no control comparison. Instead, interviews at three and six months after the intervention were analysed, together with notes and diaries. The carers appreciated information regarding resources and coping strategies, emotional support, affirmation and positive feedback. The intervention also bolstered their self-esteem and confidence, reduced burden and improved their ability to cope. The peers also offered companionship, understanding and sharing of feelings. However, the study found that some visitor–carer dyads were not well matched, and that similarity was a major factor in success. Some of the survivors were uncomfortable with the visits or jealous of the attention given to the carer. While these results suggest a number of positive benefits, the absence of a control group and the lack of standardised measures are major limitations.

Hartke and King (2003) conducted a more rigorous study, a randomised controlled trial of eight, one-hour structured telephone conferences during which stroke caregivers received support from caregiver peers and one or two professional facilitators. Eighty-eight participants, all over 60 years of age, were randomised to control and treatment conditions and were assessed at the start of the study, at the end of the intervention (experimental group only), and at six months follow-up. Objective measures, using validated scales, showed a reduction in stress for those who received peer support over the intervention and follow-up periods, but there were no significant benefits on self-ratings of depression, burden, loneliness or competence, and the positive change in stress scores for the intervention group did not differ significantly from that of the control group. However, the control group exhibited increased burden and deceased competence between the first and final assessments. Compared with this declining pattern for the control group, the treatment group did show significantly better outcomes for burden and competence, but not for depression, loneliness or stress. About one-third of the treatment group contacted other group members outside of sessions, and satisfaction ratings for all aspects of the intervention were high with 93% expressing 'good-excellent' overall satisfaction.

These findings demonstrate the acceptability of this kind of intervention, and that, despite a lack of positive improvements in many measures, peer support may still exert a protective function for stroke carers when compared to the decline that occurs in those who do not receive it. In a further study relevant to peer support, King and Semik (2006) studied carers in the first two years after stroke, and obtained evidence about the help that carers can offer to their peers. They achieved this by collecting samples of guidance and advice that experienced stroke carers said would be useful to offer to new carers. The outcome was 26 statements covering three principal domains: preparation for caring, enhancing the survivor's function and sustaining self and family. As well as providing assistance to carers (and survivors), peer support interventions also have benefits for the psychological adjustment and well-being of the peer supporters themselves (Arnstein, Vidal, Wells-Federman, Morgan & Caudill, 2002), but to date such benefit has been demonstrated only for conditions other than stroke.

Feeling that you have got someone out there that is in the same position, or you know that in the group you can ask for ideas and help. (Wife of survivor)
Well almost extended another group of friends I suppose ... we've got things in common and therefore there's another contact. (Husband of survivor)

While peer support shows some promise, such interventions are complex. Peer supporters require careful selection, preparation and support for their role. Mowbray, Moxley, Thrasher, Bybee, McCrohan, Harris and Clover (1996) discussed large-scale peer support initiatives, and concluded that successful implementation requires a mission and culture that develops the supporters' role, mentoring and supervision, and opportunities for education and advancement.

Interventions for stroke carers: summary

The fit between the interventions that have been developed and evaluated and carers' needs, as identified above, is generally good; interventions have been designed to provide information, psychological support and support after discharge. Services also provide practical home care support after discharge and respite care, but these aspects are not primarily psychological, and have not been included in the review. There are some gaps, however, and interventions focussed on more general matters, such as staff attitudes and 'holistic' care, have yet to be designed and evaluated.

In view of the many factors that complicate and obscure the outcomes of studies of interventions for carers, it is unsurprising that there is a lack of clear and consistent evidence for the efficacy of interventions. Increased satisfaction, knowledge and improvements in psychological outcomes, such as confidence and self-efficacy, are common positive outcomes. However, beneficial outcomes for functioning, quality of life and well-being are not found consistently, but training and counselling approaches seem to be the most promising for achieving gains in these areas. It is noteworthy that providing information does not generally improve outcomes, despite carers' expressed need for information. Peer support has potential to deliver broad-spectrum benefits embracing aspects that are not encompassed in programmes delivered by healthcare professionals. However, it is under-researched and the quality of such studies as exist is generally poor.

Conclusions

Unpaid carers, usually family members, make a major contribution to the care of community living stroke survivors, both practically and economically. Government policy and legislation recognise and support the carers' role, but its implementation is imperfect. Since carers are crucial in the provision of effective stroke care, it is important to understand their needs and the factors and processes involved in determining outcomes for survivors *and* carers. In recent years there has been a great deal of research into carers and the effects of caring, but the theoretical underpinning of much of the research, particularly Lazarus and Folkman's stress-coping model, has limited the scope of research. Another promising model is the theory of planned behaviour (Ajzen, 1985) which also encompasses factors that affect the motivation to care. Theoretical models to explain the benefits of caring for carers themselves have yet to be developed. Contrary to expectations, research has revealed that caring sometimes has a negative effect on survivors, although the causes of this are not well understood. A great deal of evidence has accumulated regarding the factors that affect carers; the attributes of carers, survivors, family factors and ethnicity are all clearly important. However, this research has focussed mainly on negative outcomes, and little is known about factors that enhance and maintain the positive benefits of caring for carers. Interventions to support carers have also been extensively investigated, but the focus has been on minimising negative outcomes rather than on promoting well-being and positive outcomes. There are also major methodological challenges in accomplishing this enterprise. Consequently the evidence base is incomplete and inconclusive. However, subjective psychological improvements seem to occur more reliably than improvements in function and objective measures of carers' psychological status.

Future directions

In view of the small number of models that underpin research into carers and caring (Brereton *et al.*, 2007) and the limitations of those that have been used, there should be a major effort to develop more comprehensive models encompassing the motivation for caring and its positive outcomes. This has the potential to provide a conceptual framework to underpin the development of interventions (Medical Research Council, 2008). Research into outcomes for carers themselves and research into the efficacy of interventions to support carers have been dominated by studies designed to investigate and to prevent negative impacts of caring. There is a clear need for studies that focus on the factors and interventions that promote and maintain positive outcomes for carers. The lack of strong and consistent evidence for the efficacy of specific interventions to support carers is disappointing, but perhaps not surprising given the methodological issues. It may be that successful interventions will need to be individualised and flexibly tailored to the changing needs of carers. This will require more responsive approaches to needs assessment than are currently available, with the capacity for ongoing monitoring of change. Peer support, possibly combined with professional input, may provide the necessary degree of flexibility and individuality, and this area is ripe for research. Finally, information provision has been widely studied and demonstrated to have much more limited benefits than expected on the basis of expressed need. Instead of a focus on information provision, such studies should investigate alternative approaches to managing uncertainty, such as those identified by Greenwood *et al.* (2009b).

Chapter 21

Strokes in Young People: Families and Children, Carers, Employment and Long-Term Survival

Definitions and scope

Young stroke survivors share many of the same issues as older survivors, but there are also important differences, and young survivors present special challenges to stroke services. In this chapter, a 'young' stroke survivor will be considered to be someone aged 18 to 65 years. At the lower boundary this ties in with the current dividing line between childhood and adulthood. At the upper boundary it reflects the current, normal division between working age and retirement in the United Kingdom, and also the boundary between adult and older adult services in the NHS. However, it does not map neatly onto other important demographic factors such as the likelihood of having a family with young (under 18) children at the time of stroke. Another complicating factor is that research studies variously define 'young' as under 75, 65, 50 or 40 years, or in some cases even younger. In order to clarify matters, the age ranges used in reviewed studies will be explicitly identified where this is relevant to the issue under consideration.

Stroke in children is not included in this review since it is rare with only a few hundred cases per year across the whole United Kingdom (Royal College of Physicians, 2004). Childhood stroke raises very special problems and issues, and uses a different care pathway. There are often extensive, specialist investigations to determine the cause of such an untimely event. Health services must network with education, local authority child services and third sector organisations that focus exclusively on children. There may be delicate and complex issues surrounding consent for treatment and the relative weight to place on the wishes of children and their parents, and this area is governed by special legal precedents specific to the child health field. For these reasons, there are separate guidelines

Psychological Management of Stroke, First Edition. Nadina B. Lincoln, Ian I. Kneebone, Jamie A.B. Macniven and Reg C. Morris.

for strokes in children in the United Kingdom and United States (Royal College of Physicians, 2004; Roach *et al.*, 2008) and care is provided within paediatric services, ideally a tertiary paediatric neurology service, rather than through the specialist stroke care pathway. Interested readers can find more information about childhood stroke in Biller (2009.).

Age and stroke incidence rates

The risk of stroke increases with age (Table 21.1), and the relationship between age and the incidence of stroke is universal (Feigin, Lawes, Bennett & Anderson, 2003). The number of strokes in younger people is low, but nevertheless young people with stroke present a significant demand on health services. A country the size of England, with a population of about 50 million and about 29 million under 45, would expect around 5800 new strokes in people under 45 each year. Populations usually have less people in older age groups (due to attrition through death) and proportionately more in young and middle-age groups; consequently the number of new strokes in the under 65s has been estimated as 21%, or about one in five of all new strokes, despite their much lower risk (Kersten, Low, Ashburn, George & McLellan, 2002). On average, people who have a stroke when young live for longer after their stroke than older stroke survivors, and this increases the prevalence rate for younger stroke survivors so that about 25% of community living stroke survivors are under 65 (Kersten *et al.*, 2002; Royal College of Physicians, 2008a).

Comparison of younger and older stroke survivors

Younger stroke survivors differ from their older counterparts in a number of ways. First, there are important differences in the types of stroke found in younger people; they have a proportionately higher rate of haemorrhagic

Table 21.1   Typical Incidence Rates for Stroke by Age Across World-wide Studies (Feigin *et al.*, 2003)

Age	Annual incidence per 1000
<45	0.1–0.3
45–54	1–2
55–64	2–4
65–74	5–10
75–84	12–20
85 +	15–30

strokes, particularly subarachnoid haemorrhage (Gandolofo & Conti, 2003; Teasell, McRae & Finestone, 2000). Second, ethnic differences in the risk of stroke may be accentuated in younger age groups (Jacobs, Sacco & Boden-Albala, 2003). Finally, younger stroke survivors face particular challenges linked to the life stage when the stroke occurs, and are likely to encounter marital stress, childcare problems and employment difficulties.

Young stroke survivors may well have different needs from those of their older counterparts, but we should be cautious in assuming that their outcomes are necessarily different from, or less positive than, those of older stroke survivors. Pringle, Hendry and McLafferty (2008) pointed out that older stroke survivors have generally lower quality of life and have many of the same needs and issues as younger patients. Bagg, Pombo and Hopman (2002) conducted a prospective study of 561 patients admitted to a stroke rehabilitation unit over a six-year period and assessed functional independence at admission and discharge. Age did predict absolute functional scores at discharge, but the effect of age alone on *improvement* in functioning, after adjustment for level of functioning on admission, was small and accounted for less than 2% of variation. Moreover, there is evidence demonstrating that age interacts with other factors to determine outcome; Kalra (1994), using a high threshold of 75 years to differentiate young from old, found that the younger survivors achieved better outcomes than older survivors when treated on specialist stroke units, but not when treated on general wards. Black-Schaffer and Winston (2004) reviewed 13 studies examining the influence of age on outcome and noted that results were not consistent. Black-Schaffer and Winston's own study of nearly 1000 patients aged from 20 to 98 found that younger stroke patients showed greater improvement in functional independence and were 30% more likely to return home than older patients, but this may have been influenced by younger patients receiving, on average, 23 days longer hospital treatment than older patients. Also, the relationship between age and outcome did not appear in subgroups with milder strokes. The quality of life of stroke survivors has been variously found to increase with age, decrease with age or be unaffected by age (Bays, 2001b). However, fewer studies have found higher quality of life in older patients than vice versa, and a direct comparison of 96 survivors with stroke onset between the ages of 15 and 45 with 160 matched survivors with stroke after 45 years showed that younger survivors had a higher quality of life when assessed one to five years after stroke. Moreover, quality of life was affected by different factors in the two age groups. In the both age groups, quality of life was associated with unemployment, motor impairment, aphasia, dysarthria, dysaphagia and Rankin score, while in older adults quality of life was associated with a range of additional factors including poor economic status, supratentorial versus infratentorial stroke, anterior versus posterior circulation stroke, diabetes mellitus, visual field defects, the presence of post-stroke seizures and depression (Kim, Choi-Kwon, Kwon, Lee, Park & Seo, 2005).

Experiences of young survivors

At an average interval of six years after stroke, the overall quality of life of a sample of 190 young stroke patients was moderately lower than that of age- and gender-matched controls drawn from the general population (Naess, Waje-Andreassen, Thomassen, Nyland & Myhr, 2006), and the domains of physical functioning, general health and social integration showed the greatest differences. Depression, fatigue and being unemployed showed the largest associations with reduced quality of life in the stroke survivors.

Teasell *et al.* (2000) studied 83 stroke patients under 50 years of age admitted consecutively to a Canadian stroke rehabilitation unit. The statistics produced by this study (Table 21.2) make salutary reading, and highlight the issues faced by this group. Staff were asked to rate the survivors' psychological problems and reported high rates of depression (47%) and anxiety (48%). The anxiety mainly focussed on work, but also related to recovery and childcare. Significant numbers of survivors exhibited denial (23%) and anger/frustration/hostility (31%); conflict with the spouse was common (38%), as was conflict with children (22%). Other consequences of stroke reported by Teasell *et al.* (2000) are shown in Table 21.2.

Kersten *et al.* (2002) provided general information about the experience of stroke survivors less than 65 years of age. This study analysed 315 questionnaire replies from survivors who had had strokes over a year before (median three years). Their assessment covered mobility and access, activities of daily life, social activity, employment, social status, finances, family, sex, voluntary organisations, service uptake and unmet needs. They found that 65% of those working before the stroke had to stop work altogether, and 14% reduced working hours. About 64% of the respondents reported difficulties with sex, which is much higher than in the general population where rates are around 40% for women and 30% for men (Laumann, Paik & Rosen, 1999). The results of a similar study by Low, Kersten, Ashburn, George and McLellan (2003) were concordant with those of Kersten *et al.* (2002) with regard to the experiences of young strokes. Keppel and Crowe (2000) found that body image declined following stroke in a group of 40 young men and women with a mean age of 36.7 years. This decline was most marked in those with left hemisphere strokes and was associated with a reduction in physical and global measures of self-esteem.

Table 21.2   Consequences of Stroke for Young Survivors (n = 83). Summarized from Teasell *et al.* (2000)

18.1% could not return to their original home, and 4.8% required placement with professional care.

77% were employed or students, but only 20.3% returned to work.

Only 9.4% of those in full-time employment were able to return to work.

66% had spouses at the time of the stroke, but 14.5% of these were separated within three/months of discharge.

Several in-depth qualitative studies have extended and complemented the picture emerging from the questionnaire and rating studies reviewed above. These revealed wishes, feelings and priorities of survivors and carers as well as their experiences. Roding, Lindstrom, Malm and Ohman (2003) interviewed two women and three men aged 37–54 one to two years after a first stroke. Their findings paint a graphic picture of the difficulties faced by young stroke survivors. The core theme in the accounts was 'frustrated', and there were two subthemes. 'The paralysed every day' referred to the omnipresent fatigue that affected everyday activities, work, family and social life, and in one case sexual function. This 'psychological paralysis' also influenced gender roles, particularly the roles of mother, father, provider and housekeeper. However, not all was negative, and some survivors developed new perspectives and new roles that helped them to adjust. A second theme was 'outside and invisible' and revolved around lack of information about prognosis and rehabilitation, poor motivation for rehabilitation due to the lack of personally relevant goals, a shortage of activities relevant to their needs and life stage and a sense that 'invisible' cognitive deficits were not given sufficient priority. Roding *et al.* (2003) used a very small sample, so the generality of the results may be questioned, but there is corroboration from other studies, and also a follow-up study reported in Roding (2009) and Roding, Glader, Malm and Lindstrom (2010). This study used a questionnaire to survey 1068 survivors on the Swedish stroke register aged between 18 and 55 years. The results showed that about 35% could not return to work, and that more than half perceived themselves to have enduring physical and cognitive disabilities, with women feeling more impaired than men. A total of 53% were dissatisfied with life after stroke, and impaired ability to concentrate was associated with this in both men and women, and not having a partner and not working were also associated with low satisfaction in men. Stone (2005), in an international sample of females with early strokes, also highlighted the particular issues arising from the 'invisibility' of disabilities which can predispose colleagues, family or friends to discount, ignore or even deny the 'authenticity' of the survivor's limitations. Objective evidence for cognitive difficulties in younger stroke survivors (under 45 at the time of stroke) is provided by Cao, Ferrari, Patella, Marra and Rasura (2007) in a study comparing the performance on neuropsychological tests of young stroke survivors 6–12 months after stroke with matched controls. The authors noted the marked contrast between the good recovery of function and mobility in the stroke survivors and the poor recovery of cognition. Edwards, Hahn, Baum and Dromerick (2006a) corroborated these finding in people with mild strokes and concluded that life satisfaction in this group was affected by more subtle impairments, including impaired executive function, attention and other neurological deficits. In young people with mild strokes, the rapid recovery of overt, noticeable physical functions may create a false impression of generalised recovery that is not paralleled in the less obvious cognitive domain.

A review of 78 studies of young strokes (Daniel, Wolfe, Busch & McKevitt, 2009), included studies using both qualitative and quantitative methods and highlighted reports of family, childcare, sexual, marital problems and financial difficulties in most of the studies that considered these aspects, and also noted that these problems were frequently attributed to the stroke. However, the percentage of survivors reporting problems varied considerably across studies and areas; from 5% to 54% for general family problems, 5% to 76% for sexual problems and 24% to 33% for financial problems. Four of the nine studies that examined social and leisure activities reported decreases ranging from 15% to 79%. A synthesis of four qualitative studies proposed that the experience of young stroke survivors may be encompassed by three overarching domains; 'disorientation' due to the sudden effects of stroke; 'disrupted sense of self' due to changed self-perception and loss of control, which may in turn lead to changed priorities, and finally 'roles and relationships' which frequently change due to dependency and impaired functioning (Lawrence, 2010).

Interpretation of studies of experiences

Taken together, the quantitative and qualitative studies paint a rather stark picture. Younger stroke survivors share much in common with their older counterparts, but also have special problems and needs, both practical and psychological. Some of these stem from the life stage and life tasks facing younger people with strokes: career development, child bearing and/or rearing and caring for aged parents. Others revolve around their own expectations and the normative expectations of peers with regard to engagement in social and leisure activities, employment and sexuality. The effects of the stroke may cut off a young person from peer social contact and enjoyment through sporting and physical recreations. Moreover, stroke is perceived as a disease of old age; for many people the only experience of stroke will have been in an aged grandparent or parent, where it may have led to placement in a nursing home or been the proximal cause of death. Consequently, young survivors face the added psychological task of reconciling the perceived incongruity of suffering an older person's disease at an early age (Stone, 2005). Specific issues for younger survivors are listed in Table 21.3.

Services for young stroke survivors

Young stroke survivors' access to components of stroke care, such as specialist stroke units, and their time with professional staff differ sharply between countries and world regions, as do their fatality rates and functional outcomes (Bhalla, Grieve, Rudd & Wolfe, 2008). The UK 'National Stroke Guidelines' (Royal College of Physicians, 2008a) acknowledged that younger stroke survivors have special, different needs and that 'Some younger adults feel that general

Table 21.3 Issues for Young Stroke Survivors

- Altered identity as a 'young' person
- Childcare responsibilities
- Employment needs for the survivor and their partner or carer
- Demands of the extended family (e.g. surviving dependent parents)
- 'Hidden' cognitive difficulties that impact on age-appropriate activities
- The particular impact of fatigue on tasks and activities expected of younger people
- Altered and less favourable body image
- Issues with sexual activity
- The impact of disabilities on partially fulfilled goals and life plans; the sense of lack of fulfilment
- The impact of the stroke on age-appropriate leisure and recreational activities and the social contact these afford
- Achieving an understanding of the meaning of stroke for younger people

stroke services, of which the majority of users are older adults, do not meet their needs' (p.32). The guidelines recommended that the particular needs of this group are considered, especially vocational rehabilitation and childcare, and that services are 'provided in an environment suited to their specific social needs' (p.32). In effect, this means a specialist neurological rehabilitation service with a focus on people of working age. There have also been calls for age-specific rehabilitation for young stroke survivors that does not involve separate units but nevertheless takes account of their employment and family circumstances and has links to vocational, educational and rehabilitation resources (Burgess & Mooney, 2006). Despite these exhortations, national stroke strategies around the world do not recommend specialist care services for young strokes, for example the European Stroke Initiative Executive Committee and EUSI Writing Committee (Hack, Kaste, Bogousslavsky, Brainin, Chamorro, Lees *et al.*, 2003), National Stroke Foundation (of Australia) (2005, 2010) and Canadian Stroke Strategy (Lindsay, Bayley, Hellings, Hill, Woodbury & Phillips, 2008). Consequently young stroke survivors receive treatment within stroke care services in which the majority of patients are over 65.

Research into the comparative experiences of younger and older stroke survivors *in the same service* is almost entirely absent, so studies that appear to demonstrate higher levels of unmet needs and dissatisfaction with services in young survivors may reflect difficulties with specific services rather than age-specific effects. However, the generality of this finding across many services suggests that there are age-specific differences in response to services. One study that did compare young and old people in a single service used a population attending a neurovascular clinic for people with TIAs or mild strokes (Kee, Brooks & Bhalla, 2009). They also used a high age threshold of 75 years to define 'older' and reported no difference in appointment times, preventative treatments offered, or rates of receiving CT scans. However, the younger people were more often given lifestyle advice about diet and weight, they were CT scanned sooner, and more of them received MRI scans and carotid Doppler investigations, but older people received carotid endarterectomy more rapidly. Kersten *et al.* (2002) compared two age groups (18–45 and 46–65) of community living stroke survivors in the United Kingdom and found that younger survivors had high levels of unmet needs (median 2), with the most common being personalised information about their stroke (45%,) assistance with finances (24%), help with noncare activities (19%), intellectual fulfilment (17%), assistance with adaptations and vehicles (both 16%) and social contact (15%). Those with impaired mobility and those who did not return to work reported more unmet needs. The younger group had more unmet needs in relation to holidays, intellectual fulfilment and family support, despite having the same number of unmet needs overall. On the positive side, this study found that GP services were widely used by their informants: 77% had consulted within the 12 months before the survey, 24% had utilised third sector stroke organisations (e.g. Different Strokes and The Stroke Association) and 15% to 38% received specialist rehabilitation input, with physiotherapy being the most frequent. In a study with a similar sample, Low *et al.* (2003) reported no difference in the total number of unmet needs between the same age groups (18–45 and 46–65), but did find even higher levels of unmet needs overall (median 5), and higher levels in the younger group in two of the areas identified by Kersten et al. (2002), that is, intellectual fulfilment and family support. Unfortunately, these two studies drew participants from several different services and did not report the service composition of the two age groups separately, so differences in the services they were drawn from could account for the age differences. Banks and Pearson (2003) examined responses to service provision using multimethod research to inform service development. The study was designed to cover the chronological sequence from stroke onset to returning to the community and 'moving on'. The study included 50 young stroke survivors (18–49 years old) and their partners, relatives or carers. Interviews and standard questionnaires were given twice, at 3–6 months and again at 9–15 months post discharge. The participants also kept diaries, and stroke care health professionals who supported the survivors were also interviewed. Many of the issues reported by the young survivors echoed those of older people with strokes: service variation, poor communication, lack of personalised information, lack of understanding of effects of stroke on patient and family, low involvement in decision making, gaps in post-discharge support and gaps in community support. However, a number of issues specific to the younger stroke group also emerged: problems with receiving care within services for older adults; difficulties with employment, family and other responsibilities; the need for information and support with regard to retraining, employment, welfare benefits, demands of childcare and employment for carers.

Bendz (2003) interviewed and examined the case notes of 15 stroke survivors, six women and nine men, all aged under 65 years. Average age is not reported, but the attributions for quotations indicate that most were in their later 50s or early 60s. Interviews took place at three, six and 12 months after stroke. The results suggested that rehabilitation staff in particular may not be attuned to the concerns and needs of stroke survivors aged under 65; while the survivors were preoccupied with loss of control, fatigue and fear of another stroke, the staff notes suggested a focus upon functional deficits and training. Morris, Payne and Lambert (2007) conducted qualitative analyses of separate focus groups of survivors and staff, and also identified differences between staff and survivors' perceptions of needs. This study included older as well as younger survivors, suggesting that this disparity is not unique to young survivors. Roding *et al.*'s (2003) informants were particularly vocal about services, and were critical of the lack of age-appropriate activities and environments and the lack of understanding of survivors' needs in the way that professionals formulated their problems and defined their rehabilitation goals. Despite their concerns, the informants, as in other studies, remained positive about individual staff and their commitment to help and provide care.

In summary, negative evaluations of services by younger stroke survivors may be partly attributable to:

- care within older adult services having been experienced as inappropriate,
- a perceived lack of age-appropriate goals and activities,
- feeling that the environment was not appropriate for younger people,
- feeling that professionals were not aware of the needs of younger people, and
- a sense of isolation from younger peers and lack of peer support.

Psychological consequences of stroke at an early age

The dissatisfaction and distress arising from the experiences of young stroke survivors in health services may not be entirely attributable to service shortfalls, and may be partly psychological in origin. Self-identity, or social-identity, is the way that a person views and experiences themselves and their relationships with significant others and social groups (Tajfel & Turner, 1979). It should not be confused with self-esteem, which is more narrowly focussed on the valence (positive or negative) of a person's view of themselves, and may be seen as a self-referent aspect of mood. Identity is a general, central aspect of psychological adjustment, and perceived discrepancy between the self before brain injury and after brain injury is significantly correlated with subjective distress (Cantor, Ashman, Schwartz, Gordon, Hibbard, Brown *et al.*, 2005). It is also an important factor in the efforts of brain-injured people to make sense of themselves and their circumstances (Gracey, Palmer, Rous, Psaila, Shaw, O'Dell *et al.*, 2008), and continuity in self-identity has been demonstrated to impact the psychological well-being of stroke survivors (Haslam, Holme, Haslam, Iyer, Jetten & Williams, 2008). Therefore, the distress exhibited by young stroke survivors may be exacerbated by threats to self-identity and a perceived self-discrepancy that result from the occurrence of an illness that is associated with old age and their being treated in services used predominantly by older adults. It should be noted, however, that not all psychological change resulting from stroke is detrimental to adjustment; positive gains were noted in the accounts of stroke survivors reviewed in chapter 1, and there is evidence that at least some survivors experience what has been described as 'post traumatic growth' (Gangstad *et al.*, 2009).

An important aspect of identity is self-efficacy, a person's belief about their capability to perform actions that have potentially important outcomes. Dixon, Thornton and Young (2007) interviewed 24 neurological patients, including eight with stroke, aged under 60, and found several ways in which they understood their own and others' roles in relation to rehabilitation: independence and self-reliance were important, as were motivational attributes such as determination and pushing limits. Monitoring progress and acknowledging improvements were also seen as important. Professionals and rehabilitation processes were perceived as vital factors influencing self-efficacy, as were vicarious experiences obtained via contact with other patients. However, a singular feature of the results was the way in which a higher order understanding of the purpose of rehabilitation influenced perceptions and adjustment. This may be characterised by the contrast between the view of rehabilitation as a process that leads to 'restitution' of former life, and the view of rehabilitation as a process that enables and supports adaptation, adjustment and change to meet the demands of new circumstances. Those survivors who viewed rehabilitation in terms of adaptation were considered to be better adapted and less prone to disappointment, and to hold views that were more congruent with the aims of professionals.

Implications for psychological support for young strokes

There are currently no evidence-based interventions specifically designed for young stroke survivors. However, a few general recommendations can be made on the basis of the evidence reviewed above, and these are summarised in Table 21.3. Caring for young children, relationships with spouse, sexuality, invisible cognitive disabilities, fatigue that affects engagement in activities, loss of employment, reduced intellectual fulfilment and financial problems seem to be especially salient practical issues for young stroke survivors. Addressing these adequately requires not only skilled therapists, but also networking with non-healthcare agencies such as employers, social services, job centres, marital counselling services (e.g. Relate) and community-based education or leisure facilities. Second, young stroke survivors experience major threats to their self-identity through being isolated from their peers, being unable to meet normal expectations for the leisure and employment activities of young people, having a reduced sense of self-efficacy due to their disabilities and restrictions, experiencing a sharp discontinuity between their pre-stroke self and their current self and finally having what is perceived as an 'old person's disease'. Young survivors should be afforded opportunities for psychologically oriented counselling and support when well-being is affected by a change in identity and a sense of discontinuity. Finally, young stroke survivors require help to understand the wider goal of rehabilitation as a process of adjustment and adaptation to changed capabilities and circumstances rather than simply the 'restitution' of their former patterns of activity. Peer support is widely employed by voluntary stroke groups such as Different Strokes to assist the adjustment of stroke survivors, but it has been only sparsely researched, and its benefits for stroke survivors are not fully established. However, it is included in the National Stroke Strategy for England (Department of Health, 2008), and there is some evidence for its effectiveness in supporting the psychological well-being of stroke carers (see the 'Helping Stroke Survivors Return to Work' section in this chapter.)

Work after stroke

General considerations

The total economic cost of stroke to the UK economy has been estimated as exceeding £8.9 billion per year (Saka, McGuire & Wolfe, 2009), and about £2.2 billion is due to loss of work and productivity and benefit payments. In addition to its economic importance, the benefit of work for individual health and well-being has been recognised (Waddell & Burton, 2006). This thinking now underpins the development of government policy (Black, 2008) and has led to funding for measures to bring people back into the workforce or maintain them in work. Waddell and Burton (2006) concluded that work is important as a source of income essential for material well-being and participation in society, it also meets psychosocial needs and helps in developing and maintaining individual identity, social roles and social status and finally it is associated with physical and mental health and longevity. Conversely, worklessness is associated with greater mortality, poorer mental and physical health and greater use of healthcare resources. There is, moreover, a consensus that sick and disabled people generally benefit from returning to work or remaining in work since work:

- is therapeutic;
- helps to promote recovery and rehabilitation;
- leads to better health outcomes;
- minimises the harmful physical, mental and social effects of long-term sickness absence;
- reduces the risk of long-term incapacity;
- promotes full participation in society, independence and human rights;
- reduces poverty; and
- improves quality of life and well-being (Waddell & Burton, 2006).

Work and young stroke survivors

It is not surprising that employment issues are a singular concern of younger, working-age stroke survivors. Work, or the potential to work, is valued and is a salient issue, even for those not working prior to their stroke (Alaszewski, Alaszewski, Potter & Penhale, 2007; Corr & Wilmer, 2003), and not having work after stroke is often perceived as a major problem (Corr & Wilmer, 2003). Many young stroke survivors will have been in work at the time of the stroke and, perhaps just as important, so will their partners. For some, the stroke may present an opportunity to change lifestyle, take early or medical retirement or explore eligibility for age-related benefits, such as the disability living allowance. For others, particularly those with dependent children, these routes may not be an option, and there may be significant pressure to return to work. Rates of return to work after stroke are difficult to gauge accurately due to differences in data collection methods. A review (Treger, Shames, Giaquinto & Ring, 2007) reported rates ranging from 14% to 73% with a median value of around 50% in 16 studies conducted in 12 developed countries. Most of those returning to work did so quickly, usually in 3–6 months, but there were reports of a second peak at 12–18 months, perhaps at a time when the consequences of long-term unemployment begin to impact. Daniel *et al.* (2009) reviewed 70 studies of stroke in working-age adults and found the mean percentage returning to work to be 44% (range 0 to 100%) across the studies. Three studies in this review that specifically examined return to work over a six- to 12-month period found the rate to be slightly over 50%.

Several studies have attempted to discover factors that influence return to work after stroke. Black-Schaffer and Osberg (1990) studied return to work at 3.1 months after discharge in a group of 79 survivors who had received a vocational stroke rehabilitation programme. Multiple regression analysis showed that successful return was predicted by absence of dysphasia, shorter rehabilitation stay, higher functioning on discharge (Barthel Index) and low alcohol intake prior to the stroke. A study of 183 stroke survivors of working age in Japan (Saeki, Ogata, Okubo, Takahashi & Hoshuyama, 1995) found that return to work was influenced by physical disability (weakness) and apraxia, as well as type of employment; blue-collar workers returned sooner, but white-collar workers were more likely to return to work in the long-term. Saeki and Hachisuka (2004) confirmed these findings and also demonstrated that stroke location was not predictive of the resumption of work. Similarly, Gabriele and Renate (2009) found that functional ability was the strongest predictor of return to work at 12 months, but also reported an association between higher quality of life and return to work. A review of studies by Saeki (2000) also concluded that functional ability and disability were major factors in return to work, as was length of hospital stay.

Neau, Ingrand, Mouille-Brachet, Rosier, Couderq, Alvarez *et al.* (1998) conducted a study in France of 71 consecutive admissions of young stroke patients (aged 15–45) who had been discharged from hospital for at least a year. They found an exceptionally high proportion returned to work (73%), but 26% changed aspects of their occupation, and post stroke depression occurred in 48% and was more prevalent amongst those who did not return of work. Glozier Hackett, Parag and Anderson (2008) studied young stroke patients in Auckland, New Zealand and found that 53% returned to full-time employment after their first stroke event. As in the study by Neau *et al.* (1998), being free from mental illness was associated with resumption of work, and having full-time paid employment prior to stroke also predicted return to work.

Vestling, Tufvesson and Iwarsson (2003) examined medical records and gave questionnaires to 120 stroke survivors, finding that 41% returned to work, although often with new employers and different working hours. Factors associated with successful return were the ability to walk, white-collar work and preserved cognitive abilities. Return to work was associated with higher well-being and life satisfaction. The results of Vestling *et al.* (2003) are concordant with those of Leung and Man (2005) in Hong Kong. This study included 79 brain injured people,45% with cerebral haemorrhage. Of these, 50% returned to work and return to work in the same or a different job was associated with overall disability score, the attention subtest of the neuro-cognitive status examination and type of pre-stroke employment (manual workers were less likely to return). A review of earlier studies (Saeki, 2000) also concluded that impaired cognition and memory restricted return to work. Finally, two very large scale surveys based on stroke registers have provided data on return to work. A survey in Sweden (Lindstrom, Roding & Sundelin, 2009) included 1631 stroke survivors age 18–55 years and obtained 1068 self-report questionnaire responses. They reported high rates of return to work of 65%, and that higher socioeconomic status, support from others, and a positive attitude to work were most strongly associated with return. High-level physical ability (being able to run) was predictive of return, and self-reported ability to concentrate was also associated with return, but less strongly than the other factors. Busch, Coshall, Heuschmann, McKevitt and Wolfe (2009) conducted a survey of return to work with 266 survivors on the South London Stroke Register who had been working prior to their stroke. Functional level (Barthel Index) at one week and one year was the strongest predictor of return to work, but, black ethnicity, female gender and being older were also associated with lower odds of returning to work. Despite the strong association between functional level and return to work, 53% of those classified as independent on the Barthel Index did not resume work. The role of male gender in earlier return to work has also been reported by Saeki & Toyonaga (2010), but age is not consistently associated with return to work across studies (Saeki, 2000). In their document 'Getting back to work after a stroke,' the Stroke Association and Different Strokes reported a questionnaire survey by the 'Work After Stroke Project' (Barker, 2006; Different Strokes, undated). A total of 3,000 stroke survivors from the Different Strokes' mailing list were contacted and there were 672 replies. The low response rate may have introduced bias, so the results cannot be generalised to all stroke survivors, but they are probably illustrative of the views of a large 'concerned' minority. Forty-three percent had not been able to return to work and 31% had worked since their stroke. Of those replying 75% said they wanted to return to work, but 48% of these (36% of the total) felt that they could not. The observed proportion returning to work could well be due to the self-selected sample that responded to the questionnaire; the same document reported a return to work rate of only 17% in another less selective sample of 339 stroke survivors in London. Despite being higher than the 9.4% figure for return to work reported six years earlier by Teasell *et al.* (2000), the large proportion who want to return to work, but cannot still represents a major unresolved problem. Reasons given for not returning to work (respondents could cite more than one) included; forced to retire by employer (18.5%), can't meet expectations (30.2%), can't drive/use public transport (30.6%), afraid of losing benefits (31.9%), not fit enough to work (60.7%), can no longer do previous job (62.0%).

Questionnaire studies, such as those described above, do not necessarily provide information about issues that are particularly salient for the target group. Several studies have used qualitative methods to explore the return to work of stroke survivors. Locka, Jordan, Bryanc and Maxima (2005) studied focus groups of 37 stroke survivors and 12 carers recruited through the UK-based 'Different Strokes' support organisation. The participants were highly variable in terms of time since stroke, with an average of 3.9 years, and information about level of disability and type of stroke was not given. They found that 52% returned to work when voluntary work was included, and four principal themes of relevance to work emerged; rehabilitation process, employer agency, social and structural factors and personal factors. Rehabilitation process was seen as being focussed on minimal recovery, time-limited and not sufficiently oriented to employment. The Disability Discrimination Act (1995) and sick leave arrangements were considered to be facilitating factors in the employer domain, but inflexibility and negative attitudes were barriers. Employers' ignorance about stroke and its effects was another barrier. Participants felt that the benefits system was a structural factor that militated against return to work and that information about support and opportunities for returning to work were limited. Fatigue was seen as the major personal factor in returning to work (as also observed by Roding *et al.*, 2003), and cognitive impairments were also implicated. Locka *et al.* (2005) also identified the intrinsic rewards of work as an incentive for survivors to take voluntary employment, and this accords with the results of a Scandinavian study (Vestling, Ramel & Iwarsson, 2005) which reported that those who valued the intrinsic rewards of work were also the most satisfied. Some of these findings were also echoed by another Scandinavian study (Medin, Barajas & Ekberg, 2006), in which six young stroke survivors (aged 30–65) were interviewed. As in the Locka *et al.* (2005) study, the participants felt that rehabilitation emphasised physical recovery, and low priority was given to returning to work and this did not meet their expectations or needs in rehabilitation. Several responded to the shortfall in rehabilitation by taking control and pursuing their own goals, but also acknowledged the importance of family support and support from coworkers.

Another qualitative study with 43 survivors under 60 (Alaszewski *et al.*, 2007) used diaries and four interviews conducted over an 18 month period. Participants who were working at the time of their stroke were included along with some who were not, and around 40% of those who had been in work had not returned by the end of the study. Returning to work was a salient issue for the participants and a benchmark for successful recovery. All the participants valued work and its benefits, including those not working before their stroke. They saw return to work as hinging upon the relative impact of barriers and facilitators; stress and its possible consequences for health was one such factor, as were past experiences with working or not working and severe residual disabilities which could make working impossible. Flexible, sympathetic work environments and practices, and supportive social networks helped in returning to work.

Koch, Egbert, Coeling and Ayers (2005) also used interviews to explore the work-related experiences of 12 right hemisphere stroke survivors and their primary carers, at least six months after discharge from hospital. The stroke precipitated employment changes for all, and these employment changes had a substantial psychosocial impact on both the stroke survivor and the carer. Successful return to work was associated with; personal attributes (patience, determination, sense of humour), resources located in families and social networks (support from caregivers, family, and friends), healthcare services (emotional and instrumental support from healthcare professionals), and attributes of the employment itself (employer flexibility). Weakness, fatigue and cognitive impairments were cited as barriers to return. A similar small-scale retrospective interview study of 13 stroke survivors, 24 to 64 years old and including six females, all of whom were working at the time of their stroke, identified a number of salient areas (Gilworth, Sansam & Kent, 2009). Concern about symptoms that prevented working was a prominent theme. Another theme was the timing of the return to work and the guidance and advice received about this. Once back at work, support, including support from colleagues and managers, was a major factor. Several participants discussed the challenges and benefits of changing careers, while others did not attempt to return to work, and in some cases felt resentful and demoralised as a consequence. In all stages, information and involvement in decision making were seen as crucial.

On the basis of the research reviewed above, the positive and negative factors associated with return to work are summarised in Table 21.4.

Helping stroke survivors return to work: the evidence and its implications

It is evident that work is a major issue for younger stroke survivors and their carers. Consequently, survivor-centred rehabilitation should adapt goals to meet their needs and aspirations in this area. There are several general

Table 21.4 Facilitators and Barriers for Return to Work

Facilitators	Barriers
Positive personal attributes (patience, determination)	Impaired functional abilities
Support from families and social networks	Cognitive impairments
Support from healthcare professionals	Fatigue
Sympathetic, flexible employer	More severe weakness and paralysis
Employment tasks that can be flexibly configured	Previous poor experiences with work
Previous positive experience of work	Perceived stressfulness of work
Disability legislation and statutory sick leave	Inflexible attitudes of employers
Valuing work and its intrinsic rewards	Benefits systems that encourage nonreturn to work
Preserved cognitive ability	Lack of understanding of stroke by employers
Being able to walk	Lack of information about returning to work
Having an office-based rather than a manual job	Psychological disorders
Support from workmates	Lack of employment focus in rehabilitation

employment-related considerations and influential factors that those involved in service development and rehabilitation should consider (Table 21.5). It is likely that the factors illustrated in Table 21.5 interact, and case studies and in-depth interviews (Chan, 2008; Corr & Wilmer, 2003) illustrate how outcomes depended on the interplay of individual factors such as the perception of work, hidden psychosocial needs, disaffection with alternatives to not working, financial incentives, and job characteristics.

In addition to the recommendations in Table 21.5, Wolfenden and Grace (2009) made 13 recommendations for facilitating the return to work of high-functioning working-age stroke survivors. These are based on a review of the literature and the experiences of one of the authors who was a stroke survivor. These recommendations call for education to raise awareness of the aspirations of stroke survivors, a greater focus on rehabilitation directed towards nonmedical needs such as returning to work, and for rehabilitation to continue for longer after discharge. They also target the workplace and propose that greater consideration is given to the special needs of the survivor.

The recommendations in Table 21.5 do not map clearly on the current roles and responsibilities of multiprofessional stroke rehabilitation teams in the United Kingdom, and involve areas of expertise and a degree of inter-agency working that has not been developed within health services. One promising approach is the development of vocational rehabilitation programmes designed for those with neurological impairments, and encompassing the needs of young

Table 21.5 Service Issues in Promoting Return to Work

Consideration or factor	Evidence	Implications
A very high proportion of young survivors wish to return to work. Employment is a central life role, bringing intrinsic rewards. Return to work is associated with better life satisfaction and quality of life.	Alaszewski, *et al.*, 2007; Vestling *et al.*,2003, 2005; Corr and Wilmer, 2003	• Consider employment in rehabilitation goal planning for all working-age stroke survivors.
A significant proportion of those working before stroke will not return to work. Many of these will want to return.	Teasell *et al.*, 2000; Koch *et al.*, 2005; Kersten *et al.*, 2002; Barker, 2006; Glozier *et al.*, 2008; Corr and Wilmer, 2003	• Psychological therapy should consider this as a major and sudden 'loss'. • Such survivors and their carers may require help with adjustment to new circumstances. • Encourage survivors to explore creative approaches to developing alternative activities.
Many survivors return to different types of work, including voluntary work.	Locka *et al.*, 2005; Kersten *et al.*, 2002; Vestling, 2003; Neau *et al.*, 1998; Gilworth *et al.*, 2009	• Provide vocational advice on suitable types of work. • Stroke service should network with agencies that find employment, retrain or support employment. • Encourage flexibility and exploration of options in survivors. • Develop awareness of the Disability Discrimination Act and flexible provisions for disabled employees.

(Continued)

Table 21.5 (*Continued*)

Consideration or factor	Evidence	Implications
A positive attitude to return to work is important.	Lindstrom et al., 2009; Medin et al., 2006; Alaszewski et al., 2007	• Develop connections with potential employers including voluntary organisations. • Individual and group therapeutic interventions to promote the benefits of work and influence attitudes may be beneficial.
Social, demographic and economic factors are important.	Wide variation in return rates between different countries (Treger et al., 2007). Socioeconomic status predicts return to work (Lindstrom et al., 2009). Gender, ethnicity and age are associated with return (Busch et al., 2009; Saeki & Toyonaga, 2010)	• Professionals require good awareness of national employment disability legislation, benefits systems and employment practices. • Individual demographic and socioeconomic factors and should be considered when planning support.
Employers' attitude and support are important determinants of return.	Lindstrom et al., 2009; Medin et al., 2006; Corr and Wilmer, 2003; Alaszewski et al., 2007; Koch et al., 2005	• Advocacy should be available for those who wish to return to work. • Network with employers and/or human resources departments to build support for return to work.
Residual disabilities, physical ability and especially weakness are related to return.	Black-Schaffer and Osberg, 1990; Saeki et al., 1995; Saeki, 2000; Saeki and Hachisuka, 2004; Saeki and Toyonaga, 2010; Koch et al., 2005; Lindstrom et al., 2009; Corr and Wilmer, 2003; Gilworth et al., 2009	• Return to original employment may not be realistic in all cases. • Professionals should provide realistic feedback, considering the survivors readiness to accept it. Premature pessimistic prognosis should be avoided. • Flexible, phased return may be helpful. • Long-term support may be required.

Fatigue is an important factor in return.	Roding *et al.*, 2003; Locka *et al.*, 2005; Koch *et al.*, 2005; Corr and Wilmer, 2003	• Recognise fatigue as a common barrier to returning to work. • Consider fatigue management as part of psychological therapy. • Plan return to work allowing for effects of fatigue. A phased return may be helpful.
'Hidden' cognitive deficits are a concern for survivors.	Saeki, 2000; Roding *et al.*, 2003; Locka *et al.*, 2005; Koch *et al.*, 2005; Stone, 2005; Lindstrom *et al.*, 2009; Vestling *et al.*, 2003; Leung and Man, 2005	• Cognitive assessment for all intending to return to work. • Consider cognitive rehabilitation. • Consider 'information prosthesis' and compensatory measures (diaries, pagers and electronic aids). • Incorporate consideration of cognition into psychological therapy to develop insight and promote adjustment.
Stress due to work is a factor when survivors consider return.	Alaszewski *et al.*, 2007	• Concern about work stress and its possible effects on health should be addressed through psychological therapy. • A cognitive behaviour approach may be helpful in addressing unrealistic anxieties.
Assets and resources are influential factors in return.	Alaszewski *et al.*, 2007; Kock, 2005; Locka, 2005	• Encourage survivors and carers to 'audit' their assets and incorporate into their plans. • Assets may include family and social networks, healthcare agencies, employers (managers and human resources/personnel occupational health).
Psychological disorders are a factor in stroke patients' return to work.	Glozier *et al.*, 2008; Neau *et al.*, 1998	• Offer treatment for any psychological conditions such as depression, anxiety or PTSD.

stroke survivors. Radford and Walker's (2008) review of work and stroke included studies of vocational rehabilitation for brain injured people and concluded that it has considerable potential both in terms of individual and cost benefit, but that its application to stroke is under-researched and current service provision is patchy, poorly organised and meets only a fraction of the need.

One further encouraging development, with relevance to the employment of stroke survivors and their carers, is the incorporation of peer support into the 10 point plan and four of the quality markers of the National Stroke Strategy for England (Department of Health, 2007a). Peer support for stroke survivors has not been studied, but it has been used successfully with stroke carers (Stewart *et al.*, 1998; Hartke & King, 2003), and been shown to be beneficial for other health conditions (Doull *et al.*, 2008; Dennis, 2003). As well as enhancing the experience of new stroke survivors and their carers, participation as a peer supporter fulfils the intrinsic functions of work, and has considerable potential for enhancing quality of life and re-engaging participants in the benefit and challenges of employment (Pillemer, Landreneau & Suitor, 1996; Mowbray, Moxley, Thrasher, Bybee, McCrohan, Harris *et al.*, 1996).

Finally, the use of internet-based resources may help to encourage stroke survivors and inform employers about the potential of stroke survivors through the publication of survivors' stories about their return to work. These resources may also serve to inform survivors, employers and carers about how to approach this goal, how to support survivors, and where to turn for advice and assistance. Such information is published on the Different Strokes website in three 'Returning to Work after Stroke' documents, one for survivors, one for families and friends and one for employers (see http://www.differentstrokes.co.uk).

Experiences of carers of young stroke survivors

Chapter 20 reviews the evidence relating to stroke carers in general, but in the following section some specific issues for carers of young stroke survivors are outlined.

We have seen that the psychological impact of stroke for young stroke survivors differs from that for their older counterparts in several important ways, and we might suspect that the same is true of the carers of younger survivors. Age-comparative research studies of carers are limited and small scale, but there is some evidence that bears this out. Younger carers experienced considerably more lifestyle change and strain, and they engaged in more coping activities and demonstrated less acceptance than older carers (Periard & Ames, 1993). Several studies reviewed by Greenwood *et al.* (2008b) also found greater psychological morbidity in younger carers than in older carers; lower psychological well-being, higher strain and higher burnout risk were all noted. In one study, younger female carers were less satisfied with care and communication with staff than their older counterparts, and younger carers of both genders experienced greater difficulty in talking things over with staff (McKenzie, Perry, Lockhart, Cottee, Cloud & Mann, 2007). There are also demographic differences between young and old stroke survivors that affect patterns of caregiving. Younger survivors are more likely to have living parents who can resume aspects of their former parental caregiving activities. They are also more likely to have a living spouse and less likely to have grown children. Consequently, they will probably have a greater proportion of spouse carers and a much lower proportion of offspring carers than the ratios of 55% and 20%, respectively, that are reported in general population surveys (Hirst, 2002). Young carers are also more likely to become very long-term carers due to the longer life span of survivor and carer, and the role of long-term psychological adjustment is therefore important (Buschenfeld, Morris & Lockwood, 2009).

Several studies have focussed on young carers, or identified them as a separate subgroup, and their findings show considerable overlap and will be discussed together. Banks and Pearson (2004) considered the impact of stroke on the lives of 38 survivors under 50 and their partners 12–15 months after stroke. Forsberg-Warleby, Moller & Blomstrand (2004) studied life satisfaction in partners of stroke survivors at 4–12 months after stroke, but this study was heterogeneous with respect to age because 'young' was defined as under 75. Periard and Ames (1993) grouped a sample of carers into age cohorts, but each cohort contained offspring carers as well as partners and some of the young offspring carers were caring for older survivors. Buschenfeld *et al.* (2009) conducted an in-depth qualitative study of seven spouses of young stroke survivors, aged 49 to 62 between two and seven years post stroke.

Banks and Pearson (2004) and Buschenfeld *et al.* (2009) highlighted changes in roles, responsibilities and the carers' active efforts to adjust and cope with the changes and demands of caring. Buschenfeld *et al.* (2009) also identified the ways in which life changes had enduring effects on the self-image of long-term carers, and found that carers used a number of specific coping mechanisms; recourse to previous experience, comparison with others, problem-focussed coping and social support. Although burden and strain was an enduring theme, some young carers did report positive benefits of caring and eventually achieved a positive psychological adjustment through re-appraisal of their lives. Employment was an important factor for carers in both studies, and was a protective factor for carers, providing respite from caring. One further study (Visser-Meily *et al.*, 2009), although not explicitly designated as a study of young carers, did include a group of 211 spouses with a mean age of only 54 years and followed them up over three-years post-stroke. The results showed a reduction in burden and depression in the post-stroke period, but also a reduction in the harmony of the relationship and in social relationships. This quantitative study also complemented the qualitative findings of Buschenfeld *et al.* (2009) by demonstrating that more active coping and less passive coping was associated with better outcomes for burden, depression, relationship to survivor and social relations.

A stroke in a young person with a young family can create apparently incongruous patterns of parent–child interaction, and result in children adopting precocious caring roles which may impact psychologically on the children (Daniel *et al.*, 2009). Dearden and Becker (1998; 2004) reported studies of over 6,000 young carers ranging from those as young as three years old up to eighteen. This work was not specific to stroke, but contained many findings applicable across health conditions, and many specific findings were congruent with the results of van de Port *et al.*'s (2007) small scale study of 44 children of stroke survivors. In Dearden and Becker's studies, more than half the young carers lived with a lone parent, usually the mother, and therefore most cared for their mothers. The caring tasks encompassed domestic chores (66%), emotional support and supervision (82%), general and nursing-type care (48%), intimate personal care (18%) and care for siblings (11%). Dearden and Beckers' work included many families with nonphysical illness where physical care would not have been required, and therefore more children of stroke victims may provide personal care than the 18% found by Dearden and Becker (1998; 2004). Caring activity was often long-term, with 65% caring for longer than three years and 18% for longer than six years. Time spent caring also increased with age and this increase was more pronounced for girls than boys. In Black and Asian families care was more often provided for extended family members. Caring impacted on the young carers in a number of ways. Some suffered health problems or fatigue as a consequence of the physical demands of their caring role. Dearden and Becker (2004) found a high rate of educational difficulties in young carers, but the proportion with such difficulties declined from 33% to 22% between 1995 and 2003. Restricted social contacts and friends' lack of understanding of their caring roles were additional problems and emotional issues also occurred, centring around fears for the future and parental health, and concerns about the responsibility of caring.

Interventions for carers of young stroke survivors

Carer support has been the subject of recent UK government policy ('Carers at the heart of 21st-century families and communities', Department of Health, 2008a). Several supportive interventions have been developed and evaluated for adult stroke carers; carer education, training and counselling and the provision of family support workers. None have been specifically designed for adult carers of young stroke survivors, and therefore they are reviewed in chapter 20, which considers stroke carers in general.

The United Kingdom policy referred to above does specifically recognise the role of childhood carers and makes funding available to develop services that protect children from unreasonable demands, and to ensure that they are able to develop and thrive. The Department of Health (1996) have formulated practice guidelines for working with young carers as follows.

- Listen to the child and respect their views.
- Allow private time for children who need to talk about their situation.
- Acknowledge that involvement of a young carer is the family's way of coping.
- Acknowledge the parents' strengths.
- Avoid undermining parenting capacity.
- Consider what support of parenting roles is needed. (In the United Kingdom this should form a part of social services assessment).
- Consider the needs of the child arising from their caring role.
- Consider whether caring is impacting on the child's education.
- Consider whether the child's emotional or social development are being impaired.
- Remember children should be able to be children.
- Provide information about support services.

Dependent children

Many young stroke survivors and their spouses have dependent children. The need to consider and care for children while recovering from a serious illness is a major factor in the lives of survivors and their partners. Banks and Pearson (2004) included 22 households with dependent children, and four of Buschenfeld *et al.*'s (2009) seven families had dependent children. In both studies the presence of children in the family added to practical tasks and created responsibilities that were sometimes difficult to fulfil in the context of reduced functioning and the care needs of the stroke survivor. In some families the stroke was a catalyst for a reversal of the roles of the two partners with respect to childcare and employment. For example, in a family where the father worked and the mother cared for children prior to stroke, the father relinquished work and became the children's main carer while the mother obtained employment. Families in these studies also expressed unease about young, dependent children providing care for the survivor, and concern about the effects on their children of firsthand experience of a major and sudden illness. Stroke service professionals tend to be most familiar with the needs and circumstances of older people, who inevitably comprise the majority of their clients. Consequently, they may not be attuned to meeting the needs of parents of young, dependent children. For example, it is not widely appreciated that disabled people with children under 18 years of age in the United Kingdom should be assessed for the support they require to fulfil their parenting needs, as well as the support required to meet their own needs.

One large-scale study by Visser-Meily's group in the Netherlands (Visser-Meily *et al.*, 2005a, 2005b; Visser-Meily & Meijer, 2006; van de Port *et al.*, 2007) investigated the impact of parental stroke on children. The original study enrolled 82 children in 55 two-parent families (mean age 13.3 years and 51% girls). Interviews were conducted and/or psychological measures were taken at four stages after the stroke; as soon as possible after the stroke, two months after discharge from rehabilitation, one year post stroke and three years post stroke. The psychometric measures of children's functioning tapped behaviour problems, depression, health and daily hassles. In order to explore factors predicting the children's adjustment, the characteristics and functioning of the stroke survivor and their spouse were also recorded. The results showed a stark elevation in the frequency of children exhibiting behaviour problems and depression soon after the stroke (54% with elevated scores and 21% in the clinical range) compared with the second assessment (23% with elevated scores, 12% in clinical range) and the third assessment (29% with elevated scores with 20% in the clinical range).The biggest improvement was between the first measurement, soon after the stroke, and the second measurement, 2-months after discharge. The only measure not to show improvement was externalising problem behaviours (delinquent and aggressive behaviours). In general, children with most problems at the first measurement stage continued to show the most problems in the subsequent stages. Depression of the healthy parent at the first measurement period, and their perception of the marital relationship, also predicted children's problem behaviour scores, but surprisingly the seriousness of the stroke was not a significant factor in predicting children's adjustment. One phase of the study, which included children of people with Parkinson's disease as well as stroke, demonstrated that children may continue to be affected by parental distress and relationships for several years, and may continue to experience concerns about the future and harbour feelings of resentment about lack of recognition for their role in supporting parents. These studies found that rehabilitation teams provided support for only 54% of the children, and this support included consultation with rehabilitation specialists or the social worker and attending a therapy day for the parent. Surprisingly, those children with more behaviour problems did not receive more support, but more support was given to children of more disabled parents.

A long-term, three-year follow-up using the same sample as Visser-Meily's earlier studies (van de Port, 2007) focussing on 44 children of young stroke survivors (mean age 47). This study demonstrated that, while most of the children adjusted well, about one third had behaviour problems and clinical or subclinical externalising problems, even after this length of time post-stroke. Girls were more affected by stress than boys, and depression and low life satisfaction in the parent with stroke were associated with stress in the children. In contrast to the findings of detrimental effects, some children also reported long-term positive changes; 56% felt more needed, 72% felt that they had more responsibilities and 81% felt more mature. Moreover, 24% said that parents spent more time with them and 43% felt that their parents were more positive towards them. An unfortunate limitation of all these studies is that there were no matched control groups, while the studies do demonstrate the levels of clinical problems and benefits that can be expected in the children of stroke survivors, they do not tell us by how much they are elevated compared with children of similar parents who have not had a stroke.

Taken together, these findings suggest that screening children and the healthy parent soon after the stroke can identify those most in need of psychological support. It is reassuring that stroke rehabilitation units, in the Netherlands at least, targeted those children with the most disabled parent. However, it is concerning that nearly half the children received no support from the rehabilitation service. It may be that for these children support was available elsewhere, but this point requires further research within relevant countries. It is noteworthy that the National Clinical Stroke Guidelines for the United Kingdom (Royal College of Physicians, 2008a) make no specific recommendations for the care of children of young stroke survivors, although they do recommend considering the childcare needs of younger survivors in section 3.5.1. To date no specific psychological interventions have been developed to support the children of stroke survivors, and further research is clearly needed.

Long-term survivors

People who survive strokes when young may live for many years after their first stroke, and such long-term survival may engender special psychological and social issues that are not faced in the first few years following stroke. These include living with the risk of further strokes, the need for protracted medical investigations and treatments, and implications for social life and employment. These issues, and others, are vividly illustrated in Greg's story, shown in Table 21.6.

The literature contains many studies of 'long-term' stroke survivors and their carers, but the definition of 'long term' is highly variable and can refer to periods from three months to over 20 years after stroke. Even reviews are heterogeneous with regard to the timing of included studies: one review of 23 qualitative studies of 'longer-term' problems for stroke survivors and their carers (Murray, Young, Forster & Ashworth, 2003) included studies that ranged from a few hours after stroke to six years. For the current purposes a period of three years and above will be considered as 'long term', but many studies have broad inclusion criteria (e.g. 1 to 16 years post stroke), so some studies with thresholds of less than three years are included.

Several studies of long-term survival have been published. Two, Drummond, Pearson, Lincoln, and Berman, (2005) and Indredavik, Bakke, Slordahl, Rokseth and Haheim (1999), were 10-year follow-ups of randomised controlled trials comparing outcomes of those who had been treated in stroke units, with the outcomes of those who had been treated on conventional wards. Both studies reported that survival rates were better for those treated on stroke units, and combined risks of death, disability and institutional care were reduced.

Table 21.6   Greg's Story

Strokes that afflict the "younger" person can be both less debilitating from a physical
point of view, and yet more of a psychological problem. In my case, I first suffered a
stroke when I was 14. I remember brushing my school jacket in the morning, when I
suddenly had a severe headache. This rapidly developed on the right-hand side of my
head. I could tell that there was something seriously wrong. I went out into the garden,
sat down and tried to relax. I was quickly losing the use of my right arm, and discovered
that my right leg was also rapidly becoming numb. My mother helped me back indoors.
The doctor was contacted, came, and I heard him say that I had had a stroke. As a result,
I had to immediately go into hospital.

While there I had to have extensive tests. The stroke was in the sub-arachnoid region of
the brain stem. It would be unwise to try any form of treatment, except for a type of
X-ray therapy. I was sent to Velindre Hospital in Cardiff, a specialised cancer hospital,
for the treatment. I had to rest at home for some three months or so. I then returned to
school. I remember telling my headmaster that I had to have my hair long to cover the
bald patches left by the therapy. He was not pleased, and told me so. I think that that
was another sign that the illness problem not only lay in the fact that I had had a serious
physical problem from the stroke, but also that I would also have to cope with a
growing social problem. Most of my school "friends" kept away from me, increasing
the big factor of not having anyone to sit with me and try to overcome the problem. I
had decided to return to school, and try and carry on, but I had to face myself what
problems there are in teenage life.

However, my mother, a widow since I was three, was a wonderful, caring, loving person,
who really helped me overcome the various problems, with her strong determination
that I should deal adequately with them. This showed itself when I suffered a second
stroke during the vacation after my second year at university. Again, it occurred
suddenly, whilst I was reading a newspaper. This time I spent several weeks in severe pain
in bed, because my own doctor was on leave. The replacement said that I would not
suffer another stroke. It was probably stress. My doctor eventually returned, and
confirmed that I had had another stroke. As a consequence, I spent some time in hospital
again, though the consultant did not change his assessment of my condition. I had had a
lumber puncture, and the position was that I would have to lead my life knowing that I
could have more strokes at any time. This was very hard, for anyone leading a normal life,
but for a young man trying to succeed both at university and life itself.

I went to work in London, and whilst there I had the first of a series of minor strokes.
Again, I was told during my stay in St. Bartholomews that it was most unusual for a
person of my age to have a stroke, and it was just bad luck that I had had this recurring
problem. I had little or no sympathy at work because of the illness. I had another full
stroke a year after I returned to Cardiff. I had to recuperate for a few weeks, and spent
some time in hospital. Instead of being given help to recover, and work my way back
gradually, the people at work, again, gave the impression that I was just annoying to
them, and that they had decided that I should "retire" when I had another stroke,
some time later. At the time I had not only the physical aspects of the strokes to contend
with, but also the trauma of such occurrences was difficult to cope with.

I had another minor stroke in the next year, followed by a much more major stroke. While
in hospital, my consultant had suggested that I go to the Royal Hallamshire Hospital in
Sheffield, for a treatment that was called stereotactic radiosurgery. This was 201 laser

Table 21.6 (*Continued*)

beams zeroed in to my brain stem while I lay in a CAT scanner. Two items of interest developed from this, in that six months after the treatment I rapidly developed the physical traits of a person who has suffered from a stroke. This had not happened to me before; I had recovered from the physical effects of each stroke. Now – and the condition is now permanent – I have to essentially stagger around as if I have just had a stroke. However, two years subsequent to the treatment, I had the angiogram to assess whether the treatment had effectively worked, and it had. That was 19 years ago, and I am still enjoying life. I am blinded on the right-hand side in both eyes, and hence cannot drive, and cannot use the right-hand side of my body. I learned to write with my left hand, and in fact I can do most things normally. I feel very fit, and life is most enjoyable. I thank the various people in the health professions who have helped me overcome any difficulties, and especially my mother, without whom my recovery to cope with life in general would not have been possible.

On average, about 80% of the patients had died within ten years, but the impact of stroke on mortality cannot be assessed since many of the participants were elderly when they had strokes, and age-adjusted comparisons with nonstroke populations were not provided.

Gresham, Kelly-Hayes, Wolf, Beiser, Kase and D'Agostino (1998) conducted a 20-year follow-up of a cohort of 147 stroke patients, ten of whom survived for the whole 20-year follow-up period. The mean age at stroke was 56.0 years for those still living, and 66.3 for those who had died. The whole cohort was compared with a group of age and gender-matched nonstroke controls. The stroke patients had an elevated mortality rate over this period, but the independence and mobility of survivors were similar to those of the controls. The numbers were too low for statistical comparison, but there was a trend for stroke patients to have more other illnesses, higher blood pressure and to take more medications. On the positive side, they also used less alcohol and had lower rates of depression. Anderson, Carter, Brownlee, Hackett, Broad & Bonita (2004) studied a cohort of 54 people (average age at stroke 49.1 years) in Auckland, New Zealand, who had survived for at least 21 years post stroke. As in the Gresham study, the stroke patients showed a much higher mortality rate, almost twice the average for age. However, also in accordance with the Gresham study, their health-related quality of life measured over eight domains (physical functioning, role limitations resulting from physical problems, bodily pain, general health, vitality, social functioning, role limitations attributable to emotional problems and mental health) were comparable with those of the general population, with the exception of vitality, which was lower. This contrasts with data from Norway collected at an average of six years after stroke which demonstrated moderately lower quality of life scores in stroke survivors than in matched general population controls (Naess *et al.*, 2006). This difference may reflect positive changes that occur after six years, or variations between the two countries. The elevated mortality rate of stroke patients, even those who had stroke at a young age, is a robust finding (e.g. Dennis, Burn, Sandercock, Bamford, Wade & Warlow, 1993), but the mortality figures for cohorts that had strokes in the 1980s and 1970s may present an overly pessimistic picture. Survival rates may well have improved markedly due to the advent of better standards of secondary prevention, and the availability of new medical approaches to prevention of clotting and the control of blood pressure.

Greveson *et al.* (1991) followed up a large cohort of stroke patients, most of whom lived at home, and reported major service shortfalls. The mean time since stroke was 42 months and most of the survivors were over 60 at the time of the stroke. Over one third of those living at home had not seen their GP for at least 6 months, and GPs were less likely to have seen the more severely disabled survivors. Increased level of dependence of the survivor was not matched by increased service input as might be expected if services were properly targeted. An inevitable consequence of long-term survival is that the information given to survivors and carers during the treatment and its immediate follow-up becomes out-dated. Hare, Rogers, Lester, McManus and Mant (2006) found that long-term survivors and their carers were unaware of relevant services, local support providers, the roles of professionals or where to turn for advice. Similar findings have been reported by Murray *et al.* (2003).

Buschenfeld *et al.* (2009) studied carers of young stroke survivors up to seven years post stroke and noted how families adjusted to a stroke in one of their members. The stroke started a process of active coping and adaptation over a long period. This often involved an extended family, and led to re-constituted family relationships and roles coupled with acceptance of the consequences of the stroke. In some cases there was a positive reappraisal of the outcome and the family's endeavours to adapt and adjust.

Finally, little is known about how long term survivors' experience of the effects of ageing on psychological adjustment and whether the experience of stroke and its treatment earlier in life inoculate or sensitise such people to the inevitable effects of ageing and the onset of other age-related conditions

Psychological support of long-term survivors and their families

The findings of higher mortality rates, that dependence is not correlated with service inputs, and that stroke survivors have low levels of contact with health professionals despite a high prevalence of risk factors, suggests a requirement for increased awareness of the needs of this group by health professionals, and a more proactive approach by the survivors and their families themselves. The theory of planned behaviour (Ajzen, 1985) can be used to develop psychological interventions that raise awareness and increase health-enhancing behaviours in professionals and their patients. This approach identifies attitudes towards the provision of care for a particular group, encouragement and expectations of others, and the degree of perceived control with respect to care, as important determinants of health behaviours.

It is also important to ensure that long-term survivors continue to be monitored and provided with up-to-date information about new developments in stroke care and in stroke support services. Finally, survivors and their families may need help in understanding the long-term nature of adjustment to stroke in a family member, and its implications for the family system as a whole. Psychologists and others with an understanding of systemic approaches will be of value, and in some cases formal family therapy may be applicable. For example, when families are disrupted or de-stabilised by the need to take in and care for a parent/grandparent, or by a major role reversal due to disability in a previously active and influential family member, or when communication patterns are affected by aphasia.

Conclusions

Strokes can occur at any age and have similar physical and neurological effects irrespective of age. Every stroke survivor is an individual with their own particular aspirations and needs, but, in general, there are crucial differences in the psychological challenges facing young and old stroke survivors. Younger survivors and their partners are likely to have different family configurations and family responsibilities to older survivors, and will have more unfulfilled or partially fulfilled life tasks. They are more likely to work, have partners that work and to have young school-age children for whom they have responsibilities, and from whom they may sometimes seek care. Work and employment are very salient concerns for many young survivors, and they typically feel unsupported by health services in relation to this crucial need. They are likely to live with the after-effects of stroke for longer than their older counterparts, in some cases for several decades. Young survivors also face the incongruity of having a condition that is predominantly an older persons' illness, and of being treated in services that are predominantly used by older people. This presents particular challenges to their self-identity which require special consideration. They may also require help in accepting that the goals of rehabilitation are concerned with adaptation and the maximisation of potential, rather than the restitution of former capabilities.

Individual young stroke survivors should be assessed with regard to the special factors that are prominent in younger survivors (Table 21.3 above), and the psychological significance and ramifications of these factors for each person should be assessed and taken into account when planning treatment. Health service providers should liaise with the full range of services and agencies relevant to young survivors' needs, particularly those concerned with employment.

Because of their special needs and circumstances some younger stroke survivors in the United Kingdom have formed an organisation called "Different

Strokes" [http://www.differentstrokes.co.uk/] which provides networking, support and exercise groups, post-discharge information and support for survivors and their carers. As noted above, peer support has been shown to have psychological benefit for those affected by conditions other than stroke (e.g. Dennis, 2003; Doull *et al.*, 2005) and is helpful for stroke carers (Hartke & King, 2003; Stewart *et al.*, 1998), and it is encouraging that the new stroke strategy for England makes reference to this form of support.

Future research

Studies of the experiences of stroke survivors and carers in existing stroke services suggest that they have particular needs that are often unrecognised and unmet. Since special pathways for young strokes are unlikely to be developed, research is required into methods of assessment that capture individual needs of young stroke survivors and inform the provision of services. There is an urgent and clear need for research into the vocational rehabilitation of working-age stroke survivors and into the development of integrated service models that allow wider access to this provision. At present there are no specific psychological interventions designed for young stroke survivors or their carers, despite many studies that suggest they have special psychological needs that are not well met by existing services. While it may not be practicable to develop age-specific and stroke-specific therapies, there is the potential to develop guidelines for adapting psychological approaches for this group in a way that ensures their needs are fully assessed and addressed. The provision of peer support has the potential to meet the needs of recovering stroke survivors, and of those who have completed their recovery (through their involvement as volunteers or paid supporters). Peer support has been recommended in stroke strategies, but it is under-researched and there is a need for research into its application in stroke. Little is known about the effects of parental stroke on young children in the United Kingdom, and consequently there are no guidelines for supporting children of stroke survivors, other than those involved in caring. Research to support the development of guidelines is urgently required.

Chapter 22

Prevention of Stroke

Introduction

Stroke prevention encompasses a very wide range of interventions, medical and nonmedical, applied at various stages of the life span and at different points in relation to the stroke itself. Strokes generally have a sudden onset, with a full range of symptoms from the outset, and consequently there is usually no post-diagnostic period during which symptoms are mild when patients and health practitioners can focus on reducing risks and halting progression. Prevention efforts therefore rely on reducing incidence through increasing public awareness of lifestyle risk factors and mass screening programmes. There exist major variations in trends for stroke incidence, and a tenfold difference in incidence rates, between richer and poorer countries (Feigin, Lawes, Bennett, Barker-Collo & Parag, 2009; Johnston, Mendis & Mathers 2009). In view of this, it is important that research into stroke prevention relevant to poorer countries is undertaken as a priority.

Primordial prevention (Schwamm, Pancioli, Acker, Goldstein, Zorowitz, Shephard *et al.*, 2005) takes the form of public health campaigns and work with communities and groups to ameliorate lifestyle-related risk factors, such as smoking, obesity and alcohol abuse. Primary prevention aims to reduce the risk of first strokes by intervening with individuals at high risk of stroke, due to genetic conditions such as Fabry disease and Marfan syndrome, congenital conditions such as patent foramen ovale, acquired conditions including hypertension, obesity and atrial fibrillation or stroke indicators such as transient ischemic attacks. Secondary prevention is designed to reduce the risk of further strokes in those who have had one or more strokes and usually requires them to adhere to a medication regime to control blood pressure or blood clotting, as well as adopt health promoting diets and lifestyles. The facilitation of rapid access to emergency treatment sits at the interface of prevention and treatment. It occurs after initial symptoms of stroke have developed, but may prevent the

Psychological Management of Stroke, First Edition. Nadina B. Lincoln, Ian I. Kneebone, Jamie A.B. Macniven and Reg C. Morris.

progression of the stroke, as well as reversing some of its affects, and is therefore properly considered as an aspect of prevention.

Stroke prevention guidelines

The American Stroke Association has formulated guidelines for stroke that include prevention measures aimed at primordial, primary and secondary prevention, as well as emergency treatment (Schwamm *et al.*, 2005). These guidelines recognise the importance of education programmes in promoting awareness and improving public health. The guidance recommends that local stroke strategies should:

- support educational programs that target high-risk populations and their families;
- ensure that educational efforts include community-based organizations, policymakers, and other stakeholders;
- include processes that provide rapid access to emergency medical services for patients with acute stroke; and
- ensure the direct involvement of emergency physicians and stroke experts in the development of stroke education materials.

The recommendations for improving access to treatment in the early stages of stroke are echoed in the specific guidelines for the early management of stroke published by the American Stroke Association Stroke Council (Adams, del Zoppo, Alberts, Bhatt, Brass, Furlan *et al.*, 2007) and in the European Stroke Guidelines (European Stroke Organization Executive Committee and ESO Writing Committee, 2008; Hacke, 2008). Together with the United Kingdom's 'National Clinical Guidelines for Stroke' (Royal College of Physicians, 2008a), the American and European guidelines endorse the utilisation of public awareness campaigns to improve rapid access to emergency services and reduce lifestyle related risk factors. In addition, the 'National Clinical Guidelines' provide specific guidance for secondary prevention following a first stroke or TIA. As well as surgery and pharmaceutical treatments, the recommendations for secondary prevention highlight lifestyle factors that reduce risk, such as abstaining from smoking tobacco, taking exercise and a eating a healthy diet.

Finally, the National Stroke Strategy for England (Department of Health, 2007a) prominently features prevention and early treatment in its quality standards, although these fall short of recommending national screening programmes for risk factors. Some relevant examples are:

- **Primordial prevention:**
    - o **Awareness of stroke symptoms.** Members of the public and health and care staff are able to recognise and identify the main symptoms of stroke and know it needs to be treated as an emergency.

o **Awareness of risk factors and treatments.** Increased awareness of risk factors in the public and healthcare staff; including awareness of hypertension, obesity, high cholesterol, atrial fibrillation (irregular heartbeats) and diabetes. Awareness of management methods of risks recommended in clinical guidelines, and of appropriate action to reduce overall vascular risk.

- **Primary prevention:**
  o A system which identifies as urgent those with **early risk of potentially preventable full stroke**, to be assessed within 24 hours in high-risk cases; all other cases are assessed within seven days.
  o **Urgent response.** All patients with suspected acute stroke are immediately transferred by ambulance to a hospital providing hyper-acute stroke services that are available throughout the 24-hour period.
  o **Risk factors** are identified and assessed, and those at high risk are given information about the risk factors and lifestyle management issues (exercise, smoking, diet, weight and alcohol), and are advised and supported in possible strategies to modify their lifestyle and risk factors.
- **Secondary prevention:**
  o **Risk factors** are assessed in those who have had a stroke and they are given information about the risk factors and lifestyle management issues (exercise, smoking, diet, weight and alcohol), and are advised and supported in possible strategies to modify their lifestyle and risk factors.
  o People who have had strokes and their carers, either living at home or in care homes, are offered a **review from primary care services** … [including their] secondary prevention needs, typically within six weeks of discharge home or to care home, and again before six months after leaving hospital. (Department of Health, 2007a)

Major risk factors for stroke

Psychological and behavioural factors

Psychological distress and stress. The role of psychological distress, particularly depression, in the aetiology of stroke has received considerable attention over the past 20 years. However, studies differ regarding the type and intensity of psychological distress that is measured; ranging from low well-being through distress to clinical depression. Perhaps for this reason, the evidence is not entirely consistent. One well-designed prospective study, which controlled for other risk factors, found no association between psychological distress and stroke (Colantonio, Kasi & Ostfeld, 1992). However, a large number of prospective studies following cohorts over a period of years have found an association between measures of psychological distress and stroke when other risk factors were controlled for (Jonas & Mussolino, 2000; Larson, Owens, Ford & Eaton, 2001; Ostir, Markides, Peek & Goodwin, 2001; Simons, McCallum,

Friedlander & Simons, 1998; Salaycik, Kelly-Hayes, Beiser, Nguyen, Brady, Kase & Wolf, 2007; Surtees, Wainwright, Luben Wareham, Bingham & Khaw, 2008). These studies all found an association between psychological morbidity and the incidence of fatal and nonfatal stroke, but several studies have found this association to hold only for fatal strokes. May, McCarron, Stansfeld, Ben-Shlomo, Gallacher, Yarnell *et al.* (2002) followed up 2201 men in the United Kingdom aged 49–64 over a 14-year period and found that both fatal and nonfatal strokes occurred more often in people who scored high on the General Health Questionnaire (GHQ-30), a measure of psychological distress, at the initial assessment. But the comparison was significant only for fatal stroke (risk ratio 3.36). Gump, Matthews, Eberly, Chang and MRFIT Research Group (2005) found that, amongst 11,216 men with elevated risk factors for cardio-vascular disease, those with greater depressive symptoms at the start of an 18-year follow-up period were more likely to have fatal strokes. Surtees *et al.* (2008) reported a very large-scale prospective study of 20,627 participants, aged 41 to 80 years, who were stroke free at enrolment. The study investigated the association between stroke and episodes of major depressive disorder (self-reported in a Health and Life Experiences Questionnaire) and mental health well-being (Mental Health Inventory, or MHI-5). During an 8.5-year follow-up, there were 595 strokes. Episodes of major depression were not associated with stroke, but a one-standard deviation decrease in mental health well-being increased stroke risk significantly by 11%. This increased risk was found in both men and women, and occurred after other risk factors were controlled for. One prospective study of 2478 people in the United States over six years (Ostir *et al.*, 2001) extended the evidence for the impact of psychological distress on stroke by demonstrating that positive affect, as measured by the positive affect subscale of the Centre for Epidemiological Studies Depression Scale (CES-D), was associated with a reduced risk of stroke and was a protective factor for both men and women. However, this association may be have been mediated by protective lifestyle factors, such as higher levels of exercise or better diet, in 'happier' people.

The relationship between stress and stroke has been less well studied than that between depression and stroke. An association between the intensity and frequency of self-reported stress and risk of fatal stroke was found in a prospective study of over 12,000 men and women in Copenhagen over 13-year follow-up period (Truelsen, Nielsen, Boysen & Grønbæk, 2003). This association may have been affected by other related factors, but a retrospective case control study in Sweden did find evidence for an independent effect of self-perceived stress on the risk of ischaemic stroke (Jood, Redfors, Rosengren, Blomstrand & Jern, 2009). A further prospective study of occupational stress in Japan found that occupational strain increased stroke risk in men, and this association persisted after other factors had been controlled. But no such increase in risk was evident in women workers. These rather mixed findings indicate that further research is needed into the relationship between stress and stroke risk.

A number of explanations for the association between psychological morbidity and stroke have been proposed. One explanation proposes that the increased risk of stroke in people who experience depression occurs because they exhibit poor blood pressure control and have more lifestyle risks, such as smoking, poor diet and lack of exercise (May *et al.*, 2002). However, this explanation was not borne out by studies in which the association between depression and the incidence of stroke persisted despite controls for physiological and behavioural risk factors including age, sex, systolic blood pressure, cholesterol, smoking, diet, lack of exercise, Body Mass Index, diabetes history and antihypertensive medication (Jonas & Mussolino, 2000; Joubert, Cumming & McLean, 2007). The majority of biological explanations for the association propose that long-term psychological distress may have physiological effects on the cardiovascular system or on blood clotting, which in turn predisposes people to stroke (Carod-Artal, 2007). If this were the case, then prevention and treatment of psychological distress would indirectly reduce the incidence of stroke. However, an alternative account suggests that psychological morbidity does not itself cause stroke, but a type of depression ('vascular depression'), in both young and older people, is caused by subclinical cerebral-vascular disease resulting from 'silent' infarcts (Fujikawa, Yamawaki & Touhouda, 1993). Since the association between depression and vascular disease is not the result of shared risk factors (Teper & O'Brien, 2008), it is proposed that 'hidden', subclinical, cerebral-vascular disease is a common cause for both depressive symptoms and stroke.

Physical inactivity. Despite some negative findings in studies conducted prior to 2000, recent evidence supports the notion that exercise reduces the risk of a first stroke. A meta-analysis of 23 studies (18 cohort studies and five case control studies) concluded that moderate and high levels of physical activity were associated with reduced risk of *ischemic stroke* (caused by blood clots) and *haemorrhagic stroke* (caused by burst blood vessels) (Lee, Folsom & Blair, 2003). A similar meta-analysis of 31 studies confirmed that moderate exercise was sufficient to reduce stroke risk (Wendel-Vos, Schuit, Feskens, Boshuizen, Verschuren, Saris *et al.*, 2004). Subsequent evidence from a large-scale prospective study of 3298 healthy people also supported this conclusion for men. This study demonstrated that moderate to heavy physical activity at baseline protected against the risk of ischemic stroke, independently of other stroke risk factors, over a median follow-up period of nine years (Willey, Moon, Paik, Boden-Albala, Sacco & Elkind, 2009). A prospective study of running over a 7.7 year follow-up period recruited 29,279 men and 12,123 women and found that running one kilometre per day reduced the risk of stroke by 11% in men and women combined. The protective effect was greatest for those who exceeded recommended daily distances and ran for more than 8 kilometres per day on average. Men and women who ran these distances had a 60% risk reduction compared with those who ran less than 2 kilometres per day (Williams, 2009).

Evidence for the benefit of exercise in the secondary prevention of second and subsequent stroke is lacking, although there is evidence that it is beneficial for improving the mobility of stroke survivors (Saunders, Greig, Young & Mead, 2010). Despite the lack of specific evidence, the United Kingdom National Clinical Guidelines for Stroke (Royal College of Physicians, 2008a) recommend exercise as one of the lifestyle measures aimed at improving secondary prevention, as well as for the prevention of first stroke.

All patients should be advised to take regular exercise as far as they are able:

- The aim should be to achieve moderate physical activity (sufficient to become slightly breathless) for 20–30 minutes each day.
- Exercise programmes should be considered, and tailored to the individual following appropriate assessment, starting with low-intensity physical activity and gradually increasing to moderate levels. (Royal College of Physicians, 2008a)

However, advice about exercise alone may be insufficient. Secondary prevention measures need to educate stroke survivors about safe levels of exercise since a questionnaire survey of 867 young stroke survivors demonstrated that 72% felt they do not know the 'safe' limits for exercise and were constrained by fear of over-exertion (Roding, 2009).

Alcohol and drugs. The relationship between alcohol consumption and the risk of stroke has been extensively studied. Reynolds, Lewis, Nolen, Kinney, Sathya and He (2003) conducted a meta-analysis of epidemiological studies encompassing 19 cohort studies and 16 case control studies of the relationship between alcohol intake and the incidence of stroke. Most controlled for major stroke risk factors such as obesity, age, smoking, hypertension and so on. The included studies reported data from over 450,000 cases in total. Reynolds *et al.* (2003) concluded that an intake of more than 60 g (7.7 United Kingdom units) of alcohol per day was associated with an increased relative risk for all kinds of stroke of 1.64, for ischemic stroke of 1.69 and for hemorrhagic stroke of 2.18. All these increases were statistically dependable. Consumption of less than 12 g (1.5 United Kingdom units) per day was associated with a reduced relative risk for all kinds of stroke of 0.83, and for ischemic stroke of 0.80. However, the relationship between alcohol intake and ischemic stroke was nonlinear; moderate consumption reduced risk so that drinking between 12 g (1.5 United Kingdom units) and 24 g (3.1 United Kingdom units) each day was associated with a reduced relative risk of ischemic stroke of 0.72. A subsequent prospective cohort study over eight years (Elkind, Sciacca, Boden-Albala, Rundek, Paik & Sacco, 2006) also found that moderate alcohol consumption (one drink in the past month to two drinks per day) was associated with reduced risk of ischemic stroke compared with those who had not drunk in the past year or had never drunk. The association between stroke and alcohol intake occurred despite controlling for other stroke risk factors including age, gender, race/ethnicity, hypertension, diabetes, atrial fibrillation, lipid (fat) levels and current smoking. However, some studies have failed to find a protective effect of moderate drinking (Bazzano, Gu, Reynolds, Wu, Chen, Duan *et al.*, 2007), and the relationship between consumption and risk is complex and has been shown to be moderated by type of drink (red wine may reduce risk) and drinking pattern (Mukamal, Ascherio, Mittleman, Conigrave, Camargo, Kawachi *et al.*, 2005). Binge drinking, defined as six or more drinks of the same beverage in the same session for men, and four or more for women, was found to significantly increase stroke risk in a large, prospective cohort study in Finland (Sundell, Salomaa, Vartiainen, Poikolainen & Laatikainen, 2008). The relative risk for binge drinkers compared to nonbinge drinkers for all stroke types was 1.85, and for ischemic strokes was 1.99. A review and meta-analysis by Patra, Taylor, Irving, Roerecke, Baliunas, Mohapatra and Rehm (2010) identified that the risk of haemorrhagic stroke increased as alcohol consumption rose. For ischaemic stroke only, a protective effect of low to moderate consumption was evident. These authors concluded that to benefit from the protective effects of alcohol, and to avoid an increased risk of stroke, alcohol intake should be limited to 2 United Kingdom standard units per day (16 g of alcohol).

Psychoactive, mind-altering substances other than alcohol have been less extensively studied, but there is evidence from case control studies of substantially increased stroke risk amongst users of cocaine and amphetamines. One such study of women aged 15–44 years showed that those who reported cocaine or amphetamine use had a sevenfold increase in stroke incidence compared with non-users, after other factors were controlled for (Petitti, Sidney, Quesenberry & Bernstein, 1998). A cross-sectional study of young people with haemorrhagic and ischemic stroke discharged from hospitals in the United States over a three-year period showed that amphetamine abuse was associated with a marked increased risk of haemorrhagic stroke (odds ratio 4.95), but not ischemic stroke. Cocaine use was associated with a moderate increase in the incidence of ischemic stroke (odds ratio 2.03) and haemorrhagic stroke (odds ratio 2.33) (Westover, McBride, Robert & Haley, 2007). Treadwell and Robinson (2007) reviewed several case studies and case series of stroke occurring soon after cocaine use in young people. They concluded that cocaine use was temporally associated with the occurrence of both haemorrhagic and ischemic strokes.

Cannabis use may also be temporally associated with stroke. Thanvi and Treadwell (2009) identified ten studies, reporting a total of 14 individual cases, in which cannabis use preceded ischemic strokes. In one case, a 36-year-old man had three strokes over a two-and-a-half-year period, each one after heavy cannabis use. However, these were all uncontrolled case studies, and other risk factors such as smoking, other drugs and alcohol may also have been implicated in many of the cases. Thanvi and Treadwell (2009) noted several putative mechanisms by which cannabis might cause stroke, but acknowledged that causation is uncertain, and that the link between cannabis and stroke, while plausible, is not established.

Diet and obesity. Diet exerts an important influence upon several risk factors for stroke: blood pressure, obesity, levels of cholesterol and other fats and the blood sugar levels of diabetics. A review by Bazzano, Serdula and Liu (2003) concluded that eating certain foods, especially fruit and vegetables, had a protective effect for stroke. A study of health professionals' eating habits demonstrated that the effect was enhanced by increased intake of these foods; each increase of a single serving per day in fruit and vegetable intake reduced stroke risk by 6% (Joshipura, Ascherio, Manson, Stampfer, Rimm, Speizer *et al.*, 1999). Fung, Chiuve, McCullough, Rexrode, Logroscino and Hu (2008) examined the benefits of the 'Dietary Approaches to Stop Hypertension' (DASH)-style diet in a cohort of nurses over a 24-year follow-up. This study found a reduction in risk for those whose diets most closely resembled the DASH recommendations. Goldstein, Adams, Alberts, Appel, Brass, Bushnell *et al.* (2006) reviewed prospective cohort studies and concluded that eating salt (sodium) produced an increased stroke risk in a linear fashion, and that eating foods rich in potassium had a protective effect. The review proposed that the effect on stroke risk was primarily mediated by the effects of these electrolytes on blood pressure.

The routes by which diet may exert its effect have been extensively studied. Galimanis, Mono, Arnold, Nedeltchev and Mattle (2009) reviewed the evidence for the effects of the constituents of foods on stroke risk. These included vitamins, Omega 3 fatty acids, anti-oxidants and electrolytes. They concluded that the evidence for the benefit of Omega 3 fatty acids was equivocal, and that randomised controlled trials of antioxidants (vitamin C, beta-carotene/vitamin A and vitamin E) showed no benefits for vitamin C or beta-carotene, and only weak evidence for a benefit of vitamin E. The studies of the effects of dietary electrolytes (magnesium, calcium, potassium and sodium) on stroke risk showed some evidence for a beneficial effect of magnesium in a particular sample (male smokers). These findings also echoed the conclusions of Goldstein *et al.* (2006) with regard to the risk increasing effect of sodium and the protective effect of potassium. Galimanis *et al.* (2009) highlighted the inconsistency of the evidence regarding the risk reducing effect of the B group of vitamins, including folic acid (Vitamin B9). Evidence from programmes that enhance vitamin B in foodstuffs, and a meta-analysis of eight randomised controlled trials (Wang, Qin, Demirtas, Li, Mao, Huo *et al.*, 2007), showed a stroke risk reduction of 18%, but other well-controlled trials found no benefit. A meta-analysis of 13 randomised controlled trials of folic acid supplements, including large trials with over 39,000 participants in total, concluded that folic acid alone did not have a major effect on stroke risk reduction (Lee, Hong, Chang & Saver, 2010).

In addition to the role of specific foodstuffs in determining the risk of stroke, overall calorie intake is a risk factor if it contributes to obesity. Several large-scale prospective studies have demonstrated that obesity increases stroke risk (Suk, Sacco, Boden-Albala, Cheun, Pittman, Elkind *et al.*, 2003; Wilson, Bozeman, Burton, Hoaglin, Ben-Joseph & Pashos, 2008; Hu, Tuomilehto, Silventoinen, Sarti, Männistö & Jousilahti, 2007; Kurth, Gaziano, Berger, Kase, Rexrode, Cook *et al.*, 2002; Song, Sung, Davey-Smith & Ebrahim, 2004), and a review by Goldstein *et al.* (2006) concluded that increasing degrees of obesity cumulatively increase stroke risk. However, there have been no controlled studies of the impact of weight reduction on the risk of stroke, though such prospective trials are currently underway (Selwyn, 2007).

On the basis of the evidence, the European Stroke Organisation (ESO), the UK guidelines for secondary prevention of stroke and the US guidelines for primary prevention, all recommend healthy diets. These should contain daily portions of fruit and vegetables and weekly portions of oily fish, combined with reduced salt and saturated fats and a moderate overall calorie intake to prevent or reduce obesity (Royal College of Physicians, 2008a; Goldstein *et al.*, 2006; European Stroke Organisation, 2008).

Smoking. Smoking doubles the risk of ischemic stroke and increases the risk of haemorrhagic stroke by between two and four times. It has been estimated to cause between 12% and 14% of stroke deaths in the United States, and the evidence for its impact on stroke risk has been described as 'consistent and overwhelming' (Goldstein *et al.*, 2006). Data from the United Kingdom support the findings in the United States; smoking has been found to increase the risk of stroke independent of other risk factors, and the risk increases with the number of cigarettes smoked per day (Wolf, D'Agostino, Kannel, Bonita & Belanger, 1988). A meta-analysis of 16 studies, seven of which were prospective, suggested that passive smoking may also increase the risk of stroke (Lee & Forey, 2006). The main biological mechanisms by which smoking predisposes to stroke are through the impairment of the functioning of arteries and the heart, increased blood clotting and a greater likelihood of atherosclerosis due to a build-up of fatty deposits in the arteries (Goldstein *et al.*, 2006).

Giving up smoking has been shown significantly to reduce the risk of stroke after two years (Wolf *et al.*, 1988). For men who were light smokers, the risk declined to that of nonsmokers after five years, but for heavy smokers it declined from being 3.7 times higher than nonsmokers to being only 2.2 times as high (Wannamethee, Shaper, Whincup & Walker, 1995). Unfortunately, many stroke survivors are not successful in quitting smoking. Ives, Heuschmann, Wolfe and Redfern (2008) found that while 71% of their cohort of 363 stroke survivors attempted to stop smoking, only 30% had stopped smoking and maintained cessation at one and three years after their stroke.

On the basis of this evidence, the US primary prevention guidelines (Goldstein *et al.*, 2006) recommended abstention or cessation of smoking and cited counselling, nicotine replacement and oral smoking cessation medications as effective aids to cessation. The UK 'Guidelines' (Royal College of Physicians,

2008a) similarly recommend smoking cessation as an important secondary prevention measure:

> All patients who smoke should be advised to stop smoking:
> o Smoking cessation should be promoted at every opportunity using individualised strategies which may include pharmacological agents and/or psychological support.

Biological risk factors

The American Heart Association/American Stroke Association Stroke Council (Goldstein *et al.*, 2006) reviewed the literature on risk factors in stroke and identified a range of biological risk factors which they classified as modifiable or nonmodifiable. These are summarised in Table 22.1.

The UK 'National Clinical Guidelines for Stroke' (Royal College of Physicians, 2008a) identified a similar range of physical risk factors, and both guidelines make detailed and specific recommendations about approaches for reducing biological risk factors. These measures emphasise pharmacological and surgical interventions.

From a psychological perspective, the key targets in preventing strokes stemming from biological risk factors are the application of psychology in:

o endeavours to increase awareness of risks and promote behaviour to reduce risks in the general public (see 'Knowledge and Education about Stroke Prevention', below);
o the promotion of knowledge of, and adherence to, guidelines by professionals (see the 'Knowledge Translation, Implementation of Guidelines and Audit' section in chapter 2, 'Clinical Stroke Services'); and
o enhancing the uptake of treatments and adherence to treatment regimes once they are started (see 'Improving Adherence to Treatments', below).

Table 22.1 Biological Risk Factors for Stroke

Nonmodifiable	*Modifiable*
Age, gender, low birth weight, race/ethnicity and genetic factors.	Hypertension, diabetes, atrial fibrillation and other cardiac conditions such as patent foramen ovale, dyslipidemia, carotid artery stenosis, sickle cell disease, postmenopausal hormone therapy, obesity and body fat distribution, the metabolic syndrome, oral contraceptive use, sleep-disordered breathing, migraine headache, hyperhomocysteinemia, elevated lipoprotein (a), elevated lipoprotein-associated phospholipase, hypercoagulability, inflammation and infection.

Models of health behaviour and stroke prevention

A significant amount of research into the psychological approaches to reducing the incidence of disease has been informed by theories of health behaviour. These theories typically invoke health-related beliefs, and propose processes that govern the translation of beliefs into behaviours that preserve health, prevent disease or lead to help seeking.

The health locus of control theory (Wallston & Wallston, 1978) proposes that people differ in the way they attribute causation of disease. This depends on whether they see the disease as determined by their own behaviour (internal attribution), by external factors or chance (external or chance attributions) or by the influence of other people (powerful others attributions). The type of attribution determines a person's behaviour with regard to prevention, treatment and help seeking. For example, a person with internal attributions about the cause of a first stroke is more likely to change their own behaviour to prevent further strokes than a person who attributes their stroke to external factors which are beyond their control. People with internal attributions (internal locus of control) have better outcomes for prevention and recovery in a range of health conditions including stroke (Partridge & Johnston, 1989; Morrison, Johnston & MacWalter, 2000). However, the model focuses on beliefs about causation and where the responsibility for change is located (e.g. in self or in others), and it fails to consider other important beliefs about vulnerability to a health condition, or beliefs about the likelihood of changing matters though action. Its limitations are illustrated by a study using a self-management intervention for stroke that demonstrated significant improvements in self-efficacy and in internal locus of control, without there being any significant changes in mood, activity or participation (Jones, Mandy & Partridge, 2009). Similarly, Bonetti and Johnston (2008) found that locus of control did not predict walking recovery or walking limitations in a sample of 203 stroke survivors, whereas self-efficacy and perceived behavioural control were predictive. Morrison *et al.* (2000) also noted that the reported associations between locus of control and outcome variables found in studies prior to 2000 were usually small, and in their own study general locus of control did not emerge as a predictor of anxiety or depression in a regression analysis.

The health beliefs model (Becker & Maiman, 1975) proposed that health-related behaviours are determined by beliefs about susceptibility to a condition, the severity of the condition, the benefits of actions to prevent the condition and any perceived barriers or costs associated with preventative measures. Janz and Becker (1984) reviewed 46 studies of the model and concluded that there was broad support for the predictive power of its elements, especially 'perceived barriers'. Sullivan, White, Young, Chang, Roos and Scott (2008a) also reviewed the application of the health beliefs model across a range of health conditions and noted that while it was predictive of health behaviours, the strength of predictions were not strong. Consequently, Sullivan *et al.* (2008a) extended the model by adding the concept of self-efficacy from Bandura's (1977) social cognitive theory, and the notions of 'subjective norm', or the expectations of others, from Azjen's (1991) theory of planned behaviour (see Figure 20.2). This extended model was subsequently used in two studies examining behaviours associated with stroke risk factors in community samples of people at risk of stroke. The first study (Sullivan *et al.*, 2008a) was cross-sectional and reported that the perceived seriousness of stroke and susceptibility to stroke, perceived benefits of exercise, barriers to exercise, self-efficacy and subjective norm were all associated with measures of intention to exercise. This extended model demonstrated greater predictive power than the standard health beliefs model for intention to exercise within six months, but not for a measure of general intention to exercise. In a second study of the extended health beliefs model (Sullivan, White, Young & Scott, 2009), researchers used a longitudinal design in which measures of the theory's constructs were used to predict risk-related intentions and behaviours one month later. The results of regression analyses indicated that the extended model had greater predictive power than the standard model, and that different risk-related behaviours were differentially predicted. Exercise behaviour at one month was predicted by only self-efficacy, but exercise intention at one month was predicted by perceived benefits and subjective norm. On the other hand, intention to lose weight at one month was predicted only by perceived barriers. Further support for the value of the theory of planned behaviour in predicting the behaviour of stroke patients was provided by a study of walking limitations and walking recovery (Bonetti & Johnston, 2008) which showed that perceived behavioural control was a better predictor of behavioural measures of outcome than self-efficacy and locus of control.

Another variant of the health beliefs model is Leventhal's self-regulation theory (Leventhal, Diefenbach & Leventhal, 1992). The application of this theory to disease prevention involves enhancing the understanding of factors affecting treatment compliance (Leventhal & Cameron, 1987). This model proposes that people hold a commonsense theory about their condition and its treatment. This is founded on a number of key health beliefs that shape the experience of the condition and determine help seeking, prevention and treatment related behaviour.

1. *Identity*: the name or label for the illness and ideas about its associated symptoms,
2. *Timeline*: beliefs about the duration of the condition, and its course (e.g. acute or chronic),
3. *Consequences*: ideas about the implications of the illness in terms of shorter and longer term outcomes,
4. *Cause*: beliefs about what may have led to the illness, and
5. *Cure–control*: ideas about how amenable the illness is to management and what the person can do to get over their illness.

Support for the role of the cure–control construct in stroke is evident in the results of a study of medication adherence in 180 stroke patients with a mean age of 69 one year after a first stroke (O'Carroll, Hamilton, Whittaker, Dennis, Johnston, Sudlow & Warlow, 2008). Compliance with prescribed medication regimes, as measured by the Medication Adherence Report Scale (Horne, 2004), revealed very high levels of adherence, with over 90% of the sample scoring between 23 and the maximum score of 25. The primary reason given for non-adherence was forgetting due to poor memory. However, regression analysis showed that about 30% of the variance in self-reported adherence was predicted by four variables, and the last two of these were both related to intentional non-adherence: younger age, cognitive impairment, lower perceptions about medication benefits, and specific concerns about medications (dependence, toxicity and too many tablets). The highest single correlate of the adherence scale was a measure of concerns about medication, and this attests to the importance of Leventhal's cure–control beliefs as determinants of compliance. A further finding of this study was that interviews suggested that people with a clear medication taking routine were more adherent.

Motivational interviewing (Miller & Rollnick, 2002) is an approach to accomplishing behaviour change that is less concerned with beliefs about health conditions than with the processes and mechanisms involved in achieving change. Its theoretical roots are in the transtheoretical model of Prochaska and DiClemente (1984). Within this model, motivation is viewed as a state that is amenable to change and recovery, and change and growth are considered to be natural aspects of human nature. Therapists and patients join in a shared endeavour to help patients to recognise the gap between their present state and their ideal state. They then work towards goals that reduce this gap. The six stages of behaviour change proposed by the model are (1) *precontemplation* in which the individual does not perceive a need for change, (2) *contemplation* during which a person experiences a need to change their behaviour and seriously considers making some changes in the near future, (3) *preparation* in which a person indicates their intention to change and begins to act to bring about change, (4) *action* in which concrete steps are taken to change behaviour or the environment, (5) *maintenance* during which there are active efforts to sustain the changes, and finally (6) a *relapse* stage when the individual is unable to sustain change. The individual may re-enter the change cycle at any point and could, for example, fail to maintain an action and return to the contemplation stage before resuming action, possibly after reviewing their expectations and goals. The motivational interviewing approach is unique amongst models of behaviour change in that it offers specific guidance on how processes that occur within therapeutic encounters can be harnessed to promote positive change. Therapists are encouraged to create 'free and friendly' therapeutic space, to view clients as allies in the therapeutic endeavour and to identify resistance and understand its causes, working with and through its sources rather than challenging and seeking to overcome it. Ambivalence towards change is seen as a natural part of a therapeutic process, reflecting a gap between a person's current state and their personal goals and values. Focus upon ambivalence can be helpful in therapy to promote behaviour change because it highlights and encourages a person to consider factors that are psychologically significant for them and determine their stance and actions. This process enables them to evaluate the personal costs and benefits of change, and to promote their sense of self-efficacy. The model also offers specific guidance about techniques that are useful in therapy:

- Open-ended questions: this allows clients to express views.
- Affirmations: acknowledge strengths and build confidence.
- Reflective listening: whenever you are in doubt, listen.
- Facilitate: by repeating, seeking meaning and identifying feelings.
- Summaries: identify significant processes such as ambivalence.

Martins and McNeil (2009) reviewed 37 studies of the use of motivational interviewing for a range of activities and conditions including exercise, diet, diabetes and oral health, and they concluded that it promotes health enhancing behaviours and adherence to advice. A meta-analysis of 119 studies of behaviours important in health and welfare demonstrated that motivational interviewing significantly enhanced intention to change and engagement with treatment (Lundahl, Kunz, Brownell, Tollefson & Burke, 2010). There is also a body of evidence demonstrating its effectiveness with older adults (Cummings, Cooper & Cassie, 2008), and it has been applied in an educational intervention addressing stroke risk factors in a study that is described below (Green, Haley, Eliasziw & Hoyte, 2007).

   Another stage model, the health action process approach (HAPA), was developed by Schwarzer (1992), and it provides a more detailed and sophisticated account of the cognitive processes involved in each stage than the transtheoretical model. This model makes a distinction between pre-intentional motivation processes that engender behavioural intention, and post-intentional volitional action processes that facilitate the adoption and maintenance of health behaviours. In the pre-intentional phase, perceptions about the risks of behaviours, outcomes of preventative actions and self-efficacy are all implicated in the development of intentions in the form of personal goals to reduce risks and obtain desirable outcomes. In the volitional phase, the goal intentions are translated into plans of action to meet those goals. The translation of plans into action is affected by beliefs about the ability to initiate the action and beliefs (action self-efficacy) about the ability to persevere and maintain the action (maintenance self-efficacy). Goal intentions alone do not guarantee goal attainment. Implementation intentions, encompassing plans for the actions required to attain a goal (when, where and how), are also important determinants of goal attainment (Gollwitzer & Sheeran, 2006), as is the ability to control and monitor actions (awareness of own standards, self-monitoring and self-regulation). Beliefs about recovery are also important, and affect the way in which relapses and setbacks are dealt with. The HAPA model has been tested in a number of domains, some of which, like lack of exercise and alcohol use, are risk factors for stroke, but it has not yet been applied specifically to stroke survivors or those at high risk of stroke. Studies have demonstrated its predictive validity, and their results highlight the importance of outcome expectancies and self-efficacy in the formation of intentions, and also the role of intentions, self-efficacy and action planning in the initiation and maintenance of health-related behaviours (Scholz, Keller & Perren, 2009: Schwarzer, Luszczynska, Ziegelmann, Scholz & Lippke, 2008). However, risk perception has not proved predictive of outcome in a number of studies. Despite this, the identification of specific psychological processes that contribute to risk reducing behaviours makes it a promising addition to the conceptual frameworks applicable to stroke prevention.

Psychological models and stroke prevention: a synthesis

Arguably, the models considered above differ more in focus than in substance, and a comprehensive approach to stroke prevention may benefit from a synthesis of their main tenets. Such a synthesis requires the consideration of factors that determine both the orientation of the individual patient and the efficacy of measures to promote behaviour change. The following analysis draws upon and extends an earlier synthesis of theories of behaviour change by Fishbein, Triandis, Kanfer, Beker, Middlestadt and Eicher (2001).

The first consideration is related to a person's orientation to the condition itself. There is evidence that an individual's motivation to take measures to prevent a disease is determined by awareness of the condition, beliefs and understanding about its identity and nature, its cause(s), time course and severity, perceptions of personal susceptibility and its personally relevant consequences. Perceptions of the expectations and beliefs of other significant people are also important. The second group of factors are related to the individual's views about the preventative measures themselves, and include beliefs about their utility, disadvantages, limitations, acceptability and congruence with personal standards, obstacles, costs, practicality and tractability. Once again, the perceived beliefs and expectations of significant others about prevention measures are also influential. The third set of considerations concerns perceptions of the person's own capability to implement the preventative measures, and includes a person's belief that they can perform the necessary actions and maintain them (self-efficacy or perceived behavioural control). As well as beliefs, practical aspects are also important, including having the necessary knowledge and skills to carry out activities and procedures, having access to support, the necessary resources, encouragement and guidance, being able to hold and maintain goals and plans and to monitor progress, being able to remember and perform any required activities, being free from conflicting demands and having the time to implement the prevention measures.

The final domain is concerned with the way in which interventions to promote risk reduction are delivered, and the subtle and at times circuitous routes that enable people to change established patterns of behaviour. Most models of health behaviour identify general factors that are important determinants of behaviour change, but omit to elaborate on modes of delivery that encourage the adoption of new beliefs or attitudes and foster behaviour change. The motivational interviewing approach is one exception, and some aspects of its delivery to facilitate behaviour change were summarised above.

Tailored interventions

A promising approach that is capable of integrating psychological models is the development of individually tailored interventions. In this approach individuals, or groups, are first assessed on the dimensions that a model (or models) identifies as the important determinants of behaviour change in a particular situation. Then a tailored intervention is specifically designed to promote change in the position of individuals or groups with respect to the identified determinants. The rationale is that change in behaviour will flow from alterations in the factors that determine behaviour change (Kozub, 2010; Wallston & Wallston, 1978). For example, the theory of planned behaviour postulates that a person's beliefs about an illness (e.g. how severe it is or whether it is amenable to treatment), and their beliefs about their ability to complete a treatment, separately determine the person's intention to adopt the treatment. A tailored approach would assess these beliefs in an individual, and, for example, if a person believed that their illness was serious and capable of being treated, but did not believe in the efficacy of the available treatments, then the intervention would be aimed at changing beliefs about treatments rather than beliefs about the illness.

Three broad strategies have been used to tailor messages: personalisation of messages, individual feedback about perceptions and intentions and matching of message content to an individuals' position on key determinants of behaviour change (Hawkins, Kreuter, Resnicow, Fishbein & Dijkstra, 2008). Tailoring can target processes related to the reception and registration of a message in order to capture attention, or, alternatively, may target processes that determine the impact of the message and thereby enhance its effect on behaviour. The reception of a message depends on its capacity to capture an individual's attention, the way it is elaborated through cognitive processing and its personal significance for an individual. A message that is relevant to a particular individual is more likely to be noticed, processed and remembered. In contrast, a message that matches an individual's stage in the change process, or their status in the key domains important to behaviour change, such as perceived susceptibility or sense of self-efficacy, is more likely to produce behaviour change. Many tailored health interventions have been based upon the transtheoretical stage model, where the message is determined by the person's position in the stages from precontemplation to maintenance. But other models such as health locus of control have also been used, and there is the potential to apply any relevant model. A meta-analysis of 57 studies of tailored print messages, using a variety of models, demonstrated their effectiveness in promoting health behaviour change (Noar, Benac & Harris, 2007), and this approach has potential for application in stroke prevention.

Strategies for risk reduction

Several broad approaches to the reduction of health risks have been extensively evaluated with respect to stroke. It is evident that the psychological theories reviewed above have yet to permeate thinking about risk reduction in the stroke domain. While there are many hundreds of trials of medications that reduce stroke risk, few risk reduction approaches have considered the impact of poor uptake and adherence, and even fewer have systematically utilised psychological models of behaviour change to improve effectiveness.

Knowledge and education about stroke prevention

A primary aim of all psychological approaches to stroke prevention is to increase knowledge and raise awareness of risk factors, particularly in those at high risk of stroke. It is vital that this is achieved in a way that does not create fear and avoidance. When there is awareness, the next goal is to promote action to ameliorate the risk by enhancing self-efficacy for change or adherence. Support for the importance of knowledge of risk factors comes from a large-scale Australian study of 1253 patients (Samsa, Cohen, Goldstein, Bonito, Duncan, Enarson *et al.*, 1997). This study demonstrated that people who were aware of their risk were more likely to follow stroke prevention regimes. A review of 39 studies by Jones, Jenkinson, Leathley and Watkins (2010) revealed that most of these studies found substantially less than half the sample knew the major symptoms or risk factors of stroke. Being older, belonging to an ethnic minority and having a lower educational level were all associated with poorer knowledge of stroke risk factors. Jones *et al.* (2010) concluded that knowledge about stroke risk factors and the recognition of stroke were both poor, and, surprisingly, neither previous experience of a stroke or having a higher risk were associated with increased knowledge. Sullivan, White, Young, Scott and Mulgrew (2008b), using focus groups of people at risk of stroke, found that group members were often unaware of gaps in their knowledge of stroke and failed to identify themselves as at risk. In England, a survey of 760 patients and carers found that 20% of respondents were not aware that lack of exercise increased risk of stroke, and 37% and 44% were unaware of the risks associated with diabetes and atrial fibrillation, respectively (National Audit Office, 2010). Lack of awareness of being at risk is exacerbated by the fact that some of the risk factors, particularly hypertension, are symptom free; a large-scale survey in the United States found that 30% of those with high blood pressure were unaware of it (Chobanian, Bakris, Black, Cushman, Green, Izzo *et al.*, 2003; National Heart, Lung and Blood Institute, 2003). Further data from the United States demonstrated that 46% of people with at least three risk factors did not perceive themselves as at risk. In a sample of people who had had a stroke, only 60.5% were able to accurately identify one stroke risk factor. Moreover, only 55.3% were able to identify one stroke symptom (Lloyd-Jones, Adams, Carnethon, De Simone, Ferguson, Flegal *et al.*, 2009). Samsa *et al.* (1997) found that 59% of their sample who were at high risk of stroke were nevertheless unaware of their elevated risk, and lack of awareness was associated with greater age, not recalling being told about their risk by their GP, lower depression score, better health and lower physical functioning. Taken together, these data highlight the need to educate people, not only about risk factors themselves and their role in predisposing to stroke, but also about the signs that enable the identification of the risk factors. National population screening programmes for 'silent' risk factors might help to achieve higher levels of awareness in those at risk, but the evidence for effectiveness of screening alone is equivocal (see the 'Complex Interventions' section in this chapter).

The effect of information provision on increasing knowledge about stroke, including knowledge of risk factors, has been amply confirmed by a systematic Cochrane review of randomised controlled trials (Smith, Forster, House, Knapp, Wright & Young, 2008). A meta-analysis of data from 536 stroke participants in six trials showed a large and significant effect of information upon knowledge of stroke. A similar meta-analysis of 469 participants from four trials found a smaller, but still significant, effect of information for carers' knowledge of stroke. However, Smith *et al.* (2008) failed to confirm the translation of knowledge into behaviour change and risk reduction. Two trials showed no benefit of the provision of information by itself (medical records and leaflets) on blood pressure or medication compliance. Even when information presentation was followed with help in assimilating the information and a plan for clarification and consolidation, two further trials found no evidence for decreased smoking or improved blood pressure control compared with the control groups. A review of 19 studies of complex interventions for primary and secondary stroke prevention (Redfern, McKevitt & Wolfe, 2006) included seven studies that used education without enhanced care as well. Most of these studies of educational interventions demonstrated benefits for knowledge and changed beliefs or attitudes, but the majority of the 'education only' studies measured only psychological outcomes and none of them demonstrated enduring improvement in risky behaviours or physical outcomes. A further randomised controlled trial enrolled 200 stroke survivors and employed an educational counselling intervention based upon motivational interviewing and the stage model of change (Green *et al.*, 2007). Knowledge of stroke risk factors was measured by a questionnaire incorporating questions about causes of stroke, warning signs, symptoms, risk factors, outcomes, and actions to take on experiencing symptoms. The results showed a statistically greater improvement in knowledge about stroke for the intervention group. There was also a large and significant move towards the active stages of behaviour change in behaviours such as smoking, diet, exercise and alcohol intake across both groups combined, but surprisingly this shift did not significantly favour the intervention group. However, the intervention was relatively brief, and consisted of motivational interviewing as part of only a single 15–20-minute one-to-one interview with a nurse and one 3-hour interactive group session. Moreover, there are no details about the training in motivational interviewing received by the nurse. A quasi-experimental study by Sullivan and Katajamaki (2009a) compared the effects of reading a brochure with a focus on risk factors for stroke across high and low-risk groups for stroke. Unfortunately, the groups were not matched for age, with the low-risk group being considerably younger, but nevertheless the study did demonstrate that knowledge about stroke in both groups improved and that the improvement was maintained over a period of one week. However, behaviour change was not assessed. A further study (Sullivan & Katajamaki, 2009b) assessed change in stroke knowledge in two groups of older people following an intervention based upon the health beliefs model. One group read a brochure and engaged in activities that were not about stroke; the other read the brochure and had activities designed to enhance beliefs about stroke. Both groups showed changes in beliefs about perceived susceptibility to stroke and the perceived benefit of exercise to reduce risk. But there were no differences between the groups. Beliefs about benefits were strongly and positively associated with intention to exercise.

In summary, the evidence points to the effectiveness of educational interventions in improving knowledge of stroke risk factors and in changing beliefs and possibly also intentions. However, despite the evidence that those with greater awareness of having elevated risk factors are more adherent to stroke prevention measures (Samsa *et al.*, 1997), there is a surprising lack of evidence that educational interventions, even when supplemented by active learning techniques, produce any practical reduction in stroke risk. The failure of educational programmes may be attributable to a number of factors. Only one study (Green *et al.*, 2007) utilised an approach based upon an evidence-based psychological model that addressed a range of psychological processes determining the inception and maintenance of behaviour change. Information about risks and treatments alone may be effective in promoting the early stages of change (pre-intentional, pre-contemplation and contemplation). But more individualised approaches may be required for the post-intentional action phases in which intentions are translated into behaviour and specific barriers to implementation and maintenance may be encountered. In addition to the lack of psychological sophistication, most of the interventions studied were brief, and several assessed only change in knowledge and therefore could not detect any behaviour change that did occur.

One apparent discrepancy that remains to be explained is that, whilst the educational interventions described above were not effective in reducing stroke risks such as smoking and medication compliance, there is evidence that education alone has can be effective in changing eating habits and reducing risk factors caused by poor diet (Brunner, Rees, Ward, Burke & Thorogood, 2007; and see below).

Improving adherence to treatments

The World Health Organisation (2003) estimated that only 50% of patients with chronic conditions, including stroke and stroke risk factors, follow recommended treatments, and that low rates of adherence to treatments may significantly increase the incidence of strokes in developed countries. Fortunately, studies of adherence following a stroke suggest that rates are higher than 50%, but nevertheless fall short of 100%, and rates vary widely across studies conducted in Europe and Australia. The study by O'Carroll *et al.* (2008) described above was conducted in the United Kingdom and found that over 90% of a sample of 180 stroke patients one year after stroke had adherence scores within the top three scale points of the Medication Adherence Report Scale. Hamann, Weimar, Glahn, Busse and Diener (2003) reported a one-year follow-up of 2640 stroke patients in Germany and found that 96% adhered to at least one stroke medical prevention measure, but that adherence varied across treatments; 84% were still taking aspirin, 77% continued to take oral anticoagulants but only 62% adhered to the recommendation to take clopidogrel. A second study from Germany also followed up stroke patients for a year (Sappok, Faulstich, Stuckert, Kruck, Marx, Koennecke *et al.*, 2001) and found that 87.6% were still on antithrombotic medication, but that continuance of treatment varied across stroke risk factors, and was 90.8% for hypertension, 84.9% for diabetes but only 70.2% for hyperlipidemia. De Schryver, Van Gijn, Kappelle, Koudstaal and Algra (2005) reported adherence rates for stroke survivors enrolled in two prospective clinical trials in the Netherlands. Aspirin was prescribed to 3796 people, and over a mean follow–up of 2.1 years, 18% prematurely stopped taking it and 8% stopped without a clear medical reason. Of 651 patients who were prescribed oral anticoagulation, 22% had stopped after a mean follow-up of 1.0 years, and half of these (10%) did so without a medical reason. Coetzee, Andrewes, Khan, Hale, Jenkins, Lincoln and Disler (2008) conducted a small-scale study in Australia that compared the adherence rates of 29 stroke patients and 29 amputees in the first year after discharge and found that stroke patients exhibited significantly poorer adherence rates, and that their rates were generally much lower than in the European studies. However, variability in rates of adherence to treatments for different stroke risk factors was also evident in this study: diabetes 66.5%; hypercholestrolaemia 58.3%; hypertension 59.1% and unspecified heart conditions 60.4%. This study also examined reasons for non-adherence. These were collected by both self-reports and objective measures of cognition, emotional problems, social and professional support and beliefs about medication.

Self-reported reasons for non-adherence included poor organisation (36%), not being reminded (28%), forgetting (16%), feeling it is unnecessary (12%), too many medications (4%) and not understanding the reasons for taking medicines (4%). Objective measures of cognitive and emotional dysfunction, level of social and professional support and, crucially, beliefs about medication (such as necessity, efficacy and side effects), were all significantly associated with adherence in stroke patients. Together, these measures explained 77.7% of variance in adherence in a multiple regression. These results were echoed by a larger study in Australia with 136 stroke patients (Andrewes, Coetzee, Jenkins, Finch, Hale, Khan & Lincoln, in preparation) which found a mean adherence rate of 69.9% only six weeks after discharge, and identified two additional predictors of non-adherence: level of dependency and having a right hemisphere lesion. This study concluded that 'the majority of stroke patients are taking medications at subtherapeutic levels' and that interventions to improve adherence in this group are urgently required.

Interventions for increasing compliance with therapy, particularly pharmacological treatments, have been very extensively studied over the past five decades. Van Dulmen, Sluijs, Van Dijk, De Ridder, Heerdink and Bensing (2007) conducted a review of reviews that encompassed 38 reviews of adherence to a variety of treatments for a range of conditions, including stroke, and stroke risk factors, such as hypertension. Some conclusions stemming from this review were:

- Adherence was better for simpler medication regimes, particularly those with fewer daily doses, and technical measures to simplify medication taking increased adherence.
- Reminders via post, phone, computer or visits were effective in improving adherence to medication and attendance at treatment and assessment sessions.
- Interventions to enhance self-efficacy, skill-training and self-monitoring improved adherence to therapies in patients with cardiovascular conditions.
- Education and modification of health beliefs improved knowledge of treatments and adherence to treatments across a range of conditions.
- Practical social support with a treatment regime increased adherence, and was more effective than emotional or undifferentiated support.
- Programmatic interventions to improve adherence were not always successful, and interventions that had broad focus, high intensity and long duration were more likely to be effective.

Van Dulmen, Sluijs, Van Dijk, De Ridder, Heerdink, Bensing and the International Expert Forum on Patient Adherence (2008) followed up their 2007 study by convening 20 of the authors of the reviews in an International Expert Forum on Patient Adherence. The conclusion was that adherence could best be enhanced by the development of simple, practical interventions including a multidisciplinary perspective and patients' input. The latter should focus on patients' expectations, needs and experiences in taking medication, and what might help them to be more adherent. O'Carroll, Dennis, Johnston and Sudlow (2010) developed a trial protocol to assess whether such simple interventions to help stroke patients establish and maintain a medication taking routine will promote better adherence. Based on evidence that stroke patients' concerns about their medication (e.g. dependence, toxicity and too many tablets) affect adherence, it was proposed that a trial to investigate approaches to modifying erroneous beliefs would be of value. In addition, since patients report that their adherence is affected by forgetting to take their medication, it was proposed that an 'implementation intention model' could be trialled. Simply put, this involves a patient stating clearly when and where they will take their medication with the goal that this will be incorporated into their day-to-day regime. Support that such an intervention might succeed comes from evidence of its usefulness with epilepsy (Brown, Sheeran & Reuber, 2009) and evidence that routine improves medication adherence (O'Carroll *et al.*, 2008). A particular strategy to enhance the adherence of stroke patients may be to start secondary prevention treatments early, during the hospital phase. This was found to be associated with very high rates of adherence to medications at 90 days post discharge (Ovbiagele, Saver, Fredieu, Suzuki, Selco, Rajajee *et al.*, 2004). However, this study did not compare early and late start in a randomised controlled trial.

Psychological interventions for specific risk-related behaviours

The section on risk factors for stroke earlier in the chapter described research showing that smoking is a major risk to cardiovascular health, and that cessation is beneficial (Wannamethee *et al.*, 1995). Fifty randomised controlled trials of the benefits of psychological interventions to stop or reduce smoking were reviewed by Mottillo Filion, Belisle, Joseph, Gervais, O'Loughlin *et al.* (2009). The conclusion was that a substantial increase in smoking abstinence was achieved by behavioural interventions for smoking, including one-to-one counselling, telephone-based counselling and group therapies, in which the commitment of time was greater than 20 minutes, and in which there was more than one follow-up visit. While the behavioural interventions were defined broadly, cognitive-behavioural therapy was one example that appeared specifically to prevent relapse (Killen, Fortmann, Schatzberg, Arredondo, Greer Murphy, Hayward *et al.*, 2008).

The section on stroke risk factors above also outlined the increased risk attributable to a diet containing certain foods, for example those high in sodium (salt), and also the beneficial effects of foods such as fresh fruit and vegetables and of regular exercise. Therefore, changing diet and exercise behaviour offers the opportunity of reducing stroke risk. A Cochrane review by Brunner *et al.* (2007)

included 38 trials that addressed cardiovascular risk through the provision of dietary advice to healthy adults. The conclusions were that dietary advice presented verbally, in writing, in person or over the phone, to individuals or small groups, was moderately effective in reducing cardiovascular risk factors, including some markers for cholesterol, blood pressure and sodium intake. There was also evidence that it improved diet and healthy eating, but the review was unable to draw conclusions about reduction of in the incidence of stroke and other cardiovascular events. Obesity is another well-established risk factor for stroke. Curioni, André and Veras (2006) conducted a literature search to identify trials in which weight loss programmes were used to reduce the incidence of primary stroke. Unfortunately, no relevant trials were found. However, studies were found to show that weight loss reduced the risk of mortality from diabetes through reducing the incidence of stroke and other conditions. Behavioural weight loss programmes have been shown to be effective in adults with Type II diabetes, along with diet and exercise programmes (Norris, Zhang, Avenell, Gregg, Brown, Schmid & Lau, 2005). Typically, weight loss interventions entail reducing calories and increasing activity levels. Behavioural principles incorporated in such interventions most often include self-monitoring, stimulus control, the use of cues to support regular exercise and problem solving and assertiveness skills to deal with challenging situations. There is also goal setting, and a consideration of the thoughts and emotions related to overeating and inactivity, and the management of these (Smith & Wing, 2000). Rejeski, Brawley, Ambrosius, Brubaker, Focht, Foy and Fox (2003) compared group-mediated cognitive-behavioural therapy with other approaches to reducing inactivity and increasing exercise in people with cardiovascular disease, or at high risk of such disease, and an average age of 65 years. The group-mediated cognitive-behavioural therapy included developing self-responsibility for exercise, self-monitoring, exploring motivations, providing education regarding harm risk, problem solving barriers to maintenance, the use of cues, goal setting, relapse prevention and follow-up trouble shooting. The group-mediated cognitive-behavioural therapy was more effective than other treatments in changing self-reports of physical activity, fitness and self-efficacy in dealing with 'barriers to an active lifestyle'. A similar intervention was also effective in promoting health enhancing behaviours in populations without such specific risks (Cramp & Brawley, 2006).

With the exception of diet, where the provision of information and advice alone was effective in changing behaviour and reducing risk, it will be evident that all the successful interventions described here included features that had the potential to address the principal processes identified by the psychological models of behaviour change outlined above (the health locus of control, health beliefs, transtheoretical model and health action process approach). For example, individual or group therapy and counselling potentially enabled people to explore important pre-intentional aspects such as beliefs about illness, susceptibility, efficacy of risk reduction methods and the locus of responsibility for effecting change. Goal setting, problem solving, rehearsal, and advice about maintenance and relapse had the potential to address aspects of post-intentional action stages including the enhancement of self-efficacy and barriers to implementation and adherence.

Complex interventions and community programmes

Multifaceted interventions, delivered in communities, may be beneficial in reducing stroke risk, although few have yet been tested. In one such trial, a community intervention incorporating screening for risk factors and education about risk factors and stroke recognition demonstrated large gains in knowledge of stroke symptoms (59% to 77%) that were maintained over three months. The trial found that 27% of participants changed their lifestyle. However, 64% made no changes to their behaviour at all, only 9% saw a doctor and none stopped smoking (DeLemos, Atkinson, Croopnick, Wentworth & Akins, 2003).

Redfern *et al.* (2006) reviewed trials of complex, multifaceted interventions in stroke care. Nineteen of the reviewed articles were concerned with primary or secondary prevention of stroke. The majority of the studies used education combined with care enhancements, such as risk factor screening and monitoring, improved access to treatments, individual goal setting and monitoring, regular visits for support and monitoring by professionals, peer support and counselling. Twelve of the 19 studies were successful in terms of changing behavioural intention to reduce risky behaviour. Of these, one (McAlister, Man-Son-Hing, Straus, Ghali, Anderson, Majumdar *et al.*, 2005) failed to find enduring change. Six of the studies were fully successful and demonstrated change in actual behavioural or physical outcomes, such as reduction in stroke incidence, mortality, risky behaviours or physiological risk factors. All of the studies that succeeded in promoting behavioural or physical changes utilised multiple approaches that included additional professional involvement and enhanced access to health monitoring and treatment; for example screening combined with detailed risk-assessment, an action plan, health counselling by a nurse and access to other relevant professionals such as a dietician and pharmacist (Willoughby, Sanders & Privette, 2001). Five of the studies were partially successful, and, once again, improvement in behavioural and physical outcomes occurred only when there was enhanced care as well as screening and education. As for interventions for specific risk behaviours, the success of these complex interventions depended on their potential to influence a wide range of pre- and post-intentional factors identified as important determinants of behaviour change by psychological models.

Other multifaceted interventions applicable to stroke risk factors are the Alcoholics Anonymous abstinence-based approach to alcohol abuse and similar 12-step programmes. However, their efficacy in reducing alcohol dependence remains to be proven (Ferri, Amato & Davoli, 2006). In contrast, there is evidence for the efficacy of brief interventions based in primary care (Kaner,

Dickinson, Beyer, Campbell, Schlesinger, Heather *et al.*, 2007), and of cognitive-behavioural therapy incorporating the principles of motivational interviewing, the stages of change model and relapse prevention (Magill & Ray, 2009). Brief interventions in primary care can be for as little as five minutes, and may be provided by medical doctors, nurses or psychologists. Patients identified as drinking excessively are offered feedback on their level of alcohol use and its potential harm, and high-risk situations for drinking are noted, as are useful coping and motivational strategies. These are usually integrated into a personal plan to reduce alcohol use. Cognitive-behavioural interventions are typically much longer, and can include social skills training, self-control and self-efficacy training, stress management, community reinforcement, behavioural marital therapy, covert sensitisation and contracting (Parks, Marlatt & Anderson, 2004). An interesting and novel approach to community interventions was adopted by Sullivan *et al.* (2008b) and used focus groups of people at risk of stroke to explore what they wanted from risk reduction programmes. Four elements identified as attributes of potentially successful interventions were:

1. integration with health services such as general practitioners to reinforce change in beliefs and behaviours and extend commitment;
2. a social component that enhances participants' self-efficacy to change risky behaviours;
3. education to promote the perceived probability of long-term benefits; and
4. an education component to provide personally significant and practical information for achieving change.

The importance accorded to integration with health services and to self-efficacy demonstrated that service users themselves did not view education alone as sufficient to produce dependable behaviour change and benefit, unless it was combined with programme elements supporting the wider range of psychological processes and needs implicated in behaviour change. This resonates with the conclusion, arrived at previously, that the success of interventions depends upon engagement with the broad framework of psychological processes articulated in the models of behaviour change described above. It is significant that this position was endorsed by service users, as well as being supported by the outcomes of trails of interventions discussed above.

Emergency treatment

Prompt and successful emergency treatment requires good, widespread public and professional knowledge that enables the recognition of the onset of stroke as well as knowledge of appropriate action to take when a stroke is suspected. A study of approaches to increase public awareness of stroke symptoms in Canada (Silver, Rubini, Black & Hodgson, 2003) compared people's knowledge before and after advertising campaigns in experimental and control communities.

The results showed that television advertising was effective in improving knowledge of stroke symptoms, while print advertising did not produce gains. The improvements in knowledge were consistent across gender and educational level, but were not found in those over 65 years of age. The primacy of television was echoed in a survey of the sources of information about stroke that found television (32%) was the most common source of information followed by magazines (24%), newspapers (22%), physicians (20%), a family member with stroke (19%), medical books (9%), a friend with stroke (7%) and 'word of mouth' (5%) (Schneider, Pancioli, Khoury, Rademacher, Tuchfarber & Miller, 2003). It is notable that the internet did not feature in these results, but the situation may have changed in the decade since the data were collected.

Jones *et al.* (2010) reviewed 20 studies of people's knowledge about what action to take when stroke symptoms occur. The outcomes of the studies showed considerable variation with between 53% and 98% of participants indicating that they would call the emergency services on 911/999. Six of the studies found that over 20% of the sample would phone their GP, and one study (Carroll, Hobart, Fox, Teare & Gibson, 2004) found that only 18% of stroke survivors would call the emergency services while 80% would call their GP. In view of finding such as these, and to improve access to rapid emergency care, the UK government funded a 'Stroke – Act FAST (**F**ace. **A**rms. **S**peech. **T**elephone)' campaign that used newspapers, magazines, posters and television. Initial comparisons for the same three months in the year preceding and after the campaign in four ambulance services showed a 54% increase in stroke calls (10,922 from 7079). In one service, the number of stroke patients presenting for treatment within three hours increased by 171% over a six-month comparison period (National Audit Office, 2010). A survey of nearly 2000 people before and after the campaign showed a considerable increase in numbers who would call 999 on seeing stroke symptoms: slumped face from 64% to 87%, unable to lift arms from 46% to 72% and slurred speech from 46% to 74% (National Audit Office, 2010).

Muller-Nordhorn, Nolte, Rossnagel, Jungehülsing, Reich, Roll, Villringer and Willich (2009) reported a trial of a low-cost educational intervention to reduce the time taken for stroke patients to reach hospital. This cluster randomised trial included 48 postal code areas in the catchment of three inner-city hospitals. Over 75,000 people in the experimental postal code areas received an intervention comprising an educational letter describing stroke symptoms and emphasizing the importance of calling the emergency medical service. There was also a free bookmark and sticker with the emergency medical services' telephone number. A total of 1,388 people in the control and experimental postal code areas had strokes in a two-year period, and compared with control areas, there was a 27% improvement in the time taken to reach hospital for women, but, puzzlingly, no effect for men.

In summary, there is some evidence that public awareness campaigns, based on advertising-type interventions, can increase rates of appropriate behaviour in the general public when a single response to an incident is required.

A case example: preventing a second stroke

Rachel's account highlights the dramatic onset of stroke and the quest to identify and understand the causes of her stroke against the backdrop of family life for a single mum. Her story is shown in Table 22.2. Rachel's story demonstrates how stroke may occur in an apparently health person without their being aware of underlying, latent risk factors. However, once the stroke occurred, she describes the vigorous efforts to determine why it happened so that secondary prevention measures could be put in place.

Table 22.2 Rachel's Story: Prevention of a Second Stroke

My name is Rachel and I was born on 9th April 1964 with a hole in my heart that didn't close up as it should have done. I found this out on 25th January 2008.
The 7th of September 2006 was a Thursday like any other for a single working mum. Got everyone up, children off to school, work, home, supper, children to bed, relaxing with glass of wine in front of TV, fell asleep on sofa. Woke up about 2 a.m., got up went into kitchen to have a glass of water. Started walking up the stairs … got about three quarters of the way up and I stopped. I heard a low roaring in my ears that got louder and louder and I got dizzier and dizzier until it was deafening. I got down on my hands and knees as I thought I was fainting, and I blacked out. I woke up some hours later at the bottom of the stairs and made it upstairs to my bedroom. I have no idea how, but I remember calling a friend from my bed, probably the last number I had dialled; he since told me that I said I wasn't very well, but wasn't really making sense. He then called NHS Direct (a 24-hour National Health helpline and information service), who called me back. All I remember saying was that I can't go to hospital because my children were here and have school in the morning. Whether that is what they heard or not, I don't know, but they immediately called an ambulance. I crawled from my bedroom into Georgia's bedroom (my 14-year-old daughter) to tell her I was going to hospital. She got up, and helped me with my clothes; not really understanding what was going on, almost carried me down stairs and waited with me till the ambulance arrived. She called her dad and told him what was happening and said she would get Oliver (12) up as Mum had to go to hospital. (He later came over and took them to school.) The ambulance arrived, and to hospital I went.

Hospital
This next bit is blurry. I remember lying on a bed in A&E with an excruciating headache and turning to the left to vomit on the floor over and over again, much to the nurse's exasperation as she had to clean it up. 'It would help if you could do that in the bowl provided!!' she said …. I didn't know they had put a bowl in my right hand. I couldn't see it or feel it. It didn't register to me that I had lost all feeling on my right and was almost completely blind. I was like a zombie … nothing going on in my head at all. She then mentioned something to her colleague about 'drinking'. Later on I realised she had assumed I was drunk. The next thing I remember is someone swishing by the end of my bed, and saying 'this one's just having a migraine, give her a few hours to sleep it off and

(Continued)

Table 22.2 (*Continued*)

send her home'. I wanted to scream at him 'it's not a migraine!!!!!!' but nothing would come out.

There then followed a series of memories. Intravenous acyclovir for a possible virus infection; a lumbar puncture; a CT scan; an MRI scan; Mum and Dad; Georgia and Oliver; family and friends' faces; being wheeled onto different wards, but always this massive pain in my head, growling in my ears and regular vomiting. The next memory is a huge one. I was in a room by myself with the usual hustle and bustle noises of the ward outside not making sense to me, when through the noise was a man's voice talking about a patient like he was dictating a letter. He was saying the scans had come back and the patient had a brain tumour, Frenchay Hospital, which has a specialist neurological unit, had been contacted and was standing by and an ambulance had been called. He then said my name. I was shocked, but not devastated as you would expect. He then came in to my room, and the same words came out, he told me they would drain the fluid from around the tumour and I would feel normal again. This weirdly made me very happy, and all I could think about was that I was going to feel normal again, but I was concerned about how to tell the children and he said the hospital would help.

He went and left me on my own waiting for the ambulance. I was told I got a message (I think by phone) to my mum and dad that I had a brain tumour and was moving hospitals. They had gone back home for a few days. Apparently my dad cried but I don't remember.

While I was waiting for my ambulance, the hospital was emailing my notes and scans to Frenchay ready for my arrival. The consultants at Frenchay immediately called to say it was not a tumour, but a stroke. Amazingly this hadn't been diagnosed by the neurologist in my local hospital.

I had had a stroke on 8th September 2006 in the early hours of the morning. I was 42.

On 13th September I was given an aspirin … after five days, though, the damage was already done. I lost all use of and feeling in my right side, couldn't walk, lost most of my vision, my speech was affected by my inability to think and put words together, rather than loss of voice, my hearing was much muffled and I was very confused.

Being (relatively) young with low blood pressure, low cholesterol, average weight, fit and healthy, I didn't fit the profile of most stroke survivors so the hospital didn't know what to do with me. I was not given any rehabilitation, no speech and language therapy, no occupational therapy, no physiotherapy … nothing! I was in hospital for two weeks where I regained movement of my right side fairly quickly and my speech improved too. (Oliver has just seen me writing this and added that he phoned me once and I was able to tell him I was eating a sandwich and it was horrible!)

I left hospital and was moved to Wales to be looked after by my parents at their home initially (my children had to suddenly go and live with their father) I was there for about 6 weeks before I slowly moved back home, and it was my GP who eventually managed to get me some help about four months later via the head trauma unit at another hospital. The speech and language therapist helped me communicate with my children and my parents and helped them understand my difficulties and what I needed from them to be able to communicate properly. It was really helpful.

(*Continued*)

Table 22.2 (*Continued*)

My neurologist at the hospital then discharged me, still insisting that as they couldn't find a cause, it must have been a migraine that did it, even though I told him I wasn't actually having one when I had my stroke!

The occupational therapist tried to help me at home to organise myself and my children, but being on my own I felt I couldn't manage and made the very, very difficult decision to sell my house, where I had lived for the last 17 years, and move to Wales to be near my family. Oliver came with me, and Georgia moved in with her Dad, staying to finish her GCSEs. (I miss her terribly.)

More tests

On moving I had to do all the usual things, one of them was to register with a new GP. He then referred me to Dr Shetty, the neurologist at the University Hospital in Cardiff. I duly went along, ready to tell him I had had lots of tests and they couldn't find anything. He gave me a lovely smile, said 'we are going to start again, and get to the bottom of this' and arranged for me to have a series of tests. Bloods, scans, ECGs, you name it. Once again I heard negative, negative, negative . . . . I was getting very disillusioned, but like a good girl I continued to trudge along to see every '-ologist' in the hospital (well, I wasn't exactly busy). On one visit I was taken into a room where I was to see my favourite cardiologist and was asked by the nurses to remove my clothes from the waist up which I duly did. I was then covered in electric wires and attached to a monitor. In came my cardiologist, who injected me with teeny bubbles and watched them travel through my heart with an ultrasound scanner. He then did it again, but asked me to strain as if I were doing a poo!! (Very ladylike.) I duly did. We watched the screen . . . nothing. He said 'one more'. We repeated the procedure, and he said 'there it is'.

I was stunned, after one and a half years of hearing 'negative' I had an answer. I had a hole in my heart.

Normally, being a healthcare professional myself, I would want to find out the ins and outs of the test. The whats, the whys and the wherefores, ask all the pertinent questions. What I actually did was burst into tears, not little tears, oh no. There I was, half naked, boobs out, sobbing with big fat blubbering uncontrollable tears and snot pouring out of me! The poor man didn't know where to look, and, nervously coughing and mumbling, he slowly made his excuses and sidled out of the room to leave me with the nurses.

Steps were taken quickly to organise the closure, and during this time I was found to have a clotting disorder too. I had the procedure to close the hole on Tuesday 16th September 2008.

I am now almost back. I still have loss of my right visual field and I am registered partially sighted so can no longer drive. I still can't be in a noisy environment comfortably, my memory is appalling and I lose what I am talking about a lot of the time, but I am learning various procedures to try to manage these problems. I can walk and talk like before, and I have full use of my right side, although the numbness and weakness are still there.

I have met some lovely people through my stroke, and I am lucky to have the most wonderful children, family and friends. I am looking forward now to the rest of my life, and I am trying to see my stroke as a unique opportunity to change it. I mean, what's the worst that could happen?

Conclusions

General conclusions about stroke prevention must take account of the large differences between countries and the paucity of research evidence from less wealthy countries. In wealthy countries the incidence of stroke has declined dramatically, by 42%, between the 1970s and 2008, but in poorer countries it has increased by 100% in the same period (Feigin *et al.*, 2009). In 2009 there was a tenfold difference in stroke mortality and burden between the best and worst countries (Johnston *et al.*, 2009). The decrease in incidence in wealthy nations is very encouraging, but on a global scale stroke prevention efforts will have the greatest impact on mortality and disease burden if targeted to high-incidence, poorer countries.

The evidence shows that the success of community stroke prevention programmes in enabling people to accomplish and sustain risk factor reduction depends on the adoption of long-term, individualised, multifaceted approaches. These approaches incorporate measures to promote awareness of individual risk factors, enhanced access to care and repeated follow-up as well as education. However, long-term reduction in specific risk factors, such as alcohol abuse, smoking and poor diet, may be amenable to more circumscribed, targeted psychological approaches for selected, motivated individuals. On the other hand, public awareness campaigns alone, using multiple media and carefully constructed messages, improve public awareness and increase appropriate behaviour where a single response is required to an event.

It is clear that psychological models of behaviour change have only recently begun to permeate thinking about stroke risk reduction, and have yet to be used widely in planning interventions. Most current approaches are simple and direct, relying on providing people with information about the efficacy of an approach and the assumption that they will demonstrate common sense and comply with professional 'authority'. Little attention is given to improving motivation, or to assisting with perceived barriers to adherence. The lack of psychological sophistication of many educational interventions to reduce risky behaviours may be implicated in their failure, and may be the reason that only interventions incorporating expensive, long-term measures to enhance care have been shown to be generally reliable in changing behaviour and improving health outcomes.

The psychological models of health behaviour emphasise that motivation to engage in risk reduction depends crucially on an individual's representation of the illness and the threat it poses. This representation is more or less malleable, determined by multiple experiences and sources of information operating over the life span, as well as information imparted by health care professionals. The representation, combined with beliefs about the efficacy of risk reduction methods, including medicines, determines a person's 'stage' in relation to change, how they address risk reduction and the risk reduction targets that they choose. The maintenance of these risk reduction targets depends in turn on the person's appraisal of the ease and practicability of achieving them, and the appraisal of their effectiveness in promoting desirable outcomes. Health representations do not exist in isolation, but form part of a person's overall belief system, and must be congruent with it and with a person's personality and cognitive style (Leventhal *et al.*, 1992). Individual psychological factors in the form of long-term traits and belief structures, as well as current concerns and awareness of symptoms, are all instrumental in the uptake and maintenance of risk reduction. An understanding of these dimensions of individual variation relevant to risk reduction provides an excellent basis for improving the uptake and maintenance of risk-reducing behaviours through adapting or tailoring interventions to achieve congruence with an individual's stage, predispositions and belief system (Hawkins *et al.*, 2008).

Future research

On a global scale, there is a clear need for more research into prevention in those poorer countries where the incidence of stroke is greatly elevated and increasing. The approach adopted by Sullivan (2008b), of convening community groups to gain an understanding of their needs and expectations and the perceived barriers and facilitators to risk reduction, has the potential for gathering relevant information to assist in adapting approaches to local conditions.

Whilst there has been a dramatic decrease in stroke incidence in wealthy countries, the reasons for this require further investigation. There is a need for longitudinal studies to assess the relative contribution of different sources of information (media, professionals and education), and the stage of life at which it should be presented for maximum impact. There is also a need to examine the extent to which the reduction in incidence stems from change in individual behaviour as a result of changes in awareness and service provision and access, or from corporate measures, such as changing regulations about salt in foodstuff, managing drug use, restricting alcohol consumption and banning smoking in public. The outcome of such research is vital in determining health policy and the apportioning of effort between public awareness campaigns, service enhancements and corporate and legislative measures to reduce risks. The sparse application of psychological models of health behaviour in programmes designed to prevent stroke is a concern. A possible reason is the plurality of models and the lack of a single agreed framework. An important contribution would be to continue the work of Fishbein *et al.* (2001) and convene a panel of experts to develop an overarching psychological framework applicable to the specific requirements of stroke prevention.

Chapter 23

Conclusions and Future Directions

The range of topics reviewed clearly demonstrates the diversity of psychological aspects of stroke management. Traditionally concerns have been about cognitive problems and depression, but the scope is much greater than this. With respect to cognition, psychological management encompasses far more than identifying whether cognitive problems are present and need to be taken into consideration during rehabilitation planning and making discharge decisions. At the milder end of the scale, cognitive impairments will affect return to work and the ability to drive. They may require specific rehabilitation. At the more severe end, there are considerations about patients' capacity and their ability to make decisions which affect their future care. A comprehensive stroke rehabilitation programme will require policies for the management of all these aspects. Cognitive assessment is skilled and complex activity and must be conducted by those qualified to interpret the assessments and to translate the findings into clinical recommendations. Simply administering a test and obtaining a score will not serve to either to identify or manage cognitive problems and comprise an ineffective use of resources.

In relation to mood, there is more to consider than just identifying and treating depression. Various mood states are affected, including anxiety, emotionalism, frustration, apathy and anger. Each may require specific treatment. They may also lead to behavioural changes, which affect the ability of patients to engage in a rehabilitation programme. However, it may be better to address the emotional effects of stroke before mood problems arise. This will require specific preventative strategies as well as ensuring the delivery of an active and focussed rehabilitation programme. Care pathways for psychological aspects of stroke will differ according to the setting. So the procedures and policies appropriate in an acute care setting may be very different from that in a rehabilitation unit or provided by a community stroke team. It is also impotant to consider the attributes of patients, especially age, family composition, employment status and ethnicity. The psychological effects of stroke last for many years, and therefore the care plans need to encompass provision for the long-term effects of stroke. In

Psychological Management of Stroke, First Edition. Nadina B. Lincoln, Ian I. Kneebone, Jamie A.B. Macniven and Reg C. Morris.
© 2012 John Wiley & Sons, Ltd. Published 2012 by John Wiley & Sons, Ltd.

addition, many will be at risk of further stroke, and therefore psychological factors that will influence the adoption of secondary prevention measures need to be considered. It is also not only the stroke survivors that are affected; carers and family members may also experience major life changes. Psychological services for the management of the consequences of stroke therefore need to have the capacity to address all aspects.

Various chapters have highlighted what can be achieved by appropriate psychological assessment and intervention. However, most of the good practice identified is available only in a few centres for a few people. This is partly due to lack of available expertise and resources as well as lack of psychological awareness. Although would be desirable to improve provision, to do so requires a major shift in emphasis on the part of health care commissioners. However, by summarising the research literature on the psychological management after stroke, it may be possible to improve awareness of what is needed as the first step to improving health care outcomes.

In a resource-limited health care system, it is important that the effectiveness of interventions is established and only those interventions which improve outcome are provided. To do this requires evidence of the effectiveness of psychological interventions, and this is not easy to obtain. Psychological interventions are complex with multiple components and multifaceted outcomes that are difficult to capture. A key element is often the interpersonal relationship in which the intervention is provided. Therapist effects may be as great as the effects derived from the specific techniques delivered, and different measurement approaches and instruments may produce differing outcomes. Although there are some excellent examples of randomised controlled trials which have led to improved clinical practice, such trials are not always easy to conduct to answer the questions which need answering and most lead to many more questions that need to be answered. It is therefore necessary to rely on a wide range of research methods to determine procedures and polices that are likely to be beneficial. Management of the psychological consequences of stroke must be underpinned by a solid research base. To do this requires close collaboration between academic psychologists and the commissioners and providers of psychological support in health care settings. The evidence base is constantly changing, and health care staff need to be regularly updated on developments in service provision through the development and revision of clinical practice guidelines. The dissemination and adoption of such guidelines could greatly enhance psychological outcomes, without any need for extra resources.

The aim of this book was to review the evidence base to increase understanding and to optimise psychological outcomes after stroke. It is hoped by increasing awareness of the range of procedures and the relevance of psychological aspects at every stage in the stroke care pathway that improvements to service provision will emerge. There are positive aspects to stroke as well as negative, and the challenge is to maximise the positive. The last word should go to the stroke survivors themselves.

The Devastation of a Stroke: Roger Few

"I won't be long walking the dogs, it's too cold to hang about!" I shouted as I went into the field near my house. Ten minutes later, my daughter noticed both dogs waiting at the field gate without me. Instinctively she knew I was in trouble, saw me on the ground and rushed to my side. I was unable to get up, and when my daughter noticed my mouth had dropped on one side, she dialled 999 immediately.

My wife soon joined us and as we waited for a "first response vehicle" I tried to explain what had happened. My head felt muzzy and my vision became blurred and dusky. My legs had seemed to gather pace but it was difficult walking, like something wrapping around my feet. I fell to the ground, I couldn't get up but tried to turn over onto my hands and knees. When this didn't work either, I realised I was in real trouble. My family tried to make me warm and comfortable on the ice-cold ground until the "first response" took over. As soon as the paramedic arrived, I was wrapped in foil and given oxygen. We waited for a road ambulance and then an air ambulance but as neither was readily available, the paramedic drove me to hospital. That was an hour's journey and a very uncomfortable one, made worse by my sickness.

Following a short wait in the hospital corridor, I was fast-tracked to the emergency ward where I seemed to be bombarded by people asking me questions and doing tests. I was bewildered, anxious and slowly realising that my left arm and leg felt heavy and hard. I was unable to move either of them! This was a traumatic moment. I had never been a hospital patient until now and as my family left me around midnight, I wondered what the morning would bring.

How relieved I was when daylight broke and I was comfortably installed in a ward with five other patients. I was not allowed out of bed, but was rolled onto a stretcher to be taken for X-rays and more tests. I could only take liquids from a beaker whilst my ability to swallow was monitored. Slowly I was allowed liquidised food. For a further 12 days I had numerous tests and consultations from which, in my bewildered state, I began to realise the seriousness of my condition. However, I was very relieved that my speech was almost normal and that I was allowed to sit out in an arm chair briefly by the use of a hoist. But the regular visits of family and friends were my greatest relief.

My next move was to a stroke rehab hospital. Getting used to the new environment and routine was very tiring. By now I could sit out in an arm chair for a little longer time but one day I sat out too long. The result was that I became over-tired and exhausted. This made me angry with myself because I hadn't realised a stroke can have this effect. Everything you do requires much more effort and concentration. I was frustrated at this finding and foolishly thought I would be better at home and wanted to be discharged. The hospital staff and my daughter made me see sense. No way could I have managed at home yet. I moved to a smaller ward to help me settle, and my rehab started in earnest with 2–3 physio sessions per week. The benefits were soon obvious which boosted my morale greatly. It was so good to be able to do more normal things, like partly washing oneself and being wheeled to the dining room to eat together. One thing that really made me feel I was back in the real world was when I stood up for the first time. All this was possible because the staff were so understanding and dedicated; the range of equipment was superb for our needs and the achievable goals set each week per patient increased our motivation. Three months after my stroke, I was able to make a few faltering steps with the aid of a handrail and close supervision. I could partially wash and dress myself. Preparations for returning home were started. The necessary equipment was supplied, adaptations to the house made, and any necessary aftercare was put in place. Now, 18 months from my stroke, I am able to walk with a stick and an orthotic aid. It has not been easy to come to terms with this life-changing episode, but it has helped enormously to find ways to keep busy and interested. There are plenty of clubs and amenities available to us, and it is good to share ideas and experiences with friends. It is true that every task is hard work and improvement slow. Each small achievement is so rewarding and optimism is a MUST.

Appendix 1

Stroke strategy documents for the UK home nations

Department of Health, Social Services and Public Safety (2008) *Improving stroke services in Northern Ireland*. Belfast: Department of Health, Social Services and Public Safety.

Department of Health (2007) *National Stroke Strategy (England)*. London: Department of Health.

Welsh Assembly Government (2007) *Improving Stroke Services: A Programme of Work* [WHC (2007) 08]. Cardiff: Welsh Assembly Government.

Chest, Heart and Stroke, Scotland (2003) *Stroke: A strategy for Scotland*. Edinburgh: Chest, Heart and Stroke, Scotland.

Scottish Executive Health Department (2002) *Coronary heart disease and stroke strategy for Scotland*. Edinburgh: Scottish Executive Health Department.

Worldwide service and treatment guidelines for stroke

Department of Health (2005) *The National Service Framework for Long-term Conditions*. London: Department of Health.

Division of Clinical Psychology/Division of Neuropsychology (2010) *Briefing Paper 19: Psychological Services for Stroke Survivors and Their Families*. Leicester: British Psychological Society.

Royal College of Physicians (2008a) *National Clinical Guidelines for Stroke*. London: RoyalCollege of Physicians (3rd edn).

National Collaborating Centre for Chronic Conditions/Royal College of Physicians (2008) *Stroke: National clinical guideline for diagnosis and initial management of acute stroke and transient ischaemic attack (TIA)*. London: RoyalCollege of Physicians.

Department of Health (2001) Stroke. In: *National service framework for older people*. Chap. 5. London: Department of Health.

Paediatric Stroke Working Group Royal College of Physicians (2004) *Stroke in childhood: Clinical guidelines for diagnosis, management and rehabilitation*. London: RCP.

Psychological Management of Stroke, First Edition. Nadina B. Lincoln, Ian I. Kneebone, Jamie A.B. Macniven and Reg C. Morris.
© 2012 John Wiley & Sons, Ltd. Published 2012 by John Wiley & Sons, Ltd.

Lindsay, P., Bayley, M., Hellings, C., Hill, M., Woodbury, E. and Phillips, S. (2008) Stroke rehabilitation and community reintegration. Components of inpatient stroke rehabilitation. In: Canadian best practice recommendations for stroke care. *Canadian Medical Association Journal*, **179** (12 Suppl), E56–58.

National Stroke Foundation (2010) *Clinical Guidelines for Stroke Management 2010.* Melbourne: National Stroke Foundation.

Adams, H.P., Jr., del Zoppo, G., Alberts, M.J., Bhatt, D.L., Brass, L., Furlan, A., Grubb, R.L., Higashida, R.T., Jauch, E.C., Kidwell, C., Lyden, P.D., Morgenstern, L.B., Qureshi, A.I., Rosenwasser, R.H., Scott, P.A. and Wijdicks, E.F. (2007) Guidelines for the early management of adults with ischemic stroke: a guideline from the American Heart Association/American Stroke Association Stroke Council, Clinical Cardiology Council, Cardiovascular Radiology and Intervention Council, and the Atherosclerotic Peripheral Vascular Disease and Quality of Care Outcomes in Research Interdisciplinary Working Groups: the American Academy of Neurology affirms the value of this guideline as an educational tool for neurologists. *Circulation*, **115**, e478–e534.

Hack, W., Kaste, M., Bogousslavsky, J., Brainin, M., Chamorro, A., Lees, K., et al (2003) European Stroke Initiative Executive Committee and Writing Committee. The European Stroke Initiative recommendations for stroke management: update 2003. *Cerebrovascular Disease*, **16**, 311–318.

Goldstein, L.B., Adams, R., Alberts, M.J., et al (2006) Primary prevention of ischemic stroke: a guideline from the American Heart Association/American Stroke Association Stroke Council: cosponsored by the Atherosclerotic Peripheral Vascular Disease Interdisciplinary Working group; Cardiovascular Nursing Council; Clinical Cardiology Council; Nutrition, Physical Activity, and Metabolism Council; and the Quality of Care and Outcomes Research Interdisciplinary Working group: the American Academy of Neurology affirms the value of this guideline. *Stroke*, **3**, 1583–1633.

Steiner, T., Kaste, M., Forsting, M., Mendelow, D., Kwiecinski, H., Szikora, I., Juvela S., Marchel, A., Chapot, R., Cognard, C., Unterberg, A. and Hacke, W. (2006).

Recommendations for the management of intracranial haemorrhage – part I: spontaneous intracerebral haemorrhage. The European Stroke Initiative Writing Committee and the Writing Committee for the EUSI Executive Committee. *CerebrovascularDisease*, **22**, 294–316.

Graham, I., Atar, D., Borch-Johnsen, K., Boysen, G., Burell, G., Cifkova, R., Dallongeville, J., et al (2007) Fourth Joint Task Force of the European Society of Cardiology and Other Societies on Cardiovascular Disease Prevention in Clinical Practice (Constituted by representatives of nine societies and by invited experts) European guidelines on cardiovascular disease prevention in clinical practice: executive summary. *European Heart Journal*, **28**, 2375–2414.

National Board of Health and Welfare (Sweden). *National guidelines on stroke care* [URL]. http://www.socialstyrelsen.se/nationellariktlinjerforstrokesjukvard. [accessed 14/09/2010].

Worldwide stroke treatment guidelines are available by searching:

Agency for Healthcare Research and Quality. *National Guideline Clearing House* [URL]. http://www.guideline.gov/index.aspx [accessed 30/07/2011].

References

Aben, I., Verhey, F., Lousberg, R., Lodder, J. and Honig, A. (2002) Validity of the Beck Depression Inventory, Hospital Anxiety and Depression Scale, SCL-90, and Hamilton Depression Rating Scale as screening instruments for depression in stroke patients. *Psychosomatics, 43*, 386–393.

Aben, L., Kessel, M. A., Duivenvoorden, H. J., Busschbach, J. J., Eling, P. A., Bogert, M. A., *et al.* (2009) Metamemory and memory test performance in stroke patients. *Neuropsychological Rehabilitation, 19*, 742–753.

Ablinger, I. and Domahs, F. (2009) Improved single-letter identification after whole-word training in pure alexia. *Neuropsychological Rehabilitation, 19*, 340–363.

Abraham, E., Axelrod, B. N. and Ricker, J. H. (1996) Application of the oral trail making test to a mixed clinical sample. *Archives of Clinical Neuropsychology, 11*, 697–701.

Adair, J. C. and Barrett, A. M. (2008) Spatial neglect: Clinical and neuroscience review: A wealth of information on the poverty of spatial attention. *Annals of the New York Academy of Sciences, 1142*, 21–43.

Adams, H. P., del Zoppo, G., Alberts, M. J., Bhatt, D. L., Brass, L., Furlan, A., *et al.* (2007) Guidelines for the early management of adults with ischemic stroke: A guideline from the American Heart Association/American Stroke Association Stroke Council, Clinical Cardiology Council, Cardiovascular Radiology and Intervention Council, and the atherosclerotic peripheral vascular disease and quality of care outcomes in research interdisciplinary working groups. *Stroke, 38*, 1655–1711.

Adams, J. R. and Drake, R. E. (2006) Shared decision-making and evidence-based practice. *Community Mental Health Journal, 42*, 87–105.

Adamson, J. and Donovan, J. (2005) 'Normal disruption': South Asian and African/Caribbean relatives caring for an older family member in the UK. *Social Science and Medicine, 60*, 37–48.

Adshead, F., Cody, D. D. and Pitt, B. (1992) BASDEC: a novel screening instrument for depression in elderly medical inpatients. *British Medical Journal, 305*, 397.

Afiya Trust and the National Black Carers and Carers Workers Network. (2002) *We Care Too: A Good Practice Guide for People Working with Black Carers.* London: Afiya Trust and the National Black Carers and Carers Workers Network.

Agrell, B. and Dehlin, O. (1989) Comparison of six depression rating scales in geriatric stroke patients. *Stroke, 20*, 1190–1194.

Psychological Management of Stroke, First Edition. Nadina B. Lincoln, Ian I. Kneebone, Jamie A.B. Macniven and Reg C. Morris.
© 2012 John Wiley & Sons, Ltd. Published 2012 by John Wiley & Sons, Ltd.

Ajzen, I. (1985) From intentions to action: A theory of planned behaviour. In B. J. Kuhl (ed), *Action control: From cognitions to behaviors* (pp. 11–39) Springer.

Akinsanya, J., Diggory, P., Heitz, E. and Jones, V. (2009) Assessing capacity and obtaining consent for thrombolysis for acute stroke. *Clinical Medicine, 9*, 239–241.

Akinwuntan, A. E., De Weerdt, W., Feys, H., Pauwels, J., Baten, G., Arno, P. *et al.* (2005a) Effect of simulator training on driving after stroke: A randomized controlled trial. *Neurology, 65*, 843–850.

Akinwuntan, A. E., De Weerdt, W., Feys, H., Baten, G., Arno, P. and Kiekens, C. (2005b) The validity of a road test after stroke. *Archives of Physical Medicine and Rehabilitation, 86*, 421–426.

Akinwuntan, A. E., Devos, H., Feys, H., Verheyden, G., Baten, G., Kiekens, C. *et al.* (2007) Confirmation of the accuracy of a short battery to predict fitness-to-drive of stroke survivors without severe deficits. *Journal of Rehabilitation Medicine, 39*, 698–702.

Akinwuntan, A. E., Feys, H., De Weerdt, W., Baten, G., Arno, P. and Kiekens, C. (2006) Prediction of driving after stroke: A prospective study. *Neurorehabilitation and Neural Repair, 20*, 417–423.

Akinwuntan, A. E., Feys, H., DeWeerdt, W., Pauwels, J., Baten, G. and Strypstein, E. (2002) Determinants of driving after stroke. *Archives of Physical Medicine and Rehabilitation, 83*, 334–341.

Alaszewski, A., Alaszewski, H. and Potter, J. (2004) The bereavement model, stroke and rehabilitation: a critical analysis of the use of a psychological model in professional practice. *Disability and Rehabilitation 26*, 1067–1078.

Alaszewski, A., Alaszewski, H., Potter, J. and Penhale, B. (2007) Working after a stroke: Survivors' experiences and perceptions of barriers to and facilitators of the return to paid employment. *Disability and Rehabilitation, 29*, 1858–1869.

Alawneh, J., Clatworthy, Morris, R. and Warburton, E. (2010) Stroke management Clinical Evidence, 04 (201), 1–18.

Alderman, N. (2001) Managing challenging behaviour. In T. M. Wood (ed), *Neurobehavioural Disability and Social Handicap Following Traumatic Brain Injury* (pp. 175–208) Hove: Psychology Press.

Alderman, N., Burgess, P. W., Knight, C. and Henman, C. (2003) Ecological validity of a simplified version of the multiple errands shopping test. *Journal of the International Neuropsychological Society, 9*, 31–44.

Alexander, M. P., Stuss, D. T. and Fansabedian, N. (2003) California Verbal Learning Test: performance by patients with focal frontal and non-frontal lesions. *Brain, 126*, 1493–1503.

Alexandrov, A. V., Molina, C. A., Grotta, J. C., Garami, Z., Ford, S. R., Varez-Sabin, J., *et al.* (2004) Ultrasound-enhanced systemic thrombolysis for acute ischemic stroke. *New England Journal of Medicine, 351*, 2170–2178.

Al-Khawaja, I., Wade, D. T. and Collin, F. (1996) Bedside screening for aphasia: a comparison of two methods. *Journal of Neurology, 243*, 201–204.

Allen, D. (2008) The relationship between challenging behaviour and mental ill-health in people with intellectual disabilities: A review of current theories and evidence. *Journal of Intellectual Disabilities, 12*, 267–294.

Altenmüller, E., Marco-Pallares, J., Munte, T. F. and Schneider, S. (2009) Neural reorganization underlies improvement in stroke-induced motor dysfunction by music-supported therapy. In S. DallaBella, N. Kraus, C. Overy, C. Pantev, J. S. Snyder, M. Tervaniemi, B. Tillmann and G. Schlaug (eds), *Neurosciences and*

Music III: Disorders and Plasticity (Vol. 1169, pp. 395–405). Oxford: Blackwell Publishing.

American Psychiatric Association. (1994) *Diagnostic and Statistical Manual of Mental Disorders*, 4th ed. Washington, DC: American Psychiatric Association.

Andersen, G., Vestergaard, K., Ingeman-Nielsen, M. and Lauritzen, L. (1995) Risk factors for post-stroke depression. *Acta Psychiatrica Scandinavia*, *92*, 193–198.

Anderson, C. S., Carter, K. N., Brownlee, W. J., Hackett, M. L., Broad, J. B. and Bonita, R. (2004) Very long-term outcome after stroke in Auckland, *New Zealand. Stroke*, *35*, 1920–1924.

Anderson, C. S., Linto, J. and Stewart-Wynne, E. G. (1995) A Population-Based Assessment of the Impact and Burden of Caregiving for Long-term Stroke Survivors. *Stroke*, *26*, 843–849.

Anderson, J. F. I., Augoustakis, L. V., Holmes, R. J. and Chambers, B. R. (2009) End-of-life decision-making in individuals with Locked-in syndrome in the acute period after brainstem stroke. *Internal Medicine Journal*, *40*, 61–65.

Andersson, A. G., Kamwendo, K. and Appelros, P. (2008) Fear of falling in stroke patients: Relationship with previous falls and functional characteristics. *International Journal of Rehabilitation Research*, *31*, 261–264.

Andrasik, F. (2007) What does the evidence show? Efficacy of behavioural treatments for recurrent headaches in adults. *Neurological Sciences*, *28*, S70–S77.

Andrewes, D. G., Coetzee, N., Jenkins L., Finch, S., Hale, T., Khan, F., *et al.* (Submitted) The psychometric identification of stroke and amputee patients who are at risk of non-adherence.

Angelelli, P., Paolucci, S., Bivona, U., Piccardi, L., Ciurli, P., Cantagallo, A., *et al.* (2004) Development of neuropsychiatric symptoms in poststroke patients: a cross-sectional study. *Acta Psychiatrica Scandinavica*, *110*, 55–63.

Annoni, J., Staub, F., Bruggiman, L., Gragmina, S. and Bogousslavsky, J. (2006) Emotional disturbances after stroke. *Clinical and Experimental Hypertension*, *28*, 243–249.

Appelbaum, P. S. (1998) Ought we to require emotional capacity as part of decisional competence? *Kennedy Institute of Ethics Journal*, *8*, 377–388.

Appelbaum, P. S. (2007) Assessment of patients' competence to consent to treatment. *New England Journal of Medicine*, *357*, 1834–1840.

Arai, T., Ohi, H., Sasaki, H., Nobuto, H. and Tanaka, K. (1997) Hemispatial sunglasses: Effect on unilateral spatial neglect. *Archives of Physical Medicine and Rehabilitation*, *78*, 230–232.

Arean, P., Hegel, M., Vannoy, S., Fan, M. Y. and Unuzter, J. (2008) Effectiveness of problem-solving therapy for older, primary care patients with depression: Results from the IMPACT project. *Gerontologist*, *48*, 311–323.

Arfken, C. L., Lach, H. W., Birge, S. J. and Miller, J. P. (1994) The prevalence and correlates of fear of falling in elderly persons living in the community. *American Journal of Public Health*, *84*, 565–570.

Armitage, C. J. and Conner, M. (2001) Efficacy of the theory of planned behaviour: A meta-analytic review. *British Journal of Social Psychology*, *40*, 471–499.

Arno, P. S., Levine, C. and Memmott, M. M. (1999) The economic value of informal caregiving. *Health Affairs*, *18*, 182–188.

Arnstein, P., Vidal, M., Wells-Federman, C., Morgan, B. and Caudill, M. (2002) From chronic pain patient to peer: Benefits and risks of volunteering. *Pain Management Nursing*, *3*, 94–103.

Arts, S. E., Francke, A. L. and Hutten, J. B. (2000) Liaison nursing for stroke patients: Results of a Dutch evaluation study. *Journal of Advanced Nursing, 32,* 292–300.

Ashburn, A., Hyndman, D., Pickering, R., Yardley, L. and Harris, S. (2008) Predicting people with stroke at risk of falls. *Age and Ageing, 37,* 270–276.

Aspinall, P. and Jacobson, B. (2004) *Ethnic disparities in health and health care: A focused review of the evidence and selected examples of good practice.* London: London Health Observatory.

Åström, M. (1996) Generalised anxiety disorder in stroke patients. *Stroke, 27,* 270–275.

Aybek, S., Carotal, A., Ghika-Schmid, F., Berney, A., Van Melle, G., Guex, P., *et al.* (2005) Emotional behavior in acute stroke: The Lausanne emotion in stroke study. *Cognitive and Behavioral Neurology, 18,* 37–44.

Ayers, C. R., Sorrell, J. T., Thorp, S. R. and Wetherell, J. L. (2007) Evidence-based psychological treatments for late-life anxiety. *Psychology and Aging, 22,* 8–17.

Azouvi, P., Samuel, C., Louis-Dreyfus, A., Bernati, T., Bartolomeo, P., Beis, J. M., *et al.* (2002) Sensitivity of clinical and behavioural tests of spatial neglect after right hemisphere stroke. *Journal of Neurology, Neurosurgery and Psychiatry, 73,* 160–166.

Backe, M., Larsson, K. and Fridlund, B. (1996) Patients' conceptions of their life situation within the first week after stroke event: A qualitative analysis. *Intensive and Critical Care Nursing, 12,* 285–294.

Bäckman, L. (2008) Memory and cognition in preclinical dementia: What we know and what we do not know. *Canadian Journal of Psychiatry-Revue Canadienne De Psychiatrie, 53,* 354–360.

Bäckman, L. and Small, B. J. (2007) Cognitive deficits in preclinical Alzheimer's disease and vascular dementia: Patterns of findings from the Kungsholmen Project. *Physiology and Behavior, 92,* 80–86.

Bacon, F. (1625/2009) *Essayes or Counsels, Civill and Morall/The Essays of Sir Francis Bacon.* San Diego: Book Tree.

Baddeley, A., Emslie, H. and Nimmo-Smith, I. (1992) *Speed and Capacity of Language Processing Test (SCOLP)* London: Harcourt Assessment.

Baddeley, A. D., Emslie, H. and Nimmo-Smith, I. (1994) *Doors and People: A Test of Visual and Verbal Recall and Recognition.* Bury St Edmunds: Thames Valley Test Company.

Baddeley, A. D. and Hitch, G. J. (1974) Working memory. In G. H. Bower (ed), *The Psychology of Learning and Motivation,* vol. 8. New York: Academic Press.

Bagg, S., Pombo, A. P. and Hopman, W. (2002) Effect of age on functional outcomes after stroke rehabilitation. *Stroke, 33,* 179–185.

Baier, B. and Karnath, H. O. (2005) Incidence and diagnosis of anosognosia for hemiparesis revisited. *Journal of Neurology Neurosurgery and Psychiatry, 76,* 358–361.

Baier, B. and Karnath, H. O. (2008) Tight link between our sense of limb ownership and self-awareness of actions. *Stroke, 39,* 486–488.

Bailey, M. J., Riddoch, M. J. and Crome, P. (2000) Evaluation of a test battery for hemineglect in elderly stroke patients for use by therapists in clinical practice. *Neurorehabilitation, 14,* 139–150.

Bakas, T., Austin, J. K., Okonkwo, K. F., Lewis, R. R. and Chadwick, L. (2002) Needs, concerns, strategies, and advice of stroke caregivers the first 6 months after discharge. *Journal of Neuroscience and Nursing, 34,* 242–251.

Bakheit, A. M. O., Barrett, L. and Wood, J. (2004) The relationship between the severity of post-stroke aphasia and state self-esteem. *Aphasiology, 18,* 759–764.

Bakheit, A. M. O., Shaw, S., Barrett, L., Wood, J., Carrington, S., Griffiths, S., *et al.* (2007) A prospective, randomized, parallel group, controlled study of the effect of intensity of speech and language therapy on early recovery from poststroke aphasia. *Clinical Rehabilitation, 2,* 885–894.

Ball, K. K., Beard, B. L., Roenker, D. L., Miller, R. L. and Griggs, D. S. (1988) Age and visual search: Expanding the useful field of view. *Journal of the Optical Society of the America A, 5,* 2210–2219.

Ballard, C., Stephens, S., Kenny, R., Kalaria, R., Tovee, M. and O'Brien, J. (2003) Profile of neuropsychological deficits in older stroke survivors without dementia. *Dementia and Geriatric Cognitive Disorders, 16,* 52–56.

Ballard, K. J., Granier, J. P. and Robin, D. A. (2000) Understanding the nature of apraxia of speech: Theory, analysis, and treatment. *Aphasiology, 14,* 969–995.

Ballard, K. J. and Robin, D. A. (2002) Assessment of AOS for treatment planning. *Seminars in Speech and Language, 23,* 281–291.

Bamford, J., Sandercock, P., Jones, L. and Warlow, C. (1987) The natural history of lacunar infarction: The Oxfordshire Community Stroke Project. *Stroke, 18,* 545–551.

Bandelow, B., Zohar, J., Hollander, E., Kasper, S. and Moller, H. (2002) World Federation of Societies of Biological Psychiatry (WFSBP) guidelines for pharmacological treatment of anxiety, obsessive compulsive disorder and post-traumatic stress disorders. *World Journal of Biological Psychiatry, 3,* 171–199.

Bandura, A. (1997) *Self–efficacy: The exercise of control.* New York: W. H. Freeman.

Banks, P. and Pearson, C. (2003) *Improving services for younger stroke survivors and their families.* Edinburgh: Chest, Heart and Stroke, Scotland.

Banks, P. and Pearson, C. (2004) Parallel lives: Younger stroke survivors and their partners coping with crisis. *Sexual and Relationship Therapy, 19,* 413–429.

Barber, M. and Stott, D. J. (2004) Validity of the Telephone Interview for Cognitive Status (TICS) in post-stroke subjects. *International Journal of Geriatric Psychiatry, 19,* 75–79.

Barker, G. (2006) *Getting back to work after a stroke.* London and Milton Keynes: Stroke Association/Different Strokes.

Barker-Collo, S. and Feigin, V. (2006) The impact of neuropsychological deficits on functional stroke outcomes. *Neuropsychology Review, 16,* 53–64.

Barker-Collo, S. L. (2007) Depression and anxiety 3 months post stroke: Prevalence and correlates. *Archives of Clinical Neuropsychology, 22,* 519–531.

Barker-Collo, S. L., Feigin, V. L., Lawes, C. M. M., Parag, V., Senior, H. and Rodgers, A. (2009) Reducing attention deficits after stroke using attention process training: A randomized controlled trial. *Stroke, 40,* 3293–3298.

Barrett, A. M., Buxbaum, L. J., Coslett, H. B., Edwards, E., Heilman, K. M., Hillis, A. E., *et al.* (2006) Cognitive rehabilitation interventions for neglect and related disorders: Moving from bench to bedside in stroke patients. *Journal of Cognitive Neuroscience, 18,* 1223–1236.

Barton, J. (2010) Interdisciplinary approaches to the assessment and management of well-being. In S. E. Brumfitt (ed), Psychological well-being and acquired communication impairments. Chichester, UK: Wiley.

Barton, J., Miller, A. and Chanter, J. (2002) Emotional adjustment to stroke: a group therapeutic approach. *Nursing Times, 98,* 33–35.

Basso, A., Capitani, E., Dellasala, S., Laiacona, M. and Spinnler, H. (1987) Recovery from ideomotor apraxia: A study on acute stroke patients. *Brain, 110,* 747–760.

Basso, M. R., Bornstein, R. A., Roper, B. L. and McCoy, V. L. (2000) Limited accuracy of premorbid intelligence estimators: A demonstration of regression to the mean. *The Clinical Neuropsychologist, 14,* 325–340.

Batchelor, S., Thompson, E. O. and Miller, L. A. (2008) Retrograde memory after unilateral stroke. *Cortex, 44,* 170–178.

Bateman, A. (2009) Is this approach effective? Outcome measurement at the Oliver Zangwill Centre. In F. G. B.A. Wilson, J.J. Evans and A. Bateman (ed), *Neuropsychological Rehabilitation: Theory, Models, Therapy and Outcome* (pp. 334–349). Cambridge: Cambridge University Press.

Batt, K., Shores, E. A. and Chekaluk, E. (2008) The effect of distraction on the Word Memory Test and Test of Memory Malingering performance in patients with a severe brain injury. *Journal of the International Neuropsychological Society, 14,* 1074–1080.

Bauby, J. D. (2002) *The Diving Bell and the Butterfly.* Paris: Harper Perennial.

Bauby, J. D. and Schnable, J. (Writers) (2008) *The Diving Bell and the Butterfly* [Motion picture]. Pathe Distribution.

Bayley, M. T., Hurdowar, A., Teasell, R., Wood-Dauphinee, S., Korner-Bitensky, N., Richards, C. L., *et al.* (2007) Priorities for stroke rehabilitation and research: Results of a 2003 Canadian Stroke Network Consensus Conference. *Archives of Physical Medicine and Rehabilitation, 88,* 526–528.

Bays, C. (2001a) Older adults' descriptions of hope after stroke. *Rehabilitation Nursing, 26,* 18–27.

Bays, C. L. (2001b) Quality of life of stroke survivors: a research synthesis. *Journal of Neuroscience Nursing, 33,* 310–316.

Bazzano, L., Gu, D., Reynolds, K., Wu, X., Chen, C., Duan, X., *et al.* (2007) Alcohol consumption and risk for stroke among Chinese men. *Annals of Neurology, 62,* 569–578.

Bazzano, L. A., Serdula, M. K. and Liu, S. (2003) Dietary intake of fruits and vegetables and risk of cardiovascular disease. *Current Atherosclerosis Reports, 5,* 492–499.

Bean, G., Nishisato, S., Rector, N. A. and Glancy, G. (1994) The psychometric properties of the competency interview schedule. *Canadian Journal of Psychiatry, 39,* 368–376.

Beck, A. T. (1979) *Cognitive therapy of depression.* New York: Guilford.

Beck, A. T. and Steer, R. A. (1987) *Beck Depression Inventory Manual.* San Antonio, TX: The Psychological Corporation.

Beck, A. T. and Steer, R. A. (1993) *Beck Anxiety Inventory Manual.* San Antonio, TX: Psychological Corporation.

Beck, A. T., Steer, R. A. and Brown, G. K. (1996) *Beck Depression Inventory-II (BDI-II).* San Antonio, TX: Psychological Corporation.

Beck, A. T., Steer, R. A. and Brown, G. K. (2000) *BDI-FastScreen for medical patients manual.* San Antonio, TX: Psychological Corporation.

Beck, A. T., Ward, C. H., Mendelson, M., Mock, J. and Erbaugh, J. (1961) An inventory for measuring depression. *Archives of General Psychiatry, 4,* 561–571.

Becker, G. and Kaufman, S. (1995) Managing an uncertain illness trajectory after stroke: Patients' and physicians' views of stroke. *Medical Anthropology Quarterly, 9,* 165–187.

Becker, M. H. and Maiman, L. A. (1975) Sociobehavioral determinants of compliance with health and medical care recommendations. *Medical Care, 13,* 10–24.

Bederson, J. B., Connolly, E. S., Jr., Batjer, H. H., Dacey, R. G., Dion, J. E., Diringer, M. N., *et al.* (2009) Guidelines for the management of aneurysmal subarachnoid hemorrhage: A statement for healthcare professionals from a special writing group of the Stroke Council, *American Heart Association. Stroke, 40,* 994–1025.

Beeman, M. (1993) Semantic processing in the right hemisphere may contribute to drawing inferences from discourse. *Brain and Language, 44,* 80–120.

Beis, J. M., Andre, J. M., Baumgarten, A. and Challier, B. (1999) Eye patching in unilateral spatial neglect: Efficacy of two methods. *Archives of Physical Medicine and Rehabilitation, 80,* 71–76.

Belcher, V. N., Fried, T. R., Agostini, J. V. and Tinetti, M. E. (2006) Views of older adults on patient participation in medication-related decision making. *Journal of General Internal Medicine, 21,* 298–303.

Belgen, B., Beninato, M., Sullivan, P. E. and Narielwalla, K. (2006) The association of balance capacity and falls self-efficacy with history of falling in community-dwelling people with chronic stroke. *Archives of Physical Medicine and Rehabilitation, 87,* 554–561.

Bellhouse, J., Holland, A., Clare, I. and Gunn, M. (2001) Decision-making capacity in adults: Its assessment in clinical practice. *Advances in Psychiatric Treatment, 7,* 294–301.

Benaim, C., Cailly, B., Perennou, D. and Pelissier, J. (2004) Validation of the Aphasic Depression Rating Scale. *Stroke, 35,* 1692–1696.

Benaim, C., Decavel, P., Bentabet, M., Froger, J., Pelissier, J. and Perennou, D. (2010) Sensitivity to change of two depression rating scales for stroke patients. *Clinical Rehabilitation, 24,* 251–257.

Bendz, M. (2003) The first year of rehabilitation after a stroke: From two perspectives. *Scandinavian Journal of Caring Sciences, 17,* 215–222.

Bennett, B. (1996) How nurses in a stroke rehabilitation unit attempt to meet the psychological needs of patients who become depressed following a stroke. *Journal of Advanced Nursing, 23,* 314–321.

Bennett, H. E. and Lincoln, N. B. (2006) Potential screening measures for depression and anxiety after stroke. *International Journal of Therapy and Rehabilitation, 13,* 401–406.

Bennett, H. E., Thomas, S. A., Austen, R., Morris, A. M. S. and Lincoln, N. B. (2006) Validation of screening measures for assessing mood in stroke patients. *British Journal of Clinical Psychology, 45,* 367–376.

Bennett, P. C., Ong, B. and Ponsford, J. (2005) Assessment of executive dysfunction following traumatic brain injury: Comparison of the BADS with other clinical neuropsychologiacl measures. *Journal of the International Neuropsychological Society, 11,* 606–613.

Bennett, S. J. (1993) Relationships among selected antecedent variables and coping effectiveness in postmyocardial infarction patients. *Research in Nursing and Health, 16,* 131–139.

Benowitz, L. I. and Carmichael, S. T. (2010) Promoting axonal rewiring to improve outcome after stroke. *Neurobiology of Disease, 37,* 259–266.

Ben-Sira, Z. and Eliezer, R. (1990) The structure of readjustment after heart attack. *Social Science & Medicine, 30,* 523–536.

Benton, A. L. and Hamsher, K. (1983) *Controlled Oral Word Association Test.* Iowa City: AJA Associates.

Benton, A. L., Hamsher, K. and Sivan, A. B. (1994) *Multilingual Aphasia Examination*. Iowa City, IA: AJA Associates.

Benton, A. L., Sivan, A. B., Hamsher, K., Varney, R. and Spreen, O. (1994) *Contributions to Neuropsychological Assessment: A Clinical Manual*, 2nd ed. New York: Oxford University Press.

Benton, A. L., Varney, N. R. and Hamsher, K. (1978) Visuospatial judgement: A clinical test. *Archives of Neurology*, 35, 364–367.

Berg, A., Lönnqvist, J., Palomäki, H. and Kaste, M. (2009) Assessment of depression after stroke: A comparison of different instruments. *Stroke*, 40, 523–529.

Berg, A., Palomaki, H., Loonnqvist, J., Lehtihalmes, M. and Kast, M. (2005) Depression among caregivers of stroke survivors. *Stroke*, 36, 639–643.

Bergersen, H., Froslie, K., Sunnerhagen, K. and Schanke, A. (2010) Anxiety, depression, and psychological well-being 2 to 5 years poststroke. *Journal of Stroke and Cerebrovascular Diseases*, 19, 364–369.

Berghmans, R., Dickenson, D. and Ter Meulen, R. (2004) Mental capacity: In search of alternative perspectives. *Health Care Analysis*, 12, 251–263.

Bero, L. A., Grilli, R., Grimshaw, J. M., Harvey, E., Oxman, A. D., Thomson, M. A., *et al.* (1998) Getting research findings into practice: Closing the gap between research and practice: An overview of systematic reviews of interventions to promote the implementation of research findings. *British Medical Journal*, 317 (7156), 465–468.

Bhalla, A., Grieve, R., Rudd, A. G. and Wolfe, C. D. A. (2008) Stroke in the young: access to care and outcome: A Western versus eastern European perspective. *Journal of Stroke & Cerebrovascular Disease*, 17, 360–365.

Bham, Z. and Ross, E. (2005) Traditional and Western medicine: Cultural beliefs and practices of South African Indian Muslims with regard to stroke. *Ethnicity & Disease*, 15, 548–554.

Bhavnani, G., Cockburn, J., Whiting, S. and Lincoln, N. B. (1983) The reliability of the Rivermead Perceptual Assessment and its implications for some commonly used tests of perception. *British Journal of Occupational Therapy*, 46, 17–19.

Bhogal, S. K., Teasell, R. and Speechley, M. (2003) Intensity of aphasia therapy, impact on recovery. *Stroke*, 34, 987–992.

Bielby, P. (2005) The conflation of competence and capacity in English medical law: A philosophical critique. *Medicine, Health Care and Philosophy 8*, 357–369.

Biller, J. (ed), (2009) *Stroke in Children and Young Adults*, 2nd ed. New York: Saunders Elsevier.

Bird, C. M. and Cipolotti, L. (2007) The utility of the recognition memory test and the graded naming test for monitoring neurological patients. *British Journal of Clinical Psychology*, 46, 223–234.

Bird, C. M., Malhotra, P., Parton, A., Coulthard, E., Rushworth, M. F. S. and Husain, M. (2006) Visual neglect after right posterior cerebral artery infarction. *Journal of Neurology Neurosurgery and Psychiatry*, 77, 1008–1012.

Bird, C. M., Papadopoulou, K., Ricciardelli, P., Rossor, M. N. and Cipolotti, L. (2004) Monitoring cognitive changes: Psychometric properties of six cognitive tests. *British Journal of Clinical Psychology*, 43, 197–210.

Bisiach, E. and Luzzatti, C. (1978) Unilateral neglect of representational space. *Cortex*, 14 (1), 129–133.

Bisiach, E., Perani, D., Vallar, G. and Berti, A. (1986) Unilateral neglect: Personal and extra-personal. *Neuropsychologia*, 24, 759–767.

Bisiach, E., Vallar, G., Perani, D., Papagno, C. and Berti, A. (1986) Unawareness of disease following lesions of the right hemisphere: Anosognosia for hemiplegia and anosognosia for hemianopia. *Neuropsychologia*, *24*, 471–482.

Bisson, J. and Andrew, M. (2007) Psychological treatment of post-traumatic stress disorder (PTSD). *Cochrane Database Systematic Reviews* (3), CD003388.

Bisson, J. I., Hampton, V., Rosser, A. and Holm, S. (2009) Developing a care pathway for advance decisions and powers of attorney: Qualitative study. *British Journal of Psychiatry*, *194*, 55–61.

Black, C. (2008) *Working for a Healthier Tomorrow*. London.

Blackhall, L. J., Murphy, S. T., Frank, G., Michel, V. and Azen, S. (1995) Ethnicity and attitudes toward patient autonomy. *Journal of the American Medical Association*, *274*, 820–825.

Black-Schaffer, R. M. and Osberg, J. S. (1990) Return to work after stroke: Development of a predictive model. *Archives of Physical Medicine and Rehabilitation*, *71*, 285–290.

Black-Schaffer, R. M. and Winston, C. (2004) Age and functional outcome after stroke. *Topics in Stroke Rehabilitation*, *11*, 23–32.

Blake, H. and Lincoln, N. (2000) Factors associated with strain in co-resident spouses of stroke patients. *Clinical Rehabilitation*, *14*, 307–314.

Blake, H., McKinney, M., Treece, K., Lee, E. and Lincoln, N. B. (2002) An evaluation of screening measures for cognitive impairment after stroke. *Age and Ageing*, *31*, 451–456.

Blaser, T., Hofmann, K., Buerger, T., Effenberger, O., Wallesch, C. W. and Goertler, M. (2002) Risk of stroke, transient ischemic attack, and vessel occlusion before endarterectomy in patients with symptomatic severe carotid stenosis. *Stroke*, *33*, 1057–1062.

Bogousslavsky, J. (2003) William Feinberg lecture 2002. Emotions, mood, and behavior after stroke. *Stroke*, *34*, 1046–1050.

Bogousslavsky, J. and Caplan, L. R. (2001) *Uncommon Causes of Stroke*. Cambridge: Cambridge University Press.

Bogousslavsky, J., Vanmelle, G. and Regli, F. (1988) The Lausanne stroke registry: Analysis of 1, 000 consecutive patients with first stroke. *Stroke*, *19*, 1083–1092.

Bolte-Taylor, J. (2008) *My Stroke of Insight*. London: Hodder & Stoughton.

Bond, J., Gregson, B., Smith, M., Rousseau, N., Lecouturier, J. and Rodgers, H. (1998) Outcomes following acute hospital care for stroke or hip fracture: How useful is an assessment of anxiety or depression for older people? *International Journal of Geriatric Psychiatry*, *13*, 601–610.

Bonetti, D. and Johnston, M. (2008) Perceived control predicting the recovery of individual-specific walking behaviours following stroke: Testing psychological models and constructs. *British Journal of Health Psychology*, *13*, 463–478.

Boone, K. B. (ed) (2007) *Assessment of Feigned Cognitive Impairment: A Neuropsychological Perspective*. New York: Guilford Press.

Borkman, T. (1976) Experiential knowledge: A new concept for the analysis of self-help groups. *Social Service Review*, *50*, 445–456.

Botez, S. A., Carrera, E., Maeder, P. and Bogousslavsky, J. (2007) Aggressive behavior and posterior cerebral artery stroke. *Archives of Neurology*, *64*, 1029–1033.

Botner, E. M., Miller, W. C. and Eng, J. J. (2005) Measurement properties of the Activities-specific Balance Confidence Scale among individuals with stroke. *Disability and Rehabilitation*, *27*, 156–163.

Bouska, M. J. and Kwatny, E. (1982) *Manual for the Application of the Motor-Free Visual Perception Test to the Adult Population.* Philadelphia: Temple University Rehabilitation Research and Training Center.

Bouwmeester, L., Heutink, J. and Lucas, C. (2007) The effect of visual training for patients with visual field defects due to brain damage: A systematic review. *Journal of Neurology Neurosurgery and Psychiatry*, 78, 555–564.

Bowen, A., Hesketh, A., Patchick, E., Young, A., Davies, L., Vail, A., Long, A., Watkins, C., Wilkinson, M., Pearl, G., Lambon Ralph, M., Tyrrell, P.on behalf of the ACT NoW investigators. (2011) Clinical effectiveness, cost effectiveness and service users' perceptions of early, intensively resourced communication therapy following a stroke, a randomised controlled trial (The ACT NoW Study) Health Technology Assessment, in press.

Bowen, A., Knapp, P., Hoffman, A. and Lowe, D. (2005) Psychological assessment and treatment after stroke: What services are provided for people admitted to hospital in the UK? *Clinical Rehabilitation*, 19, 323–330.

Bowen, A. and Lincoln, N. B. (2007a) Rehabilitation for spatial neglect improves test performance but not disability. *Stroke*, 38, 2869–2870.

Bowen, A. and Lincoln, N. B. (2007b) Cognitive rehabilitation for spatial neglect following stroke. *Cochrane Database Systematic Reviews* (2), CD003586.

Bowen, A., McKenna, K. and Tallis, R. C. (1999) Reasons for variability in the reported rate of occurence of unilateral spatial neglect after stroke. *Stroke*, 30, 1196–1202.

Bowen, A., West, C., Hesketh, A. and Vail, A. (2009) Rehabilitation for apraxia evidence for short-term improvements in activities of daily living. *Stroke*, 40, E396–E397.

Bowlby, J. (1973) Attachment and Loss: Vol. *2 Separation: Anxiety and Anger.* New York: Basic Books.

Bowling, A. (1995) *Measuring Disease.* Buckingham: Open University Press.

Bradbury, C. L., Christensen, B. K., Lau, M. A., Ruttan, L. A., Arundine, A. L. and Green, R. E. (2008) The efficacy of cognitive behavior therapy in the treatment of emotional distress after acquired brain injury. *Archives of Physical Medicine and Rehabilitation*, 89, S61–S68.

Brandt, J., Spencer, M. and Folstein, M. (1988) The Telephone Interview for Cognitive Status. *Neuropsychiatry, Neurospychology and Behavioural Neurology*, 1, 111–117.

Brazzelli, M., Sandercock, P. A. G., Chappell, F. M., Celani, M. G., Righetti, E., Arestis, N., *et al.* (2009) Magnetic resonance imaging versus computed tomography for detection of acute vascular lesions in patients presenting with stroke symptoms. *Cochrane Database of Systematic Reviews* (4), CD007424.

Breden, T. M. and Vollmann, J. (2004) The cognitive based approach of capacity assessment in psychiatry: A philosophical critique of the MacCAT-T. *Health Care Analysis*, 12, 273–284.

Brereton, L., Carroll, C. and Barnston, S. (2007) Interventions for adult family carers of people who have had a stroke: A systematic review. *Clinical Rehabilitation*, 21, 867–884.

Brereton, L. and Nolan, M. (2000) 'You do know he's had a stroke, don't you?' Preparation for family care-giving: The neglected dimension. *Journal of Clinical Nursing*, 9, 498–506.

Brereton, L. and Nolan, M. (2002) 'Seeking': A key activity for new family carers of stroke survivors. *Journal of Clinical Nursing*, 11, 22–31.

British Psychological Society (2007) *New Ways of Working for Applied Psychologists in Health and Social Care: Organising, Managing, and Leading Psychological Services.* Leicester: British Psychological Society

Broadbent, D. E., Cooper, P. F., Fitzgerald, P. and Parkes, K. R. (1982) The Cognitive Failures Questionnaire and its correlates. *British Journal of Clinical Psychology, 21*, 1–16.

Broderick, J. P., Brott, T. G., Duldner, J. E., Tomsick, T. and Leach, A. (1994) Initial and recurrent bleeding are the major causes of death following subarachnoid hemorrhage. *Stroke, 25*, 1342–1347.

Brown, G. K. and Nicassio, P. M. (1987) Development of a questionnaire for the assesment of active and passive coping strategies in chronic pain patients. *Pain, 31*, 53–64.

Brown, I., Sheeran, P. and Reuber, M. (2009) Enhancing antiepileptic drug adherence: A randomized controlled trial. *Epilepsy & Behavior, 16*, 634–639.

Brown, R. A. and Lewinsohn, P. M. (1984) A psychoeducational approach to the treatment of depression: Comparison of group, individual and minimal contact procedures. *Journal of Consulting and Clinical Psychology, 52*, 774–783.

Bruce, D. G., Devine, A. and Prince, R. L. (2002) Recreational physical activity levels in healthy older women: The importance of fear of falling. *Journal of the American Geriatrics Society, 50*, 84–89.

Brugger, P., Regard, M., Landis, T. and Oelz, O. (1999) Hallucinatory experiences in extreme-altitude climbers. *Neuropsychiatry Neuropsychology and Behavioral Neurology, 12*, 67–71.

Bruggimann, L., Annoni, J. M., Staub, F., von Steinbuchel, N., Van der Linden, M. and Bogousslavsky, J. (2006) Chronic posttraumatic stress symptoms after nonsevere stroke. *Neurology, 66*, 513–516.

Brumfitt, S. and Barton, J. (2006) Evaluating wellbeing in people with aphasia using speech therapy and clinical psychology. *International Journal of Therapy and Rehabilitation, 13*, 305–310.

Brumfitt, S. and Sheeran, P. (1999a) The development and validation of the Visual Analogue Self-Esteem Scale. *British Journal of Clinical Psychology, 38*, 387–400.

Brumfitt, S. and Sheeran, P. (1999b) *VASES: Visual Analogue Self-Esteem Scale.* Bicester: Winslow Press Ltd.

Brunila, T., Lincoln, N. B., Lindell, A., Tenovuo, O. and Hämäläinen, H. (2002) Experiences of combined visual training and arm activation in the rehabilitation of unilateral visual neglect: A clinical study. *Neuropsychological Rehabilitation, 12*, 27–40.

Brunner, E., Rees, K., Ward, K., Burke, M. and Thorogood, M. (2007) Dietary advice for reducing cardiovascular risk. *Cochrane Database Systematic Reviews* (2), CD002128.

Buckner, L. and Yeandle, S. (2007) *Valuing Carers: Calculating the Value of Unpaid Care.* London: Carers UK.

Bull, M. J. and Roberts, J. (2001) Components of a proper hospital discharge for elders. *Journal of Advanced Nursing, 35*, 571–581.

Bunton, P. J. C., An evaluation of screening measures for detecting low mood and cognitive impairment in acute stroke patients. DClinPsychol Thesis, University of Liverpool, UK.

Burgess, M. and Chalder, T. (2005) *Overcoming Chronic Fatigue.* London. Constable & Robinson.

Burgess, M. and Mooney, E. (2006) Stroke rehabilitation for the young: Age-specific rehabilitation. *British Journal of Neuroscience Nursing, 2*, 6–8.

Burgess, P. W., Alderman, N., Evans, J., Emslie, H. and Wilson, B. A. (1998) The ecological validity of tests of executive function. *Journal of the International Neuropsychological Society, 4*, 547–558.

Burgess, P. W. and Shallice, T. (1997) *The Hayling and Brixton Tests.* Bury St Edmunds: Thames Valley Test Company.

Burns, A., Lawlor, B. A. and Craig, S. (1999) *Assessment Scales in Old Age Psychiatry.* London: Martin Dunitz.

Burton, C. and Gibbon, B. (2005) Expanding the role of the stroke nurse: A pragmatic clinical trial. *Journal of Advanced Nursing, 52*, 640–650.

Burton, C. R. (2000a) A description of the nursing role in stroke rehabilitation. *Journal of Advanced Nursing, 32*, 174–181.

Burton, C. R. (2000b) Living with stroke: A phenomenological study. *Journal of Advanced Nursing, 32*, 301–309.

Burton, C. R. (2000c) Re-thinking stroke rehabilitation: The Corbin and Strauss chronic illness trajectory framework. *Journal of Advanced Nursing, 32*, 595–602.

Burvill, P., Johnson, G. A., Jamrozik, K., Anderson, C. and Stewart-Wynne, E. (1997) Risk factors for poststroke depression. *International Journal of Geriatric Psychiatry, 12*, 219–226.

Burvill, P. W., Johnson, G. A., Jamrozik, K. D., Anderson, C. S., Stewart-Wynne, E. G. and Chakera, T. M. H. (1995) Anxiety disorders after stroke: Results from the Perth Community Stroke Study. *British Journal of Psychiatry, 166*, 328–332.

Busch, F. N. (2009) Anger and depression. *Advances in Psychiatric Treatment, 15*, 271–278.

Busch, M. A., Coshall, C., Heuschmann, P. U., McKevitt, C. and Wolfe, C. D. A. (2009) Sociodemographic differences in return to work after stroke: the South London Stroke Register (SLSR). *Journal of Neurology Neurosurgery and Psychiatry, 80*, 888–893.

Buschenfeld, K., Morris, R. and Lockwood, S. (2009) The experience of partners of young stroke survivors. *Disability and Rehabilitation, 31*, 1643–1651.

Butler, A. C., Chapman, J. E., Forman, E. M. and Beck, A. T. (2005) The empirical status of cognitive behaviour therapy: A review of meta-analyses. *Clinical Psychology Review, 1*, 17–31.

Caeiro, L., Ferro, J., Santos, C. and Figueira, M. (2006) Depression in acute stroke. *Journal of Psychiatry and Neuroscience, 31*, 377–383.

Calvert, T., Knapp, P. and House, A. (1998) Psychological associations with emotionalism after stroke. *Journal of Neurology Neurosurgery and Psychiatry, 65*, 928–929.

Cameron, J. and Gignac, M. (2008) 'Timing it right': A conceptual framework for addressing the support needs of family caregivers to stroke survivors from the hospital to the home. *Patient Education and Counselling, 70*, 305–314.

Cantor, J., Ashman, T., Schwartz, M. E., Gordon, W. A., Hibbard, M. R., Brown, M., *et al.* (2005) The role of self-discrepancy theory in understanding post-traumatic brain injury affective disorders: A pilot study. *Journal of Head Trauma Rehabilitation, 20*, 527–543.

Cao, M., Ferrari, M., Patella, R., Marra, C. and Rasura, M. (2007) Neuropsychological findings in young-adult stroke patients. *Archives of Clinical Neuropsychology, 22*, 133–142.

Cappa, S. F., Benke, T., Clarke, S., Rossi, B., Stemmer, B. and Heugten, C. M. (2005) EFNS guidelines on cognitive rehabilitation: Report of an EFNS task force. *European Journal of Neurology, 12*, 665–680.

Carers UK. (2006) *In the Know: The Importance of Information for Carers.* London: Carers UK.

Carers UK. (2008) *Carers' Voices: Shaping the 2008 National Strategy for Carers.* London: Carers UK.

Carlomagno, S., Pandolfi, M., Labruna, L., Colombo, A. and Razzano, C. (2001) Recovery from moderate aphasia in the first year poststroke: Effect of type of therapy. *Archives of Physical Medicine and Rehabilitation, 82,* 1073–1080.

Carmichael, S. T., Tatsukawa, K., Katsman, D., Tsuyuguchi, N. and Kornblum, H. I. (2004) Evolution of diaschisis in a focal stroke model. *Stroke, 35,* 758–763.

Carnwath, T. and Johnson, D. (1987) Psychiatric morbidity among spouses of patients with stroke. *British Medical Journal, 14,* 409–411.

Carod-Artal, F. J. (2007) Are mood disorders a stroke risk factor? *Stroke, 38,* 1–3.

Carota, A., Berney, A., Aybek, S., Iaria, G., Staub, F., Ghika-Schmid, F., *et al.* (2005) A prospective study of predictors of poststroke depression. *Neurology, 64,* 428–438.

Carota, A. and Bogousslavsky, J. (2003) Poststroke depression. *Advances in Neurology, 92,* 435–445.

Carota, A., Rossetti, A. O., Karapanayiotides, T. and Bogousslavsky, J. (2001) Catastrophic reaction in acute stroke: A reflex behavior in aphasic patients. *Neurology, 57,* 1902–1905.

Carota, A., Staub, F. and Bogousslavsky, J. (2002) Emotions, behaviours and mood changes in stroke. *Current Opinion in Neurology, 15,* 57–69.

Carpenter, M. G., Adkin, A. L., Brawley, L. R. and Frank, J. S. (2006) Postural, physiological and psychological reactions to challenging balance: Does age make a difference? *Age and Ageing, 35,* 298–303.

Carr, E. G., Robinson, S., Taylor, J. C. and Carlson, J. I. (1990) Positive approaches to the treatment of severe behaviour problems in persons with developmental disabilities: A review and analysis of reinforcement and stimulus-based procedures. Monograph of the Association for Persons with Severe Handicaps No. 4. Seattle, WA: TASH.

Carrhill, R. A. (1992) The measurement of patient satisfaction. *Journal of Public Health Medicine, 14,* 236–249.

Carroll, C., Hobart, J., Fox, C., Teare, L. and Gibson, J. (2004) Stroke in Devon: Knowledge was good, but action was poor. *Journal of Neurology, Neurosurgery & Psychiatry, 75,* 567–571.

Carson, A., MacHale, S., Allen, K., Lawrie, S., Dennis, M., House, A., *et al.* (2000) Depression after stroke and lesion location: A systematic review. *Lancet, 356,* 122–126.

Cartoni, A. and Lincoln, N. B. (2005) The sensitivity and specificity of the Middlesex Elderly Assessment of Mental State (MEAMS) for detecting cognitive impairment after stroke. *Neuropsychological Rehabilitation, 15,* 55–67.

Carver, C. S. (1997) You want to measure coping but your protocol's too long: Consider the Brief COPE. *International Journal of Behavioural Medicine, 4,* 92–100.

Carver, C. S., Scheier, M. F. and Weintraub, J. K. (1989) Assessing coping strategies: A theoretically based approach. *Journal of Personality and Social Psychology, 56,* 267–283.

Castillo, C. S., Schultz, S. K. and Robinson, R. G. (1995) Clinical correlates of early-onset and late-onset poststroke generalized anxiety. *American Journal of Psychiatry, 152,* 1174–1179.

Chakrabarty, A. and Shivane, A. (2008) Pathology of intracerebral haemorrhage. *Advances in Clinical Neuroscience and Rehabilitation, 8* (1), 20–21.

Chan, M. L. (2008) Description of a return-to-work occupational therapy programme for stroke rehabilitation in Singapore. *Occupational Therapy International*, 15, 87–99.

Charland, L. C. (1998) Appreciation and emotion: Theoretical reflections on the MacArthur Treatment Competence Study. *Kennedy Institute of Ethics Journal*, 8, 359–376.

Charles, C., Gafni, A. and Whelan, T. (1997) Shared decision-making in the medical encounter: What does it mean? (Or it takes at least two to tango). *Social Science & Medicine*, 44, 681–692.

Chatterjee, A. (1994) Picturing unilateral spatial neglect: Viewer versus object centered reference frames. *Journal of Neurology Neurosurgery and Psychiatry*, 57 (10), 1236–1240.

Chavez, J. C., Hurko, O., Barone, F. C. and Feuerstein, G. Z. (2009) Pharmacologic interventions for stroke looking beyond the thrombolysis time window into the penumbra with biomarkers, not a stopwatch. *Stroke*, 40, E558–E563.

Chest Heart and Stroke Scotland. (2003a) *Improving Stroke Services: Patients' and carers' views.* Edinburgh: Chest, Heart & Stroke Scotland.

Chest Heart and Stroke Scotland. (2003b) *Stroke: A Strategy for Scotland.* Edinburgh: Chest, Heart and Stroke, Scotland.

Chest Heart and Stroke Scotland (CHSS) Scottish Association of Health Councils. (2001) *Improving Stroke Services: Patients' and Carers' Views.* Edinburgh: CHSS.

Childs, L. and Kneebone, I. I. (2002) Falls, fear of falling and psychological management. *International Journal of Therapy and Rehabilitation*, 9, 225–231.

Ch'Ng, A., French, D. and Mclean, N. (2008) Coping with the challenges of recovery from stroke: Long term perspectives of stroke support group members. *Journal of Health Psychology*, 13, 1136–1146.

Chobanian, A., Bakris, G., Black, H., Cushman, W., Green, L., Izzo Jr, J., *et al.* (2003) National Heart, Lung, and Blood Institute Joint National Committee on Prevention, Detection, Evaluation, and Treatment of High Blood Pressure; National High Blood Pressure Education Program Coordinating Committee: The Seventh Report of the Joint National Committee on Prevention, Detection, Evaluation, and Treatment of High Blood Pressure: the JNC 7 report. *Journal of the American Medical Association*, 289, 2560–2572.

Choi-Kwon, S., Choi, J., Kwon, S. U., Kang, D. W. and Kim, J. S. (2007) Fluoxetine is not effective in the treatment of poststroke fatigue: A double-blind, placebo-controlled study. *Cerebrovascular Diseases*, 23, 103–108.

Chriki, L. S., Bullain, S. S. and Stern, T. A. (2006) The recognition and management of psychological reactions to stroke. *Primary Care Companion to the Journal of Clinical Psychiatry*, 8, 234–240.

Church, M. (1986) Issues in psychological therapy with elderly people. In I. Hanley and M. Gilhooly (eds), *Psychological Therapies for the Elderly*. Beckenham: Croom Helm.

Cicerone, K., Levin, H., Malec, J., Stuss, D. and Whyte, J. (2006) Cognitive rehabilitation interventions for executive function: Moving from bench to bedside in patients with traumatic brain injury. *Journal of Cognitive Neuroscience*, 18, 1212–1222.

Cicerone, K. D., Dahlberg, C., Kalmar, K., Langenbahn, D. M., Malec, J. F., Bergquist, T. F., *et al.* (2000) Evidence-based cognitive rehabilitation: recommendations for clinical practice. *Archives of Physical Medicine and Rehabilitation*, 81, 1596–1615.

Cicerone, K. D., Dahlberg, C., Malec, J. F., Langenbahn, D. M., Felicetti, T., Kneipp, S., *et al.* (2005) Evidence-based cognitive rehabilitation: Updated review of the literature from 1998 through 2002. *Archives of Physical and Medical Rehabilitation*, *86*, 1681–1692.

Cleary, P. D., Edgmanlevitan, S., Roberts, M., Moloney, T. W., McMullen, W., Walker, J. D., *et al.* (1991) Patients evaluate thier hospital care: A national survey. *Health Affairs*, *10*, 254–267.

Closs, S. J. and Tierney, A. J. (1993) The complexities of using a structure, process and outcome framework: The case of an evaluation of discharge planning for elderly patients. *Journal of Advanced Nursing*, *18*, 1279–1287.

Cockburn, J., Bhavnani, G., Whiting, S. and Lincoln, N. B. (1982) Normal performance on some tests of perception in adults. *British Journal of Occupational Therapy*, *45*, 67–68.

Coetzee, N., Andrewes, D., Khan, F., Hale, T., Jenkins, L., Lincoln, N., *et al.* (2008) Predicting compliance with treatment following stroke: A new model of adherence following rehabilitation. *Brain Impairment*, *9*, 122–139.

Cohen, S. and Wills, T. A. (1985) Stress, social support, and the buffering hypothesis. *Psychological Bulletin*, *98*, 310–357.

Colantonio, A., Kasl, S. V. and Ostfeld, A. M. (1992) Depressive symptoms and other psychosocial factors as predictors of stroke in the elderly. *American Journal of Epidemiology*, *136*, 884–894.

Colarusso, R. R. and Hammill, D. D. (1996) *Motor Free Visual Perception Test Revised*. San Rafael, CA: Academic Therapy Publications.

Collin, C., Wade, D. T., Davies, S. and Horne, V. (1988) The Barthel Index: A reliability study. *International Journal of Disability Studies*, *10*, 61–63.

Coltheart, M. (ed) (1987) *The Psychology of Reading (Attention and Performance XII)*. Hove: Lawrence Erlbaum Associates.

Coltheart, M. and Byng, S. (1989) A treatment for surface dyslexia. In G. D. X Seron (ed), *Cognitive Approaches in Neuropsychological Rehabilitation* (pp. 159–174). Hillsdale, NJ: Lawrence Erlbaum Associates.

Commission for Health Improvement (2004) *Unpacking the Patient's Perspective: Variations in NHS Patient Experience in England*. London: Commission for Health Improvement.

Committeri, G., Pitzalis, S., Galati, G., Patria, F., Pelle, G., Sabatini, U., *et al.* (2007) Neural bases of personal and extrapersonal neglect in humans. *Brain*, *130*, 431–441.

Cornish, I. M. (2000) Factor structure of the Everyday Memory Questionnaire. *British Journal of Psychology*, *91*, 427–438.

Corr, S. and Wilmer, S. (2003) Returning to work after a stroke: An important but neglected area. *British Journal of Occupational Therapy*, *66*, 186–192.

Corwin, J. and Bylsma, F. W. (1993) Psychological examination of traumatic encephalopathy. *The Clinical Neuropsychologist*, *7*, 3–21.

Coughlan, A. K. and Storey, P. (1988) The Wimbledon Self-Report Scale: Emotional and mood appraisal. *Clinical Rehabilitation*, *2*, 207–213.

Coulthard, E., Parton, A. and Husain, M. (2006) Action control in visual neglect. *Neuropsychologia*, *44*, 2717–2733.

Coward, L. J., Featherstone, R. L. and Brown, M. M. (2005) Safety and efficacy of endovascular treatment of carotid artery stenosis compared with carotid endarterectomy: A Cochrane systematic review of the randomized evidence. *Stroke*, *36*, 905–911.

Cox, E., Dooley, A., Liston, M. and Miller, M. (1998) Coping with stroke: Perceptions of elderly who have experienced stroke and rehabilitation interventions. *Topics in Stroke Rehabilitation*, *4*, 76–88.

Coyne, J. C. (1976) Toward an interactional description of depression. *Psychiatry, 39,* 28–40.

Cramer, S. C. (2008) Repairing the human brain after stroke: I. Mechanisms of spontaneous recovery. *Annals of Neurology, 63,* 272–287.

Cramp, L. R. and Brawley, A. G. (2006) Moms in motion: A group-mediated cognitive-behavioral physical activity intervention. *Journal of Behavioral Nutrition and Physical Activity, 3,* 23.

Crasilneck, H. B. and Hall, J. A. (1979) The use of hypnosis in the rehabilitation of complicated vascular and post-traumatic neurological patients. *International Journal of Clinical and Experimental Hypnosis, 18,* 145–159.

Creed, A., Swanwick, G. and O'Neill, D. (2004) Screening for post stroke depression in patients with acute stroke including those with communication disorders. *International Journal of Geriatric Psychiatry, 19,* 594–599.

Croquelois, A., Wintermark, M., Reichhart, M., Meuli, R. and Bogousslavsky, J. (2003) Aphasia in hyperacute stroke: Language follows brain penumbra dynamics. *Annals Neurology, 54,* 321–329.

Crotty, M. and George, S. (2009) Retraining visual processing skills to improve driving ability after stroke. *Archives of Physical Medicine and Rehabilitation, 90,* 2096–2102.

Cruice, M., Worrall, L., Hickson, L. and Murison, R. (2003) Finding a focus for quality of life with aphasia: Social and emotional health, and psychologiacl well-being. *Aphasiology, 17,* 333–353.

Cruice, M., Worrall, L., Hickson, L. and Murison, R. (2005) Measuring quality of life: Comparing family members' and friends' ratings with those of their aphasic partners. *Aphasiology, 19,* 111–129.

Cuijpers, P., van Straten, A., Andersson, G. and van Oppen, P. (2008) Psychotherapy for depression in adults: A meta-analysis of comparative outcome studies. *Journal of Consulting and Clinical Psychology, 76,* 909–922.

Cullen, B., O'Neill, B., Evans, J. J., Coen, R. F. and Lawlor, B. A. (2007) A review of screening tests for cognitive impairment. *Journal of Neurology Neurosurgery and Psychiatry, 78,* 790–799.

Cumming, R. G., Salkeld, G., Thomas, M. and Szonyi, G. (2000) Prospective study of the impact of fear of falling on activities of daily living, SF-36 scores, and nursing home admission. *Journals of Gerontology Series A: Biological Sciences and Medical Sciences, 55,* M299–M305.

Cumming, T., Churilov, L., Skoog, I., Blomstrand, C. and Linden, T. (2010) Little evidence for different phenomenology in poststroke depression. *Acta Psychiatrica Scandinavica, 121,* 424–430.

Cummings, J. L., Arciniegas, D. B., Brooks, B. R., Herndon, R. M., Lauterbach, E. C., Pioro, E. P., et al. (2006) Defining and diagnosing involuntary emotional expression disorder. *CNS Spectrums, 11,* A1–A7.

Cummings, S., Cooper, R. and Cassie, K.M. (2011) Motivational interviewing to affect behavioral change in older adults. *Research on Social Work Practice,* in press.

Cunningham, R. and Ward, C. D. (2003) Evaluation of a training programme to facilitate conversation between people with aphasia and their partners. *Aphasiology, 17,* 687–707.

Curioni, C., André, C. and Veras, R. (2006) Weight reduction for primary prevention of stroke in adults with overweight or obesity. *Cochrane Database of Systematic Reviews* (4), CD006062.

Currier, M. B., Murray, G. B. and Welch, C. C. (1992) Electroconvulsive therapy for poststroke geriatric patients. *Journal of Neuropsychiatry and Clinical Neurosciences*, *4*, 140–144.

Czernuszenko, A. and Czlonkowska, A. (2009) Risk factors for falls in stroke patients during inpatient rehabilitation. *Clinical Rehabilitation*, *23*, 176–188.

D'Elia, L. F., Satz, P., Uchiyama, C. L. and White, T. (1996) *Color Trails Test: Professional Manual*. Odessa, FL: Psychological Assessment Resources.

Dabul, B. (2000) *Apraxia Battery for Adults*, 2nd ed. Austin, TX: Pro-Ed.

Daffertshofer, M., Mielke, O., Pullwitt, A., Felsenstein, M. and Hennerici, M. (2004) Transient ischemic attacks are more than 'ministrokes'. *Stroke*, *35*, 2453–2458.

Dagnan, D., Trower, P. and Smith, R. (1998) Care staff responses to people with learning disabilities and challenging behaviour: A cognitive-emotional analysis. *British Journal of Clinical Psychology*, *37*, 59–68.

Dai, Y. T., Chang, Y., Hsieh, C. Y. and Tai, T. Y. (2003) Effectiveness of a pilot project of discharge planning in Taiwan. *Research in Nursing and Health*, *26*, 53–63.

Dam, H. (2001) Depression in stroke patients 7 years following stroke. *Acta Psychiatrica Scandanavica*, *103*, 287–293.

Dam, H., Pederson, H. E. and Ahlgren, P. (1989) Depression among patients with stroke. *Acta Psychiatrica Scandinavica*, *80*, 118–124.

Damecour, C. L. and Caplan, D. (1991) The relationship of depression to symptomatology and lesion site in aphasic patients. *Cortex*, *27*, 385–401.

Dani, K. A., McCormick, M. T. and Muir, K. W. (2008) Brain lesion volume and capacity for consent in stroke trials: Potential regulatory barriers to the use of surrogate markers. *Stroke*, *39* (8), 2336–2340.

Daniel, H. C. and Van der Merwe, J. D. (2006) Cognitive behavioural approaches and neuropathic pain In F. Cevero and T. S. Jensen (ed), *Handbook of Clinical Neurology* (Vol. 81, pp. 855–868) Amsterdam: Elsevier.

Daniel, K., Wolfe, C. D. A., Busch, M. A. and McKevitt, C. (2009) What are the social consequences of stroke for working-aged adults? A systematic review. *Stroke*, *40*, E431–E440.

Darlington, A. S. E., Dippel, D. W. J., Ribbers, G. M., van Balen, R., Passchier, J. and Busschbach, J. J. V. (2009) A prospective study on coping strategies and quality of life in patients after stroke, assessing prognostic relationships and estimates of cost-effectiveness. *Journal of Rehabilitation Medicine*, *41*, 237–241.

Darzi, L. (2007) *NHS Next Stage Review Interim Report*. London: TSO.

Das, A. K., Das, L. and Mulley, G. P. (2006) Awareness of living wills in the United Kingdom. *Age and Ageing*, *35*, 543–543.

das Nair, R. and Lincoln N. (2007) Cognitive rehabilitation for memory deficits following stroke. *Cochrane Database of Systematic Reviews* (3), CD002293.

das Nair, R. and Lincoln, N. (2008) Effectiveness of memory rehabilitation after stroke. *Stroke*, *39*, 516–516.

das Nair, R. and Lincoln, N. B. (Submitted) Evaluation of rehabilitation of memory in people with neurological disabilities: A randomised trial. *Archives of Physical Medicine and Rehabilitation*.

David, R., Enderby, P. and Bainton, D. (1982) Treatment of acquired aphasia: Speech threapists and volunteers compared. *Journal of Neurology Neurosurgery and Psychiatry*, *45*, 957–961.

Davidson, A. and Young, C. (1985) Repatterning of stroke rehabilitation clients following return to life in the community. *Journal of Neurosurgical Nursing 17*, 123–128.

Davidson, B., Worrall, L. and Hickson, L. (2003) Identifying the communication activities of older people with aphasia: Evidence from naturalistic observation. *Aphasiology, 17*, 243–264.

Davis, A. M., Cockburn, J. M., Wade, D. T. and Smith, P. T. (1995) A subjective memory assessment questionnaire for use with elderly people after stroke. *Clinical Rehabilitation, 9*, 238–244.

Davis, C., Bradshaw, C. M. and Szabadi, E. (1999) The Doors and People memory test: Validation of norms and some new correction formulae. *British Journal of Clinical Psychology, 38*, 305–314.

Davis, C., Farias, D. and Baynes, K. (2009) Implicit phoneme manipulation for the treatment of apraxia of speech and co-occurring aphasia. *Aphasiology, 23*, 503–528.

Davis, S. J. C. and Coltheart, M. (1999) Rehabilitation of topographical disorientation: An experimental single case study. *Neuropsychological Rehabilitation, 9*, 1–30.

Davous, P. (1998) CADASIL: A review with proposed diagnostic criteria. *European Journal of Neurology, 5*, 219–233.

de Coster, L., Leentjens, A. F. G., Lodder, J. and Verhey, F. R. J. (2005) The sensitivity of somatic symptoms in post-stroke depression: A discriminant analytic approach. *International Journal of Geriatric Psychiatry, 20*, 358–362.

de Frietas, G. R. and Bogousslavsky, J. (2002) Thalamic infarcts. In G. Donnan, B. Norrving, J. Bamford and J. Bogousslavsky (eds), *Subcortical Stroke*, 2nd ed. (pp. 255–286) Oxford: Oxford University Press.

de Groot, M. H., Phillips, S. J. and Eskes, G. A. (2003) Fatigue associated with stroke and other neurologic conditions: Implications for stroke rehabilitation. *Archives of Physical Medicine and Rehabilitation, 84*, 1714–1720.

de Koning, I., Dippel, D. W. J., van Kooten, F. and Koudstaal, P. J. (2000) A short screening instrument for poststroke dementia: The R-CAMCOG. *Stroke, 31*, 1502–1508.

de Koning, I., van Kooten, F., Dippel, D. W. J., van Harskamp, F., Grobbee, D. E., Kluft, C., *et al.* (1998) The CAMCOG: A useful screening instrument for dementia in stroke patients. *Stroke, 29*, 2080–2086.

de Koning, I., van Kooten, F., Koudstaal, P. J. and Dippel, D. W. J. (2005) Diagnostic value of the Rotterdam-CAMCOG in post-stroke dementia. *Journal of Neurology Neurosurgery and Psychiatry, 76*, 263–265.

De Leon, J., Gottesman, R. F., Kleinman, J. T., Newhart, M., Davis, C., Heidler-Gary, J., *et al.* (2007) Neural regions essential for distinct cognitive processes underlying picture naming. *Brain, 130*, 1408–1422.

De Renzi, E. and Faglioni, P. (1978) Normative data and screening power of a shortened version of the Token Test. *Cortex, 14*, 41–49.

De Renzi, E., Faglioni, P. and Sorgato, P. (1982) Modality-specific and supramodal mechanisms of apraxia. *Brain, 105*, 301–312.

De Renzi, E. and Lucchelli, F. (1988) Ideational apraxia. *Brain, 111*, 1173–1186.

De Renzi, E., Motti, F. and Nichelli, P. (1980) Imitating gestures. A quantitative approach to ideomotor apraxia. *Archives of Neurology, 37*, 6–10.

De Renzi, E. and Vignolo, L. A. (1962) The Token Test: A sensitive test to detect disturbances in aphasics. *Brain, 85*, 665–678.

De Schryver, E. L., Van Gijn, J., Kappelle, L. J., Koudstaal, P. J. and Algra, A. (2005) Nonadherence to aspirin or oral anticoagulants in secondary prevention after ischemic stroke. *Journal of Neurology* 252, 1316–1321.

De Sepulveda, L. I. B. and Chang, B. (1994) Effective coping with stroke disability in a community setting: the development of a causal model. *Journal of Neuroscience Nursing*, 26, 193–203.

De Wit, L., Putman, K., Baert, I., Lincoln, N. B., Angst, F., Beyens, H., *et al.* (2008) Anxiety and depression in the first six months after stroke. A longitudinal multi-centre study. *Disability & Rehabilitation*, 30, 1858–1866.

De Wit, L., Putman, K., Dejaeger, E., Baert, I., Berman, P., Bogaerts, K., *et al.* (2005) Use of time by stroke patients: A comparison of four European rehabilitation centers. *Stroke*, 36, 1977–1983.

Dearden, C. and Becker, S. (2004) *Young Carers in the UK: The 2004 Report.* London: Carers UK.

Dearden, D. and Becker, S. (1998) *Young Carers in the United Kingdom: A Profile.* Young Carers' Research Group, Loughborough University.

Dees, M., Vernooij-Dassen, M., Dekkers, W. and van Weel, C. (2010) Unbearable suffering of patients with a request for euthanasia or physician-assisted suicide: An integrative review. *Psychooncology*, 19, 339–352.

DeLaune, M. and Brown, S. C. (2001) Spousal responses to role changes following a stroke. *Medical and Surgical Nursing*, 10, 79–82.

Delbaere, K., Crombez, G., Vanderstraeten, G., Willems, T. and Cambier, D. (2004) Fear-related avoidance of activities, falls and physical frailty: A prospective community-based cohort study. *Age and Ageing*, 33, 368–373.

DeLemos, C. D., Atkinson, R. P., Croopnick, S. L., Wentworth, D. A. and Akins, P. T. (2003) How effective are 'community' stroke screening programs at improving stroke knowledge and prevention practices? Results of a 3-month follow-up study. *Stroke*, 34, E247–E249.

Delis, D. C., Kaplan, E. and Kramer, J. (2001) *Delis-Kaplan Executive Function System.* San Antonio, TX: The Psychological Corporation.

Delis, D. C., Kaplan, E., Kramer, J. and Ober, B. (2000) *California Verbal Learning Test-II.* San Antonio, TX: The Psychological Corporation.

Della Sala, S., Laiacona, M., Spinnler, H. and Trivelli, C. (1993) Autobiographical recollection and frontal damage. *Neuropsychologia*, 31, 823–839.

Dempster, C., Knapp, P. and House, A. (1998) The collaboration of carers during psychological therapy. *Mental Health Nursing*, 18, 24–27.

Dennis, C. L. (2003) Peer support within a health care context: a concept analysis. *International Journal of Nursing Studies*, 40, 321–332.

Dennis, M., O'Rourke, S., Slattery, J., Staniforth, T. and Warlow, C. (1997) Evaluation of a stroke family care worker: Results of a randomised controlled trial. *British Medical Journal*, 314, 1071–1076.

Dennis, M. S., Burn, J. P. S., Sandercock, P. A. G., Bamford, J. M., Wade, D. T. and Warlow, C. P. (1993) Long-term survival after first-ever stroke: The Oxfordshire Community Stroke Project. *Stroke*, 24, 796–800.

Dennis, M. S., Lo, K. M., McDowall, M. and West, T. (2002) Fractures after stroke: Frequency, types, and associations. *Stroke*, 33, 728–734.

Department for Constitutional Affairs. (2005) The Mental Capacity Act 2005. Norwich: TSO.

Department for Constitutional Affairs. (2007) *Mental Capacity Act 2005: Code of Practice*. Norwich: TSO.

Department of Health. (1996) *Carers (Recognition and Services) Act 1995 Policy Guidance and Practice Guide*. London: Department of Health.

Department of Health. (1997) *White Paper: The New NHS: Modern. Dependable. Norwich: TSO.*

Department of Health. (1998) *White Paper: Saving Lives*. Norwich: TSO.

Department of Health. (1999) *Caring about Carers: A National Strategy for Carers*. London: Department of Health.

Department of Health. (2000) *The NHS Plan: A Plan for Investment: A Plan for Reform*. Norwich: TSO.

Department of Health. (2001) Stroke. In *National Service Framework for Older People* (chap. 5). London: Department of Health.

Department of Health. (2005) *The National Service Framework for Long-Term Conditions*. London: Department of Health.

Department of Health. (2006) *Our Health, Our Care Our Say: A New Direction for Community Services*. Norwich: TSO.

Department of Health. (2007a) *National Stroke Strategy (England)* London: Department of Health.

Department of Health. (2007b) *Independence, Choice and Risk: A Guide to Supported Decision Making*. London: Department of Health.

Department of Health. (2007c) *Deprivation of Liberty Safeguards. Briefing sheet*. London: Department of Health.

Department of Health. (2008a) *Carers at the Heart Of 21st-Century Families and Communities: 'A Caring System on Your Side. A Life of Your Own'*. London: Department of Health.

Department of Health. (2008b) *Improving Access to Psychological Therapies Implementation Plan: National Guidelines for Regional Delivery*. London: Department of Health.

Department of Health. (2009a) *The Stroke Specific Education Framework*. http://www.dh.gov.uk/prod_consum_dh/groups/dh_digitalassets/@dh/@en/@ps/@sta/@perf/documents/digitalasset/dh_116343.pdf

Department of Health. (2009b) The NHS Constitution for England. Leeds: Department of Health.

Department of Health. (2009c) *The New Revised Essence of Care: A Consultation on the New Benchmark on Pain*. Leeds: Department of Health.

Department of Health, Social Services and Public Safety. (2008) *Improving Stroke Services in Northern Ireland*. Belfast: Department of Health, Social Services and Public Safety.

Derogatis, L. R., Lipman, R. S. and Covi, L. (1973) SCL-90: An outpatient psychiatric rating scale – preliminary report. *Psychopharmacol Bull, 9*, 13–28.

Desmond, D. W., Tatemichi, T. K. and Hanzawa, L. (1994) The Telephone Interview for Cognitive Status (TICS): Reliability and validity in a stroke sample. *International Journal of Geriatric Psychiatry, 9*, 803–807.

DeVecchio, T. and O'Leary, K. D. (2004) Effectiveness of anger treatments for specific anger problems: A meta-analytic review. *Clinical Psychology Review, 24*, 15–34.

Devos, H., Akinwuntan, A., Nieuwboer, A., Ringoot, I., Van Berghen, K., Tant, M., *et al.* (2010) Effect of simulator training on fitness-to-drive after stroke: A 5-year follow-up of a randomized controlled trial. *Neurorehabilitation & Neural Repair.* ePub ahead of print 23 July.

Devos, H., Akinwuntan, A., Nieuwboer, A., Truijen, S., Tant, M. & De Weerdt, W. (2011) Screening for fitness to drive after stroke: A systematic review and meta-analysis. *Neurology 76*, 747–756.

Dewey, H. M., Thrift, A. G., Mihalopoulos, C., Carter, R., Macdonell, R. A. L., McNeil, J. J., *et al.* (2002) Informal care for stroke survivors: Results from the North East Melbourne Stroke Incidence Study (NEMESIS). *Stroke, 33*, 1028–1033.

Dickson, S., Barbour, R. S., Brady, M., Clark, A. M. and Paton, G. (2008) Patients' experiences of disruptions associated with post–stroke dysarthria. *International Journal of Language and Communication Disorders, 43*, 135–153.

Dieguez, S., Staub, F., Bruggimann, L. and Bogousslavsky, J. (2004) Is poststroke depression a vascular depression? Proceedings paper. *Journal of the Neurological Sciences, 226*, 53–58.

Different Strokes. (2009) *Survivors Stories: Adulthood, Childhood and Adolescence, Achievements.* [http://www.differentstrokes.co.uk/research/was.htm]. Accessed 18-02-2009.

DiGiuseppe, R. and Tafrate, R. C. (2007) Anger treatment for adults: A meta-analytic review. *Clinical Psychology: Science and Practice, 10*, 70–84.

Diller, L. and Weinberg, J. (1977) Hemi-inattention in rehabilitation: The evolution of a rational remediation program. *Advances in Neurology, 18*, 63–82.

Directgov. (2009) *Caring and Support Services.* http://www.direct.gov.uk/en/CaringForSomeone/CaringAndSupportServices/DG_10016779

Division of Clinical Psychology. (2007) *Marketing Strategy for Clinical Psychologists.* Leicester: British Psychological Society.

Division of Clinical Psychology/Division of Neuropsychology. (2010) *Briefing Paper 19: Psychological Services for Stroke Survivors and Their Families.* Leicester: British Psychological Society.

Dixon, G., Thornton, E. W. and Young, C. A. (2007) Perceptions of self-efficacy and rehabilitation among neurologically disabled adults. *Clinical Rehabilitation, 21*, 230–240.

Donabedian, A. (1993) Quality in health care: Whose responsibility is it? *American Journal of Medical Quality, 8*, 32–36.

Dong, Y., Sharma, V. K., Chan, B. P., Venketasubramanian, N., Teoh, H. L., Seet, R. C. *et al.* (2010) The Montreal Cognitive Assessment (MoCA) is superior to the Mini-Mental State Examination (MMSE) for the detection of vascular cognitive impairment after acute stroke. *Journal of the Neurological Sciences, 299*, 15–18.

Donkervoort, M., Dekker, J. and Deelman, B. T. (2006) The course of apraxia and ADL functioning in left hemisphere stroke patients treated in rehabilitation centres and nursing homes. *Clinical Rehabilitation, 20*, 1085–1093.

Donkervoort, M., Dekker, J., Stehmann-Saris, F. C. and Deellman, B. G. (2001) Efficacy of strategy training in left hemisphere stroke patients with apraxia: A randomised clinical trial. *Neuropsychological Rehabilitation, 11*, 549–566.

Donkervoort, M., Dekker, J., van den Ende, E., Stehmann-Saris, J. C. and Deelman, B. G. (2000) Prevalence of apraxia among patients with a first left hemisphere stroke in rehabilitation centres and nursing homes. *Clinical Rehabilitation, 14*, 130–136.

Donnan, G., Norrving, B., Bamford, J. and Bogousslavsky, J. (eds) (2002) *Subcortical Stroke,* 2nd ed. Oxford: Oxford University Press.

Donnellan, C., Hevey, D., Hickey, A. and O'Neill, D. (2006) Defining and quantifying coping strategies after stroke: A review. *Journal of Neurology Neurosurgery and Psychiatry, 77,* 1208–1218.

Doolittle, N. (1992) The experience of recovery following lacunar stroke. *Rehabilitation Nursing, 17,* 122–125.

Doornhein, K. and de Haan, E. (1998) Cognitive training for memory deficits in stroke patients. *Neuropsychological Rehabilitation, 8,* 393–400.

Douglas, K. (2002) *My Stroke of Luck.* London: Little, Brown.

Doull, M., O'Connor, A. M., Welch, V., Tugwell, P. and Wells, G. A. (2005) Peer support strategies for improving the health and wellbeing of individuals with chronic diseases [Protocol]. *Cochrane Database of Systematic Reviews* (3).

Dowswell, G., Lawler, J., Dowswell, T., Young, J., Forster, A. and Hearn, J. (2000) Investigating recovery from stroke: A qualitative study. *Journal of Clinical Nursing, 9,* 507–515.

Dowswell, G., Lawler, J., Young, J., Forster, A. and Hearn, J. (1997) A qualitative study of specialist nurse support for stroke patients and care-givers at home. *Clinical Rehabilitation, 11,* 293–301.

Doyle, P. J. (2002) Measuring health outcomes in stroke survivors. *Archives of Physical Medicine and Rehabilitation, 83,* S39–S43.

Doyle, P. J., McNeil, M. R. and Hula, W. D. (2003) The Burden of Stroke Scale (BOSS): Validating patient-reported communication difficulty and associated psychological distress in stroke survivors. *Aphasiology, 17,* 291–304.

Draper, B., Bowring, G., Thompson, C., Van Heyst, J., Conroy, P. and Thompson, J. (2007) Stress in caregivers of aphasic stroke patients: a randomized controlled trial. *Clinical Rehabilitation, 21,* 122–130.

Draper, P. and Brocklehurst, H. (2007) The impact of stroke on the well-being of the patient's spouse: An exploratory study. *Journal of Clinical Nursing, 16,* 264–271.

Dromerick, A., Edwards, D. and Kumar, A. (2008) Hemiplegic shoulder pain syndrome: Frequency and characteristics during inpatient stroke rehabilitation. *Archives of Physical Medicine and Rehabilitation, 89,* 1589–1593.

Dronkers, N. F. (1996) A new brain region for coordinating speech articulation. *Nature, 384* (6605), 159–161.

Drummond, A. and Walker, M. (1996) Generalisation of the effects of leisure rehabilitation for stroke patients. *British Journal of Occupational Therapy, 59,* 330–334.

Drummond, A. E. R., Pearson, B., Lincoln, N. B. and Berman, P. (2005) Ten year follow-up of a randomised controlled trial of care in a stroke rehabilitation unit. *British Medical Journal, 331,* 491–492.

Dubler, N. N. (1985) Some legal and moral issues surrounding informed consent for treatment and research involving the cognitively impaired elderly. In H. E. P. M. B. Kapp and A. E. Doudera (eds), *Legal and Ethical Aspects of Health Care.* Ann Arbor: Health Administration Press.

Dumoulin, C., Korner-Bitensky, N. and Tannenbaum, C. (2005) Urinary incontinence after stroke: does rehabilitation make a difference? A systematic review of the effectiveness of behavioral therapy. *Topics in Stroke Rehabilitation, 12,* 66–76.

Duncan, P. W., Horner, R. D., Reker, D. A., Samsa, G. P., Hoenig, H., Hamilton, B., *et al.* (2002) Adherence to postacute rehabilitation guidelines is associated with functional recovery in stroke. *Stroke, 33,* 167–177.

Duncan, P. W., Samsa, G. P., Weinberger, M., Goldstein, L. B., Bonito, A., Witter, D. M., *et al.* (1997) Health status of individuals with mild stroke. *Stroke, 28,* 740–745.

Duncan, P. W., Zorowitz, R., Bates, B., Choi, J. Y., Glasberg, J. J., Graham, G. D., *et al.* (2005) Management of adult stroke rehabilitation care: A clinical practice guideline. *Stroke, 36*, E100–E143.

Dunn, L. B., Nowrangi, M. A., Palmer, B. W., Jeste, D. V. and Saks, E. R. (2006) Assessing decisional capacity for clinical research or treatment: A review of instruments. *American Journal of Psychiatry, 163*, 1323–1334.

Dunn, M. C., Clare, I. C. H. and Holland, A. J. (2008) Substitute decision-making for adults with intellectual disabilities living in residential care: Learning through experience. *Health Care Analysis, 16*, 52–64.

Dunn, M. C., Clare, I. C. H., Holland, A. J. and Gunn, M. J. (2007) Constructing and reconstructing 'best interests': An interpretative examination of substitute decision-making under the Mental Capacity Act 2005. *Journal of Social Welfare & Family Law, 29*, 117–133.

Dymek, M. P., Atchison, P., Harrell, L. and Marson, D. C. (2001) Competency to consent to medical treatment in cognitively impaired patients with Parkinson's disease. *Neurology, 56*, 17–24.

Early Supported Discharge Trialists (2005) Services for reducing duration of hospital care for acute stroke patients. *Cochrane Database Systematic Reviews* (2), CD000443.

Earnst, K. S., Marson, D. C. and Harrell, L. E. (2000) Cognitive models of physicians' legal standard and personal judgments of competency in patients with Alzheimer's disease. *Journal of the American Geriatrics Society, 48*, 919–927.

Eaves, Y. (2002) Rural African American caregivers' and stroke survivors' satisfaction with health care. *Topics in Geriatric Rehabilitation 17*, 72–84.

Ebrahim, S. (1996) Caring for older people: Ethnic elders. *British Medical Journal, 313*, 610–613.

Eccles, S., House, A. and Knapp, P. (1999) Psychological adjustment and self reported coping in stroke survivors with and without emotionalism. *Journal of Neurology, Neurosurgery and Psychiatry, 67*, 125–126.

Eccleston, C., Williams, A. C. D. and Morley, S. (2009) Psychological therapies for the management of chronic pain (excluding headache) in adults. *Cochrane Database of Systematic Reviews* (2), CD007407.

Edgworth, J., Robertson, I. H. and MacMillan, T. (1998) *The Balloons Test: A Screening Test for Visual Inattention.* Bury St Edmunds: Thames Valley Test Company.

Edmans, J.A. and Lincoln, N.B. (1987) The frequency of perceptual deficits after stroke. *Clinical Rehabilitation, 1*, 273–281.

Edmans, J. A., Webster, J. and Lincoln, N. B. (2000) A commparison of two approaches in the treatment of perceptual problems after stroke. *Clinical Rehabilitation, 14*, 230–243.

Edmonds, L. A., Nadeau, S. E. and Kiran, S. (2009) Effect of Verb Network Strengthening Treatment (VNeST) on lexical retrieval of content words in sentences in persons with aphasia. *Aphasiology, 23*, 402–424.

Edwards, C. L., Sudhakar, S., Scales, M. T., Applegate, K. L., Webster, W. and Dunn, R. H. (2000) Electromyographic (EMG) biofeedback in the comprehensive treatment of central pain and ataxic tremor following thalamic stroke. *Applied Psychophysiology and Biofeedback, 25*, 229–240.

Edwards, D. F., Hahn, M., Baum, C. and Dromerick, A. W. (2006a) The impact of mild stroke on meaningful activity and life satisfaction. *Journal of Stroke and Cerebrovascular Diseases, 15*, 151–157.

Edwards, D. F., Hahn, M. G., Baum, C. M., Perlmutter, M. S., Sheedy, C. and Dromerick, A. W. (2006b) Screening patients with stroke for rehabilitation needs: Validation of the post-stroke rehabilitation guidelines. *Neurorehabilitation and Neural Repair, 20,* 42–48.

Eilertsen, G., Kirkevold, M. and Bjørk, I. (2010) Recovering from a stroke: A longitudinal, qualitative study of older Norwegian women. *Journal of Clinical Nursing, 19,* 2004–2013.

Elkind, M., Sciacca, R., Boden-Albala, B., Rundek, T., Paik, M. and Sacco, R. (2006) Moderate alcohol consumption reduces risk of ischemic stroke: The Northern Manhattan Study. *Stroke, 37,* 13–19.

Elliott, M. A. and Armitage, C. J. (2009) Promoting drivers' compliance with speed limits: Testing an intervention based on the theory of planned behaviour. *British Journal of Psychology, 100,* 111–132.

Ellis, A. (1991) Using RET effectively: reflections and interview. In M. E. Bernard (ed), *Using Rational Emotive Therapy Effectively* (pp. 1–33). New York: Plenum.

Ellis, G. (2006) On behalf of the Stroke Liaison Workers Collaboration. Meta-analysis of stroke liaison workers for patients and carers: Results by intervention characteristic. *Cerebrovascular Disease, 21* (Suppl. 4), 120.

Ellis, G. (2008) *Stroke Liaison Workers for Patients and Carers.* MD thesis, University of Glasgow.

Ellis, G., Mant, J., Langhorne, P., Dennis, M. and Winner, S. (2010) Stroke liaison workers for stroke patients and carers: An individual patient data meta-analysis. *Cochrane Database of Systematic Reviews* (5), CD005066.

Ellis-Hill, C., Payne, S. and Ward, C. (2000) Self-body split: Issues of identity in physical recovery following a stroke. *Disability and Rehabilitation, 22,* 725–733.

Ellis-Hill, C. S. and Horn, S. (2000) Change in identity and self-concept: A new theoretical approach to recovery following a stroke. *Clinical Rehabilitation, 14,* 279–287.

Elwyn, G. (2006) Idealistic, impractical, impossible? Shared decision making in the real world. *British Journal of General Practice, 56,* 403–404.

Emerson, E. (1995) *Challenging Behaviour: Analysis and Intervention in People with Learning Disabilities.* Cambridge: Cambridge University Press.

Emerson, E. (1998) Working with people with challenging behaviour. In C. H. E. Emerson, J. Bromley, and A. Caine (ed), *Clinical Psychology and People with Intellectual Disabilities* (pp. 127–153). Chichester: UK: John Wiley & Sons Ltd.

Enderby, P. (1983) *Frenchay Dysarthria Assessment and Computer Differential Analysis.* Oxford: NFER-Nelson.

Enderby, P. and Palmer, R. (2008) *Frenchay Dysarthria Assessment,* 2nd ed. Austin, TX: Pro-Ed.

Enderby, P., Wood, V. and Wade, D. (1997) *Frenchay Aphasia Screening Test.* Oxford: Whurr Publishers.

Enderby, P. M., John, A. and Petheram, B. (2006) *Therapy Outcome Measures for Rehabilitation.* Chichester, UK: Wiley.

Engberg, W., Lind, A., Linder, A., Nilsson, L. and Sernert, N. (2008) Balance-related efficacy compared with balance function in acute stroke. *Physiotherapy Theory and Practice, 24,* 105–111.

Engel, G. L. (1977) The need for a new medical model: A challenge for biomedicine. *Science, 196,* 129–136.

Engell, B., Hutter, B-O., Willmes, K. and Huber, W. (2003) Quality of life in aphasia: Validation of a pictorial self-rating procedure. *Aphasiology*, 17, 383–396.

Enterlante, T. M. and Kern, J. M. (1995) Wives' reported role changes following a husband's stroke: A pilot study. *Rehabilitation Nursing*, 20, 155–160.

Etchells, E., Darzins, P., Silberfeld, M., Singer, P. A., McKenny, J., Naglie, G., *et al.* (1999) Assessment of patient capacity to consent to treatment. *Journal of General Internal Medicine*, 14, 27–34.

European Stroke Organisation (ESO) Executive Committee and ESO Writing Committee. (2008) Guidelines for management of ischaemic stroke and transient ischaemic attack. *Cerebrovascular Diseases*, 25 (5), 457–507.

Evans, J. J. (2006) Theoretical influences on brain injury rehabilitation. Paper presented at the Oliver Zangwill Centre 10th Anniversary Conference, Cambridge, UK.

Evans, J. J., Wilson, B. A. and Emslie, H. (1996) *Selecting, Administering and Interpreting Cognitive Tests*. Bury St Edmunds: Thames Valley Test Company.

Evans, K., Warner, J. and Jackson, E. (2007) How much do emergency healthcare workers know about capacity and consent? *Emergency Medicine Journal*, 24, 391–393.

Evans, S., Fishman, B., Spielman, L. and Haley, A. (2003) Randomized trial of cognitive behavior therapy versus supportive psychotherapy for HIV-related peripheral neuropathic pain. *Psychosomatics*, 44, 44–50.

Faircloth, C., Boylstein, C., Rittman, M., Young, M. and Gubrium, J. (2004) Sudden illness and biographical flow in narratives of stroke recovery. *Sociology of Health and Illness*, 26, 242–261.

Faircloth, C. A., Boylstein, C., Rittman, M. and Gubrium, J. F. (2005) Constructing the stroke: sudden-onset narratives of stroke survivors. *Qualitative Health Research*, 15, 928–941.

Fang, J. and Cheng, Q. (2009) Etiological mechanisms of post-stroke depression: A review. *Neurological Research*, 31, 904–909.

Fassassi, S., Bianchi, Y., Stiefel, F. and Waeber, G. (2009) Assessment of the capacity to consent to treatment in patients admitted to acute medical wards. *Medical Ethics*, 10, 15.

Fazel, S., Hope, T. and Jacoby, R. (1999) Dementia, intelligence, and the competence to complete advance directives. *Lancet*, 354 (9172), 48–48.

Feibel, J. H. and Springer, C. J. (1982) Depression and failure to resume social activities after stroke. *Archives of Physical Medicine and Rehabilitation*, 63, 276–278.

Feigin, V. L., Lawes, C. M. M., Bennett, D. A. and Anderson, C. S. (2003) Stroke epidemiology: A review of population based studies of incidence, prevalence, and case-fatality in the late 20th century. *Lancet Neurology*, 2, 43–53.

Feigin, V. L., Barker-Collo, S., Krishnamurthi, R., Theadom, A. and Starkey, N. (2009) Epidemiology of ischaemic stroke and traumatic brain injury. *Best Practice & Research Clinical Anaesthesiology*, 24 (4), 485–494.

Ferber, S. and Karnath, H. (2001) How to assess spatial neglect-line bisection or cancellation tasks? *Journal of Clinical and Experimental Neuropsychology*, 23, 599–607.

Ferri, M., Amato, L. and Davoli, M. (2006) Alcoholics Anonymous and other 12-step programmes for alcohol dependence. *Cochrane Database of Systematic Reviews* (3), CD005032.

Ferster, C. B. (1973) A functional analysis of depression. *American Psychologist* 28, 857–870.

Festa, J. R., Lazar, R.M. and Marshall, R.S. (2008) Ischemic stroke and aphasic disorders. In J. E. Morgan and J. H. Ricker (ed), *Textbook of Clinical Neuropsychology*. New York: Taylor and Francis.

Field, E. L., Norman, P. and Barton, J. (2008) Cross-sectional and prospective associations between cognitive appraisals and posttraumatic stress disorder symptoms following stroke. *Behaviour Research and Therapy, 46,* 62–70.

Filiatrault, J. and Desrosiers, J. (2010) Coping strategies used by seniors going through the normal aging process: Does fear of falling matter? *Gerontology.* ePub ahead of print 6 May.

Filley, C. M. (2008) Neuroanatomy for the neuropsychologist. In J. E. Morgan and J. H. Ricker (eds), *Textbook of Clinical Neuropsychology* (pp. 61–82) New York: Taylor and Francis.

Finset, A. and Andersson, S. (2000) Coping strategies in patients with acquired brain injury: Relationships between coping, apathy, depression and lesion location. *Brain Injury, 14,* 887–905.

Fish, J., Evans, J. J., Nimmo, M., Martin, E., Kersel, D., Bateman, A., *et al.* (2007) Rehabilitation of executive dysfunction following brain injury: 'Content-free' cueing improves everyday prospective memory performance. *Neuropsychologia, 45,* 1318–1330.

Fish, J., Manly, T., Emslie, H., Evans, J. J. and Wilson, B. A. (2008) Compensatory strategies for acquired disorders of memory and planning: Differential effects of a paging system for patients with brain injury of traumatic versus cerebrovascular aetiology. *Journal of Neurology Neurosurgery and Psychiatry, 79,* 930–935.

Fishbein, M., Triandis, H. C., Kanfer, F. H., Beker, M., Middlestadt, S. E. and Eicher, A. (2001) Factors influencing behavior and behavior change. In A. Baum, T. A. Reveson and J. E. E. Singer (eds), *Handbook of Health Psychology* (pp. 3–17). Mahwah, NJ: Lawrence Erlbaum Associates.

Fisher, C. M. (2002) Commentary on subcortical strokes. In G. Donnan, B. Norrving, J. Bamford & J. Bogousslavsky (eds), *Subcortical Stroke,* 2nd ed. (pp. 17–26) Oxford: Oxford University Press.

Fisk, G. D., Owsley, C. and Pulley, L. V. (1997) Driving after stroke: Driving exposure, advice, and evaluations. *Archives of Physical Medicine and Rehabilitation, 78,* 1338–1345.

Fitzpatrick, R. (1990) Measurement of patient satisfaction. In A. Hopkins & D. Costain (ed), *Measuring the Outcomes of Medical Care.* London: Royal College of Physicians.

Flaherty-Craig, C. V., Barrett, A. M. and Eslinger, P. J. (2002) Emotion-related processing impairments. In P. J. Eslinger (ed), *Neuropsychological Interventions: Clinical Research and Practice.* New York: The Guilford Press.

Fleet, W. S. and Heilman, K. M. (1986) The fatigue effect in hemispatial neglect [Abstract]. *Neurology, 36,* 258.

Flory, J. and Emanuel, E. (2004) Interventions to improve research participants' understanding in informed consent for research: A systematic review. *Journal of the American Medical Association, 292,* 1593–1601.

Folden, S. L. (1994) Managing the effects of a stroke: The first months. *Rehabilitation Nursing Research Fall, 24,* 79–85.

Folkman, S. and Lazarus, R. (1988) *Ways of Coping Questionnaire.* Palo Alto, CA: Consulting Psychologists Press.

Folkman, S., Lazarus, R. S., Gruen, R. J. and DeLongis, A. (1986) Appraisal, coping, health status, and psychological symptoms. *Journal of Personality and Social Psychology*, 50, 571–579.

Folstein, M., Folstein, S. and McHugh, P. (1975) Mini-Mental State: A practical method for grading the cognitive state of patients for the clinician. *Journal of Psychiatric Research*, 12, 189–198.

Ford, H. and Foley, L. (2008) *Regaining Confidence after Stroke*. London: Sutton & Merton PCT. http://www.southwestlondoncardiacnetwork.nhs.uk/Events/ Events.html

Forsberg-Warleby, G., Moller, A. and Blomstrand, C. (2001) Spouses of first-ever stroke patients: Psychological well-being in the first phase after stroke. *Stroke*, 32, 1646–1651.

Forsberg-Warleby, G., Moller, A. and Blomstrand, C. (2004) Life satisfaction in spouses of patients with stroke during the first year after stroke. *Journal of Rehabilitation Medicine*, 36, 4–11.

Forsblom, A., Laitinen, S., Sarkamo, T. and Tervaniemi, M. (2009) Therapeutic role of music listening in stroke rehabilitation. *Neurosciences and Music III: Disorders and Plasticity*, 1169, 426–430.

Forster, A. and Young, J. (1995) Incidence and consequences of falls due to stroke: A systematic enquiry. *British Medical Journal*, 311 (6997), 83–86.

Forster, A. and Young, J. (1996) Specialist nurse support for patients with stroke in the community: A randomised controlled trial. *British Medical Journal*, 312 (7047), 1642–1646.

Fosbinder, D. (1994) Patient perceptions of nursing care: An emerging theory of interpersonal competence. *Journal of Advanced Nursing*, 20, 1085–1093.

Foundas, A. L., Macauley, B. L., Raymer, A. M., Maher, L. M., Heilman, K. M. and Gonzalez, R. L. J. (1995) Ecological implications of limb apraxia: Evidence from mealtime behavior. *International Journal of the Neuropsychological Society 1* (1), 62–66.

Fox, C. J., Iaria, G. and Barton, J. J. S. (2008) Disconnection in prosopagnosia and face processing. *Cortex*, 44, 996–1009.

Franzen-Dahlin, A., Larson, J., Murray, V., Wredling, R. and Billing, E. (2008) A randomized controlled trial evaluating the effect of a support and education programme for spouses of people affected by stroke. *Clinical Rehabilitation*, 22, 722–730.

Fraser, C. J., Christensen, H. and Griffiths, K. M. (2005) Effectiveness of treatments for depression in older people. *Medical Journal of Australia*, 182, 627–632.

Frassinetti, F., Angeli, V., Meneghello, S., Avanzi, S. and Ladavas, E. (2002) Long-lasting amelioration of visuospatial neglect by prism adaptation. *Brain*, 125, 608–623.

Frattali, C., Thompson, C., Holland, A., Wohl, C. and Ferketic, M. (1995) *ASHA Functional Assessment of Communication Skills (FACS)*. Rockville, MD: American Speech-Language-Hearing Association.

Freedman, M., Stuss, D. T. and Gordon, M. (1991) Assessment of competency: The role of neurobehavioral deficits. *Annals of Internal Medicine*, 115, 203–208.

French, B., Leathley, M. J., Radford, K., Dey, M. P., McAdam, J., Marsden, J., *et al.* (2009) *UK Stroke Survivor Needs Survey Information Mapping Exercise*. Report to the Stroke Association, London.

References

Friederici, A. D., Fiebach, C. J., Schlesewsky, M., Bornkessel, I. D. and von Cramon, D. Y. (2006) Processing linguistic complexity and grammaticality in the left frontal cortex. *Cerebral Cortex, 16,* 1709–1717.

Frisk, V. and Milner, B. (1990) The role of the left hippocampal region in the acquisition and retention of story content. *Neuropsychologia, 28,* 349–359.

Fucetola, R., Connor, L. T., Perry, J., Leo, P., Tucker, F. M. and Corbetta, M. (2006) Aphasia severity, semantics, and depression predict functional communication in acquired aphasia. *Aphasiology, 20,* 449–461.

Fuchs-Lacelle, S. and Hadjistavropoulos, T. (2004) Development and preliminary validation of the pain assessment checklist for seniors with limited ability to communicate (PACSLAC). *Pain Management Nursing, 5,* 37–49.

Fujikawa, T., Yamawaki, S. and Touhouda, Y. (1993) Incidence of silent cerebral infarction in patients with major depression. *Stroke, 24,* 1631.

Fung, T., Chiuve, S., McCullough, M., Rexrode, K., Logroscino, G. and Hu, F. (2008) Adherence to a DASH-style diet and risk of coronary heart disease and stroke in women. *Archives of Internal Medicine, 168,* 713.

Fure, B., Wyller, T. B., Engedal, K. and Thommessen, B. (2006) Cognitive impairments in acute lacunar stroke. *Acta Neurologica Scandinavica, 114,* 17–22.

Gaber, T. A. Z. K. (2008) Evaluation of the Addenbrooke's Cognitive Examination's validity in a brain injury rehabilitation setting. *Brain Injury, 22,* 589–593.

Gabriele, W. and Renate, S. (2009) Work loss following stroke. *Disability and Rehabilitation, 31,* 1487–1493.

Gainotti, G., Azzoni, A., Razzano, C., Lanzillotta, M. and Marra, C. (1997) The Post-Stroke Depression Rating Scale: A test specifically devised to investigate affective disorders of stroke patients. *Journal of Clinical and Experimental Neuropsychology, 19,* 340–356.

Galimanis, A., Mono, M.-L., Arnold, M., Nedeltchev, K. and Mattle, H. P. (2009) Lifestyle and stroke risk: A review. *Current Opinion in Neurology 22,* 60–68.

Galski, T., Bruno, R. L. and Ehle, H. T. (1993) Prediction of behind-the-wheel driving performance in patients with cerebral brain damage: A discriminant function analysis. *American Journal of Occupational Therapy, 47,* 391–396.

Gamble, G. E., Barberan, E., Laasch, H. U., Bowsher, D., Tyrrell, P. J. and Jones, A. K. (2002) Poststroke shoulder pa in: A prospective study of the association and risk factors in 152 patients from a consecutive cohort of 205 patients presenting with stroke. *European Journal of Pain, 6,* 467–474.

Gandolfo, C. and Conti, M. (2003) Stroke in young adults: Epidemiology. *Neurological Sciences, 24,* S1–S3.

Gangstad, B., Norman, P. and Barton, J. (2009) Cognitive processing and posttraumatic growth after stroke. *Rehabilitation Psychology, 54,* 69–75.

Ganti, A. K., Lee, S. J., Vose, J. M., Devetten, M. P., Bociek, R. G., Armitage, J. O., *et al.* (2007) Outcomes after hematopoietic stem-cell transplantation for hematologic malignancies in patients with or without advance care planning. *Journal of Clinical Oncology, 25,* 5643–5648.

Ganzini, L., Volicer, L., Nelson, W. A., Fox, E. and Derse, A. R. (2004) Ten myths about decision-making capacity. *Journal of American Medical Directors Association, 5,* 263–267.

Gauggel, S. and Fischer, S. (2001) The effect of goal setting on motor performance and motor learning in brain-damaged patients. *Neuropsychological Rehabilitation, 11,* 33–44.

General Medical Council (2008) Consent: patients and doctors making decisions together. London: General Medical Council.

George, S. and Crotty, M. (2010) Establishing criterion validity of the Useful Field of View assessment and Stroke Drivers' Screening Assessment: Comparison to the result of on-road assessment. *American Journal of Occupational Therapy, 64,* 114–122.

Gerritsen, M. J., Berg, I. J., Deelman, B. G., Visser-Keizer, A. C. and Meyboom-de Jong, B. (2003) Speed of information processing after unilateral stroke. *Journal of Clinical Experimental Neuropsychology, 25,* 1–13.

Gerstmann, J. (1940) Syndrome of finger agnosia, disorientation for right and left, agraphia and acalculia: Local diagnostic value. *Archives of Neurology & Psychiatry, 44,* 398.

Geschwind, N. (1975) The apraxias: Neural mechanisms of disorders of learned movement. *American Scientist, 63,* 188–195.

Geurts, A. C. H., Haart, M., van Nes, I. J. and Duysens, J. (2005) A review of standing balance recovery from stroke. *Gait Posture, 22,* 267–281.

Geusgens, C., van Heugten, C., Donkervoort, M., van den Ende, E., Jolles, J. and van den Heuvel, W. (2006) Transfer of training effects in stroke patients with apraxia: An exploratory study. *Neuropsychological Rehabilitation, 16,* 213–229.

Ghose, S. S., Williams, L. S. and Swindle, R. W. (2005) Depression and other mental health diagnoses after stroke increase inpatient and outpatient medical utilization three years poststroke. *Medical Care, 43,* 1259–1264.

Giacobbe, P. and Flint, A. (2007) Pharmacological treatment of poststroke pathological laughing and crying. *Journal of Psychiatry & Neuroscience, 32* (5), 384.

Gilewski, M. J., Zelinski, E. M. and Schaie, K. W. (1990) The Memory Functioning Questionnaire for assessment of memory complaints in adulthood and old age. *Psychology and Aging, 5,* 482–490.

Gillen, R., Tennen, H., McKee, T. E., Gernert-Dott, P. and Affleck, G. (2001) Depressive symptoms and history of depression predict rehabilitation efficiency in stroke patients. *Archives of Physical Medicine and Rehabilitation, 82,* 1645–1649.

Gillen, G. (2005) Brief report: Positive consequences of surviving a stroke. *American Journal of Occupational Therapy, 59,* 346–350.

Gillespie, D. C., Bowen, A. and Foster, J. K. (2006) Memory impairment following right hemisphere stroke: A comparative meta-analytic and narrative review. *The Clinical Neuropsychologist, 20,* 59–75.

Gillick, M. R. (2004) Advance care planning. *New England Journal of Medicine, 350,* 7–8.

Gilworth, G., Phil, M., Cert, A., Sansam, K. A. J. and Kent, R. M. (2009) Personal experiences of returning to work following stroke: An exploratory study. *Work: A Journal of Prevention Assessment & Rehabilitation, 34,* 95–103.

Giroud, M., Czlonkowska, A., Ryglewicz, D. and Wolfe, C. (2002) The problem of interpreting variations in health status (morbidity and mortality) in Europe. In C. M. A. R. C. Wolfe (ed), *Stroke services: Policy and practice across Europe.* Oxford: Radcliffe Medical Press.

Glader, E. L., Stegmayr, B. and Asplund, K. (2002) Poststroke fatigue: A 2-year follow-up study of stroke patients in Sweden. *Stroke, 33* (5), 1327–1333.

Glancy, G. P. and Knott, T. F. (2003) Part III: The psychopharmacology of long term aggression: Towards an evidenced based algorithm. *Canadian Psychiatric Association Bulletin (February)*, 13–18.

Glass, T. A., Matchar, D. B., Belyea, M. and Feussner, J. R. (1993) Impact of social support on outcome in first stroke. *Stroke, 24,* 64–70.

Glozier, N., Hackett, M. L., Parag, V. and Anderson, C. S. (2008) The influence of psychiatric morbidity on return to paid work after stroke in younger adults: The Auckland Regional Community Stroke (ARCOS) study, 2002 to 2003. *Stroke, 39,* 1526–1532.

Glueckauf, R. L., Blonder, L. X., Ecklund-Johnson, E., Maher, L., Crosson, B. and Gonzalez-Rothi, L. (2003) Functional Outcome Questionnaire for Aphasia: Overview and preliminary psychometric evaluation. *Neurorehabilitation, 18,* 281–290.

Godefroy, O., Dubois, C., Debachy, B., Leclerc, M. and Kreisler, A. (2002) Vascular aphasias main characteristics of patients hospitalized in acute stroke units. *Stroke, 33,* 702–705.

Gold, J. J. and Squire, L. R. (2006) The anatomy of amnesia: Neurohistological analysis of three new cases. *Learning & Memory, 13,* 699–710.

Goldberg, D. (1992) *General Health Questionnaire (GHQ-12)*. Windsor: NFER-Nelson.

Goldberg, D. and Hillier, V. F. (1979) A scaled version of the General Health Questionnaire. *Psychological Medicine, 9,* 139–145.

Goldberg, D. and Williams, P. (1988) *A user's guide to the General Health Questionnaire.* Windsor: NFER-Nelson.

Goldberg, G., Segal, M. E., Berk, S. N. and Gershkoff, A. M. (1997) Stroke transition after inpatient rehabilitation. *Topics in Stroke Rehabilitation, 4,* 64–79.

Goldenberg, G. (1996) Defective imitation of gestures in patients with damage in the left or right hemispheres. *Journal of Neurology Neurosurgery and Psychiatry, 61,* 176–180.

Goldenberg, G. (1999) Matching and imitation of hand and finger postures in patients with damage in the left or right hemispheres. *Neuropsychologia, 37,* 559–566.

Goldenberg, G. (2003) Apraxia and beyond: Life and work of Hugo Liepmann. *Cortex, 39,* 509–524.

Goldenberg, G., Daumuller, M. and Hagman, S. (2001) Assessment and therapy of complex activities of daily living in apraxia. *Neuropsychological Rehabilitation, 11,* 147–169.

Goldenberg, G. and Hagman, S. (1998) Therapy of activities of daily living in patients with apraxia. *Neuropsychological Rehabilitation, 8,* 123–141.

Golding, E. (1989) *Middlesex Elderly Assessment of Mental State.* Suffolk, UK: Thames Valley Test Company.

Goldstein, K. (1942) *After effects of brain injuries in war: Their evaluation and treatment: The application of psychological methods in the clinic.* New York: Grune and Stratton.

Goldstein, L., Adams, R., Alberts, M., Appel, L., Brass, L., Bushnell, C., *et al.* (2006) Primary prevention of ischemic stroke: A guideline from the American Heart Association/American Stroke Association Stroke Council: Cosponsored by the Atherosclerotic Peripheral Vascular Disease Interdisciplinary Working Group; Cardiovascular Nursing Council; Clinical Cardiology Council; Nutrition, Physical Activity, and Metabolism Council; and the Quality of Care and Outcomes Research

Interdisciplinary Working Group: The American Academy of Neurology affirms the value of this guideline. *Stroke*, *37*, 1583.

Gollwitzer, P. and Sheeran, P. (2006) Implementation intentions and goal achievement: A meta-analysis of effects and processes. *Advances in Experimental Social Psychology*, *38*, 69–119.

Goodglass, H., Kaplan, E. and Barresi, B. (2001) *Boston Diagnostic Aphasia Examination*, 3rd ed. Upper Saddle River, NJ: Pearson Assessment.

Goodyear, K. and Roseveare, C. (2003) Driving restrictions after stroke: Doctors' awareness of DVLA guidelines and advice given to patients. *Clinical Medicine*, *3*, 86–87.

Gordon, W. A., Hibbard, M., Egelko, S., Diller, L., Shaver, M., Lieberman, A., *et al.* (1985) Perceptual remediation in patients with right brain damage: A comprehensive program. *Archives of Physical Medicine and Rehabilitation*, *66*, 353–359.

Gordon, W. A. and Hibbard, M. R. (1997) Poststroke depression: An examination of the literature. *Archives of Physical Medicine and Rehabilitation*, *78*, 658–663.

Gorelick, P. B., Amico, L. L., Ganellen, R. and Benevento, L. A. (1988) Transient global amnesia and thalamic infarction. *Neurology*, *38*, 496–499.

Gormsen, L., Rosenberg, R., Bach, F. and Jensen, T. (2010) Depression, anxiety, health-related quality of life and pain in patients with chronic fibromyalgia and neuropathic pain. *European Journal of Pain*, *14*, 127e1–127e8.

Gottfries, G. G., Noltorp, S. and Norgaard, N. (1997) Experience with a Swedish version of the Geriatric Depression Scale in primary care centres. *International Journal of Geriatric Psychiatry*, *12*, 1029–1034.

Gracey, F., Palmer, S., Rous, B., Psaila, K., Shaw, K., O'Dell, J., *et al.* (2008) 'Feeling part of things': Personal construction of self after brain injury. *Neuropsychological Rehabilitation*, *18*, 627–650.

Graham, I., Atar, D., Borch-Johnsen, K., Boysen, G., Burell, G., Cifkova, R., *et al.* (2007) European guidelines on cardiovascular disease prevention in clinical practice: Executive summary. *European Heart Journal*, *28*, 2375.

Graham, N. L., Emery, T. and Hodges, J. R. (2004) Distinctive cognitive profiles in Alzheimer's disease and subcortical vascular dementia. *Journal of Neurology, Neurosurgery and Psychiatry*, *75*, 61–71.

Granholm, E., McQuaid, J. R., McClure, F. S., Pedrelli, P. and Jeste, J. V. (2002) A randomised controlled pilot study of cognitive behavioural social skills training for older patients with schizophrenia. *Schizophrenia Research*, *53*, 167–169.

Grant, J. S. (1999) Social problem-solving partnerships with family caregivers. *Rehabilitation Nursing*, *24*, 254–260.

Grant, J. S., Elliott, T. R., Weaver, M., Bartolucci, A. A. and Giger, J. N. (2002) Telephone intervention with family caregivers of stroke survivors after rehabilitation. *Stroke*, *33*, 2060–2065.

Grant, J. S., Weaver, M., Elliott, T. R., Bartolucci, A. A. and Giger, J. N. (2004) Family caregivers of stroke survivors: Characteristics of caregivers at risk for depression. *Rehabilitation Psychology*, *49*, 172–179.

Grau-Olivares, M., Arboix, A., Bartres-Faz, D. and Junque, C. (2007) Neuropsychological abnormalities associated with lacunar infarction. *Journal of the Neurological Sciences*, *257*, 160–165.

Gravel, K., Legare, F. and Graham, I. D. (2006) Barriers and facilitators to implementing shared decision-making in clinical practice: A systematic review of health professionals' perceptions. *Implementation Science*, *1*, 16.

Gray, J. M., Robertson, I., Pentland, B. and Anderson, S. (1992) Microcomputer-based attentional retraining after brain damage: A randomised group controlled trial. *Neuropsychological Rehabilitation, 2*, 97–115.

Green, P. (2003) *Manual for the Word Memory Test.* Edmonton: Green's Publishing.

Green, T., Haley, E., Eliasziw, M. and Hoyte, K. (2007) Education in stroke prevention: Efficacy of an educational counselling intervention to increase knowledge in stroke survivors. *Canadian Journal of Neuroscience Nursing, 29*, 13–20.

Greener, J., Enderby, P. and Whurr, R. (2000) Speech and language therapy for aphasia following stroke. *Cochrane Database Systematic Reviews* (2), CD000425.

Greenhalgh, T., Robert, G., Macfarlane, F., Bate, P. and Kyriakidou, O. (2004) Diffusion of innovations in service organizations: Systematic review and recommendations. *Milbank Quarterly, 82*, 581–629.

Greenwood, N., Mackenzie, A., Cloud, G. C. and Wilson, N. (2008b) Informal carers of stroke survivors – factors influencing carers: A systematic review of quantitative studies. *Disability and Rehabilitation, 30*, 1329–1349.

Greenwood, N., Mackenzie, A., Cloud, G. C. and Wilson, N. (2009a) Informal primary carers of stroke survivors living at home – challenges, satisfactions and coping: A systematic review of qualitative studies. *Disability and Rehabilitation, 31*, 337–351.

Greenwood, N., Mackenzie, A. and Harris, R. (2008a) New Deal for Carers or unfair deal: What is in it for informal carers of stroke survivors? *Policy and Politics, 36*, 299–303.

Greenwood, N., Mackenzie, A., Wilson, N. and Cloud, G. (2009b) Managing uncertainty in life after stroke: A qualitative study of the experiences of established and new informal carers in the first 3 months after discharge. *International Journal of Nursing Studies, 46*, 1122–1133.

Gresham, G. E., Kelly-Hayes, M., Wolf, P. A., Beiser, A. S., Kase, C. S. and D'Agostino, R. B. (1998) Survival and functional status 20 or more years after first stroke: The Framingham Study. *Stroke, 29*, 793–797.

Greveson, G. C., Gray, C. S., French, J. M. and James, O. F. W. (1991) Long-term outcome for patients and carers following hospital admission for stroke. *Age and Ageing, 20*, 337–344.

Grisso, T. and Appelbaum, P. S. (1998) *Assessing competence to consent to treatment: A guide for physicians and other health professionals.* New York: Oxford University Press.

Grisso, T., Appelbaum, P. S. and HillFotouhi, C. (1997) The MacCAT-T: A clinical tool to assess patients' capacities to make treatment decisions. *Psychiatric Services, 48*, 1415–1419.

Grol, R., Bosch, M. C., Hulscher, M., Eccles, M. P. and Wensing, M. (2007) Planning and studying improvement in patient care: The use of theoretical perspectives. *Milbank Quarterly, 85*, 93–138.

Grol, R. and Grimshaw, J. (2003) From best evidence to best practice: Effective implementation of change in patients' care. *Lancet, 362* (9391), 1225–1230.

Guadagnoli, E. and Ward, P. (1998) Patient participation in decision-making. *Social Science & Medicine, 47*, 329–339.

Guerrini, C., Berlucchi, G., Bricolo, E. and Aglioti, S. M. (2003) Temporal modulation of spatial tactile extinction in right-brain-damaged patients. *Journal of Cognitive Neuroscience, 15*, 523–536.

Gump, B., Matthews, K., Eberly, L. and Chang, Y. (2005) Depressive symptoms and mortality in men: Results from the Multiple Risk Factor Intervention Trial. *Stroke*, *36*, 98–102.

Gurr, B. (2009a) Emotional support for stroke survivors: Share Your Story Group. *International Journal of Therapy and Rehabilitation*, *16*, 564–570.

Gurr, B. (2009b) A psychological well-being group for stroke patients. *Clinical Psychology Forum*, *202*, 12–17.

Gurrera, R. J., Moye, J., Karel, M. J., Azar, A. R. and Armesto, J. C. (2006) Cognitive performance predicts treatment decisional abilities in mild to moderate dementia. *Neurology*, *66*, 1367–1372.

Haaland, K. Y. and Flaherty, D. (1984) The different types of limb apraxia error made by patients with left vs. right hemisphere damage. *Brain and Cognition*, *3*, 370–384.

Haaland, K. Y., Harrington, D. L. and Knight, R. T. (2000) Neural representations of skilled movement. *Brain*, *123*, 2306–2313.

Haas, M. (1999) A critique of patient satisfaction. *Health Information Management*, *29*, 9–13.

Hack, W., Kaste, M., Bogousslavsky, J., Brainin, M., Chamorro, A., Lees, K., *et al.* (2003) European Stroke Initiative Executive Committee and the EUSI Writing Committee. European Stroke Initiative recommendations for stroke management: Update 2003. *Cerebrovascular Diseases*, *16*, 311–337.

Hacke, W. (2008) Guidelines for management of ischaemic stroke and transient ischaemic attack 2008: The European Stroke Organisation (ESO) Executive Committee and the ESO Writing Committee. *Cerebrovascular Diseases*, *25*, 457–507.

Hacker, V. L. and Jones, C. (2009) Detecting feigned impairment with the word list recognition of the Wechsler Memory Scale, 3rd ed. *Brain Injury*, *23*, 243–249.

Hacker, V. L., Stark, D. and Thomas, S. (2010) Validation of the Stroke Aphasic Depression Questionnaire using the brief assessment schedule depression cards in an acute stroke sample. *British Journal of Clinical Psychology*, *49*, 123–127.

Hackett, M., Anderson, C., House, A. and Xia, J. (2009) Interventions for treating depression after stroke. *Stroke*, *40*, e487.

Hackett, M. L. and Anderson, C. S. (2005) Predictors of depression after stroke: A systematic review of observational studies. *Stroke*, *36*, 2296–2301.

Hackett, M. L., Anderson, C. S., House, A. and Halteh, C. (2008a) Interventions for preventing depression after stroke. *Cochrane Database of Systematic Reviews* (3), CD003689.

Hackett, M. L., Anderson, C. S., House, A. and Xia, J. (2008b) Interventions for treating depression after stroke. *Cochrane Database of Systematic Reviews*, (4), CD003437.

Hackett, M. L., Hill, K. M., Hewison, J., Anderson, C. S. and House, A. O. (2010) Stroke survivors who score below threshold on standard depression measures may still have negative cognitions of concern. *Stroke*, *41*, 478–481.

Hackett, M. L., Yang, M., Anderson, C. S., Horrocks, J. A. and House, A. (2010) Pharmaceutical interventions for emotionalism after stroke. *Cochrane Database of Systematic Reviews* (2), CD003690.

Hackett, M. L., Yapa, C., Parag, V. and Anderson, C. S. (2005) Frequency of depression after stroke: A systematic review of observational studies. *Stroke*, *36*, 1330–1340.

Hadidi, N., Treat-Jacobson, D. J. and Lindquist, R. (2009) Poststroke depression and functional outcome: A critical review of literature. *Heart and Lung*, *38*, 151–162.

Hafsteinsdóttir, T. B. and Grypdonck, M. (1997) Being a stroke patient: A review of the literature. *Journal of Advanced Nursing*, *26*, 580–588.

Haggstrom, T., Axelsson, K. and Norberg, A. (1994) The experience of living with stroke sequelae illuminated by means of stories and metaphors. *Qualitative Health Research, 4*, 321–337.

Haley, W. E., Allen, J. Y., Grant, J. S., Clay, O. J., Perkins, M. and Roth, D. L. (2009) Problems and benefits reported by stroke family caregivers results from a prospective epidemiological study. *Stroke, 40*, 2129–2133.

Halligan, P. W., Manning, L. and Marshall, J. C. (1990) Individual variation in line bisection: A study of four patients with right hemisphere damage and normal controls. *Neuropsychologia, 28*, 1043–1051.

Halligan, P. W. and Marshall, J. C. (1991) Left neglect for near but not far space in man. *Nature, 350* (6318), 498–500.

Halligan, P. W. and Marshall, J. C. (1995) Supernumerary phantom limb after right hemispheric stroke. *Journal of Neurology Neurosurgery and Psychiatry, 59*, 341–342.

Halligan, P. W., Marshall, J. C. and Wade, D. T. (1989) Visuospatial neglect: Underlying factors and test sensitivity. *Lancet, 2* (8668), 908–911.

Halligan, P. W., Marshall, J. C. and Wade, D. T. (1993) 3 arms: A case study of supernumerary phantom limb after right-hemisphere stroke. *Journal of Neurology Neurosurgery and Psychiatry, 56*, 159–166.

Hamann, G. F., Weimar, C., Glahn, J., Busse, O. and Diener, H. C. (2003) Adherence to secondary stroke prevention strategies: Results from the German Stroke Data Bank. *Cerebrovascular Disease, 15*, 282–288.

Hammarberg, M. (1992) PENN inventory for posttraumatic stress disorder: psychometric properties. *Psychological Assessment, 4*, 67–76.

Hammond, M. F., O'Keefe, S. T. and Barer, D. H. (2000) Development and validation of a brief observer-rated screening scale for depression in elderly medical patients. *Age and Ageing, 29*, 511–515.

Hamsher, K., Levin, H. S. and Benton, A. L. (1979) Facial recognition in patients with focal brain lesions. *Archives of Neurology, 36*, 837–839.

Han, B. and Haley, W. E. (1999) Family caregiving for patients with stroke: Review and analysis. *Stroke, 30*, 1478–1485.

Hand, P. J., Kwan, J., Lindley, R. I., Dennis, M. S. and Wardlaw, J. M. (2006) Distinguishing between stroke and mimic at the bedside: The brain attack study. *Stroke, 37* (3), 769–775.

Hanks, R. A., Rapport, L. J., Millis, S. R. and Deshpande, S. A. (1999) Measures of executive functioning as predictors of functional ability and social integration in a rehabilitation sample. *Archives of Physical Medicine and Rehabilitation, 80* (9), 1030–1037.

Hanna-Pladdy, B., Heilman, K. M. and Foundas, A. L. (2003) Ecological implications of ideomotor apraxia: Evidence from physical activities of daily living. *Neurology, 60*, 487–490.

Hansard, L. I. (2007) *New Deal for Carers.* London: TSO.

Hanson, L. C. and Rodgman, E. (1996) The use of living wills at the end of life: A national study. *Archives of Internal Medicine, 156* (9), 1018–1022.

Hanssen, I. (2005) From human ability to ethical principle: An intercultural perspective on autonomy. *Medicine, Health Care and Philosophy, 7* (3), 269–279.

Hardeman, W., Johnston, M., Johnston, D. W., Bonetti, D., Wareham, N. J. and Kinmonth, A. L. (2002) Application of the theory of planned behaviour in behaviour change interventions: A systematic review. *Psychology & Health, 17* (2), 123–158.

Hardy, S. and Joyce, T. (2009) The Mental Capacity Act: Practicalities for health and social care professionals. *Advances in Mental Health and Learning Disabilities*, *3* (1), 9–14.

Hare, R., Rogers, H., Lester, H., McManus, R. J. and Mant, J. (2006) What do stroke patients and their carers want from community services? *Family Practice*, *23* (1), 131–136. doi: 10. 1093/fampra/cmi098.

Harris, L. E., Luft, F. C., Rudy, D. W. and Tierney, W. M. (1995) Correlates of health care satisfaction in inner-city patients with hypertension and chronic renal insufficiency. *Social Science & Medicine*, *41* (12), 1639–1645.

Hart, S. and Morris, R. (2008) Screening for depression after stroke: an exploration of professionals' compliance with guidelines. *Clinical Rehabilitation*, *22* (1), 60–70.

Hartke, R. J. and King, R. B. (2003) Telephone group intervention for older stroke caregivers. *Topics in Stroke Rehabilitation*, *9* (4), 65–81.

Hartman, J. and Landau, W. M. (1987) Comparison of formal language therapy with supportive counseling for aphasia due to acute vascular accident. *Archives of Neurology*, *44*, 646–649.

Hartman-Maeir, A. and Katz, N. (1995) Validity of the Behavioural Inattention Test (BIT): Relationships with functional tasks. *American Journal of Occupational Therapy*, *49*, 507–516.

Harvey, A., Watkins, E., Mansell, W. and Shafran, R. (2004) *Cognitive Behavioural Processes across Psychological Disorders: A Transdiagnostic Approach to Research and Treatment*. Oxford: Oxford University Press.

Haselkorn, J. K., Mueller, B. A. and Rivara, F. A. (1998) Characteristics of drivers and driving record after traumatic and nontraumatic brain injury. *Archives of Physical Medicine and Rehabilitation*, *79* (7), 738–742.

Hashimoto, H., Iida, J., Kawaguchi, S. and Sakaki, T. (2004) Clinical features and management of brain arteriovenous malformations in elderly patients. *Acta Neurochirurgica*, *146* (10), 1091–1098.

Haslam, C., Holme, A., Haslam, S. A., Iyer, A., Jetten, J. and Williams, W. H. (2008) Maintaining group memberships: Social identity continuity predicts well-being after stroke. *Neuropsychological Rehabilitation*, *18* (5–6), 671–691.

Hatcher, B. J., Durham, J. D. and Richey, M. (1985) Overcoming stroke-related depression. *Journal of Gerontological Nursing*, *11*, 35–39.

Hawkins, R. P., Kreuter, M., Resnicow, K., Fishbein, M. and Dijkstra, A. (2008) Understanding tailoring in communicating about health. *Health Education Research*, *23* (3), 454–466.

Hawley, C. A. (2010) *The Attitudes of Health Professionals to Giving Advice on Fitness to Drive*. Road Safety Research Report No. 91. London: Department for Transport.

Healey, A. K., Kneebone, II, Carroll, M. and Anderson, S. J. (2008) A preliminary investigation of the reliability and validity of the Brief Assessment Schedule Depression Cards and the Beck Depression Inventory-Fast Screen to screen for depression in older stroke survivors. *International Journal of Geriatric Psychiatry*, *23* (5), 531–536.

Healthcare Commission. (2005) *Stroke Survey of Patients 2005*. London: Healthcare Commission.

Healthcare Commission. (2006) *Survey of Patients 2006: Caring for People after They Have Had a stroke: A Follow-Up Survey of Patients*. London: Healthcare Commission.

Heath, M., Roy, E. A., Westwood, D. and Black, S. E. (2001) Patterns of apraxia associated with the production of intransitive limb gestures following left and right hemisphere stroke. *Brain and Cognition, 46* (1–2), 165–169.

Heaton, R. K., Chelune, G. J., Talley, J. L., Kay, G. G. and Curtiss, G. (1993) *Wisconsin Card Sorting (WCST) Manual Revised and Expanded.* Odessa, FL: Psychological Assessment Resources.

Heilman, K. M., Bowers, D., Coslett, H. B., Whelan, H. and Watson, R. T. (1985) Directional hypokinesia: Prolonged reaction-times for leftward movements in patients with right hemisphere lesions and neglect. *Neurology, 35* (6), 855–859.

Heilman, K. M., Rothi, L. J. and Valenstein, E. (1982) Two forms of ideomotor apraxia. *Neurology, 32,* 342–346.

Heimer, L. and Van Hoesen, G.W. (2006) The limbic lobe and its output channels: Implications for emotional functions and adaptive behaviour. *Neuroscience & Biobehavioral Reviews, 30,* 126–147.

Helfand, M. and Freeman, M. (2009) Assessment and management of acute pain in adult medical inpatients: A systematic review. *Pain Medicine, 10,* 1183–1199.

Hellstrom, K. and Lindmark, B. (1999) Fear of falling in patients with stroke: A reliability study. *Clinical Rehabilitation, 13,* 509–517.

Hénon, H., Durieu, I., Guerouaou, D., Lebert, F., Pasquier, F. and Leys, D. (2001) Poststroke dementia: Incidence and relationship to prestroke cognitive decline. *Neurology, 57,* 1216–1222.

Henry, J. D. and Crawford, J. R. (2004) A meta-analytic review of verbal fluency performance following focal cortical lesions. *Neuropsychology, 18,* 284–295.

Her Majesty's Government. (1995) Carers (Recognition and Services) Act 1995. London: TSO.

Her Majesty's Government. (2000) Carers and Disabled Children Act 2000. London: TSO.

Her Majesty's Government. (2001) Health and Social Care Act, 2001. London: HMSO.

Her Majesty's Government. (2004) Carers (Equal Opportunities) Act 2004. London: TSO.

Her Majesty's Government. (2005) Mental Capacity Act, 2005. London: HMSO.

Her Majesty's Government. (2006) Work and Families Act, 2006. London: TSO.

Her Majesty's Government. (2007a) Local Government and Public Involvement in Health Act, 2007. London: HMSO.

Her Majesty's Government. (2007b) Mental Health Act, 2007. London: HMSO.

Hermsdorfer, J., Hentze, S. and Goldenberg, G. (2006) Spatial and kinematic features of apraxic movement depend on the mode of execution. *Neuropsychologia, 44,* 1642–1652.

Herr, K., Bjoro, K. and Decker, S. (2006) Tools for assessment of pain in nonverbal older adults with dementia: A state-of-the-science review. *Journal of Pain and Symptom Management, 31,* 170–192.

Herrera-Guzman, I., Pena-Casanova, J., Lara, J. P., Gudayol-Ferre, E. and Bohm, P. (2004) Influence of age, sex, and education on the Visual Object and Space Perception Battery (VOSP) in a healthy normal elderly population. *The Clinical Neuropsychologist, 18,* 385–394.

Herrmann, M., Curio, N., Petz, T., Synowitz, H., Wagner, S., Bartels, C., *et al.* (2000) Coping with illness after brain diseases: A comparison between patients with malignant brain tumors, stroke, Parkinson's disease and traumatic brain injury. *Disability and Rehabilitation, 22,* 539–546.

Herrmann, M., Freyholdt, U., Fuchs, G. and Wallesch, C-W. (1997) Coping with chronic neurological impairment: A contrastive analysis of Parkinson's disease and stroke. *Disability and Rehabilitation, 19*, 6–12.

Herrmann, N., Black, S. E., Lawrence, J., Szekely, C. and Szalai, J. P. (1998) The Sunnybrook stroke study: A prospective study of depressive symptoms and functional outcome. *Stroke, 29*, 618–624.

Hesketh, A., Long, A., Patchick, E., Lee, J. and Bowen, A. (2008) The reliability of rating conversation as a measure of functional communication following stroke. *Aphasiology, 22*, 970–984.

Hibbard, M. R., Grober, S., Gordon, W. A. and Aletta, E. G. (1990a) Modification of cognitive psychotherapy for the treatment of post-stroke depression. *The Behavior Therapist, 13*, 15–17.

Hibbard, M. R., Grober, S. E., Gordon, W. A., Aletta, E. G. and Freeman, A. (1990b) Cognitive therapy and the treatment of poststroke depression. *Topics in Geriatric Rehabilitation, 5*, 43–55.

Hibbard, M. R., Grober, S. E., Stein, P. N. and Gordon, W. A. (1992) Post-stroke depression. In A. Freeman & F. M. Dattilio (eds), *Comprehensive Casebook of Cognitive Therapy* (pp. 303–310). New York: Plenum.

Hickok, G. and Poeppel, D. (2000) Towards a functional neuroanatomy of speech perception. *Trends in Cognitive Sciences, 4*, 131–138.

Higgins, J., Salbach, N. M., Wood-Dauphinee, S., Richards, C. L., Côotée, R. and Mayo, N. E. (2006) The effect of a task-oriented intervention on arm function in people with stroke: A randomized controlled trial. *Clinical Rehabilitation, 20*, 296–310.

Hilari, K. and Byng, S. (2001) Measuring quality of life in people with aphasia: The Stroke Specific Quality of Life Scale. *International Journal of Language & Communication Disorders, 36*, 86–91.

Hilari, K., Byng, S., Lamping, D. L. and Smith, S. C. (2003) Stroke and aphasia quality of life scale-39 (SAQOL-39): Evaluation of acceptability, reliability, and validity. *Stroke, 34*, 1944–1950.

Hilari, K., Northcott, S., Roy, P., Marshall, J., Wiggins, R., Chataway, J., *et al.* (2010) Psychological distress after stroke and aphasia: The first six months. *Clinical Rehabilitation, 24*, 181–190.

Hilari, K., Owen, S. and Farrelly, S. J. (2007) Proxy and self-report agreement on the Stroke and Aphasia Quality of Life Scale-39. *Journal of Neurology Neurosurgery and Psychiatry, 78*, 1072–1075.

Hillis, A. E. (2007) Aphasia: Progress in the last quarter of a century. *Neurology, 69*, 200–213.

Hillis, A. E., Barker, P. B., Beauchamp, N. J., Gordon, B. and Wityk, R. J. (2000) MR perfusion imaging reveals regions of hypoperfusion associated with aphasia and neglect. *Neurology, 55*, 782–788.

Hillis, A. E., Gold, L., Kannan, V., Cloutman, L., Kleinman, J. T., Newhart, M., *et al.* (2008) Site of the ischemic penumbra as a predictor of potential for recovery of functions. *Neurology, 71*, 184–189.

Hillis, A. E., Work, M., Barker, P. B., Jacobs, M. A., Breese, E. L. and Maurer, K. (2004) Re-examining the brain regions crucial for orchestrating speech articulation. *Brain, 127*, 1479–1487.

Hirst, M. (2002) Transitions to informal care in Great Britain during the 1990s. *Journal of Epidemiology and Community Health, 56*, 579–587.

Hochstenbach, J., Mulder, T., van Limbeek, J., Donders, R. and Schoonderwaldt, H. (1998) Cognitive decline following stroke: A comprehensive study of cognitive decline following stroke. *Journal of Clinical and Experimental Neuropsychology, 20*, 503–517.

Hochstenbach, J. B., Anderson, P. G., van Limbeek, J. and Mulder, T. T. (2001) Is there a relation between neuropsychologic variables and quality of life after stroke? *Archives of Physical Medicine and Rehabilitation, 82*, 1360–1366.

Hochstenbach, J. B., Den Otter, R. and Mulder, T. W. (2003) Cognitive recovery after stroke: A 2-year follow-up. *Archives of Physical and Medical Rehabilitation, 84*, 1499–1504.

Hodgkinson, H. M. (1972) Evaluation of a mental test score for assessment of mental impairment in the elderly. *Age and Ageing, 1*, 233–238.

Hoffmann, M., Schmitt, F. and Bromley, E. (2009) Comprehensive cognitive neurological assessment in stroke. *Acta Neurologica Scandinavica, 119*, 162–171.

Hoffmann, T. and McKenna, K. (2001) Prediction of outcome after stroke. *Physical & Occupational Therapy in Geriatrics, 19*, 53–75.

Holbrook, M. (1982) Stroke: Social and emotional outcome. *Journal of the Royal College of Physicians of London, 16*, 100–104.

Holland, A. L., Frattali, C. M. and Fromm, D. (1999) *Communication Activities for Daily Living*, 2nd ed. Austin, TX: Pro-Ed.

Holliday, R. C., Ballinger, C. and Playford, E. D. (2007) Goal setting in neurological rehabilitation: Patients' perspectives. *Disability and Rehabilitation, 29*, 389–394.

Hommel, M., Miguel, S. T., Naegele, B., Gonnet, N. and Jaillard, A. (2009) Cognitive determinants of social functioning after a first ever mild to moderate stroke at vocational age. *Journal of Neurology Neurosurgery and Psychiatry, 80*, 876–880.

Hopko, D. R., Lejuez, C. W., Ruggiero, K. J. and Eifert, G. H. (2003) Contemporary behavioral activation treatments for depression: Procedures, principles, and progress. *Clinical Psychology Review, 23*, 699–717.

Hopper, T., Holland, A. and Rewega, M. (2002) Conversational coaching: Treatment outcomes and future directions. *Aphasiology, 16*, 745–761.

Horne, R. (2004) Measuring adherence: The case for self-report. *International Journal of Behavioral Medicine 11*, 75.

Horner, M. D. and Hamner, M. B. (2002) Neurocognitive functioning in posttraumatic stress disorder. *Neuropsychology Review, 12*, 15–30.

Horowitz, M. J., Wilner, N. and Alvarez, W. (1979) Impact of Event Scale: A measure of subjective stress. *Psychosomatic Medicine, 41*, 209–218.

House, A. (2000) The treatment of depression after stroke. *Journal of Psychosomatic Research, 48*, 235.

House, A. (2003) Problem-solving therapy improves psychological outcome after stroke: A randomised controlled trial. Unpublished.

House, A., Dennis, M., Hawton, K. and Warlow, C. (1989b) Methods of identifying mood disorder in stroke patients: Experience in the Oxfordshire Community Stroke Project. *Age and Ageing, 18*, 371–379.

House, A., Dennis, M., Mogridge, L., Warlow, C., Hawton, K. and Jones, L. (1991) Mood disorders in the year after 1st stroke. *British Journal of Psychiatry, 158*, 83–92.

House, A., Dennis, M., Molyneux, A., Warlow, C. and Hawton, K. (1989a) Emotionalism after stroke. *British Medical Journal, 298*, 991–994.

House, A., Knapp, P., Bamford, J. and Vail, A. (2001) Mortality at 12 and 24 months after stroke may be associated with depressive symptoms at 1 month. *Stroke, 32,* 696–701.

House, J. S., Landis, K. R. and Umberson, D. (1988) Social relationships and health. *Science, 241,* 540–545.

House of Lords. (2005) *Assisted Dying for the Terminally Ill Bill (HL), Volume 1 Report.* London: TSO.

Howard, D. and Patterson, K. (1992) *Pyramids and Palm Trees: A Test of Semantic Access from Pictures and Words.* Bury St Edmunds: Thames Valley Test Company.

Howard, D., Swinburn, K. and Porter, G. (2009) Putting the CAT out: What the Comprehensive Aphasia Test has to offer. *Aphasiology, 24,* 56–74.

Howland, J., Lachman, M. E., Peterson, E. W., Cote, J., Kasten, L. and Jette, A. (1998) Covariates of fear of falling and associated activity curtailment. *Gerontologist, 38,* 549–555.

Hu, G., Tuomilehto, J., Silventoinen, K., Sarti, C., Mannisto, S. and Jousilahti, P. (2007) Body mass index, waist circumference, and waist-hip ratio on the risk of total and type-specific stroke. *Archives of Internal Medicine, 167,* 1420–1427.

Hull, S., Hartigan, N. and Kneebone, I. (2007) Is bingo a psychological intervention? Developing a support group for stroke survivors and carers. *Clinical Psychology Forum, 180* (December), 27–29.

Hull, S. and Kneebone, I. (2007) Revision and assessment of the evidence for a revised cognitive behavioural model for fear of falling. Paper presented at the World Congress of Behavioural and Cognitive Therapies, Barcelona, Spain.

Hunot, V., Churchill, R., Teixeira, V. and Silva de Lima, M. (2007) Psychological therapies for generalised anxiety disorder. *Cochrane Database of Systematic Reviews* (1), CD001848.

Hunt, D. and Smith, J. A. (2004) The personal experience of carers of stroke survivors: An interpretative phenomenological analysis. *Disability and Rehabilitation, 26,* 1000–1011.

Huppert, F., Brayne, C., Gill, C., Paykel, E. and Beardsall, L. (1995) CAMCOG- a concise neuropsychological test to assist dementia diagnosis: Socio-demographic determinants in an elderly population sample. *British Journal of Clinical Psychology, 34,* 529–541.

Hurdowar, A., Graham, I. D., Bayley, M., Harrison, M., Wood-Dauphinee, S. and Bhogal, S. (2007) Quality of stroke rehabilitation clinical practice guidelines. *Journal of Evaluation in Clinical Practice, 13,* 657–664.

Hurn, J., Kneebone, I. and Cropley, M. (2006) Goal setting as an outcome measure: a systematic review. *Clinical Rehabilitation, 20,* 756–772.

Husain, M., Mannon, S., Mort, D., Hodgson, T., Driver, J. and Kennard, C. (2002) Impaired spatial memory contributes to unilateral neglect. *Journal of Neurology Neurosurgery and Psychiatry, 73,* 221–221.

Husain, M. and Rorden, C. (2003) Non-spatially lateralized mechanisms in hemispatial neglect. *Nature Reviews Neuroscience, 4,* 26–36.

Husband, H. J. and Tarbuck, A. F. (1994) Cognitive rating scales: A comparison of the Mini-Mental State Examination and the Middlesex Elderly Assessment of Mental State. *International Journal of Geriatric Psychiatry, 9,* 797–802.

Hussian, R. A. and Lawrence, P. S. (1981) Social reinforcement of activity in the treatment of depressed institutionalised elderly patients. *Cognitive Therapy and Research, 5,* 57–69.

Hyndman, D. and Ashburn, A. (2003) People with stroke living, in the community: Attention deficits, balance, ADL ability and falls. *Disability and Rehabilitation, 25,* 817–822.

Hyndman, D., Pickering, R. M. and Ashburn, A. (2008) The influence of attention deficits on functional recovery post stroke during the first 12 months after discharge from hospital. *Journal of Neurology, Neurosurgery and Psychiatry, 79,* 656–663.

Ilse, I. B., Feys, H., de Wit, L., Putman, K. and de Weerdt, W. (2008) Stroke caregivers' strain: Prevalence and determinants in the first six months after stroke. *Disability and Rehabilitation, 30* (7), 523–530.

Indredavik, B., Bakke, F., Slordahl, S. A., Rokseth, R. and Haheim, L. L. (1999) Stroke unit treatment: 10-year follow-up. *Stroke, 30,* 1524–1527.

Ingles, J. L., Eskes, G. A. and Phillips, S. J. (1999) Fatigue after stroke. *Archives of Physical Medicine and Rehabilitation, 80,* 173–178.

Ingram, B. L. (2006) *Clinical Case Formulations: Matching the Integrative Treatment Plan to the Client.* Hoboken, NJ: John Wiley & Sons Inc.

Isozumi, K. (2004) Obesity as a risk factor for cerebrovascular disease. *Keio Journal of Medicine., 53,* 7–11.

Ives, S., Heuschmann, P., Wolfe, C. and Redfern, J. (2008) Patterns of smoking cessation in the first 3 years after stroke: The South London Stroke Register. *European Journal of Cardiovascular Prevention & Rehabilitation, 15,* 329–335.

Ivnik, R. J., Malec, J. F., Smith, G. E., Tangalos, E. G., Peterson, R. C., Kokmen, E., *et al.* (1992) Mayo's older Americans Normative Studies: WAIS-R norms for ages 56 to 97. *Clinical Neuropsychologist, 6,* 1–30.

Jackson, E. and Warner, J. (2002) How much do doctors know about consent and capacity? *Journal of the Royal Society of Medicine, 95* (12), 601–603.

Jacob, R. G., Furman, J. M. R., Clark, D. B. and Durrant, J. D. (1992) Vestibular symptoms, panic, and phobia. *Annals of Clinical Psychiatry, 4,* 163–174.

Jacobs, B. S., Boden-Albala, B., Lin, I. F. and Sacco, R. L. (2002) Stroke in the young in the Northern Manhattan Stroke Study. *Stroke, 33,* 2789–2793.

Jacobs, B. S., Sacco, R. L. and Boden-Albala, B. (2003) Epidemiology of stroke in the young: Response. *Stroke, 34,* E13–E14.

Jaillard, A., Naegele, B., Trabucco-Miguel, S., LeBas, J. F. and Hommel, M. (2009) Hidden dysfunctioning in subacute stroke. *Stroke, 40,* 2473–2479.

Jain, S. (1982) Operant conditioning for management of a non-compliant rehabilitation case after stroke. *Archives of Physical and Medical Rehabilitation, 63,* 374–376.

Janz, N. and Becker, M. (1984) The health belief model: A decade later. *Health Education & Behavior, 11,* 1–47.

Jaster, J. H. (2001) Unexpected sudden death after lateral medullary infarction. *Journal of Neurology, Neurosurgery and Psychiatry, 70,* 137–147.

Jefferies, E. and Lambon Ralph, M. A. (2006) Semantic impairment in stroke aphasia versus semantic dementia: A case-series comparison. *Brain, 129,* 2132–2147.

Jefford, M. and Moore, R. (2008) Improvement of informed consent and the quality of consent documents. *Lancet Oncology, 9,* 485–493.

Jehkonen, M., Ahonen, J., Dastidar, P., Koivisto, A., Laippala, P. and Vilkki, J. (1998) How to detect visual neglect in acute stroke. *Lancet, 351,* 727–728.

Jehkonen, M., Ahonen, J. P., Dastidar, P., Koivisto, A. M., Laippala, P., Vilkki, J., *et al.* (2000) Visual neglect as a predictor of functional outcome one year after stroke. *Acta Neurologica Scandinavica, 101,* 195–201.

Jehkonen, M., Laihosalo, M. and Kettunen, J. (2006a) Anosognosia after stroke: Assessment, occurrence, subtypes and impact on functional outcome reviewed. *Acta Neurologica Scandinavica*, *114*, 293–306.

Jehkonen, M., Laihosalo, M. and Kettunen, J. E. (2006b) Impact of neglect on functional outcome after stroke: A review of methodological issues and recent research findings. *Restorative Neurology and Neuroscience*, *24*, 209–215.

Jehkonen, M., Laihosalo, M., Koivisto, A. M., Dastidar, P. and Ahonen, J. P. (2007) Fluctuation in spontaneous recovery of left visual neglect: A 1-year follow-up. *European Neurology*, *58*, 210–214.

Jenkinson, C., Coulter, A., Bruster, S., Richards, N. and Chandola, T. (2002) Patients' experiences and satisfaction with health care: Results of a questionnaire study of specific aspects of care. *Quality & Safety in Health Care*, *11*, 335–339.

Jennett, S. M. and Lincoln, N. B. (1991) An evaluation of the effectiveness of group therapy for memory problems. *International Disability Studies*, *13*, 83–86.

Jeste, D. V., Palmer, B. W., Golshan, S., Eyler, L. T., Dunn, L. B., Meeks, T., *et al.* (2009) Multimedia consent for research in people with schizophrenia and normal subjects: A randomized controlled trial. *Schizophrenia Bulletin*, *35*, 719–729.

Jia, H., Damush, T. M., Qin, H., Ried, L. D., Wang, X., Young, L. J., *et al.* (2006) The impact of poststroke depression on healthcare use by veterans with acute stroke. *Stroke*, *37*, 2796–2801.

Johnson, G., Burvill, P. W., Anderson, C. S., Jamrozik, K., Stewart-Wynne, E. G. and Chakera, T. M. (1995) Screening instruments for depression and anxiety following stroke: Experience in the Perth community stroke study. *Acta Psychiatrica Scandinavia*, *91*, 252–257.

Johnston, C. and Liddle, J. (2007) The Mental Capacity Act 2005: A new framework for healthcare decision making. *Journal of Medical Ethics*, *33*, 94–97.

Johnston, M., Pollard, B. and Hennessey, P. (2000) Construct validation of the hospital anxiety and depression scale with clinical populations. *Journal of Psychosomatic Research*, *48*, 579–584.

Johnston, S., Mendis, S. and Mathers, C. (2009) Global variation in stroke burden and mortality: Estimates from monitoring, surveillance, and modelling. *The Lancet Neurology*, *8*, 345–354.

Jonas, B. S. and Mussolino, M. E. (2000) Symptoms of depression as a prospective risk factor for stroke. *Psychosomatic Medicine*, *62*, 463–471.

Jones, F., Mandy, A. and Partridge, C. (2008) Reasons for recovery after stroke: A perspective based on personal experience. *Disability & Rehabilitation*, *30*, 507–516.

Jones, F., Mandy, A. and Partridge, C. (2009) Changing self-efficacy in individuals following a first time stroke: Preliminary study of a novel self-management intervention. *Clinical Rehabilitation*, *23*, 522–533.

Jones, F., Partridge, C. and Reid, F. (2008) The Stroke Self-Efficacy Questionnaire: Measuring individual confidence in functional performance after stroke. *Journal of Clinical Nursing*, *17*, 244–252.

Jones, S. P., Jenkinson, A. J., Leathley, M. J. and Watkins, C. L. (2010) Stroke knowledge and awareness: An integrative review of the evidence. *Age and Ageing 39*, 11–22.

Jonsson, A. C., Lindgren, I., Hallstrom, B., Norrving, B. and Lindgren, A. (2006) Prevalence and intensity of pain after stroke: A population based study focusing on patients' perspectives. *Journal of Neurology Neurosurgery and Psychiatry*, *77*, 590–595.

Jood, K., Redfors, P., Rosengren, A., Blomstrand, C. and Jern, C. (2009) Self-perceived psychological stress and ischemic stroke: A case-control study. *BMC Medicine, 7,* 53.

Jorgensen, L., Engstad, T. and Jacobsen, B. K. (2002) Higher incidence of falls in long-term stroke survivors than in population controls: Depressive symptoms predict falls after stroke. *Stroke, 33,* 542–547.

Jorm, A. F. (2000) Does old age reduce the risk of anxiety and depression? A review of epidemiological studies across the adult life span. *Psychological Medicine, 30,* 11–22.

Joshipura, K. J., Ascherio, A., Manson, J. E., Stampfer, M. J., Rimm, E. B., Speizer, F. E., *et al.* (1999) Fruit and vegetable intake in relation to risk of ischemic stroke. *Journal of the American Medical Assocation, 282,* 1233–1239.

Joubert, J., Cumming, T. and McLean, A. (2007) Diversity of risk factors for stroke: The putative roles and mechanisms of depression and air pollution. *Journal of the Neurological Sciences, 262,* 71–76.

Joyce, T. (2008) *Best Interests Guidance on determining the best interests of adults who lack the capacity to make a decision (or decisions) for themselves [England and Wales].* Leicester: British Psychological Society.

Juby, L. C., Lincoln, N. B. and Berman, P. (1996) The effect of a stroke rehabilitation unit on functional and psychological outcome: A randomised controlled trial. *Cerebrovascular Diseases, 6,* 106–110.

Kagan, A., Black, S. E., Duchan, J. F., Simmons-Mackie, N. and Square, P. (2001) Training volunteers as conversation partners using 'Supported Conversation for Adults with Aphasia' (SCA): A controlled trial. *Journal of Speech Language and Hearing Research, 44,* 624–638.

Kalra, L. (1994) Does age affect benefits of stroke unit rehabilitation? *Stroke, 25,* 346–351.

Kalra, L., Perez, I., Gupta, S. and Wittink, M. (1997) The influence of visual neglect on stroke rehabilitation. *Stroke, 28,* 1386–1391.

Kanagaratnam, P. and Asbjornsen, A. E. (2007) Executive deficits in chronic PTSD related to political violence. *Journal of Anxiety Disorders, 21,* 510–525.

Kane, M. J., Conway, A. R. A., Miura, T. K. and Colflesh, G. J. H. (2007) Working memory, attention control, and the N-back task: A question of construct validity. *Journal of Experimental Psychology: Learning Memory and Cognition, 33,* 615–622.

Kane, R. L., Chen, Q., Finch, M., Blewett, L., Burns, R. and Moskowitz, M. (2000) The optimal outcomes of post-hospital care under Medicare. *Health Service Research, 35,* 615–661.

Kaner, E. F., Dickinson, H. O., Beyer, F. R., Campbell, F., Schlesinger, C., Heather, N., *et al.* (2007) Effectiveness of brief alcohol interventions in primary care populations. *Cochrane Database of Systematic Reviews* (2), CD004148.

Kant, R. (1997) Rehabilitation following stroke: A participant perspective. *Disability and Rehabilitation 19,* 297–304.

Kaplan, E., Goodglass, H. and Weintraub, S. (1983) *The Boston Naming Test: Second Edition Manual.* New York: Lea & Febiger.

Kapp, M. B. and Mossman, D. (1996) Measuring decisional capacity: Cautions on the construction of a 'capacimeter'. *Psychology Public Policy and Law, 2,* 73–95.

Karelina, K., Norman, G. J., Zhang, N., Morris, J. S., Peng, H. Y. and DeVries, A. C. (2009) Social isolation alters neuroinflammatory response to stroke. *Proceedings of the National Academy of Sciences of the United States of America, 106,* 5895–5900.

Karnath, H. O., Baier, B. and Nagele, T. (2005) Awareness of the functioning of one's own limbs mediated by the insular cortex? *Journal of Neuroscience, 25,* 7134–7138.

Karnath, H. O., Ruter, J., Mandler, A. and Himmelbach, M. (2009) The anatomy of object recognition-visual form agnosia caused by medial occipitotemporal stroke. *Journal of Neuroscience*, *29*, 5854–5862.

Kaschel, R., Della Sala, S., Cantagallo, A., Fahlböck, A., Laaksonen, R. and Kazen, M. (2002) Imagery mnemonics for the rehabilitation of memory: A randomised group controlled trial. *Neuropsychological Rehabilitation*, *12*, 127–153.

Kaufman, S. (1988) Towards a phenomenology of boundaries in medicine: Chronic illness experience in the case of stroke. *Medical Anthropology Quarterly 2*, 338–354.

Kauhanen, M. L., Korpelainen, J. T., Hiltunen, P., Määttä, R., Mononen, H., Brusin, E., *et al.* (2000) Aphasia, depression, and non-verbal cognitive impairment in ischaemic stroke. *Cerebrovascular Diseases*, *10*, 455–461.

Kay, J., Lesser, R. and Coltheart, M. (1992) *Psycholinguistic Assessment of Language Processing Ability (PALPA)* Hove: Psychology Press.

Kazdin, A. E. (1977) Assessing the clinical or applied importance of behavior change through social validation. *Behavior Modification*, *1*, 427–452.

Keane, S., Turner, C., Sherrington, C. and Beard, J. R. (2006) Use of Fresnel prism glasses to treat stroke patients with hemispatial neglect. *Archives of Physical Medicine and Rehabilitation*, *87*, 1668–1672.

Kee, Y-Y. K., Brooks, W. and Bhalla, A. (2009) Do older patients receive adequate stroke care? An experience of a neurovascular clinic. *Postgraduate Medical Journal*, *85*, 115–118.

Kelley, C. G., Lipson, A. R., Daly, B. J. and Douglas, S. L. (2009) Advance directive use and psychosocial characteristics: An analysis of patients enrolled in a psychosocial cancer registry. *Cancer Nursing*, *32*, 335–341.

Kelly, H., Brady, M. C. and Enderby, P. (2010) Speech and language therapy for aphasia following stroke. Cochrane Database of Systematic Reviews (5), CD000425.

Kelson, M., Ford, C. and Rigge, M. (1998) *Stroke Rehabilitation: Patient and Carer Views: A Report of the College of Health for the Intercollegiate Working Party for Stroke.* London: Royal College of Physicians.

Kemp, B. J., Corgiat, M. and Gill, C. (1991/1992) Effects of brief cognitive-behavioral group psychotherapy on older persons with and without disabling illness. *Behaviour, Health and Ageing*, *2*, 21–28.

Kent, R. D. (2000) Research on speech motor control and its disorders: a review and prospective. *Journal of Communication Disorders*, *33*, 391–428.

Keppel, C. C. and Crowe, S. F. (2000) Changes to body image and self-esteem following stroke in young adults. *Neuropsychological Rehabilitation*, *10*, 15–31.

Kerkhoff, G., Keller, I., Ritter, V. and Marquardt, C. (2006) Repetitive optokinetic stimulation induces lasting recovery from visual neglect. *Restorative Neurology and Neuroscience*, *24*, 357–369.

Kerkhoff, G. and Rossetti, Y. (2006) Plasticity in spatial neglect: Recovery and rehabilitation. *Restorative Neurology and Neuroscience*, *24*, 201–206.

Kerns, R. D., Rosenberg, R., Jamison, R. N., Caudill, M. A. and Haythornthwaite, J. (1997) Readiness to adopt a self-management approach to chronic pain: The pain stages of change questionnaire (PSOCQ) *Pain*, *72*, 227–234.

Kerr, S. M. and Smith, L. N. (2001) Stroke: An exploration of the experience of informal caregiving. *Clinical Rehabilitation*, *15*, 428–436.

Kersten, P., Low, J. T. S., Ashburn, A., George, S. L. and McLellan, D. L. (2002) The unmet needs of young people who have had a stroke: Results of a national UK survey. *Disability and Rehabilitation*, *24*, 860–866.

Kertesz, A. (2006) *The Western Aphasia Battery Revised*. New York: Psychological Corporation.

Kertesz, A. and Ferro, J. M. (1984) Lesion size and location in ideomotor apraxia. *Brain*, 107, 921–933.

Kiernan, J. A. (2008) *Barr's The Human Nervous System: An Anatomical Viewpoint*, 9th ed. London: Lippincott Williams & Wilkins.

Kiernan, R. J., Mueller, J., Langston, J. W. and Vandyke, C. (1987) The Neurobehavioral cognitive status examination: A brief but differntiated approach to cognitive assessment. *Annals of Internal Medicine*, 107, 481–485.

Killen, J. D., Fortmann, S. P., Schatzberg, A. F., Arredondo, C., Greer Murphy, G., Hayward, C., *et al.* (2008) Extended cognitive behavior therapy for cigarette smoking cessation. *Addiction*, 103, 1381–1390.

Kim, E. J., Suh, M. K., Lee, B. H., Park, K. C., Ku, B. D., Chung, C. S., *et al.* (2009) Transcortical sensory aphasia following a left frontal lobe infarction probably due to anomalously represented language areas. *Journal of Clinical Neuroscience*, 16, 1482–1485.

Kim, H. J. (2000) Electronic memory aids for outpatient brain injury: Follow-up findings. *Brain Injury*, 14, 187–196.

Kim, H. J., Craik, F. I. M., Luo, L. and Ween, J. E. (2009) Impairments in prospective and retrospective memory following stroke. *Neurocase*, 15, 145–156.

Kim, J. S. and Choi-Kwon, S. (1999) Sensory sequelae of medullary infarction: Differences between lateral and medial medullary syndrome. *Stroke*, 30, 2697–2703.

Kim, J. S. and Choi-Kwon, S. (2000) Poststroke depression and emotional incontinence: Correlation with lesion location. *Neurology*, 54, 1805–1810.

Kim, J. S. (2003) Central post-stroke pain or paresthesia in lenticulo-capsular hemorrhages. *Neurology*, 61, 679–682.

Kim, J. S., Choi, S., Kwon, S. U. and Seo, Y. S. (2002) Inability to control anger or aggression after stroke. *Neurology*, 58, 1106–1108.

Kim, J. S., Choi-Kwon, S., Kwon, S. U., Lee, H. J., Park, K-A. and Seo, Y. S. (2005) Factors affecting the quality of life after ischemic stroke: Young versus old patients. *Journal of Clinical Neurology*, 1, 59–68.

Kim, M., Na, D. L., Kim, G. M., Adair, J. C., Lee, K. H. and Heilman, K. M. (1999) Ipsilesional neglect: behavioural and anatomical features. *Journal of Neurology, Neurosurgery and Psychiatry*, 67, 35–38.

Kim, S. J., Kim, D. H., Choi, N. K., Kim, H. C., Moon, Y. S. and Chung, C. S. (2003) Correlates of depression and anxiety in acute stroke patients. *Journal of the Korean Geriatrics Society*, 7, 230–242.

Kim, S. Y. H., Caine, E. D., Currier, G. W., Leibovici, A. and Ryan, J. M. (2001) Assessing the competence of persons with Alzheimer's disease in providing informed consent for participation in research. *American Journal of Psychiatry*, 158, 712–717.

King, R. B. and Semik, P. E. (2006) Stroke caregiving: Difficult times, resource use, and needs during the first 2 years. *Journal of Gerontological Nursing*, 32, 37–44.

Kinsbourne, M. (1993) Orientational bias model of unilateral neglect: eEvidence from attentional gradients within hemispace. In Ian H. Robertson and John C. Marshall (ed), *Unilateral Neglect: Clinical and Experimental Studies* (pp. 63–86). Hillsdale, NJ: Lawrence Erlbaum Associates.

Kinsella, G., Murtagh, D., Landry, A., Honfray, K., Hammond, M., O'Beirne, L., *et al.* (1996) Everyday memory following traumatic brain injury. *Brain Injury, 10,* 499–507.

Kiresuk, T. J. and Sherman, R. E. (1968) Goal attainment scaling – general method for evaluating comprehansive community mental health programs. *Community Mental Health Journal, 4,* 443–453.

Kirkevold, M. (2002) The unfolding illness trajectory of stroke. *Disability and Rehabilitation, 24,* 887–898.

Kitching, N., Salthouse, E. and Hopkins, C. (2007) A pilot study to evaluate the sensitivity and specificty of a neuropsychological screen for detecting cognitive impairment after stroke. *Clinical Psychology Forum,* 174(June), 5–8.

Kitwood, T. and Bredin, K. (1992) Towards a theory of dementia care: Personhood and well-being. *Ageing & Society, 12,* 269–287.

Kjellström, T., Norrving, B. and Shatchkute, A. (2006) *Helsingborg Declaration 2006 on European Stroke Strategies.* Copenhagen: WHO Europe.

Klavora, P., Heslegrave, R. J. and Young, M. (2000) Driving skills in elderly persons with stroke: Comparison of two new assessment options. *Archives of Physical Medicine and Rehabilitation, 81,* 701–705.

Klinedinst, N. J., Clark, P. C., Blanton, S. and Wolf, S. L. (2007) Congruence of depressive symptom appraisal between persons with stroke and their caregivers. *Rehabilitation Psychology, 52,* 215–225.

Knapp, P. and Hewison, J. (1999) Disagreement in patient and career assessment of functional abilities after stroke. *Stroke, 30,* 934–938.

Kneebone, I. (1999) Post-stroke depression and the non-mental health therapist. *British Journal of Therapy and Rehabilitation, 6,* 476–481.

Kneebone, I., Baker, J. and O'Malley, H. (2010) Screening for depression after stroke: Developing protocols for the occupational therapist. *British Journal of Occupational Therapy, 73* (2), 71–76.

Kneebone, I. and Dunmore, E. (2000) Psychological management of post-stroke depression. *British Journal of Clinical Psychology, 39,* 53–65.

Kneebone, I. and Hull, S. (2009) Cognitive behaviour therapy for post-traumatic stress symptoms in the context of hydrocephalus: A single case. *Neuropsychological Rehabilitation, 19,* 86–97.

Knight, C., Alderman, N. and Burgess, P. W. (2002) Development of a simplified version of the multiple errands test for use in hospital settings. *Neuropsychological Rehabilitation, 12,* 231–255.

Knollman-Porter, K. (2008) Acquired apraxia of speech: A review. *Topics in Stroke Rehabilitation, 15,* 484–493.

Koch, L., Egbert, N., Coeling, H. and Ayers, D. (2005) Returning to work after the onset of illness: Experiences of right hemisphere stroke survivors. *Rehabilitation Counseling Bulletin, 48,* 209–218.

Koelsch, S. (2009) A neuroscientific perspective on music therapy. In S. DallaBella, N. Kraus, K. Overy, C. Pantev, J. S. Snyder, M. Tervaniemi, B. Tillmann and G. Schlaug (eds), *Neurosciences and Music III: Disorders and Plasticity* (Vol. 1169, pp 374–384) Oxford: Blackwell Publishing.

Kohut, H. (1977) *The Restoration of the Self.* New York: International Universities Press.

Kontou, E. (2010) *Mood and Communication Problems after Stroke.* PhD diss., University of Nottingham, Nottingham, UK.

Kopelman, M. D., Wilson, B. A. and Baddeley, A. D. (1990) *The Autobiographical Memory Interview*. Bury St Edmunds: Thames Valley Test Company.

Korner-Bitensky, N., Menon-Nair, A., Thomas, A., Boutin, E. and Arafah, A. M. (2007) Practice style traits: Do they help explain practice behaviours of stroke rehabilitation professionals? *Journal of Rehabilitation Medicine, 39*, 685–692.

Korner-Bitensky, N. A., Mazer, B. L., Sofer, S., Gelina, I., Meyer, M. B., Morrison, C., et al. (2000) Visual testing for readiness to drive after stroke. *American Journal of Physical Medicine and Rehabilitation, 79*, 253–259.

Koski, L., Iacoboni, M. and Mazziotta, J. C. (2002) Deconstructing apraxia: Understanding disorders of intentional movement after stroke. *Current Opinion in Neurology, 15*, 71–77.

Kotila, M., Numminen, H., Waltimo, O. and Kaste, M. (1998) Depression after stroke: Results of the FINNSTROKE study. *Stroke, 29*, 368–372.

Kotila, M., Numminen, H., Waltimo, O. and Kaste, M. (1999) Post-stroke depression and functional recovery in a population-based stroke register: The Finnstroke study. *European Journal of Neurology, 6*, 309–312.

Kozub, E. (2010) Community stroke prevention programs: An overview. *Journal of Neuroscience Nursing, 42*, 143–149.

Krabbe-Hartkamp, M. J., van der Grond, J., de Leeuw, F. E., de Groot, J. C., Algra, A., Hillen, B., et al. (1998) Circle of Willis: Morphologic variation on three-dimensional time-of-flight MR angiograms. *Radiology, 207*, 103–111.

Kreisler, A., Godefroy, O., Delmaire, C., Debachy, B., Leclercq, M., Pruvo, J-P., et al. (2000) The anatomy of aphasia revisited. *Neurology, 54* (5), 1117–1123.

Kressig, R. W., Wolf, S. L., Sattin, R. W., O'Grady, M., Greenspan, A., Curns, A., et al. (2001) Associations of demographic, functional, and behavioral characteristics with activity-related fear of falling among older adults transitioning to frailty. *Journal of the American Geriatrics Society, 49*, 1456–1462.

Kriegsman, D. M. W., VanEijk, J. T. M., Penninx, B. W. J. H., Deeg, D. J. H. and Boeke, A. J. P. (1997) Does family support buffer the impact of specific chronic diseases on mobility in community-dwelling elderly? *Disability and Rehabilitation, 19*, 71–83.

Krupp, L. B., Larocca, N. G., Muirnash, J. and Steinberg, A. D. (1989) The Fatigue Severity Scale: Application to patients with multiple sclerosis and systemic lupus-erythematosus. *Archives of Neurology, 46*, 1121–1123.

Krynski, M. D., Tymchuk, A. J. and Ouslander, J. G. (1994) How informed can consent be: New light on comprehension among elderly people making decisions about enteral tube feeding. *Gerontologist, 34*, 36–43.

Kucharska-Pietura, K., Phillips, M. L., Gernand, W. and David, A. S. (2003) Perception of emotions from faces and voices following unilateral brain damage. *Neuropsychologia, 41*, 1082–1090.

Kulas, J. F. and Axelrod, B. N. (2002) Comparison of seven-subtest and Satz-Mogel short forms of the WAIS-III. *Journal of Clinical Psychology, 58*, 773–782.

Kumar, S., Selim, M. and Caplan, L. (2010) Medical complications after stroke. *The Lancet Neurology, 9*, 105–118.

Kunzmann, U., Little, T. and Smith, J. (2002) Perceiving control: A double-edged sword in old age. *Journals of Gerontology Series B: Psychological Sciences and Social Sciences, 57*, P484–P491.

Kuroda, Y. and Kuroda, R. (2005) The relationship between verbal communication and observed psychological status in aphasia: Preliminary findings. *Aphasiology, 19*, 849–859.

Kurth, T., Gaziano, J., Berger, K., Kase, C., Rexrode, K., Cook, N., *et al.* (2002) Body mass index and the risk of stroke in men. *Archives of Internal Medicine, 162,* 2557–2562.

Kwa, V. I. H., Limburg, M. and deHaan, R. J. (1996) The role of cognitive impairment in the quality of life after ischaemic stroke. *Journal of Neurology, 243,* 599–604.

Kwakkel, G., Kollen, B. and Lindeman, E. (2004) Understanding the pattern of functional recovery after stroke: Facts and theories. *Restorative Neurology and Neuroscience, 22,* 281–299.

Kwakkel, G., Wagenaar, R. C., Kollen, B. J. and Lankhorst, G. J. (1996) Predicting disability in stroke: A critical review of the literature. *Age and Ageing, 25,* 479–489.

Labi, M. L., Phillips, T. F. and Greshman, G. E. (1980) Psychosocial disability in physically restored long-term stroke survivors. *Archives of Physical Medicine and Rehabilitation, 61,* 561–565.

LaBresh, K. and Tyler, P. (2003) A collaborative model for hospital-based cardiovascular secondary prevention. *Quality Management in Healthcare, 12,* 20–27.

Lach, H. W. (2006) Self-efficacy theory and fear of falling: In search of a complete theory. *Journal of the American Geriatrics Society, 54,* 381–382.

Lachs, M., Feinstein, A., Cooney Jr, L., Drickamer, M., Marottoli, R., Pannill, F., *et al.* (1990) A simple procedure for general screening for functional disability in elderly patients. *Annals of Internal Medicine, 112,* 699–706.

Laeng, B. (2006) Constructional apraxia after left or right unilateral stroke. *Neuropsychologia, 44,* 1595–1606.

Lafosse, J. M., Reed, B. R., Mungas, D., Sterling, S. B., Wahbeh, H. and Jagust, W. J. (1997) Fluency and memory differences between ischemic vascular dementia and Alzheimer's disease. *Neuropsychology, 11,* 514–522.

Laidlaw, K. (2008) Post-stroke depression and CBT with older people, In Gallagher-Thompson T. D., Steffan, A. & Thompson, L.W. (eds), *Handbook of Behavioural and Cognitive Psychotherapy with Older Adults* (pp. 233–246). New York: Springer.

Lamb, S. E., Becker, C., Jørstad-Stein, E. C. and Hauer, K. (2005) Development of a common outcome data set for fall injury prevention trials: The ProFANE consensus. *Journal of American Geriatrics Society, 53,* 1618–1622.

Lammie, A. (2000) Pathology of small vessel stroke. *British Medical Bulletin, 56,* 296–306.

Lammie, G. A. (2002) Hypertensive cerebral small vessel disease and stroke. *Brain Pathology, 12,* 358–370.

Lander, Z. (2009) *A Qualitative Analysis of the Phenomena Stroke Survivors Associate with Post-Stroke Anxiety.* DClinPsy, University of Leicester, Leicester.

Landreville, P., Desrosiers, J., Vincent, C., Verreault, R. and Boudreault, V. (2009) The role of activity restriction in poststroke depressive symptoms. *Rehabilitation Psychology, 54,* 315–322.

Langhorne, P., Stott, D. J., Robertson, L., MacDonald, J., Jones, L., McAlpine, C., *et al.* (2000) Medical complications after stroke: A multicenter study. *Stroke, 31,* 1223–1229.

Langhorne, P., Taylor, G., Murray, G., Dennis, M., Anderson, C., Bautz-Holter, E., *et al.* (2005) Early supported discharge services for stroke patients: A meta-analysis of individual patients' data. *Lancet, 365* (9458), 501–506.

Langhorne, P. and Widen-Holmqvist, L. (2007) Early supported discharge trialists. *Journal of Rehabilitation Medicine, 39,* 269–269.

Lannin, N. A. and Herbert, R. D. (2003) Is hand splinting effective for adults following stroke? A systematic review and methodological critique of published research. *Clinical Rehabilitation, 17*, 807–816.

Lantz, E. R. and Meyers, P. M. (2008) Neuropsychological effects of brain arteriovenous malformations. *Neuropsychoogy Review, 18*, 167–177.

Larner, A. J. (2007) Addenbrooke's Cognitive Examination (ACE) for the diagnosis and differential diagnosis of dementia. *Clinical Neurology and Neurosurgery, 109*, 491–494.

Larrabee, G. (ed) (2007) *Assessment of Malingered Neuropsychological Deficits.* Oxford: Oxford University Press.

Larrabee, J., Ostrow, C., Withrow, M., Janney, M., Jnr, G. H. and Burant, C. (2004) Predictors of patient satisfaction with inpatient hospital nursing care. *Research in Nursing & Health, 27*, 254–268.

Larsen, T., Olsen, T. S. and Sorensen, J. (2006) Early home-supported discharge of stroke patients: A health technology assessment. *International Journal of Technology Assessment in Health Care, 22*, 313–320.

Larson, E. B., Kirschner, K., Bode, R., Heinemann, A. and Goodman, R. (2005) Construct and predictive validity of the repeatable battery for the assessment of neuropsychological status in the evaluation of stroke patients. *Journal of Clinical and Experimental Neuropsychology, 27*, 16–32.

Larson, S., Owens, P., Ford, D. and Eaton, W. (2001) Depressive disorder, dysthymia, and risk of stroke: Thirteen-year follow-up from the Baltimore epidemiologic catchment area study. *Stroke, 32*, 1979–1983.

Laska, A. C., Martensson, B., Kahan, T., von Arbin, M. and Murray, V. (2007) Recognition of depression in aphasic stroke patients. *Cerebrovascular Diseases, 24*, 74–79.

Laukka, E. J., MacDonald, S. W. S. and Bäckman, L. (2008) Terminal-decline effects for select cognitive tasks after controlling for preclinical dementia. *American Journal of Geriatric Psychiatry, 16*, 355–365.

Laumann, E. O., Paik, A. and Rosen, R. C. (1999) Sexual dysfunction in the United States: Prevalence and predictors. *Journal of the American Medical Association, 281*, 537–544.

Lawler, J., Dowswell, G., Hearn, J., Forster, A. and Young, J. (1999) Recovering from stroke: A qualitative investigation of the role of goal setting in late stroke recovery. *Journal of Advanced Nursing, 30*, 401–409.

Lawrence, M. (2010) Young adults' experience of stroke: A qualitative review of the literature [Review]. *British Journal of Nursing, 19*, 241–248.

Lazarus, R. S. (1993) Coping theory and research: past, present, and future. *Psychosomatic Medicine, 55*, 234–247.

Lazarus, R. S. and Folkman, S. (1984) *Stress, Appraisal and Coping.* New York: Springer.

Lee, A. C. K., Tang, S. W., Yu, G. K. K. and Cheung, R. T. F. (2008) The smiley as a simple screening tool for depression after stroke: A preliminary study. *International Journal of Nursing Studies, 45*, 1081–1089.

Lee, C., Folsom, A. and Blair, S. (2003) Physical activity and stroke risk: A meta-analysis. *Stroke, 34*, 2475.

Lee, J. H., Soeken, K. and Picot, S. J. (2007) A meta-analysis of interventions for informal stroke caregivers. *Western Journal of Nursing Research, 29*, 344–356.

Lee, M., Hong, K. S., Chang, S. C. and Saver, J. L. (2010) Efficacy of homocysteine-lowering therapy with folic acid in stroke prevention: A meta-analysis. *Stroke, 41*, 1205–1212.

Lee, N., Tracy, J., Bohannon, R. W. and Ahlquist, M. (2003) Driving resumption and its predictors after stroke. *Connecticut Medicine, 67,* 387–391.

Lee, P. and Forey, B. (2006) Environmental tobacco smoke exposure and risk of stroke in nonsmokers: A review with meta-analysis. *Journal of Stroke and Cerebrovascular Diseases, 15,* 190–201.

Leeds L., Meera, R. J. and Hobson, J. F. (2004) The utility of the Stroke Aphasia Depression Questionnaire in a stroke rehabilitiation unit. *Clinical Rehabilitation, 18,* 228–231.

Leeds L., Meara, R. J., Woods, R. and Hobson, J. P. (2001) A comparison of the new executive functioning domains of the CAMCOG-R with existing tests of executive function in elderly stroke survivors. *Age and Ageing, 30,* 251–254.

Legg, L., Drummond, A., Leonardi-Bee, J., Gladman, J. R. F., Corr, S., Donkervoort, M., *et al.* (2007) Occupational therapy for patients with problems in personal activities of daily living after stroke: Systematic review of randomised trials. *British Medical Journal, 335,* 922–925.

Legg, L. A., Drummond, A. E. and Langhorne, P. (2006) Occupational therapy for patients with problems in activities of daily living after stroke. *Cochrane Database of Systematic Reviews* (4), CD003585.

Legh-Smith, J., Wade, D. T. and Hewer, R. L. (1986) Driving after a stroke. *Journal of Royal Society of Medicine, 79,* 200–203.

Legh-Smith, J. A., Denis, R., Enderby, P. M., Wade, D. T. and Langton-Hewer, R. (1987) Selection of aphasic stroke patients for intensive speech therapy. *Journal of Neurology, Neurosurgery and Psychiatry, 50,* 1488–1492.

Legters, K. (2002) Fear of falling. *Physical Therapy, 82,* 264–272.

Leonard, C., Rochon, E. and Laird, L. (2008) Treating naming impairments in aphasia: Findings from a phonological components analysis treatment. *Aphasiology, 22,* 923–947.

Leppavuori, A., Pohjasvaara, T., Vataja, R., Kaste, M. and Erkinjuntti, T. (2002) Insomnia in ischemic stroke patients. *Cerebrovascular Diseases, 14,* 90–97.

Leppavuori, A., Pohjasvaara, T., Vataja, R., Kaste, M. and Erkinjuntti, T. (2003) Generalized anxiety disorders three to four months after ischemic stroke. *Cerebrovascular Diseases, 16,* 257–264.

Leskin, L. P., White, P. M. and Abdullaev, Y. (2007) Attentional networks reveal executive control deficits in posttraumatic stress disorder: An fMRI study *Psychophysiology, 44,* S46–S47.

Lesniak, M., Bak, T., Czepiel, W., Seniow, J. and Czlonkowska, A. (2008) Frequency and prognostic value of cognitive disorders in stroke patients. *Dementia and Geriatric Cognitive Disorders, 26,* 356–363.

Leung, K. L. and Man, D. W. K. (2005) Prediction of vocational outcome of people with brain injury after rehabilitation: A discriminant analysis *Work: A Journal of Prevention, Assessment and Rehabilitation 25,* 333–340.

Levack, W. M. M., Taylor, K., Siegert, R. J., Dean, S. G., McPherson, K. M. and Weatherall, M. (2006) Is goal planning in rehabilitation effective? A systematic review. *Clinical Rehabilitation, 20,* 739–755.

Leventhal, H. and Cameron, L. (1987) Behavioral theories and the problem of compliance. *Patient Education and Counseling, 10,* 117–138.

Leventhal, H., Diefenbach, M. and Leventhal, E. A. (1992) Illness cognition: Using common sense to understand treatment adherence and affect cognition interactions. *Cognitive Therapy and Research 16,* 143–163.

Levine, B., Robertson, I. H., Clare, L., Carter, G., Hong, J., Wilson, B. A., *et al.* (2000) Rehabilitation of executive functioning: An experimental-clinical validation of Goal Management Training. *Journal of the International Neuropsychological Society, 6,* 299–312.

Levy, D., Blizzard, R. A., Halligan, P. W. and Stone, S. P. (1995) Fluctuations in visual neglect after stroke. *European Neurology, 35,* 341–343.

Lewinsohn, P. M. and Graf, M. (1973) Pleasant activities and depression. *Journal of Consulting and Clinical Psychology, 41,* 261–268.

Lewis, S. C., Dennis, M. S., O'Rourke, S. J. and Sharpe, M. (2001) Negative attitudes among short-term stroke survivors predict worse long-term survival. *Stroke, 32,* 1640–1645.

Lezak, M. D., Howieson, D. B., Loring, D. W., Hannay, H. J. and Fischer, J. S. (2004) *Neuropsychological Assessment.* Oxford: Oxford University Press.

Lichtenberger, E. O. and Kaufman, A. S. (2009) *Essentials of WAIS-IV Assessment.* Hoboken, NJ: John Wiley & Sons Inc.

Lightbody, C. E. (2007) *Detecting Depression following a Stroke.* PhD diss., University of Central Lancashire, Preston, UK.

Lightbody, C. E., Baldwin, R., Connolly, M., Gibbon, B., Jawaid, N., Leathley, M., *et al.* (2007) Can nurses help identify patients with depression following stroke? A pilot study using two methods of detection. *Journal of Advanced Nursing, 57,* 505–512.

Lilley, S., Lincoln, N. and Francis, V. (2003) A qualitative study of stroke patients' and carers' perceptions of the stroke family support organizer service. *Clinical Rehabilitation, 17,* 540–547.

Lim, C. and Alexander, M. P. (2009) Stroke and episodic memory disorders. *Neuropsychologia, 47,* 3045–3058.

Lincoln, N. (1982) The speech questionnaire: An assessment of functional language ability. *Disability & Rehabilitation, 4,* 114–117.

Lincoln, N. and Clarke, D. (1987) The performance of normal elderly people on the Rivermead Perceptual Assessment Battery. *British Journal of Occupational Therapy, 50,* 156–157.

Lincoln, N., Sutcliffe, L. and Unsworth, G. (2000) Validation of the Stroke Aphasic Depression Questionnaire (SADQ) for use with patients in hospital. *Clinical Neuropsychological Assessment, 1,* 88–96.

Lincoln, N. B. (1982) The speech questionnaire: An assessment of functional language ability. *International Rehabilitation Medicine, 4,* 114–117.

Lincoln, N. B. and Bowen, A. (2006) The need for randomised treatment studies in neglect research. *Restorative Neurology and Neuroscience, 24,* 401–408.

Lincoln, N. B., Drummond, A. E. R., Edmans, J. A., Yeo, D. and Willis, D. (1998) The Rey Figure Copy as a screeening instrument of perceptual deficits after stroke. *British Journal of Occupational Therapy, 61,* 33–35.

Lincoln, N. B. and Fanthome, Y. (1994) Reliability of the Stroke Drivers Screening Assessment. *Clinical Rehabilitation, 8,* 157–160.

Lincoln, N. B. and Flannaghan, T. (2003) Cognitive behavioural psychotherapy for depression following stroke. *Stroke, 34,* 111–115.

Lincoln, N. B., Flannaghan, T., Sutcliffe, L. and Rother, L. (1997) Evaluation of cognitive behavioural treatment of depression after stroke: A pilot study. *Clinical Rehabilitation, 11,* 114–122.

Lincoln, N. B., Majid, M. J. and Weyman, N. (2000) Cognitive rehabilitation for attention deficits following stroke. *Cochrane Database of Systematic Reviews* (3), CD002842.

Lincoln, N. B., McGuirk, E., Mulley, G. P., Lendrem, W., Jones, A. C. and Mitchell, J. R. (1984) Effectiveness of speech therapy for aphasic stroke patients: a randomised controlled trial. *Lancet, 1,* 1197–1200.

Lincoln, N. B., Nicholl, C. R., Flannaghan, T., Leonard, M. and Van der Gucht, E. (2003) The validity of questionnaire measures for assessing depression after stroke. *Clinical Rehabilitation, 17,* 840–846.

Lincoln, N. B., Radford, K.A. and Nouri, F.M. (2010) *Stroke Drivers' Screening Assessment: Revised Manual.* University of Nottingham, Nottingham. http://www.nottingham.ac.uk/iwho/research/publishedassessments.aspx

Lincoln, N. B. and Tinson, D. J. (1989) The relation between subjective and objective memory impairment after stroke. *British Journal of Clinical Psychology, 28,* 61–65.

Lincoln, N. B., Whiting, S. E., Cockburn, J. and Bhavnani, G. (1985) An evaluation of perceptual retraining. *International Rehabilitation Medicine, 7,* 99–110.

Lincoln, N. B., Willis, D., Philips, S. A., Juby, L. C. and Berman, P. (1996) Comparison of rehabilitation practice on hospital wards for stroke patients. *Stroke, 27,* 18–23.

Lindgren, I., Jonsson, A. C., Norrving, B. and Lindgren, A. (2007) Shoulder pain after stroke: A prospective population-based study. *Stroke, 38,* 343–348.

Lindsay, P., Bayley, M., Hellings, C., Hill, M., Woodbury, E. and Phillips, S. (2008) Stroke rehabilitation and community reintegration: Components of inpatient stroke rehabilitation. *Canadian Medical Association Journal, 179,* E56–E58.

Lindstrom, B., Roding, J. and Sundelin, G. (2009) Positive attitiudes and preserved high level motor performance are important factors for return to work in younger persons after stroke: A national survey. *Journal of Rehabilitation Medicine, 41,* 714–718.

Lissauer, H. (1890) Ein Fall von Seelenblindheit nebst einem Beitrag zur Theorie derselben. *Archiv fur Psychiatrie, 21,* 222–270.

Liu-Ambrose, T., Pang, M. Y. C. and Eng, J. J. (2007) Executive function is independently associated with performances of balance and mobility in community-dwelling older adults after mild stroke: Implications for falls prevention. *Cerebrovascular Diseases, 23,* 203–210.

Lloyd-Jones, D., Adams, R., Carnethon, M., De Simone, G., Ferguson, T., Flegal, K., *et al.* (2009) Heart disease and stroke statistics – 2009 update: A report from the American Heart Association Statistics Committee and Stroke Statistics Subcommittee. *Circulation, 119,* e21.

Locka, S., Jordan, L., Bryanc, K. and Maxima, J. (2005) Work after stroke: Focusing on barriers and enablers. *Disability and Society, 20,* 33–47.

Locke, E. A. and Latham, G. P. (2002) Building a practically useful theory of goal setting and task motivation: A 35-year odyssey. *American Psychologist, 57,* 705–717.

Loeb, P. A. (1996) *ILS: Independent Living Scales Manual.* New York: Psychological Corporation.

Logan, P. A., Ahern, J., Gladman, J. R. F. and Lincoln, N. B. (1997) A randomized controlled trial of enhanced Social Service occupational therapy for stroke patients. *Clinical Rehabilitation, 11,* 107–113.

Logan, P. A., Dyas, J. and Gladman, J. R. F. (2004) Using an interview study of transport use by people who have had a stroke to inform rehabilitation. *Clinical Rehabilitation, 18,* 703–708.

Lomas, J., Pickard, L., Bester, S., Elbard, H., Finlayson, A. and Zoghaib, C. (1989) The communicative effectiveness index: Development and psychometric evaluation of a functional communication measure for adult aphasia. *Journal of Speech and Hearing Disorders, 54,* 113–124.

Long, A., Hesketh, A. and Bowen, A. (2009) Communication outcome after stroke: A new measure of the carer's perspective. *Clinical Rehabilitation, 23,* 383–383.

Long, A. F., Hesketh, A., Paszek, G., Booth, M. and Bowen, A. (2008) Development of a reliable self-report outcome measure for pragmatic trials of communication therapy following stroke: The Communication Outcome after Stroke (COAST) scale. *Clinical Rehabilitation, 22,* 1083–1094.

Loong, T. W. (2003) Understanding sensitivity and specificity with the right side of the brain. *British Medical Journal, 327* (7417), 716–719.

Lopez, M. A. and Mermelstein, R. J. (1995) A cognitive behavioural program to improve geriatric rehabilitation outcome. *Gerontologist, 35,* 696–700.

Lorig, K. R., Ritter, P., Stewart, A. L., Sobel, D. S., Brown, B. W., Bandura, A., *et al.* (2001) Chronic disease self-management program: 2-year health status and health care utilization outcomes. *Medical Care, 39,* 1217–1223.

Low, J. T. S., Kersen, P., Ashburn, A., George, S. and McLellan, D. L. (2003) A study to evaluate the met and unmet needs of members belonging to Young Stroke groups affiliated with the Stroke Association. *Disability and Rehabilitation, 25,* 1052–1056.

Low, J. T. S., Payne, S. and Roderick, P. (1999) The impact of stroke on informal carers: A literature review. *Social Science & Medicine, 49,* 711–725.

Luaute, J., Halligan, P., Rode, G., Rossetti, Y. and Boisson, D. (2006) Visuo-spatial neglect: A systematic review of current interventions and their effectiveness. *Neuroscience and Biobehavioral Reviews, 30,* 961–982.

Lundahl, B. W., Kunz, C., Brownell, C., Tollefson, D. and Burke, B. L. (2010) A meta-analysis of motivational interviewing twenty-five years of empirical studies. *Research on Social Work Practice, 20,* 137–160.

Lundberg, C., Caneman, G., Samuelsson, S. M., Hakamies-Blomqvist, L. and Almkvist, O. (2003) The assessment of fitness to drive after a stroke: The Nordic Stroke Driver Screening Assessment. *Scandinavian Journal of Psychology, 44,* 23–30.

Lundqvist, A., Gerdle, B. and Ronnberg, J. (2000) Neuropsychological aspects of driving after stroke: In the simulator and on the road. *Applied Cognitive Psychology, 14,* 135–150.

Luria, A. R. (1962) *Higher Cortical Functions in Man.* New York: Basic Books.

Lustman, P. J., Griffith, L. S., Freedland, K. E., Kissel, S. S. and Clouse, R. E. (1998) Cognitive behavior therapy for depression in type 2 diabetes mellitus: A randomized, controlled trial. *Annals of Internal Medicine, 129,* 613–621.

Luther, A., Lincoln, N. B. and Grant, F. (1998) Reliability of stroke patients' reports on rehabilitation services received. *Clinical Rehabilitation, 12,* 238–244.

Lynch, J., Mead, G., Greig, C., Young, A., Lewis, S. and Sharpe, M. (2007) Fatigue after stroke: The development and evaluation of a case definition. *Journal of Psychosomatic Research, 63,* 539–544.

Lynch, J. K., Hirtz, D. G., DeVeber, G. and Nelson, K. B. (2002) Report of the National Institute of Neurological Disorders and Stroke workshop on perinatal and childhood stroke. *Pediatrics, 109,* 116–123.

Lyonette, C. and Yardley, L. (2003) The influence on carer wellbeing of motivations to care for older people and the relationship with the care recipient. *Ageing and Society, 23,* 487–506.

Mackenzie, A. and Greenwood, N. (2009) Positive aspects of caregiving in stroke survivors: A systematic review of adult carers: Poster presentation. Paper presented at the 4th UK Stroke Forum Conference, Glasgow.

Mackenzie, A., Perry, L., Lockhart, E., Cottee, M., Cloud, G. and Mann, H. (2007) Family carers of stroke survivors: Needs, knowledge, satisfaction and competence in caring. *Disability and Rehabilitation, 29*, 111–121.

Mackenzie, C. and Lowit, A. (2007) Behavioural intervention effects in dysarthria following stroke: Communication effectiveness, intelligibility and dysarthria impact. *International Journal of Language and Communication Disorders, 42*, 131–153.

Mackenzie, C. and Paton, G. (2003) Resumption of driving with aphasia following stroke. *Aphasiology, 17*, 107–122.

Mackenzie, J. A., Lincoln, N. B. and Newby, G. J. (2008) Capacity to make a decision about discharge destination after stroke: A pilot study. *Clinical Rehabilitation, 22*, 1116–1126.

Mackintosh, S. F., Hill, K. D., Dodd, K. J., Goldie, P. A. and Culham, E. G. (2006) Balance score and a history of falls in hospital predict recurrent falls in the 6 months following stroke rehabilitation. *Archives of Physical Medicine and Rehabilitation, 87*, 1583–1589.

Maclean, N., Pound, P., Wolfe, C. and Rudd, A. (2000) Qualitative analysis of stroke patients' motivation for rehabilitation. *British Medical Journal, 321* (7268), 1051–1054.

Maddicks, R., Marzillier, S. L. and Parker, G. (2003) Rehabilitation of unilateral neglect in the acute recovery stage: The efficacy of limb activation therapy. *Neuropsychological Rehabilitation, 13*, 391–408.

Magill, M. and Ray, L. A. (2009) Cognitive-behavioral treatment with adult alcohol and illicit drug users: A meta-analysis of randomized controlled trials. *Journal of Studies on Alcohol and Drugs, 70*, 516–527.

Mahoney, F. I. and Barthel, D. (1965) Functional evaluation: The Barthel Index. *Maryland State Medical Journal, 14*, 56–65.

Mahoney, J., Drinka, T. J. K., Abler, R., Gunterhunt, G., Matthews, C., Gravenstein, S., *et al.* (1994) Screening for depression: Single question versus GDS. *Journal of the American Geriatrics Society, 42*, 1006–1008.

Maki, B. E., Holliday, P. J. and Topper, A. K. (1991) Fear of falling and postural performance in the elderly. *Journal of Gerontology, 46*, M123–M131.

Malouin, F., Belleville, S., Richards, C. L., Desrosiers, J. and Doyon, J. (2004) Working memory and mental practice outcomes after stroke. *Archives of Physical Medicine and Rehabilitation, 85*, 177–183.

Manes, F., Ruiz Villamil, A., Ameriso, S., Roca, M. and Torralva, T. (2009) 'Real life' executive deficits in patients with focal vascular lesions affecting the cerebellum. *Journal of the Neurological Sciences, 283*, 95–98.

Manly, T. (2002) Cognitive rehabilitation for unilateral neglect: Review. *Neuropsychological Rehabilitation, 12*, 289–310.

Manly, T., Davison, B., Gaynord, B., Greenfield, E., Parr, A., Ridgeway, V., *et al.* (2004) An electronic knot in the handkerchief: 'Content free cueing' and the maintenance of attentive control. *Neuropsychological Rehabilitation, 14*, 89–116.

Manly, T., Dove, A., Blows, S., George, M., Noonan, M. P., Teasdale, T. W., *et al.* (2009) Assessment of unilateral spatial neglect: Scoring star cancellation performance from video recordings-method, reliability, benefits, and normative data. *Neuropsychology, 23*, 519–528.

Manly, T., Hawkins, K., Evans, J., Woldt, K. and Robertson, I. H. (2002) Rehabilitation of executive function: Facilitation of effective goal management on complex tasks using periodic auditory alerts. *Neuropsychologia, 40*, 271–281.

Manthorpe, J., Rapaport, J. and Stanley, N. (2009) Expertise and experience: People with experiences of using services and carers' views of the Mental Capacity Act 2005. *British Journal of Social Work, 39*, 884–900.

Marcel, A. J., Tegner, R. and Nimmo-Smith, I. (2004) Anosognosia for plegia: Specificity, extension, partiality and disunity of bodily unawareness. *Cortex, 40*, 19–40.

Marchetti, C., Carey, D. and Della Sala, S. (2005) Crossed right hemisphere syndrome following left thalamic stroke. *Journal of Neurology, 252*, 403–411.

Marin, R. S. (1990) Differential diagnosis and classification of apathy. *American Journal of Psychiatry, 147*, 22–30.

Markson, L. J., Kern, D. C., Annas, G. J. and Glantz, L. H. (1994) Physician assessment of patient competence. *Journal of the American Geriatrics Society, 42*, 1074–1080.

Markus, H. (2007) Improving the outcome of stroke. *British Medical Journal, 335*, 359–360.

Marottolli, R. A., Mendes de Leon, C. F., Glass, T. A., Williams, C. S., Cooney, L. M. J. and Berkman, L. F. (2000) Consequences of driving cessation: Decreased out-of-home activity levels. *Journal of Gerontology B Psychology Sciences Social Science, 55*, S334–S340.

Marsden, J., Gibson, L. M., Lightbody, C. E., Sharma, A. K., Siddigi, M. and Watkins, C. (2008) Can early onset bone loss be effectively managed in post stroke patients? An integrative review. *Age and Ageing, 37*, 142–150.

Marsh, N. V. and Kersel, D. A. (1993) Screening tests for visual neglect following stroke. *Neuropsychological Rehabilitation, 3*, 245–257.

Marshall, S. C., Molnar, F., Man-Son-Hing, M., Blair, R., Brosseau, L., Finestone, H. M., *et al.* (2007) Predictors of driving ability following stroke: A systematic review. *Topics in Stroke Rehabilitation, 14*, 98–114.

Marson, D. C., Chatterjee, A., Ingram, K. K. and Harrell, L. E. (1996) Toward a neurologic model of competency: Cognitive predictors of capacity to consent in Alzheimer's disease using three different legal standards. *Neurology, 46*, 666–672.

Marson, D. C., Cody, H. A., Ingram, K. K. and Harrell, L. E. (1995a) Neuropsychologic predictors of competence in Alzheimer's disease: Using a rational reasons legal standard. *Archives of Neurology, 52*, 955–959.

Marson, D. C., Earnst, K. S., Jamil, F., Bartolucci, A. and Harrell, L. E. (2000) Consistency of physicians' legal standard and personal judgments of competency in patients with Alzheimer's disease. *Journal of the American Geriatrics Society, 48*, 911–918.

Marson, D. C., Ingram, K. K., Cody, H. A. and Harrell, L. E. (1995b) Assesing the competence of patients with Alzheimer's disease under different legal standards: A prototype instrument. *Archives of Neurology, 52*, 949–954.

Marson, D. C., McInturff, B., Hawkins, L., Bartolucci, A. and Harrell, L. E. (1997) Consistency of physician judgments of capacity to consent in mild Alzheimer's disease. *Journal of the American Geriatrics Society, 45*, 453–457.

Martin, I. and McDonald, S. (2006) That can't be right! What causes pragmatic language impairment following right hemisphere damage? *Brain Impairment, 7*, 202–211.

Martino, R., Beaton, D. and Diamant, N. (2010) Perceptions of psychological issues related to dysphagia differ in acute and chronic patients. *Dysphagia, 25*, 26–34.

Martins, R. and McNeil, D. (2009) Review of motivational interviewing in promoting health behaviors. *Clinical Psychology Review, 29*, 283–293.

Marx, J. J. and Thömke, F. (2009) Classical crossed brain stem syndromes: Myth or reality? *Journal of Neurology, 256,* 898–903.

Mateer, C. A. and Sira, C. S. (2008) Practical rehabilitation strategies in the context of clinical neuropsychology feedback. In J. E. M. J., H., Ricker (ed), *Textbook of Clinical Neuropsychology,* (pp. 996–1007)., New York: Taylor & Francis.

Mathiowetz, V., Weber, K., Kashman, N. and Volland, G. (1985) Adult norms for the Nine Hole Peg Test of Finger Dexterity. *Occupational Therapy Journal of Research, 5,* 24–38.

Mathuranath, P., Nestor, P., Berrios, G., Rakowicz, W. and Hodges, J. (2000) A brief cognitive test battery to differentiate Alzheimer's disease and frontotemporal dementia. *Neurology, 55,* 1613–1620.

May, C. P. and Hasher, L. (1998) Synchrony effects in inhibitory control over thought and action. *Journal of Experimental Psychology: Human Perception and Performance, 24,* 363–379.

May, M., McCarron, P., Stansfeld, S., Ben-Shlomo, Y., Gallacher, J., Yarnell, J., *et al.* (2002) Does psychological distress predict the risk of ischemic stroke and transient ischemic attack? The Caerphilly study. *Stroke, 33,* 7–12.

Mayer, S. A. and Rincon, F. (2005) Treatment of intracerebral haemorrhage. *Lancet Neurology, 4,* 662–672.

Mayo, N. E., Fellows, L. K., Scott, S. C., Cameron, J. and Wood-Dauphinee, S. (2009) A longitudinal view of apathy and its impact after stroke. *Stroke, 40,* 3299–3307.

Mazer, B. L., Korner-Bitensky, N. A. and Sofer, S. (1998) Predicting ability to drive after stroke. *Archives of Physical Medicine and Rehabilitation, 79,* 743–750.

Mazer, B. L., Sofer, S., Korner-Bitensky, N., Gelinas, I., Hanley, J. and Wood-Dauphinee, S. (2003) Effectiveness of a visual attention retraining program on the driving performance of clients with stroke. *Archives of Physical Medicine and Rehabilitation, 84,* 541–550.

McAlister, F., Man-Son-Hing, M., Straus, S., Ghali, W., Anderson, D., Majumdar, S., *et al.* (2005) Impact of a patient decision aid on care among patients with nonvalvular atrial fibrillation: A cluster randomized trial.2 *Canadian Medical Association Journal, 173,* 496–501.

McCaffery, M. (1968) *Nursing Practice Theories Related to Cognition, Bodily Pain, and Man–Environment Interactions.* Los Angeles: University of Los Angeles Students Store.

McCance, T. V., McKenna, H. P. and Boore, J. R. P. (1999) Caring: Theoretical perspectives of relevance to nursing. *Journal of Advanced Nursing, 30,* 1388–1395.

McCann, A. (2006) *Stroke Survivor: A Personal Guide to Recovery.* London: Jessicca Kingsley.

McCarron, M. O., Loftus, A. M. and McCarron, P. (2008) Driving after a transient ischaemic attack or minor stroke. *Emergency Medicine Journal, 25,* 358–359.

McClenahan, R. and Weinman, J. (1998) Determinants of carer distress in non-acute stroke. *International Journal of Language & Communication Disorders, 33*(Suppl.) 138–143.

McCracken, L. M. (2005) *Contextual Cognitive-Behavioral Therapy for Chronic Pain.* Seattle, WA: International Association for the Study of Pain.

McCrum, R. (1998) *My Year Off: Rediscovering Life after Stroke.* London: Picador.

McCullagh, E., Brigstocke, G., Donaldson, N. and Kalra, L. (2005) Determinants of care giving burden and quality of life in caregivers of stroke patients. *Stroke, 36,* 2181–2186.

McDowd, J. M., Filion, D. L., Pohl, P. S., Richards, L. G. and Stiers, W. (2003) Attentional abilities and functional outcomes following stroke. *Journals of Gerontology Series B: Psychological Sciences and Social Sciences, 58*, P45–P53.

McGeough, E., Pollock, A., Smith, L. N., Dennis, M., Sharpe, M., Lewis, S., *et al.* (2009) Interventions for post-stroke fatigue. *Cochrane Database of Systematic Reviews* (3), CD007030.

McGwin, G., Sims, R. V., Pulley, L. and Roseman, J. M. (2000) Relations among chronic medical conditions, medications, and automobile crashes in the elderly: A population-based case-control study. *American Journal of Epidemiology, 152*, 424–431.

McKenna, P. (2009) *Rookwood Driving Battery*. Oxford: Psychological Corporation.

McKenna, P. and Bell, V. (2007) Fitness to drive following cerebral pathology: The Rookwood Driving Battery as a tool for predicting on-road driving performance. *Journal of Neuropsychology, 1*, 85–100.

McKenna, P., Jefferies, L., Dobson, A. and Frude, N. (2004) The use of a cognitive battery to predict who will fail an on-road driving test. *British Journal of Clinical Psychology, 43*, 325–336.

McKenna, P. and Warrington, E. K. (1983) *Graded Naming Test*. Oxford: NFER-Nelson.

McKenzie, A., Perry, L., Lockhart, E., Cottee, M., Cloud, G. and Mann, H. (2007) Family carers of stroke survivors: Needs, knowledge, satisfaction and competence in caring. *Disability and Rehabilitation, 29*, 111–121.

McKevitt, C., Redfern, J., Mold, F. and Wolfe, C. (2004) Qualitative studies of stroke: A systematic review. *Stroke, 35*, 1499–1505.

McKinney, M., Blake, H., Treece, K. A., Lincoln, N. B., Playford, E. D. and Gladman, J. R. F. (2002) Evaluation of cognitive assessment in stroke rehabilitation. *Clinical Rehabilitation, 16*, 129–136.

McLean, J., Roper-Hall, A., Mayer, P. and Main, A. (1991) Service needs of stroke survivors and their informal carers: A pilot study. *Journal of Advanced Nursing, 16*, 559–564.

McLellan, D. L. (1991) Functional recovery and the principles of disability medicine. In J. O. E. M Swash (ed), *Clinical Neurology* (pp. 768–790) Edinburgh: Churchill Livingstone.

McMillan, T. M. and Sparkes, C. (1999) Goal planning and neurorehabilitation: The Wolfson Neurorehabilitation Centre approach. *Neuropsychological Rehabilitation, 9*, 241–251.

McMillan, T. M., Williams, W. H. and Bryant, R. (2003) Post-traumatic stress disorder and traumatic brain injury: A review of causal mechanisms, assessment, and treatment. *Neuropsychological Rehabilitation, 13*, 149–164.

McNair, D. M., Lorr, M. and Droppleman, L. F. (1981) *Manual for the Profile of Mood States*. Sacramento: California Educational and Industrial Testing Services.

McNeil, M. R. and Prescott, T. E. (1978) *Revised Token Test*. Austin, TX: Pro-Ed.

McNeil, M. R., Robin, D. A. and Schmidt, R. A. (1997) *Apraxia of Speech: Definition, Differentiation, and Treatment* (pp 311–344) Berlin: George Thieme Verlag.

McVicker, S., Parr, S., Pound, C. and Duchan, J. (2009) The Communication Partner Scheme: A project to develop long-term, low-cost access to conversation for people living with aphasia. *Aphasiology, 23*, 52–71.

Mead, G.E., Lewis, S.C., Wardlaw, J.M., Dennis, M.S. and Warlow, C.P. (2000) How well does the Oxfordshire Community Stroke Project classification predict the site and size of the infarct on brain imaging? *Journal of Neurology Neurosurgery and Psychiatry, 68,* 558–562.

Mead, G., Lynch, J., Greig, C., Young, A., Lewis, S. and Sharpe, M. (2007) Evaluation of fatigue scales in stroke patients. *Stroke, 38,* 2090–2095.

Meade, C. D. (1999) Improving understanding of the informed consent process and document. *Seminars in Oncology Nursing, 15,* 124–137.

Medical Research Council. (2008) *Developing and Evaluating Complex Interventions: New Guidance.* London: Medical Research Council.

Medin, J., Barajas, J. and Ekberg, K. (2006) Stroke patients' experiences of return to work. *Disability and Rehabilitation, 28,* 1051–1060.

Meichenbaum, D. (1985) *Stress Inoculation Training.* Elmsford, NY: Pergamon Press.

Meijer, R., van Limbeek, J., Kriek, B., Ihnenfeldt, D., Vermeulen, M. and de Haan, R. (2004) Prognostic social factors in the subacute phase after a stroke for the discharge destination from the hospital stroke-unit: A systematic review of the literature. *Disability and Rehabilitation, 26,* 191–197.

Melzack, R. (1975) McGill Pain Questionnaire – major properties and scoring methods. *Pain, 1,* 277–299.

Melzack, R. (1987) The short form McGill Pain Questionnaire. *Pain, 30,* 191–197.

Melzack, R. and Wall, P. D. (1965) Pain mechanisms – a new theory. *Science, 150*(3699), 971–977.

Menon, A. and Korner-Bitensky, N. (2004) Evaluating unilateral spatial neglect post stroke: Working your way through the maze of assessment choices. *Topics in Stroke Rehabilitation, 11,* 41–66.

Merriman, C., Norman, P. and Barton, J. (2007) Psychological correlates of PTSD symptoms following stroke. *Psychology, Health & Medicine, 12,* 592–602.

Merskey, H. and Bogduk, N. (1994) *Classification of Chronic Pain.* Seattle, WA: International Association for the Study of Pain.

Meterko, M., Nelson, E. C. and Rubin, H. R. (1990) Patient judgements of hospital quality: report of a pilot study. *Medical Care (Philadelphia),* 28(9 Suppl.) S1–S56.

Meyers, J. E., Volbrecht, M. and Kaster-Bundgaard, J. (1999) Driving is more than pedal pushing. *Applied Neuropsychology, 6,* 154–164.

Michie, S., Johnston, M., Abraham, C., Lawton, R., Parker, D. and Walker, A. (2005) Making psychological theory useful for implementing evidence based practice: A consensus approach. *Quality & Safety in Health Care, 14,* 26–33.

Michielsen, H. J., De Vries, J. and Van Heck, G. L. (2003) Psychometric qualities of a brief self-rated fatigue measure: The Fatigue Assessment Scale. *Journal of Psychosomatic Research, 54,* 345–352.

Miller, S. M. (1987) Monitoring and blunting – validation of a questionnaire to assess styles of information seeking under threat. *Journal of Personality and Social Psychology, 52,* 345–353.

Miller, W. R. and Rollnick, S. (2002) *Motivational Interviewing: Preparing People for Change,* 2nd ed. New York: Guilford Press.

Miltner, W. H., Bauder, H., Sommer, M., Dettmers, C. and Taub, E. (1999) Effects of constraint-induced movement therapy on patients with chronic motor deficits after stroke: A replication. *Stroke, 30,* 586–592.

Mioshi, E., Dawson, K., Mitchell, J., Arnold, R. and Hodges, J. (2006) The Addenbrooke's Cognitive Examination Revised (ACE-R): A brief cognitive test battery for dementia screening. *International Journal of Geriatric Psychiatry, 21,* 1078–1085.

Mishkin, M., Ungerleider, L. G. and Macko, K. A. (1983) Object vision and spatial vision: Two cortical pathways. *Trends in Neurosciences, 6,* 414–417.

Mitchell, A. J., Kemp, S., Benito-Leon, J. and Reuber, M. (2010) The influence of cognitive impairment on health-related quality of life in neurological disease. *Acta Neuropsychiatrica, 22,* 2–13.

Mitrushina, M., Boone, K. B., Razani, J. and D'Elia, L. F. (2005) *Handbook of Normative Data for Neuropsychological Assessment.* Oxford: Oxford University Press.

Mohr, D.C. and Goodkin, D.E., (1999) Treatment of depression in multiple sclerosis: review and meta-analysis. *Clinical Psychology: Science and Practice, 6,* 1–9.

Mohr, J. P., Pessin, M. S., Finkelstein, S., Funkenstein, H. H., Duncan, G. W. and Davis, K. R. (1978) Broca aphasia – pathological and clinical. *Neurology, 28,* 311–324.

Mok, E. and Woo, C. P. (2004) The effects of slow stroke back massage on anxiety and shoulder pain in elderly stroke patients. *Complementary Therapies in Nursing and Midwifery, 10,* 209–216.

Mok, V. C. T., Wong, A., Lam, W. W. M., Fan, Y. H., Tang, W. K., Kwok, T., *et al.* (2004) Cognitive impairment and functional outcome after stroke associated with small vessel disease. *Journal of Neurology Neurosurgery and Psychiatry, 75,* 560–566.

Mold, F., McKevitt, C. and Wolfe, C. (2003) A review and commentary of the social factors which influence stroke care: Issues of inequality in qualitative literature. *Health and Social Care in the Community, 11,* 405–414.

Molloy, D. W., Alemayehu, E. and Roberts, R. (1991) Reliability of a standardised Mini-Mental-State-Examination compared with the traditional Mini-Mental-State-Examination. *American Journal of Psychiatry, 148,* 102–105.

Molloy, G. J., Johnston, M., Johnston, D. W., Pollard, B., Morrison, V., Bonetti, D., *et al.* (2008) Spousal caregiver confidence and recovery from ambulatory activity limitations in stroke survivors. *Health Psychology, 27,* 286–290.

Monaghan, J., Channell, K., McDowell, D. and Sharma, A. K. (2005) Improving patient and carer communication, multidisciplinary team working and goal-setting in stroke rehabilitation. *Clinical Rehabilitation, 19,* 194–199.

Montgomery, S. A. and Åsberg, M. (1979) A new depression scale designed to be sensitive to change. *British Journal of Psychiatry, 134,* 382–389.

Moore, S. R., Gresham, L. S., Bromberg, M. B., Kasarkis, E. J. and Smith, R. A. (1997) A self report measure of affective lability. *Journal of Neurology Neurosurgery and Psychiatry, 63,* 89–93.

Morgan, J. and Ricker, J. (2008) *Textbook of Clinical Neuropsychology.* Boca Raton, FL: Taylor & Francis.

Morley, S., Eccleston, C. and Williams, A. (1999) Systematic review and meta-analysis of randomized controlled trials of cognitive behaviour therapy and behaviour therapy for chronic pain in adults, excluding headache. *Pain, 80,* 1–13.

Morris, K., Hacker, V. and Lincoln, N.B. (2010) The Validity of the Addenbrooke's Cognitive Examination-Revised (ACE-R) in acute stroke. Submitted for publication.

Morris, P. L. P., Raphael, B. and Robinson, R. G. (1992) Clinical depression is associated with impaired recovery from stroke. *The Medical Journal of Australia, 157,* 239–242.

Morris, P. L. P., Robinson, R. G., Andrzejewski, P., Samuels, J. and Price, T. R. (1993) Association of depression with 10-year poststroke mortality. *American Journal of Psychiatry, 150,* 124–129.

Morris, P. L. P., Robinson, R. G., Raphael, B. and Bishop, D. (1991) The relationship between the perception of social support and post-stroke depression in hospitalized patients. *Psychiatry, 54,* 306–316.

Morris, R., Payne, O. and Lambert, A. (2007) Patient, carer and staff experience of a hospital-based stroke service. *International Journal of Quality Health Care, 19,* 105–112.

Morrison, V. (1999) Predictors of carer distress following stroke. *Review of Clinical Gerontology, 9,* 265–271.

Morrison, V. and Bennett, P. (2009) *An Introduction to Health Psychology,* 2nd ed. Edinburgh: Pearson Education.

Morrison, V., Johnston, M. and MacWalter, R. (2000) Predictors of distress following an acute stroke: Disability, control cognitions and satisfaction with care. *Psychology and Health, 15,* 395–407.

Mort, D. J., Malhotra, P., Mannan, S. K., Rorden, C., Pambakian, A., Kennard, C., *et al.* (2003) The anatomy of visual neglect. *Brain, 126,* 1986–1997.

Moss, A. M. S. and Nicholas, M. (2006) Language rehabilitation in chronic aphasia and time postonset: A review of single-subject data. *Stroke, 37,* 3043–3051.

Mottillo, S., Filion, K. B., Belisle, P., Joseph, L., Gervais, A., O'Loughlin, J., *et al.* (2009) Behavioural interventions for smoking cessation: A meta-analysis of randomized controlled trials. *European Heart Journal, 30,* 718–730.

Mowbray, C. T., Moxley, D. P., Thrasher, S., Bybee, D., McCrohan, N., Harris, S., *et al.* (1996) Consumers as community support providers: Issues created by role innovation. *Community Mental Health Journal, 32,* 47–67.

Moye, J. and Marson, D. C. (2007) Assessment of decision-making capacity in older adults: An emerging area of practice and research. *Journal of Gerontology: Psychological Sciences, 62,* 3–11.

Mukamal, K., Ascherio, A., Mittleman, M., Conigrave, K., Camargo, C., Kawachi, I., *et al.* (2005) Alcohol and risk for ischemic stroke in men: The role of drinking patterns and usual beverage. *Annals of Internal Medicine, 142,* 11–19.

Müller-Nordhorn, J., Nolte, C. H., Rossnagel, K., Jungehülsing, G. J., Reich, A., Roll, S., *et al.* (2006) Knowledge about risk factors for stroke: A population-based survey with 28 090 participants. *Stroke, 37,* 946–950.

Mumby, K., Bowen, A. and Hesketh, A. (2007) Apraxia of speech: How reliable are speech and language therapists' diagnoses? *Clinical Rehabilitation, 21,* 760–767.

Mumma, C. M. (1986) Perceived losses following stroke. *Rehabilitation Nursing, 11,* 19–24.

Murphy, G. and Clare, I. (2003) Adults' capacity to make legal decisions. In C. C. R. Bull (ed), *Handbook of Psychology in Legal Contexts* (pp. 31–66). Chichester: Wiley.

Murphy, S. L., Dubin, J. A. and Gill, T. M. (2003) The development of fear of falling among community living older women: Predisposing factors and subsequent fall events. *The Journals of Gerontology, Gerontology Series A: Biological Sciences and Medical Sciences, 58A,* M943–M947.

Murray, C. D. and Harrison, B. (2004) The meaning and experience of being a stroke survivor: An interpretative phenomenological analysis. *Disability and Rehabilitation 26,* 808–816.

Murray, C. J. L. and Lopez, A. D. (1997) Mortality by cause for eight regions of the world: Global Burden of Disease Study. *Lancet, 349* (9061), 1269–1276.

Murray, J., Young, J., Forster, A. and Ashworth, R. (2003) Developing a primary care based stroke model: The prevalence of longer term problems experienced by patients and carers. *British Journal of General Practice, 53,* 803–807.

Murray Parkes, C. (1971) Psycho-social transitions: A field for study. *Social Science and Medicine*, 5, 101–115.

Murray, U. (1998) *'They Look after Their Own Don't They?' Inspection of Community Care Services for Black and Minority Ethnic Older People*. London: Department of Health.

Mynorswallis, L. M., Gath, D. H., Lloydthomas, A. R. and Tomlinson, D. (1995) Randomized controlled trial comparing problem-solving treatment with Amytriptyline and placebo for major depression in primary care. *British Medical Journal*, 310 (6977), 441–445.

Myron, R., Gillespie, S., Swift, P. and Williamson, T. (2008) *Whose Decision? Preparation for and Implementation of the Mental Capacity Act in Statutory and Non-statutory Services in England and Wales*. London: Mental Health Foundation.

Mysiw, W. J., Beegan, J. G. and Gatens, P. J. (1989) prospective cognitive assessment of stroke patients before in-patient rehabilitation. *American Journal of Physical Medicine and Rehabilitation*, 68, 168–171.

Naeser, M. A. and Palumbo, C. L. (1994) Neuroimaging and langauage recovery in stroke. *Journal of Clinical Neurophysiology*, 11, 150–174.

Naess, H., Nyland, H. I., Thomassen, L., Aarseth, J. and Myhr, K. M. (2005) Fatigue at long-term follow-up in young adults with cerebral infarction. *Cerebrovascular Diseases*, 20, 245–250.

Naess, H., Waje-Andreassen, U., Thomassen, L., Nyland, H. and Myhr, K. M. (2006) Health-related quality of life among young adults with ischemic stroke on long-term follow-up. *Stroke*, 37, 1232–1236.

Nair, R. D. (2007) *Effectiveness of Memory Rehabilitation following Brain Damage*. PhD, University of Nottingham, Nottingham.

Nakhutina, L., Borod, J. C. and Zgaljardic, D. J. (2006) Posed prosodic emotional expression in unilateral stroke patients: Recovery, lesion location, and emotional perception. *Archives of Clinical Neuropsychology*, 21, 1–13.

Nasreddine, Z. S., Phillips, N. A., Bedirian, V., Charbonneau, S., Whitehead, V., Collin, I., et al. (2005) The Montreal Cognitive Assessment, MoCA: A brief screening tool for mild cognitive impairment. *Journal of the American Geriatrics Society*, 53, 695–699.

National Audit Office. (2005) *Reducing Brain Damage: Faster Access to Better Stroke Care*. Report by the Comptroller and Auditor General, National Audit Office. London: Department of Health.

National Audit Office. (2010) *Department of Health: Progress in Improving Stroke Care*. Report by the Comptroller and Auditor General, HC 291 Session 2009–2010. London: TSO.

National Collaborating Centre for Chronic Conditions. (2008) *Stroke: National Clinical Guideline for Diagnosis and Initial Management of Acute Stroke and Transient Ischaemic Attack (TIA)* London: Royal College of Physicians.

National Conference of Commissioners on Uniform State Laws. (1993) *Uniform Health Care Decisions Act*. Chicago: National Conference of Commissioners on Uniform State Laws.

National Heart Lung and Blood Institute. (2003) *The Seventh Report of the Joint National Committee on Prevention, Detection, Evaluation, and Treatment of High Blood Pressure*. Bethesda, MD: National Heart, Lung, and Blood Institute.

National Institute for Health and Clinical Excellence (NICE). (2007) *Depression: Management of Depression in Primary and Secondary Care*. Clinical Guideline 23 (amended). London: NICE.

National Institute for Health and Clinical Excellence (NICE). (2009a) *Depression in Adults (Update).* Clinical Guideline 90. London: NICE.

National Institute for Health and Clinical Excellence (NICE). (2009b) *NICE quality standards stroke topic expert group meeting: Briefing paper.* London: NICE.

National Institute for Health and Clinical Excellence (NICE). (2011) *Anxiety (Partial Update).* NICE Clinical Guideline. London: NICE.

National Stroke Foundation. (2005) *Clinical Guidelines for Stroke Rehabilitation and Recovery.* Melbourne: National Stroke Foundation.

National Stroke Foundation. (2010) *Clinical Guidelines for Stroke Management (Draft).* Melbourne: National Stroke Foundation.

Nayak, S., Wheeler, B. L., Shiflett, S. C. and Agostinelli, S. (2000) Effect of music therapy on mood and social interaction among individuals with acute traumatic brain injury and stroke. *Rehabilitation Psychology, 45,* 274–283.

Neau, J. P., Ingrand, P., Mouille-Brachet, C., Rosier, M. P., Couderq, C., Alvarez, A., *et al.* (1998) Functional recovery and social outcome after cerebral infarction in young adults. *Cerebrovascular Diseases, 8,* 296–302.

Nelson, H. and Willison, J. (1991) *National Adult Reading Test.* Chiswick: NFER–Nelson.

Newsom, J. T. and Schulz, R. (1998) Caregiving from the recipient's perspective: Negative reactions to being helped. *Health Psychology, 17,* 172–181.

NHS Choices. (2009) *Real Stories: Stroke.* http://www.nhs.uk/Conditions/Stroke/Pages/Jimstory.aspx?url=Pages/Realstories.aspx

NHS Tayside. (2009) *Stroke Patient Stories: Heart & Stroke Information Point.* http://www.heartstroketayside.org.uk

Nicholl, C. R., Lincoln, N. B., Muncaster, K. and Thomas, S. (2002) Cognitions and post-stroke depression. *British Journal of Clinical Psychology, 41,* 221–231.

Nickels, L. (2002) Therapy for naming disorders: Revisiting, revising, and reviewing. *Aphasiology, 16,* 935–979.

Nieboer, A. P., Schulz, R., Matthews, K. A., Scheier, M. F., Ormel, J. and Lindenberg, S. M. (1998) Spousal caregivers' activity restriction and depression: A model for changes over time. *Social Science & Medicine, 47,* 1361–1371.

Niemann, H., Ruff, R. M. and Baser, C. A. (1990) Computer assisted attention retraining in head injured individuals: A controlled efficacy study of an out-patient program. *Journal of Consulting and Clinical Psychology, 58,* 811–817.

Nieuwenhuis-Mark, R., van Hoek, A. and Vingerhoets, A. (2008) Understanding excessive crying in neurologic disorders: Nature, pathophysiology, assessment, consequences, and treatment. *Cognitive and Behavioral Neurology, 21,* 111–123.

Nieuwenhuys, R., Voogd, J. and van Huijzen, C. (2008) *The Human Central Nervous System,* 4th ed. Berlin: Springer.

Nilsson, I., Jansson, L. and Norberg, A. (1997) To meet with a stroke: Patients' experiences and aspects seen through a screen of crises. *Journal of Advanced Nursing, 25,* 953–963.

Noar, S. M., Benac, C. N. and Harris, M. S. (2007) Does tailoring matter? Meta-analytic review of tailored print health behavior change interventions. *Psychological Bulletin, 133,* 673–693.

Nøkleby, K., Boland, E., Bergersen, H., Schanke, A. K., Farner, L., Wagle, J., *et al.* (2008) Screening for cognitive deficits after stroke: A comparison of three screening tools. *Clinical Rehabilitation, 22,* 1095–1104.

Norman, D. and Shallice, T. (1986) Attention to action: Willed and automatic control of behaviour. In G. E. S. R.J. Davidson and D. Shapiro (ed), *Consciousness and Self-Regulation*. New York: Plenum.

Norman, D. A. and Shallice, T. (1980) *Attention to Action: Willed and Automatic Control of Behaviour Center for Human Information Processing*. Technical Report No. 99.

Norris, G. and Tate, R. L. (2000) The behavioural assessment of the dysexecutive syndrome (BADS): Ecological, concurrent and construct validity. *Neuropsychological Rehabilitation, 10*, 33–45.

Norris, S. L., Zhang, X., Avenell, A., Gregg, E., Brown, T., Schmid, C. H., *et al.* (2005) Long-term non-pharmacological weight loss interventions for adults with type 2 diabetes mellitus. *Cochrane Database of Systematic Reviews* (2), CD004095.

Norris, S. L., Zhang, X., Avenell, A., Gregg, E., Schmid, C. H. and Lau, J. (2005) Pharmacotherapy for weight loss in adults with type 2 diabetes mellitus. *Cochrane Database of Systematic Reviews* (1), CD004096.

Nouri, F. (1988) Fitness to drive and the general practitioner. *International Disability Studies 10*, 101–103.

Nouri, F. M. and Lincoln, N. B. (1992) Validation of a cognitive assessment: Predicting driving performance after stroke. *Clinical Rehabilitation, 6*, 275–281.

Nouri, F. M. and Lincoln, N. B. (1993) Predicting driving performance after stroke. *British Medical Journal, 307*, 482–483.

Nouri, F. M. and Lincoln, N. B. (1994) *The Stroke Drivers Screening Assessment*. Nottingham: Nottingham Rehab.

Nouri, F. M., Tinson, D. J. and Lincoln, N. B. (1987) Cognitive ability and driving after stroke. *International Disability Studies, 9*, 110–115.

Novack, T. A., Caldwell, S. G., Duke, L. W., Bergquist, T. F. and Gage, R. J. (1996) Focused versus unstructured intervention for attention deficits after traumatic brain injury. *Journal of Head Trauma Rehabilitation, 11*, 52–60.

Novaco, R. W. (2010) Anger and Psychopathology. In G. S. C. S. M. Potegal (ed), *International Handbook of Anger: Constituent and Concomitant Biological, Psychological, and Social Processes* (pp 465–497). New York: Springer.

Nyberg, L. and Gustafson, Y. (1995) Patient falls in stroke rehabilitation – a challenge to rehabilitation strategies. *Stroke, 26*, 838–842.

Nys, G., van Zandvoort, M., de Kort, P., Jansen, B., De Haan, E. and Kappelle, L. (2007) Cognitive disorders in acute stroke: Prevalence and clinical determinants. *Cerebrovascular Diseases, 23*, 408–416.

Nys, G. M. S., Van Zandvoort, M. J. E., De Kort, P. L. M., Jansen, B. P. W., Van der Worp, H. B., Kappelle, L. J., *et al.* (2005a) Domain-specific cognitive recovery after first-ever stroke: A follow-up study of 111 cases. *Journal of the International Neuropsychological Society, 11*, 795–806.

Nys, G. M., van Zandvoort, M. J., de Kort, P. L., van der Worp, H. B., Jansen, B. P., Algra, A., *et al.* (2005b) The prognostic value of domain-specific cognitive abilities in acute first-ever stroke. *Neurology, 64*, 821–827.

Nys, G. M. S., van Zandvoort, M. J. E., de Kort, P. L. M., Jansen, B. P. W., Kappelle, L. J. and de Haan, E. H. F. (2005c) Restrictions of the Mini-Mental State Examination in acute stroke. *Archives of Clinical Neuropsychology, 20*, 623–629.

Nys, G. M. S., de Haan, E. H. F., Kunneman, A., de Kort, P. L. M. and Dijkerman, H. C. (2008) Acute neglect rehabilitation using repetitive prism adaptation: A randomized placebo-controlled trial. *Restorative Neurology and Neuroscience, 26*, 1–12.

Nys, G. M. S., van Zandvoort, M. J. E., van der Worp, H. B., de Haan, E. H. F., de Kort, P. L. M., Jansen, B. P. W., *et al.* (2006) Early cognitive impairment predicts long-term depressive symptoms and quality of life after stroke. *Journal of the Neurological Sciences*, 247, 149–156.

O'Connell, B., Hanna, B., Penney, W., Pearce, J., Owen, M. and Warelow, P. (2001) Recovery after stroke: A qualitative perspective. *Journal of Quality in Clinical Practice*, 21, 120–125.

O'Brien, J. T., Erkinjuntti, T., Reisberg, B., Roman, G., Sawada, T., Pantoni, L., *et al.* (2003) Vascular cognitive impairment. *Lancet Neurology*, 2, 89–98.

O'Carroll, R., Dennis, M., Johnston, M. and Sudlow, C. (2010) Improving adherence to medication in stroke survivors (IAMSS): A randomised controlled trial: Study protocol. *Neurology*, 10, 15.

O'Carroll, R. E., Hamilton, B., Whittaker, J., Dennis, M., Johnston, M., Sudlow, C., *et al.* (2008) Psychological factors which influence adherence to medication in stroke survivors. *CSO Final Report*, 4, 297.

Oddy, M. and Herbert, C. (2003) Intervention with families following brain injury: Evidence-based practice. *Neuropsychological Rehabilitation*, 13, 259–273.

Office for National Statistics. (2009) *National Statistics Online: Census 2001*. London: Office for National Statistics.

Office of Public Sector Information. (2007) Mental Health Act, 2007. Norwich: TSO.

Ogar, J., Willock, S., Baldo, J., Wilkins, D., Ludy, C. and Dronkers, N. (2006) Clinical and anatomical correlates of apraxia of speech. *Brain and Language*, 97, 343–350.

Ogden, J. A., Mee, E. W. and Utley, T. (1998) Too little, too late: Does tirilazad mesylate reduce fatigue after subarachnoid hemorrhage? *Neurosurgery*, 43, 782–787.

O'Halloran, R., Hickson, L. and Worrall, L. (2008) Environmental factors that influence communication between people with communication disability and their healthcare providers in hospital: A review of the literature within the International Classification of Functioning, Disability and Health (ICF) framework. *International Journal of Language & Communication Disorders*, 43, 601–632.

O'Halloran, R., Worrall, L. and Hickson, L. (2007a) Development of a measure of communication activity for the acute hospital setting: Part I: Rationale and preliminary findings. *Journal of Medical Speech-Language Pathology*, 15, 39–50.

O'Halloran, R., Worrall, L., Hickson, L. and Code, C. (2007b) Development of a measure of communication activity for the acute hospital setting: Part II: Item analysis, selection, and reliability. *Journal of Medical Speech-Language Pathology*, 15, 51–66.

Ohtomo, E., S., H., Terashi, A., Hasegawa, K. and Araki, K. (1991) Clinical evaluation of aniracetam on psychiatric symptoms related to cerebrovascular disease. *Journal of Clinical and Experimental Medicine*, 156, 143–187.

O'Kelly, D. (2002) Experience and perspective of the patient. *Age and Ageing*, 31, 21–23.

Okonkwo, O., Griffith, H. R., Belue, K., Lanza, S., Zamrini, E. Y., Harrell, L. E., *et al.* (2007) Medical decision-making capacity in patients with mild cognitive impairment. *Neurology*, 69, 1528–1535.

Olofsson, A., Andersson, S. O. and Carlberg, B. (2005) 'If only I manage to get home I'll get better' – interviews with stroke patients after emergency stay in hospital on their experiences and needs. *Clinical Rehabilitation*, 19, 433–440.

O'Neill, P. A., Cheadle, B., Wyatt, R., McGuffog, J. and Fullerton, K. J. (1990) The value of the Frenchay Aphasia Screening Test in screening for dysphasia: Better than the clinician? *Clinical Rehabilitation* 4, 123–128.

Onyett, S. (2007) *New Ways of Working for Applied Psychologists in Health and Social Care – Working Psychologically in Teams*. Leicester: British Psychological Society.

Orfei, M. D., Robinson, R. G., Prigatano, G. P., Starkstein, S., Rusch, N., Bria, P., *et al.* (2007) Anosognosia for hemiplegia after stroke is a multifaceted phenomenon: A systematic review of the literature. *Brain, 130,* 3075–3090.

O'Rourke, S., MacHale, S., Signorini, D. and Dennis, M. (1998) Detecting psychiatric morbidity after stroke – comparison of the GHQ and the HAD Scale. *Stroke, 29,* 980–985.

Osterrieth, P. (1944) Filetest de copie d'une figure complexe; contribution a l'etude de la perception et de la memoire (Test of copying a complex figure; contribution to the study of perception and memory). *Archives de psychologie, 30,* 206–356.

Ostir, G. V., Markides, K. S., Peek, M. K. and Goodwin, J. S. (2001) The association between emotional well-being and the incidence of stroke in older adults. *Psychosomatic Medicine, 63,* 210–215.

O'Sullivan, M., Morris, R. G. and Markus, H. S. (2005) Brief cognitive assessment for patients with cerebral small vessel disease. *Journal of Neurology, Neurosurgery and Psychiatry, 76,* 1140–1145.

Ota, H., Fujii, T., Suzuki, K., Fukatsu, R. and Yamadori, A. (2001) Dissociation of body-centered and stimulus-centered representations in unilateral neglect. *Neurology, 57,* 2064–2069.

Ovbiagele, B., Saver, J., Fredieu, A., Suzuki, S., Selco, S., Rajajee, V., *et al.* (2004) In-hospital initiation of secondary stroke prevention therapies yields high rates of adherence at follow-up. *Stroke, 35,* 2879–2883.

Owen, G. S., Freyenhagen, F., Richardson, G. and Hotopf, M. (2009) Mental capacity and decisional autonomy: An interdisciplinary challenge. *Inquiry: An Interdisciplinary Journal of Philosophy, 52,* 79–107.

Ownsworth, T. L., McFarland, K. and Young, R. M. D. (2000) Self-awareness and psychosocial functioning following acquired brain injury: An evaluation of a group support programme. *Neuropsychological Rehabilitation, 10,* 465–484.

Owsley, C., Ball, K., McGwin, G., Sloane, M. E., Roenker, D. L., White, M. F., *et al.* (1998) Visual processing impairment and risk of motor vehicle crash among older adults. *Journal of the American Medical Association, 279,* 1083–1088.

Pachalska, M., Grochmal-Bach, B., MacQueen, B. D. and Franczuk, B. (2006) Post-traumatic stress disorder in Polish stroke patients who survived Nazi concentration camps. *Medical Science Monitor, 12,* CR137–CR149.

Pachet, A., Astner, K. and Brown, L. (2009) Clinical utility of the Mini-Mental Status Examination when assessing decision-making capacity. *Journal of Geriatric Psychiatry and Neurology, 23,* 3–8.

Padovani, A., DiPiero, V., Bragoni, M., Iacoboni, M. and Gualdi, G. F. (1995) Patterns of neuropsychological impairment in mild dementia: A comparison between Alzheimer's disease and multi-infarct dementia. *Acta Neurologica Scandinavica, 92,* 433–442.

Paediatric Stroke Working Group Royal College of Physicians. (2004) *Stroke in Childhood: Clinical Guidelines for Diagnosis, Management and Rehabilitation.* London: Royal College of Physicians.

Palmer, B. W., Jeste, D. V. and Sheikh, J. I. (1997) Anxiety disorders in the elderly: DSM-IV and other barriers to diagnosis and treatment. *Journal of Affective Disorders, 46,* 183–190.

Palmer, S. and Glass, T. A. (2003) Family function and stroke recovery: A review. *Rehabilitation Psychology, 48,* 255–265.

Pambakian, A. L. M., Mannan, S. K., Hodgson, T. L. and Kennard, C. (2004) Saccadic visual search training: A treatment for patients with homonymous hemianopia. *Journal of Neurology Neurosurgery and Psychiatry*, 75, 1443–1448.

Pang, M. Y. C. and Eng, J. J. (2008) Fall-related self-efficacy, not balance and mobility performance, is related to accidental falls in chronic stroke survivors with low bone mineral density. *Osteoporosis International*, 19, 919–927.

Paolucci, S., Antonucci, G., Gialoreti, L. E., Traballesi, M., Lubich, S., Pratesi, L., *et al.* (1996) Predicting stroke inpatient rehabilitation outcome: The prominant role of neuropsychological disorders. *European Journal of Neurology*, 36, 385–390.

Paolucci, S., Antonucci, G., Pratesi, L., Traballesi, M., Lubich, S. and Grasso, M. G. (1998) Functional outcome in stroke inpatient rehabilitation: Predicting no, low and high response patients. *Cerebrovascular Disease*, 8, 228–234.

Parikh, R. M., Lipsey, J. R., Robinson, R. G. and Price, T. R. (1988) A two year longitudinal study of poststroke mood disorders: Prognostic factors related to one and two year outcome. *International Journal of Psychiatry in Medicine*, 18, 45–56.

Parikh, R. M., Robinson, R. G., Lipsey, J. R., Starkstein, S. E., Fedoroff, J. P. and Price, T. R. (1990) The impact of poststroke depression on recovery of activities of daily living over a 2-year follow-up. *Archives of Neurology*, 47, 785–789.

Parker, C. J., Gladman, J. R. F., Drummond, A. E. R., Dewey, M. E., Lincoln, N. B., Barer, D., *et al.* (2001) A multicentre randomized controlled trial of leisure therapy and conventional occupational therapy after stroke. *Clinical Rehabilitation*, 15, 42–52.

Parks, G. A., Marlatt, G. A. and Anderson, B. K. (2004) Cognitive-behavioural Alcohol Treatment. In *The Essential Handbook of Treatment and Prevention of Alcohol Problems* (pp. 69–86). Chichester: Wiley.

Parr, S., Byng, S. and Gilpin, S. (1997) *Talking about Aphasia*. Buckingham: Open University Press.

Parra, O., Arboix, A., Bechich, S., Garcia-Eroles, L., Montserrat, J. M., Lopez, J. A., *et al.* (2000) Time course of sleep-related breathing disorders in first-ever stroke or transient ischemic attack. *American Journal of Respiratory and Critical Care Medicine*, 161, 375–380.

Parton, A., Malhotra, P. and Husain, M. (2004) Hemispatial neglect. *Journal of Neurology Neurosurgery and Psychiatry*, 75, 13–21.

Partridge, C. and Johnston, M. (1989) Perceived control and recovery from disability: Measurement and prediction. *British Journal of Clinical Psychology*, 28, 53–59.

Parvizi, J., Arciniegas, D. B., Bernardini, G. L., Hoffmann, M. W., Mohr, J. P., Rapoport, M. J., *et al.* (2006) Diagnosis and management of pathological laughter and crying. *Mayo Clinic Proceedings*, 81, 1482–1486.

Patient Voices. (2009) *Reconnecting with Life: Stories of Life after Stroke*. http://www.pilgrim.myzen.co.uk/patientvoices/naoconn.htm

Patomella, A. H., Tham, K. and Kottorp, A. (2006) P-Drive: Assessment of driving performance after stroke. *Journal of Rehabilitation Medicine*, 38, 273–279.

Patra, J., Taylor, B., Irving, H., Roerecke, M., Baliunas, D., Mohapatra, S., *et al.* (2010) Alcohol consumption and the risk of morbidity and mortality for different stroke types – a systematic review and meta-analysis. *Public Health*, 10, 258.

Pazzaglia, M., Smania, N., Corato, E. and Aglioti, S. M. (2008) Neural underpinnings of gesture discrimination in patients with limb apraxia. *Journal of Neuroscience*, 28, 3030–3041.

Pearlin, L. I., Mullan, U. T., Semple, S. J. and Skaff, M. M. (1990) Caregiving and the stress process: An overview of concepts and their measures. *Gerontologist, 30,* 583–593.

Pecchioni, L. L. (2001) Implicit decision-making in family caregiving. *Journal of Social and Personal Relationships, 18,* 219–237.

Pedersen, P. M., Jorgensen, H. S., Kammersgaard, L. P., Nakayama, H., Raaschou, H. O. and Olsen, T. S. (2001) Manual and oral apraxia in acute stroke, frequency and influence on functional outcome: The Copenhagen Stroke Study. *American Journal of Physical Medical Rehabilitation, 80,* 685–692.

Pendlebury, S. T., Cuthbertson, F. C., Welch, S. J. V., Mehta, Z. and Rothwell, P. M. (2010) Underestimation of cognitive impairment by Mini-Mental State Examination versus the Montreal Cognitive Assessment in patients with transient ischemic attack and stroke: A population-based study. *Stroke, 41,* 1–4.

Penley, J. A., Tomaka, J. and Wiebe, J. S. (2002) The association of coping to physical and psychological health outcomes: A meta-analytic review. *Journal of Behavioral Medicine, 25,* 551–603.

Periard, M. E. and Ames, B. D. (1993) Lifestyle changes and coping patterns among caregivers of stroke survivors. *Public Health Nursing, 10,* 252–256.

Petitti, D., Sidney, S., Quesenberry, C. and Bernstein, A. (1998) Stroke and cocaine or amphetamine use. *Epidemiology, 9,* 596–600.

Pidikiti, R. D. and Novack, T. A. (1991) The disabled driver – an unmet challenge. *Archives of Physical Medicine and Rehabilitation, 72,* 109–111.

Pierce, L. L. (2001) Caring and expressions of spirituality by urban caregivers of people with stroke in African American families. *Qualitative Health Research, 11,* 339–352.

Pierce, S. R. and Buxbaum, L. J. (2002) Treatments of unilateral neglect: A review. *Archives of Physical Medicine and Rehabilitation, 83,* 256–268.

Pilkington, F. B. (1999) A qualitative study of life after stroke. *Journal of Neuroscience Nursing, 31,* 336–348.

Pillemer, K., Landreneau, L. T. and Suitor, J. J. (1996) Volunteers in a peer support project for caregivers: What motivates them? *American Journal of Alzheiemer's Disease, 11,* 13–19.

Ping, W. and Songhai, L. (2008) Clinical observation on post-stroke anxiety neurosis treated by acupuncture. *Journal of Traditional Chinese Medicine, 28,* 186–188.

Pinquart, M., Duberstein, P. R. and Lyness, J. M. (2006) Treatments for later-life depressive conditions: A meta-analytic comparison of pharmacotherapy and psychotherapy. *American Journal of Psychiatry, 163,* 1493–1501.

Piper, B. F. (1989) Fatigue: current bases for practice. In Funk, S. G., Tornquist, E. M., Champagne, M. T., Copp, L. A. and Wiese, R. A. (eds), *Key Sspects of Comfort: Management of Pain, Fatigue and Nausea* (pp. 187–189). New York: Springer.

Pizzamiglio, L., Fasotti, L., Jehkonen, M., Antonucci, G., Magnotti, L., Boelen, D., *et al.* (2004) The use of optokinetic stimulation in rehabilitation of the hemineglect disorder. *Cortex, 40,* 441–450.

Pizzamiglio, L., Frasca, R., Guariglia, C., Inoccia, C. and Antonucci, G. (1990) Effect of optokinetic stimulation in patients with visual neglect. *Cortex, 26,* 535–540.

Playford, E. D., Siegert, R., Levack, W. and Freeman, J. (2009) Areas of consensus and controversy about goal setting in rehabilitation: A conference report. *Clinical Rehabilitation, 23,* 334–344.

Pohjasvaara, T., Erkinjuntti, T., Ylikoski, R., Hietanen, M., Vataja, R. and Kaste, M. (1998) Clinical determinants of poststroke dementia. *Stroke, 29,* 75–81.

Pohjasvaara, T., Mäntylä, R., Ylikoski, R., Kaste, M. and Erkinjuntti, T. (2000) Comparison of Different Clinical Criteria (DSM-III, ADDTC, ICD-10, NINDS-AIREN, DSM-IV) for the Diagnosis Of Vascular Dementia. *Stroke 31*, 2952–2957.

Pohjasvaara, T., Vataja, R., Leppavuori, A., Kaste, M. and Erkinjuntti, T. (2002) Cognitive functions and depression as predictors of poor outcome 15 months after stroke. *Cerebrovascular Diseases, 14*, 228–233.

Pohjasvaara, T., Vataja, R., Leppävuori, A., Kaste, M. and Erkinjuntti, T. (2001) Depression is an independent predictor of poor long-term functional outcome post-stroke. *European Journal of Neurology, 8*, 315–319.

Poirier, J. and Derouesne, C. (1984) Cerebral lacunae: A proposed new classification. *Clinical Neuropathology, 3*, 266.

Polanowska, K., Seniow, J., Paprot, E., Lesniak, M. and Czlonkowska, A. (2009) Left-hand somatosensory stimulation combined with visual scanning training in rehabilitation for post-stroke hemineglect: A randomised, double-blind study. *Neuropsychological Rehabilitation, 19*, 364–382.

Ponsford, A. S., Viitanen, M., Lundberg, C. and Johansson, K. (2008) Assessment of driving after stroke: A pluridisciplinary task. *Accident Analysis and Prevention, 40*, 452–460.

Ponsford, J. and Kinsella, G. (1991) The use of a rating scale of attentional behaviour. *Neuropsychological Rehabilitation, 1*, 241–257.

Posner, M. I., Walker, J. A., Friedrich, F. J. and Rafal, R. D. (1984) Effects of parietal injury on covert orienting of attention. *Journal of Neuroscience, 4*, 1863–1874.

Pound, P., Gompertz, P. and Ebrahim, S. (1993) Development and results of a questionnaire to measure carer satisfaction after stroke. *Journal of Epidemiology and Community Health, 47*, 500–505.

Pound, P., Gompertz, P. and Ebrahim, S. (1998) A patient-centred study of the consequences of stroke. *Clinical Rehabilitation, 12*, 338–347.

Pound, P., Tilling, K., Rudd, A. G. and Wolfe, C. D. A. (1999) Does patient satisfaction reflect differences in care received after stroke? *Stroke, 30*, 49–55.

Powell, J., Letson, S., Davidoff, J., Valentine, T. and Greenwood, R. (2008) Enhancement of face recognition learning in patients with brain injury using three cognitive training procedures. *Neuropsychological Rehabilitation, 18*, 182–203.

Powell, L. E. and Myers, A. M. (1995) The Activities-specific Balance Confidence scale (ABC). *Journals of Gerontology Series A: Biological Sciences and Medical Sciences, 50*, M28–M34.

Pratt, C. A., Ha, L., Levine, S. R. and Pratt, C. B. (2003) Stroke knowledge and barriers to stroke prevention among African Americans: Implications for health communication. *Journal of Health Communication, 8*, 369–381.

Price, C. I. M., Curless, R. H. and Rodgers, H. (1999) Can stroke patients use visual analogue scales? *Stroke, 30*, 1357–1361.

Prigatano, G. P. (1999) *Principles of Neuropsychological Rehabilitation*. New York: Oxford University Press.

Prigatano, G. P. (2008) Neuropsychological rehabilitation and psychodynamic psychotherapy. In J. E. M. J. H. Ricker (ed), *Textbook of Clinical Neuropsychology* (pp. 985–995) New York: Taylor & Francis.

Prigatano, G. P., Klonoff, P. S., O'Brien, K. P., Altman, I. M., Amin, K., Chiapello, D. A., *et al.* (1994) Productivity after neuropsychologically oriented milieu rehabilitation. *Journal of Head Trauma Rehabilitation, 9*, 91–102.

Pringle, J., Hendry, C. and McLafferty, E. (2008) A review of the early discharge experiences of stroke survivors and their carers. *Journal of Clinical Nursing*, *17*, 2384–2397.

Prochaska, J. O. and DiClemente, C. C. (1984) *The Transtheoretical Approach: Crossing the Traditional Boundaries of Therapy*. Homewood, IL: Dow Jones/Irwin.

Pyles, D. A. M. and Bailey, J. S. (1990) Diagnosing severe behavior problems. In A. C. Repp & N. N. E. Singh (eds), *Perspectives on the Use of Nonaversive and Aversive Interventions for Persons with Developmental Disabilities* (pp. 381–401). Sycamore IL: Sycamore Publishing.

Quaranta, D., Marra, C. and Gainotti, G. (2008) Mood disorders after stroke: Diagnostic validation of the Poststroke Depression Rating Scale. *Cerebrovascular Diseases*, *26*, 237–243.

Radford, F. M. and Lincoln, N. B. (2004) Concurrent validity of the Stroke Drivers Screening Assessment. *Archives of Physical Medicine and Rehabilitation*, *85*, 324–328.

Radford, K. A. and Walker, M. F. (2008) Impact of stroke on return to work. *Brain Impairment*, *9*, 161–169.

Radloff, L. S. (1977) The CES-D scale: A self-report depression scale for research in the general population. *Applied Psychological Measurement*, *1*, 385–401.

Rahmqvist, M. (2001) Patient satisfaction in relation to age, health status and other background factors: A model for comparisons of care units. *International Journal for Quality in Health Care*, *13*, 385–390.

Randolph, C. (1998) *Repeatable Battery for the Assessment of Neuropsychological Status Manual*. San Antonio, TX: Psychological Corporation.

Rasquin, S. M. C., Lodder, J., Ponds, R., Winkens, I., Jolles, J. and Verhey, F. R. J. (2004) Cognitive functioning after stroke: A one-year follow-up study. *Dementia and Geriatric Cognitive Disorders*, *18*, 138–144.

Rasquin, S. M. C., van de Sande, P., Praamstra, A. J. and van Heugten, C. M. (2009) Cognitive-behavioural intervention for depression after stroke: Five single case studies on effects and feasibility. *Neuropsychological Rehabilitation*, *19*, 208–222.

Rath, J. F., Simon, D., Langenbahn, D. M., Sherr, R. L. and Diller, L. (2003) Group treatment of problem-solving deficits in outpatients with traumatic brain injury: A randomised outcome study. *Neuropsychological Rehabilitation*, *13*, 461–488.

Raven, J. (1998) *Manual for Raven's Progressive Matrices and Vocabulary Scales*. Oxford, UK: Oxford Psychologists Press.

Raven, J. C. (1958) *Standard Progressive Matrices*. London: H.K. Lewis.

Raven, J. C., Raven, J. and Court, J. H. (1956) *Coloured Progressive Matrices*. Oxford, UK: Oxford Psychologists Press.

Raymont, V., Buchanan, A., David, A. S., Hayward, P., Wessely, S. and Hotopf, M. (2007) The inter-rater reliability of mental capacity assessments. *International Journal of Law and Psychiatry*, *30*, 112–117.

Reddon, J. R., Gill, D. M., Gauk, S. E. and Maerz, M. D. (1988) Purdue Pegboard: Test–retest estimates. *Perceptual and Motor Skills*, *66*, 503–506.

Redfern, J., McKevitt, C. and Wolfe, C. (2006) Development of complex interventions in stroke care: A systematic review. *Stroke*, *37*, 2410–2419.

Reitan, R. M. (1955) Certain differential effects of left and right cerebral lesions in human adults. *Journal of Comparative and Physiological Psychology*, *48*, 474–477.

Rejeski, W., Brawley, L., Ambrosius, W., Brubaker, P., Focht, B., Foy, C., *et al.* (2003) Older adults with chronic disease: Benefits of group-mediated counseling in the promotion of physically active lifestyles. *Health Psychology*, *22*, 414–423.

Reker, D. M., Duncan, P. W., Horner, R. D., Hoenig, H., Samsa, G. P., Hamilton, B. B., *et al.* (2002) Postacute stroke guideline compliance is associated with greater patient satisfaction. *Archives of Physical Medicine and Rehabilitation, 83*, 750–756.

Rey, A. (1959) Le test de copie de figure complexe. *Journal of Gerontology, 38*, 344–348.

Reynolds, K., Lewis, B., Nolen, J. D., Kinney, G. L., Sathya, B. and He, J. (2003) Alcohol consumption and risk of stroke: A meta-analysis. *Journal of the American Medical Assocation, 289*, 579–588.

Richards, F. and Dale, J. (2009) The Mental Health Act 1983 and incapacity: What general hospital doctors know. *Psychiatric Bulletin 33*, 176–178.

Ricker, J. H., Axelrod, B. N. and Houtler, B. D. (1996) Clinical validation of the oral trail making test. *Neuropsychiatry Neuropsychology and Behavioral Neurology, 9*, 50–53.

Riddoch, M. and Humphreys, G. (1993) *Birmingham Object Recognition Battery.* Hove: Lawrence Erlbaum Associates.

Riddoch, M. and Humphreys, G. W. (1987) A case of integrative visual agnosia. *Brain, 110*, 1431–1462.

Riddoch, M. J. and Humphreys, G. W. E. (1994) *Cognitive Neuropsychology and Cognitive Rehabilitation.* Hove: Lawrence Erlbaum Associates.

Ripley, M. (2006) *Surviving a Stroke: Recovering and Adjusting to Living with Hypertension.* London: White Ladder Press.

Rittman, M., Faircloth, C., Boylstein, C., Gubrium, J., Williams, C., Van Puymbroeck, M., *et al.* (2004) The experience of time in the transition from hospital to home following stroke. *Journal of Rehabilitation Research and Development, 41*, 259–268.

Ro, T. and Rafal, R. (2006) Visual restoration in cortical blindness: Insights from natural and TMS-induced blindsight. *Neuropsychological Rehabilitation, 16*, 377–396.

Roach, E. S., Golomb, M. R., Adams, R., Biller, J., Daniels, S., Deveber, G., *et al.* (2008) Management of stroke in infants and children: A scientific statement from a special writing group of the American Heart Association Stroke Council and the Council on Cardiovascular Disease in the young. *Stroke, 39*, 2644–2691.

Robertson, I. H. (2005) The neural basis for a theory of cognitive rehabilitation. In P. W. Halligan and D. T. Wade (eds), *Effectiveness of Rehabilitation for Cognitive Deficits* (pp. 281–294) Oxford: Oxford University Press.

Robertson, I. H., Hogg, K. and McMillan, T. M. (1998) Rehabilitation of unilateral neglect: Improving function by contralesional limb activation. *Neuropsychological Rehabilitation, 8*, 19–29.

Robertson, I. H. and Murre, J. M. J. (1999) Rehabilitation of brain damage: Brain plasticity and principles of guided recovery. *Psychological Bulletin, 125*, 544–575.

Robertson, I. H. and North, N. (1993) Active and passive activation of left limbs: Influence on visual and sensory neglect *Neuropsychologia, 31*, 293–300.

Robertson, I. H., North, N. and Geggie, C. (1992) Spatiomotor cueing in unilateral left neglect: Three case studies of its therapeutic effects. *Journal of Neurology, Neurosurgery and Psychiatry, 55*, 799–805.

Robertson, I. H., Ridgeway, V., Greenfield, E. and Parr, A. (1997) Motor recovery after stroke depends on intact sustained attention: A 2-year follow-up study. *Neuropsychology, 11*, 290–295.

Robertson, I. H., Ward, T., Ridgeway, V. and Nimmo-Smith, I. (1994) *The Test of Everyday Attention.* Bury St Edmunds: Thames Valley Test Company.

Robey, R. R. (1994) The efficacy of treatment for aphasic persons: A meta-analysis. *Brain and Language, 47*, 582–608.

Robinson, L., Francis, J., James, P., Tindle, N., Greenwell, K. and Rodgers, H. (2005) Caring for carers of people with stroke: Developing a complex intervention following the Medical Research Council framework. *Clinical Rehabilitation, 19*, 560–571.

Robinson, R. G., Bolduc, P. L. and Price, T. R. (1987) Two-year longitudinal study of poststroke mood disorders: Diagnosis and outcome at two years. *Stroke, 18*, 837–843.

Robinson, R. G., Bolla-Wilson, K., Lipsey, J. R. and Price, T. R. (1986) Depression influences intellectual impairment in stroke patients. *British Journal of Psychiatry, 148*, 541–547.

Robinson, R. G., Jorge, R. E., Moser, D. J., Acion, L., Solodkin, A., Small, S. L., *et al.* (2008) Escitalopram and problem-solving therapy for prevention of poststroke depression: A randomized controlled trial. *Journal of the American Medical Association, 299*, 2391–2400.

Robinson, R. G., Parikh, R. M., Lipsey, J. R., Starkstein, S. E. and Price, T. R. (1993) Pathological laughing and crying following stroke; Validation of a measurement scale and a double-blind treatment study. *American Journal of Psychotherapy, 150*, 286–293.

Robinson, R. G., Starr, L. B., Kubos, K. L. and Price, T. R. (1983) A two-year longitudinal study of post-stroke mood disorders: Findings during the initial evaluation. *Stroke, 14*, 736–741.

Robson, C. (1993) *Observational Methods*. Oxford, UK: Blackwell.

Rochette, A. and Desrosiers, J. (2002) Coping with the consequences of stroke. *International Journal of Rehabilitation Research, 25*, 17–24.

Rochette, A., Tribble, D., Desrosiers, J., Bravo, G. and Bourget, A. (2006) Adaptation and coping following a first stroke: A qualitative analysis of a phenomenological orientation. *International Journal of Rehabilitation Research, 29*, 247–249.

Rode, G., Charles, N., Perenin, M. T., Vighetto, A., Trillet, M. and Aimard, G. (1992) Partial remission of hemiplegia and somatoparaphrenia through vestibular stimulation in a case of unilateral neglect. *Cortex, 28*, 203–208.

Roder, B., Stock, O., Neville, H., Bien, S. and Rosler, F. (2002) Brain activation modulated by the comprehension of normal and pseudo-word sentences of different processing demands: A functional magnetic resonance imaging study. *NeuroImage, 15*, 1003–1014.

Rodgers, H., Atkinson, C., Bond, S., Suddes, M., Dobson, R. and Curless, R. H. (1999) Randomized controlled trial of a comprehensive stroke evaluation program for patients and carers. *Stroke, 30*, 2585–2591.

Rodin, J. (1986) Aging and health – effects of sense of control. *Science, 233*, 1271–1276.

Roding, J. (2009) *Stroke in the Younger: Self-Reported Impact on Work Situation, Cognitive Function, Physical Function and Life Satisfaction: A National Survey*. New Series No. 1241. Umeå, Sweden.

Roding, J., Glader, E. L., Malm, J. and Lindstrom, B. (2010) Life satisfaction in younger individuals after stroke: Different predisposing factors among men and women. *Journal of Rehabilitation Medicine, 42*, 155–161.

Roding, J., Lindstrom, B., Malm, J. and Ohman, A. (2003) Frustrated and invisible – younger stroke patients' experiences of the rehabilitation process. *Disability and Rehabilitation, 25*, 867–874.

Roger, P. R. and Johnson-Greene, D. (2009) Comparison of assessment measures for post-stroke depression. *Clinical Neuropsychologist, 23*, 780–793.

Rogers, R. (ed) (2008) *Clinical Assessment of Malingering and Deception*, 3rd ed. New York: Guilford Press.

Rollnick, S., Miller, W. R. and Butler, C. C. (2007) *Motivational Interviewing in Health Care: Helping Patients Change Behavior*. New York: Guilford Press.

Roman, G. C., Sachdev, P., Royall, D. R., Bullock, R. A., Orgogozo, J. M., Lopez-Pousa, S., *et al.* (2004) Vascular cognitive disorder: A new diagnostic category updating vascular cognitive impairment and vascular dementia. *Journal of Clinical Neuroscience*, *226*, 81–87.

Roosink, M., Renzenbrink, G. J., Van Dongen, R. T. M., Buitenweg, J. R., Geurts, A. C. H. and IJzerman, M. J. (2008) Diagnostic uncertainties in post-stroke pain. Paper presented at the 12th World Congress on Pain, Glasgow, Scotland.

Rorden, C., Berger, M. F. and Karnath, H. O. (2006) Disturbed line bisection is associated with posterior brain lesions. *Brain Research*, *1080*, 17–25.

Rose, F., Brooks, B., Attree, E., Parslow, D., Leadbetter, A., McNeil, J., *et al.* (1999) A preliminary investigation into the use of virtual environments in memory retraining after vascular brain injury: Indications for future strategy? *Disability & Rehabilitation*, *21*, 548–554.

Rosenbaum, R. S., Moscovitch, M., Foster, J. K., Schnyer, D. M., Ga, F., Kovacevic, N., *et al.* (2008) Patterns of autobiographical memory loss in medial-temporal lobe amnesic patients. *Journal of Cognitive Neuroscience*, *20*, 1490–1506.

Ross, A., Winslow, I., Marchant, P. and Brumfitt, S. (2006) Evaluation of communication, life participation and psychological well-being in chronic aphasia: The influence of group intervention. *Aphasiology*, *20*, 427–448.

Ross, E. D. and Monnot, M. (2008) Neurology of affective prosody and its functional-anatomic organization in right hemisphere. *Brain and Language*, *104*, 51–74.

Ross, E. D., Thompson, R. D. and Yenkosky, J. (1997) Lateralization of affective prosody in brain and the callosal integration of hemispheric language functions. *Brain and Language*, *56*, 27–54.

Ross, K. B. and Wertz, R. T. (2003) Quality of life with and without aphasia. *Aphasiology*, *17*, 355–364.

Rossetti, Y., Rode, G., Pisella, L., Farne, A., Li, L., Boisson, D., *et al.* (1998) Prism adaptation to a rightward optical deviation rehabilitates left hemispatial neglect. *Nature*, *395*, 166–169.

Rossi, P. W., Kheyfets, S. and Reding, M. (1990) Fresnel prisms improve visual perception in stroke patients with homonymous hemiapnopia or unilateral visual neglect. *Neurology*, *40*, 1597–1599.

Roth, L. H., Lidz, C. W., Meisel, A., Soloff, P. H., Kaufman, K., Spiker, D. G., *et al.* (1982) Competency to decide about treatment or research: An overview of some empirical data. *International Journal of Law and Psychiatry*, *5*, 29–50.

Roth, L. H., Meisel, A. and Lidz, C. W. (1977) Tests of competency to consent to treatment. *American Journal of Psychiatry*, *134*, 279–284.

Roth, M., Huppert, F. A., Mountjoy, C. Q. and Tym, E. (1999) *CAMDEX-R: The Cambridge Examination for Mental Disorders of the Elderly–Revised* Cambridge: Cambridge University Press.

Rousseaux, M., Cabaret, M., Lesoin, F., Devos, P., Dubois, F. and Petit, H. (1986) Evaluation of the amnesia caused by restricted thalamic infarcts: 6 cases. *Cortex*, *22*, 213–228.

Rowe, F., Brand, D., Jackson, C. A., Price, A., Walker, L., Harrison, S., *et al.* (2009) Visual impairment following stroke: do stroke patients require vision assessment? *Age and Ageing*, *38*, 188–193.

Roy, E. A., Heath, M., Westwood, D., Schweizer, T. A., Dixon, M. J., Black, S. E., *et al.* (2000) Task demands and limb apraxia in stroke. *Brain and Cognition, 44,* 253–279.

Royal College of Physicians. (2000) *National Clinical Guidelines for Stroke.* London: Royal College of Physicians.

Royal College of Physicians. (2002a) *National Clinical Guidelines for Stroke: Update 2002.* London: Royal College of Physicians.

Royal College of Physicians. (2002b) *National Sentinel Stroke Audit Report 2001/2: Prepared on Behalf of the Intercollegiate Stroke Working Party.* London: Royal College of Physicians.

Royal College of Physicians. (2004) *Stroke in Childhood: Clinical Guidelines for Diagnosis, Management and Rehabilitation.* London: Royal College of Physicians.

Royal College of Physicians. (2005) *National Sentinel Stroke Audit Report 2004 Prepared on Behalf of the Intercollegiate Stroke Working Party.* London: Royal College of Physicians.

Royal College of Physicians. (2007) National Sentinel Stroke Audit Report. *Phase I (Organisational Audit) 2006 Phase II (Clinical Audit) 2006: Prepared on Behalf of the Intercollegiate Stroke Working Party.* London: Royal College of Physicians.

Royal College of Physicians. (2008a) *National Clinical Guidelines for Stroke,* 3rd ed. London: Royal College of Physicians.

Royal College of Physicians. (2008b) *National Sentinel Stroke Audit Phase I (Organisational Audit) 2008: Report for England, Wales and Northern Ireland.* London: Royal College of Physicians.

Royal College of Physicians. (2008c) *National Sentinel Stroke Audit, Phase II (Clinical Audit) 2008: Report for England, Wales and Northern Ireland: Prepared on Behalf of the Intercollegiate Stroke Working Party.* London: Royal College of Physicians.

Royal College of Physicians. (2009) *National Sentinel Stroke Audit: Phase II (Clinical Audit) 2008: Prepared on Behalf of the Intercollegiate Stroke Working Party.* London: Royal College of Physicians.

Rudd, A. G., Hoffman, A., Irwin, P., Lowe, D. and Pearson, M. G. (2005) Stroke unit care and outcome: Results from the 2001 National Sentinel Audit of Stroke (England, Wales, and Northern Ireland). *Stroke, 36,* 103–106.

Rudd, A. G., Irwin, P., Rutledge, Z., Lowe, D., Wade, D. T. and Pearson, M. (2001) Regional variations in stroke care in England, Wales and Northern Ireland: Results from the National Sentinel Audit of stroke. *Clinical Rehabilitation, 15,* 562–572.

Rusconi, E., Pinel, P., Dehaene, S. and Kleinschmidt, A. (2010) The enigma of Gerstmann's syndrome revisited: A telling tale of the vicissitudes of neuropsychology. *Brain, 133,* 320–332.

Rusconi, M. L., Meinecke, C., Sbrissa, P. and Bernardini, B. (2002) Different cognitive trainings in the rehabilitation of visuo-spatial neglect. *Europa Medicophysica, 38,* 159–166.

Rustad, R. A., DeGroot, T. L., Jungkunz, M. L., Freeberg, K. S., Borowick, G. and Wanttie, A. M. (1993) *The Cognitive Assessment of Minnesota.* Tucson, AZ: Therapy SkillBuilders.

Rutman, D. and Silberfeld, M. (1992) A preliminary report on the discrepancy between clinical and test evaluations of competence. *Canadian Journal of Psychiatry – Revue Canadienne De Psychiatrie, 37,* 634–639.

Rybarczyk, B., Winemiller, D. R., Lazarus, L. W., Haut, A. and Hartman, C. (1996) Validation of a depression screeening measure for stroke inpatients. *American Journal of Geriatric Psychiatry, 4,* 131–139.

Rycroft-Malone, J., Kitson, A., Harvey, G., McCormack, B., Seers, K., Titchen, A., *et al.* (2002) Ingredients for change: Revisiting a conceptual framework. *Quality & Safety in Health Care*, 11, 174–180.

Sabari, J. S., Meisler, J. and Silver, E. (2000) Reflections upon rehabilitation by members of a community based stroke club. *Disability and Rehabilitation*, 22, 330–336.

Sabate, E. (2003) *Adherence to Long-Term Therapies: Evidence for Action.* Geneva: World Health Organization.

Sabel, B. A. and Kasten, E. (2000) Restoration of vision by training of residual functions. *Current Opinion in Ophthalmology*, 11, 430–436.

Sabel, B. A. and Kasten, E. (2001) Rehabilitation of visual disorders after brain injury. *Neuropsychologia*, 39, 651–651.

Sabel, B. A., Kenkel, S. and Kasten, E. (2005) Vision restoration therapy. *British Journal of Ophthalmology*, 89, 522–524.

Sacco, S., Sara, M., Pistoia, F., Conson, M., Albertini, G. and Carolei, A. (2008) Management of pathologic laughter and crying in patients with locked-in syndrome: A report of 4 cases. *Archives of Physical Medicine and Rehabilitation*, 89, 775–778.

Sackley, C., Brittle, N., Patel, S., Ellins, J., Scott, M., Wright, C., *et al.* (2008) The prevalence of joint contractures, pressure sores, painful shoulder, other pain, falls, and depression in the year after a severely disabling stroke. *Stroke*, 39, 3329–3334.

Sackley, C. M., Hoppitt, T. J. and Cardoso, K. (2006) An investigation into the utility of the Stroke Aphasic Depression Questionnaire (SADQ) in care home settings. *Clinical Rehabilitation*, 20, 598–602.

Saeki, S. (2000) Disability management after stroke: its medical aspects for workplace accommodation. *Disability and Rehabilitation*, 22, 578–582.

Saeki, S. and Hachisuka, K. (2004) The association between stroke location and return to work after first stroke. *Journal of Stroke Cerebrovascular Disorders*, 13, 160–163.

Saeki, S., Ogata, H., Okubo, T., Takahashi, K. and Hoshuyama, T. (1995) Return to work after stroke: A follow-up study. *Stroke*, 26, 399–401.

Saeki, S. and Toyonaga, T. (2010) Determinants of early return to work after first stroke in Japan. *Journal of Rehabilitation Medicine*, 42, 254–258.

Saffran, E. M. (2000a) Aphasia and the relationship of language and brain. *Seminars in Neurology*, 20, 409–418.

Saffran, E. M. (2000b) The organization of semantic memory: In support of a distributed model. *Brain and Language*, 71 (1), 204–212.

Sagen, U., Finset, A., Moum, T., Morland, T., Vik, T. G., Nagy, T., *et al.* (2010) Early detection of patients at risk for anxiety, depression and apathy after stroke. *General Hospital Psychiatry*, 32, 80–85.

Sahraie, A., Trevethan, C. T., Weiskrantz, L., Olson, J., MacLeod, M. J., Murray, A. D., *et al.* (2003) Spatial channels of visual processing in cortical blindness. *European Journal of Neuroscience*, 18, 1189–1196.

Saini, M. (2009) A meta-analysis of the psychological treatment of anger: Developing guidelines for evidence-based practice. *Journal of the American Academy of Psychiatry and the Law*, 37, 473–488.

Saka, O., McGuire, A. and Wolfe, C. (2009) Cost of stroke in the United Kingdom. *Age and Ageing*, 38, 27–32.

Saka, O., Serra, V., Samyshkin, Y., McGuire, A. and Wolfe, C. C. D. A. (2009) Cost-effectiveness of stroke unit care followed by early supported discharge. *Stroke*, 40, 24–29.

Salaycik, K., Kelly-Hayes, M., Beiser, A., Nguyen, A., Brady, S., Kase, C., *et al.* (2007) Depressive symptoms and risk of stroke: The Framingham Study. *Stroke, 38,* 16–21.

Salbach, N. M., Mayo, N. E., Hanley, J. A., Richards, C. L. and Wood-Dauphinee, S. (2006) Psychometric evaluation of the original and Canadian French version of the activities-specific balance scale among people with stroke. *Archives of Physical Medicine and Rehabilitation, 87,* 1597–1604.

Salkovskis, P. M. (1989) Somatic Problems. In K. Hawton, P. M. Salkovskis, J. Kirk & D. M. Clark (eds), Cognitive Behavioural Therapy for Psychiatric Problems: A Practical Guide (pp. 235–276). Oxford: Oxford University Press.

Salter, K., Bhogal, S. K., Foley, N., Jutai, J. and Teasell, R. (2007) The assessment of poststroke depression. *Topics in Stroke Rehabilitation, 14,* 1–24.

Salter, K., Jutai, J., Foley, N., Hellings, C. and Teasell, R. (2006) Identification of aphasia post stroke: A review of screening assessment tools. *Brain Injury, 20,* 559–568.

Sampson, M. J., Kinderman, P., Watts, S. and Sembi, S. (2003) Psychopathology and autobiographical memory in stroke and non-stroke hospitalized patients. *International Journal of Geriatric Psychiatry, 18,* 23–32.

Samsa, G., Cohen, S., Goldstein, L., Bonito, A., Duncan, P., Enarson, C., *et al.* (1997) Knowledge of risk among patients at increased risk for stroke. *Stroke, 28,* 916–921.

Samuel, C., Louis-Dreyfus, A., Kaschel, R., Makiela, E., Troubat, M., Anselmi, N., *et al.* (2000) Rehabilitation of very severe unilateral neglect by visuo-spatio-motor cueing: Two single case studies. *Neuropsychological Rehabilitation, 10,* 385–399.

Samuelsson, S-M. (2005) Physicians' control of driving after stroke attacks. *Tidsskrift for den Norske Lægeforening, 125,* 2610–2612.

Sandberg, J. and Eriksson, H. (2009) From alert commander to passive spectator: Older male carers' experience of receiving formal support. *International Journal of Older People Nursing, 4,* 33–40.

Santos, C. O., Caeiro, L., Ferro, J. M., Albuquerque, R. and Figueira, M. L. (2006) Anger, hostility and aggression in the first days of acute stroke. *European Journal of Neurology, 13,* 351–358.

Santos, M., Kovari, E., Gold, G., Bozikas, V. P., Hof, P.R., Bouras, C. and Giannako-poulos, P. (2009a) The neuroanatomical model of post-stroke depression: Towards a change of focus? *Journal of the Neurological Sciences, 283,* 158–162.

Santos, M., Gold, G., Kovari, E., Herrmann, F. R., Bozikas, V. P., Bouras, C., *et al.* (2009b) Differential impact of lacunes and microvascular lesions on poststroke depression. *Stroke, 40,* 3557–3562.

Sappok, T., Faulstich, A., Stuckert, E., Kruck, H., Marx, P. and Koennecke, H. C. (2001) Compliance with secondary prevention of ischemic stroke: A prospective evaluation. *Stroke, 32,* 1884–1889.

Sarkamo, T., Tervaniemi, M., Laitinen, S., Forsblom, A., Soinila, S., Mikkonen, M., *et al.* (2008) Music listening enhances cognitive recovery and mood after middle cerebral artery stroke. *Brain, 131,* 866–876.

Sarno, M. T. (1969) *The Functional Communication Profile Manual of Directions.* New York: Institute of Rehabilitation Medicine, New York University Medical Center.

Saunders, D. H., Greig, C. A., Mead, G. E. and Young, A. (2009) Physical fitness training for stroke patients. *Cochrane Database of Systematic Reviews* (4), CD003316.

Saunders, D. H., Greig, C. A., Young, A. and Mead, G. E. (2010) Physical fitness training for patients with stroke: An updated review. *Stroke, 41,* 160–161.

Saxena, S. K., Koh, G. C. H., Ng, T. P., Fong, N. P. and Yong, D. (2007) Determinants of length of stay during post-stroke rehabilitation in community hospitals *Singapore Medical Journal 48,* 400–407.

Saxton, J. A., Ratcliff, G., Dodge, H., Pandav, R., Baddeley, A. D. and Ganguli, M. (2001) Speed and Capacity of Language Processing Test: Normative data from an older American community-dwelling sample. *Applied Neuropsychology, 8*, 193–203.

Say, R., Murtagh, M. and Thomson, R. (2006) Patients' preference for involvement in medical decision making: A narrative review. *Patient Education and Counseling, 60*, 102–114.

Sayers, G. M., Barratt, D., Gothard, C., Onnie, C., Perera, S. and Schulman, D. (2001) The value of taking an 'ethics history'. *Journal of Medical Ethics, 27*, 114–117.

Schanke, A. K. and Sundet, K. (2000) Comprehensive driving assessment: Neuropsychological testing and on-road evaluation of brain injured patients. *Scandanavian Journal of Psychology, 41*, 113–121.

Scheffer, A. C., Schuurmans, M. J., van Dijk, N., Van Der Hooft, T. and De Rooij, S. E. (2008) Fear of falling: Measurement strategy, prevalence, risk factors and consequences among older persons. *Age and Ageing, 37*, 19–24.

Schiff, R., Rajkumar, C. and Bulpitt, C. (2000) Views of elderly people on living wills: Interview study. *British Medical Journal, 320*, 1640–1641.

Schiff, R., Sacares, P., Snook, J., Rajkumar, C. and Bulpitt, C. J. (2006) Living wills and the Mental Capacity Act: A postal questionnaire survey of UK geriatricians. *Age and Ageing, 35*, 116–121.

Schindler, I., Kerkhoff, G., Karnath, H. O., Keller, I. and Goldenberg, G. (2002) Neck muscle vibration induces lasting recovery in spatial neglect. *Journal of Neurology Neurosurgery and Psychiatry, 73*, 412–419.

Schmid, A. A. and Rittman, M. (2007) Fear of falling: An emerging issue after stroke. *Topics in Stroke Rehabilitation, 14*, 46–55.

Schneider, A. T., Pancioli, A. M., Khoury, J. C., Rademacher, E., Tuchfarber, A., Miller, R., *et al.* (2003) Trends in community knowledge of the warning signs and risk factors for stroke. *Journal of the American Medical Assocation, 289*, 343–346.

Schoettke, H. (1997) Rehabilitation von Aufmerksamkeits-störungen nach einem Schlaganfall–Effektivität eines verhaltensmedizinischneuropsychologischen Aufmerksamkeitstrainings. *Verhaltenstherapie, 7*, 21–33.

Schofield, T. M. and Leff, A. P. (2009) Rehabilitation of hemianopia. *Current Opinion in Neurology, 22*, 36–40.

Scholte op Reimer, W. J., de Haan, R. J., Limburg, M. and van den Bos, G. A. (1996) Patients' satisfaction with care after stroke: Relation with characteristics of patients and care. *Quality in Health Care, 5*, 144–150.

Scholte op Reimer, W. J. M., de Haan, R. J., Rijnders, P. T., Limburg, M. and van den Bos, G. A. (1998) The burden of caregiving in partners of long-term stroke survivors. *Stroke, 29*, 1605–1611.

Scholz, U., Keller, R. and Perren, S. (2009) Predicting behavioral intentions and physical exercise: A test of the health action process approach at the intrapersonal level. *Health Psychology, 28*, 702–708.

Schramke, C. J., Stowe, R. M., Ratcliff, G., Goldstein, G. and Condray, R. (1998) Poststroke depression and anxiety: Different assessment methods result in variations in incidence and severity estimates. *Journal of Clinical and Experimental Neuropsychology, 20*, 723–737.

Schreurs, K. M. G. and de Ridder, D. T. D. (1997) Integration of coping and social support perspectives: Implications for the study of adaptation to chronic disease. *Clinical Psychology Review, 17*, 89–112.

Schreurs, K. M. G., de Ridder, D. T. D. and Bensing, J. M. (2002) Fatigue in multiple sclerosis: Reciprocal relationships with physical disabilities and depression. *Journal of Psychosomatic Research, 53,* 775–781.

Schroder, A., Wist, E. R. and Homberg, V. (2008) TENS and optokinetic stimulation in neglect therapy after cerebrovascular accident: A randomized controlled study. *European Journal of Neurology, 15,* 922–927.

Schubert, D. S., Burns, R., Paras, W. and Sioson, E. (1992) Increase of medical hospital length of stay by depression in stroke and amputation patients: A pilot study. *Psychotherapy & Psychosomatics, 57,* 61–66.

Schuell, H. (1965) *Minnesota Test for Differential Diagnosis of Aphasia.* Minneapolis: University of Minnesota Press.

Schulz, C. H. (1994) Helping factors in a peer developed support group for persons with head injury, part 2: Survivor interview perspective. *The American Journal of Occupational Therapy, 48,* 305–309.

Schwamm, L., Fonarow, G., Reeves, M., Pan, W., Frankel, M., Smith, E., *et al.* (2009) Get With the Guidelines-Stroke is associated with sustained improvement in care for patients hospitalized with acute stroke or transient ischemic attack. *Circulation, 119,* 107–115.

Schwamm, L. H., Pancioli, A., Acker, J. E., Goldstein, L. B., Zorowitz, R. D., Shephard, T. J., *et al.* (2005) Recommendations for the establishment of stroke systems of care: Recommendations from the American Stroke Association's Task Force on the Development of Stroke Systems. *Stroke, 36,* 690–703.

Schwartz, L. M., Woloshin, S., Black, W. C. and Welch, H. G. (1997) The role of numeracy in understanding the benefit of screening mammography. *Annals of internal medicine, 127,* 966–972.

Schwartzberg, S. L. (1994) Helping factors in a peer developed support group for persons with head injury, part 1: Participant observer perspective. *The American Journal of Occupational Therapy, 48,* 297–304.

Schwarzer, R. (1992) Self-efficacy in the adoption and maintenance of health behaviors: Theoretical approaches and a new model. In R. E. Schwarzer (ed), *Self-Efficacy: Thought Control of Action* (pp. 217–243). Washington, DC: Hemisphere.

Schwarzer, R., Luszczynska, A., Ziegelmann, J. P., Scholz, U. and Lippke, S. (2008) Social-cognitive predictors of physical exercise adherence: Three longitudinal studies in rehabilitation. *Health Psychology, 27,* 54–63.

Schweizer, T. A., Levine, B., Rewilak, D., O'Connor, C., Turner, G., Alexander, M. P., *et al.* (2008) Rehabilitation of executive functioning after focal damage to the cerebellum. *Neurorehabilitation and Neural Repair, 22,* 72–77.

Scogin, F. and McElreath, L. (1994) Efficacy of psychosocial treatments for geriatric depression: A quantitative review. *Journal of Consulting and Clinical Psychology, 62,* 69–74.

Scogin, F., Welsh, D., Hanson, A., Stump, J. and Coates, A. (2005) Evidence-based psychotherapies for depression in older adults. *Clinical Psychology-Science and Practice, 12,* 222–237.

Scott, S. and Barton, J. (2010) Psychological approaches to working with people in the early stages of recovery. In S. E. Brumfitt (ed), *Psychological Well-Being and Acquired Communication Impairments.* Chichester: Wiley.

Scottish Intercollegiate Guideline Network. (2003) *Management of Patients with Stroke: Rehabilitation, Prevention and Management of Complications, and Discharge Planning: A National Clinical Guideline.* Edinburgh: Royal College of Physicians.

Secretary of State for Health. (2007a) *Our Health, Our Care, Our Say: A New Direction for Community Services.* Government White Paper. London: TSO.

Secretary of State for Health. (2007b) *Trust, Assurance and Safety: The Regulation of Health Professionals in the 21st Century.* Government White Paper. London: TSO.

Seddon, D., Robinson, C. and Perry, J. (2010) Unified assessment: Policy, implementation and practice. *British Journal of Social Work, 40,* 207–225.

Seddon, D., Robinson, C., Reeves, C., Tommis, Y., Woods, B. and Russell, I. (2007) In their own right: Translating the policy of carer assessment into practice. *British Journal of Social Work, 37,* 1335–1352.

Seenan, P., Long, M. and Langhorne, P. (2007) Stroke units in their natural habitat: Systematic review of observational studies. *Stroke, 38,* 1886–1892.

Sellal, F., Wolff, V. and Marescaux, C. (2004) The cognitive pattern of vascular dementia and its assessment. *Seminars in Cerebrovascular Diseases and Stroke, 4,* 79–86.

Sellars, C., Hughes, T. and Langhorne, P. (2005) Speech and language therapy for dysarthria due to non-progressive brain damage. *Cochrane Database of Systematic Reviews* (3), CD002088.

Selwyn, A. P. (2007) Weight reduction and cardiovascular and metabolic disease prevention: Clinical trial update. *American Journal of Cardiology, 100,* S33–S37.

Sembi, S., Tarrier, N., O'Neill, P., Burns, A. and Faragher, B. (1998) Does post-traumatic stress disorder occur after stroke: A preliminary study. *International Journal of Geriatric Psychiatry, 13,* 315–322.

Sentinella, J., Sexton, B. and Inwood, C. M. (2005) *Inter-Rater Reliability of the Stroke Drivers' Screening Assessment.* Published Project Report PPR062. Crowthorne, UK: Transport Research Laboratory.

Shale, A. (2004) Beyond common sense. *RCSLT Bulletin 621,* 14–15.

Shallice, T. and Burgess, P. (1991) Higher-order cognitive impairments and frontal lobe lesions in man. In H. S. Levin, H. M. Eisenberg & A. L. Benton (eds), *Frontal Lobe Function and Dysfunction.* New York: Oxford University Press.

Shalowitz, D., Garrett-Mayer, E. and Wendler, D. (2006) The accuracy of surrogate decision makers: A systematic review. *Archives of Internal Medicine, 166,* 493–497.

Sharpe, M., Hawton, K., House, A., Molyneux, A., Sandercock, P., Bamford, J., *et al.* (1990) Mood disorders in long-term survivors of stroke: Associations with brain lesion location and volume. *Psychological Medicine, 20,* 815–828.

Sheikh, J. I. and Yesavage, J. A. (1986) Geriatric Depression Scale: Recent evidence and development of a shorter version. *Clinical Gerontology, 5,* 165–173.

Shewan, C. M. and Kertesz, A. (1984) Effects of speech and language treatment on recovery from aphasia. *Brain and Language, 23,* 272–299.

Shinar, D., Gross, C. R., Price, T. R., Banko, M., Bolduc, P. L. and Robinson, R. G. (1986) Screening for depression in stroke patients: The reliability and validity of the Center for Epidemiologic Studies Depression Scale. *Stroke, 17,* 241–245.

Silberfeld, M. and Checkland, D. (1999) Faulty judgment, expert opinion, and decision-making capacity. *Theoretical Medicine and Bioethics, 20,* 377–393.

Silver, F., Rubini, F., Black, D. and Hodgson, C. S. (2003) Advertising strategies to increase public knowledge of the warning signs of stroke. *Stroke, 34,* 1965–1968.

Simon, C. and Kumar, S. (2002) Stroke patients' carers' views of formal community support. *British Journal of Community Nursing, 7,* 158–163.

Simons, L., McCallum, J., Friedlander, Y. and Simons, J. (1998) Risk factors for ischemic stroke: Dubbo Study of the elderly. *Stroke, 29,* 1341.

Simpson, J. (1998) *Touching the Void.* London: Vintage.

Singh, A., Herrmann, N. and Black, S. E. (1998) The importance of lesion location in poststroke depression: A critical review. *Canadian Journal of Psychiatry*, *43*, 921–927.

Sinnett, S., Juncadella, M., Rafal, R., Azanon, E. and Soto-Faraco, S. (2007) A dissociation between visual and auditory hemi-inattention: Evidence from temporal order judgements. *Neuropsychologia*, *45*, 552–560.

Sisson, R. (1998) Life after a stroke: Coping with change. *Rehabilitation Nursing*, *23*, 198–203.

Sitzia, J. (1999) How valid and reliable are patient satisfaction data? *An analysis of 195 studies. International Journal for Quality in Health Care*, *11*, 319–328.

Sitzia, J. and Wood, N. (1997) Patient satisfaction: A review of issues and concepts. *Social Science & Medicine*, *45*, 1829–1843.

Sivan, A. B. (1992) *Benton Visual Retention Test*, 5th ed. San Antonio, TX: Psychological Corporation.

Skinner, B. F. (1953) *Science and Human Behavior*. New York: Macmillan.

Skinner, C., Wirz, S., Thompson, I. and Davidson, J. (1984) *The Edinburgh Functional Communication Profile*. Oxford: Winslow Press.

Small, S. L., Flores, D. K. and Noll, D. C. (1998) Different neural circuits subserve reading before and after therapy for acquired dyslexia. *Brain and Language*, *62*, 298–308.

Smania, N., Aglioti, S. M., Giradi, F., Tinazzi, S. P. M., Fiaschi, A., Consentino, A., *et al.* (2006) Rehabilitation of limb apraxia improves daily life activites in patients with stroke. *Neurology*, *67*, 2050–2052.

Smania, N., Girardi, F., Domenciali, C., Lora, E. and Aglioti, S. (2000) The rehabilitation of limb apraxia: A study in left brain damaged patients. *Archives of Physical Medicine and Rehabilitation*, *81*, 379–388.

Smith, C. A. and Lazarus, R. S. (1993) Appraisal components, core relational themes and the emotions. *Cognition & Emotion*, *7*, 233–269.

Smith, C. F. and Wing, R. R. (2000) New directions in behavioral weight-loss programs. *Diabetes Spectrum*, *13*, 142–148.

Smith, J., Forster, A., House, A., Knapp, P., Wright, J. J. and Young, J. (2008) Information provision for stroke patients and their caregivers. *Cochrane Database of Systematic Reviews* (2), CD001919.

Smith, J., Forster, A. and Young, J. (2009) Cochrane review: Information provision for stroke patients and their caregivers. *Clinical Rehabilitation*, *23*, 195–206.

Smith, L. N., Lawrence, M., Kerr, S. M., Langhorne, P. and Lees, K. R. (2004) Informal carers' experience of caring for stroke survivors. *Journal of Advanced Nursing*, *46*, 235–244.

Smith-Arena, L., Edelstein, L. and Rabadi, M. H. (2006) Predictors of a successful driver evaluation in stroke patients after discharge based on an acute rehabilitation hospital evaluation. *American Journal of Physical Medicine & Rehabilitation*, *85*, 44–52.

Snaith, R. P., Ahmed, S. N., Mehta, S. and Hamilton, M. (1971) Assessment of the severity of primary depressive illness. *Psychological Medicine*, *1*, 143–149.

Snaphaan, L. and de Leeuw, F. E. (2007) Poststroke memory function in nondemented patients: A systematic review on frequency and neuroimaging correlates. *Stroke*, *38*, 198–203.

Snaphaan, L., van der Werf, S., Kanselaar, K. and de Leeuw, F. (2009) Post-stroke depressive symptoms are associated with post-stroke characteristics. *Cerebrovascular Diseases*, *28*, 551–557.

Sneeuw, K. C. A., Aaronson, N. K., deHaan, R. J. and Limburg, M. (1997) Assessing quality of life after stroke: The value and limitations of proxy ratings. *Stroke*, *28*, 1541–1549.

Soderstrom, S. T., Pettersson, R. P. and Leppert, J. (2006) Prediction of driving ability after stroke and the effect of behind-the-wheel training. *Scandinavian Journal of Psychology*, *47*, 419–429.

Sommerfeld, D., Eek, E., Svensson, A., Holmqvist, L. and von Arbin, M. (2004) Spasticity after stroke: Its occurrence and association with motor impairments and activity limitations. *Stroke*, *35*, 134–139.

Song, Y., Sung, J., Smith, G. and Ebrahim, S. (2004) Body mass index and ischemic and hemorrhagic stroke: A prospective study in Korean men. *Stroke*, *35*, 831–836.

Sonnenblick, M., Friedlander, Y. and Steinberg, A. (1993) Dissociation between the wishes of terminally ill parents and decisions by their offspring. *Journal of the American Geriatrics Society*, *41*, 599–604.

Soo, C. and Tate, R. (2007) Psychological treatment for anxiety in people with traumatic brain injury [Review]. *Cochrane Database of Systematic Reviews* (3), CD005239.

Spalletta, G., Guida, G., De Angelis, D. and Caltagirone, C. (2002) Predictors of cognitive level and depression severity are different in patients with left and right hemispheric stroke within the first year of illness. *Journal of Neurology*, *249*, 1541–1551.

Spalletta, G., Ripa, A. and Caltagirone, C. (2005) Symptom profile of DSM-IV major and minor depressive disorders in first-ever stroke patients. *American Journal of Geriatric Psychiatry*, *13*, 108–115.

Spencer, K. A., Tompkins, C. A. and Schulz, R. (1997) Assessment of depression in patients with brain pathology: The case of stroke. *Psychological Bulletin*, *122*, 132–152.

Spitzer, R. L., Kroenke, K. and Williams, J. B. W. (1999) Validation and utility of a self-report version of PRIME-MD: The PHQ primary care study. *Journal of the American Medical Association*, *282*, 1737–1744.

Spitzer, R. L., Williams, J. B. W., Gibbon, M. and First, M. B. (1992) The structured clinical interview for DSM-III-R (SCID) .1. History, rationale and description. *Archives of General Psychiatry*, *49*, 624–629.

Spivak, B., Trottern, S. F., Mark, M., Bleich, A. and Weizman, A. (1992) Acute transient stress induced hallucinations in soldiers. *British Journal of Psychiatry*, *160*, 412–414.

Spreen, O. and Benton, A. L. (1977) *Neurosensory Center Comprehensive Examination for Aphasia (NCCEA)*. Victoria, BC: University of Victoria Neuropsychology Laboratory.

Srikanth, V., Thrift, A. G., Fryer, J. L., Saling, M. M., Dewey, H. M., Sturm, J. W., *et al.* (2006) The validity of brief screening cognitive instruments in the diagnosis of cognitive impairment and dementia after first-ever stroke. *International Psychogeriatrics*, *18*, 295–305.

Srivastava, A., Taly, A. B., Gupta, A., Murali, T., Noone, M. L., Thirthahalli, J., *et al.* (2008) Stroke with supernumerary phantom limb: Case study, review of literature and pathogenesis. *Acta Neuropsychiatrica*, *20*, 256–264.

Staekenborg, S. S., Su, T., van Straaten, E. C. W., Lane, R., Scheltens, P., Barkhof, F., *et al.* (2010) Behavioural and psychological symptoms in vascular dementia: Differences between small- and large-vessel disease. *Journal of Neurology Neurosurgery and Psychiatry*, *81*, 547–551.

Staniszewska, S. H. and Henderson, L. (2005) Patients' evaluations of the quality of care: Influencing factors and the importance of engagement. *Journal of Advanced Nursing*, *49*, 530–537.

Stanley, M. A., Diefenbach, G. J. and Hopko, D. R. (2004) Cognitive behavioral treatment for older adults with generalized anxiety disorder: A therapist manual for primary care settings. *Behavior Modification*, *28*, 73–117.

Stapleton, T., Ashburn, A. and Stack, E. (2001) A pilot study of attention deficits, balance control and falls in the subacute stage following stroke. *Clinical Rehabilitation*, *15*, 437–444.

Starkstein, S. E., Fedoroff, J. P., Price, T. R., Leigurda, R. S. and Robinson, R. G. (1993) Catastrophic reaction after cerebrovascular lesions: Frequency, correlates and validation of a scale. *Journal of Neuropsychiatry and Clinical Neuroscience*, *5*, 189–194.

Staub, F. and Bogousslavsky, J. (2001) Fatigue after stroke: A major but neglected issue. *Cerebrovascular Diseases*, *12*, 75–81.

Stein, D. J., Ipser, J. C. and Seedat, S. (2006) Pharmacotherapy for post traumatic stress disorder (PTSD). *Cochrane Database of Systematic Reviews* (1), CD002795.

Stenager, E. N., Madsen, C., Stenager, E. and Boldsen, J. (1998) Suicide in patients with stroke: Epidemiological study. *British Medical Journal*, *316* (7139), 1206–1206.

Stephen, M. (2008) *Diary of a Stroke*. London: Psychology New Press.

Stephens, S., Kenny, R. A., Rowan, E., Allan, L., Kalaria, R. N., Bradbury, M., *et al.* (2004) Neuropsychological characteristics of mild vascular cognitive impairment and dementia after stroke. *International Journal of Geriatric Psychiatry*, *19*, 1053–1057.

Stern, R. A. (1997) *Visual Analog Mood Scales Professional Manual*. Odessa, FL: Psychological Assessment Resources.

Stern, R. A., Javorsky, D. J., Singer, E. A., Harris, N. G., Somerville, J. A., Duke, L. M., *et al.* (1999) *The Boston Qualitative Scoring System for the Rey-Osterreith Complex Figure*. Odessa, FL: Psychological Assessment Resources.

Stern, R. A. and White, T. (2003) The Neuropsychological Assessment Battery (NAB): development and psychometric properties [Meeting abstract]. *Archives of Clinical Neuropsychology*, *18*, 805–805.

Stewart, J. A., Dundas, R., Howard, R. S., Rudd, A. G. and Wolfe, C. D. A. (1999) Ethnic differences in incidence of stroke: Prospective study with stroke register. *British Medical Journal*, *318*, 967–971.

Stewart, M. J., Doble, S., Hart, G., Langille, L. and MacPherson, K. (1998) Peer visitor support for family caregivers of seniors with stroke. *Canadian Journal of Nursing Research*, *30*, 87–117.

Stone, J., Townend, E., Kwan, J., Haga, K., Dennis, M. S. and Sharpe, M. (2004) Personality change after stroke: Some preliminary observations. *Journal of Neurology Neurosurgery and Psychiatry*, *75*, 1708–1713.

Stone, S. D. (2005) Reactions to invisible disability: The experiences of young women survivors of hemorrhagic stroke. *Disability and Rehabilitation*, *27*, 293–304.

Stone, S. D. (2007) Patient concerns posthaemorrhagic stroke: A study of the Internet narratives of patients with ruptured arteriovenous malformation. *Journal of Clinical Nursing*, *16*, 289–297.

Stone, S. P., Halligan, P. W. and Greenwood, R. J. (1993) The incidence of neglect phenomena and related disorders in patients with an acute right or left hemisphere stroke. *Age and Ageing*, *22*, 46–52.

Strachowski, D., Khaylis, A., Bonrad, A., Neri, E., Spiegel, D. and Taylor, C. B. (2008) The effects of cognitive behavior therapy on depression in older patients with cardiovascular risk. *Depression and Anxiety*, 25, E1–E10.

Strauss, E., Sherman, E. M. S. and Spreen, O. (2006) *A Compendium of Neuropsychological Tests: Administration, Norms, and Commentary.* New York: Oxford University Press.

Stroebe, W., Zech, E., Stroebe, M. S. and Abakoumkin, G. (2005) Does social support help in bereavement? *Journal of Social and Clinical Psychology*, 24, 1030–1050.

Stroke Alliance for Europe (SAFE) (2009) Stories from Stroke Survivors, Their Carers and Families. http://www.safestroke.org/Facts/StrokeStories/tabid/373/Default.aspx

Stroke Association. (2001) *Psychological Changes after Stroke.* London: Stroke Association.

Stroke Association. (2009) Information/It Happened to Me. http://www.stroke.org.uk/information/it_happened_to_me/index.html

Stroke Association/British Heart Foundation. (2009) *Stroke Statistics 2009 Edition.* London: Stroke Association/British Heart Foundation.

Stroke Unit Trialists Collaboration. (1999) Organised inpatient (stroke unit) care for stroke: Cochrane review. *The Cochrane Library* (1).

Stroke Unit Trialists' Collaboration. (1997) Collaborative systematic review of the randomized trials of organized inpatient (stroke unit) care after stroke. *British Medical Journal*, 314, 1157–1159.

Stroke Unit Trialists' Collaboration. (2007) Organised inpatient (stroke unit) care for stroke. *Cochrane Database of Systematic Reviews* (4).

Strudwick, A. and Morris, R. (2010) A qualitative study exploring the experiences of African-Caribbean informal stroke carers in the UK. *Clinical Rehabilitation*, 24, 159–167.

Sturm, J. W., Donnan, G. A., Dewey, H. M., Macdonell, R. A. L., Gilligan, A. K., Srikanth, V., et al. (2004a) Quality of life after stroke: The North East Melbourne Stroke Incidence Study (NEMESIS). *Stroke*, 35, 2340–2345.

Sturm, J. W., Donnan, G. A., Dewey, H. M., Macdonell, R. A. L., Gilligan, A. K. and Thrift, A. G. (2004b) Determinants of handicap after stroke: The North East Melbourne Stroke Incidence Study (NEMESIS). *Stroke*, 35, 715–720.

Sturm, W., Thimm, A., Kuest, J., Karbe, H. and Fink, G. R. (2006) Alertness-training in neglect: Behavioral and imaging results. *Restorative Neurology and Neuroscience*, 24, 371–384.

Sturm, W. and Willmes, K. (1991) Efficacy of a reaction training on various attentional and cognitive functions in stroke patients. *Neuropsychological Rehabilitation*, 1, 259–280.

Sturm, W., Wilmes, K. and Orgass, B. (1997) Do specific attention deficits need specific training? *Neuropsychological Rehabilitation*, 7, 81–103.

Sturman, E. D. (2005) The capacity to consent to treatment and research: A review of standardized assessment tools. *Clinical Psychology Review*, 25, 954–974.

Stuss, D. T. and Alexander, M. P. (2007) Is there a dysexecutive syndrome? *Philosophical Transactions of the Royal Society of London B: Biological Sciences*, 362, 901–915.

Stuss, D. T. and Knight, R. T. (2002) *Principles of Frontal Lobe Function.* Oxford: Oxford University Press.

Sugarman, J., McCrory, D. C. and Hubal, R. C. (1998) Getting meaningful informed consent from older adults: A structured literature review of empirical research. *Journal of the American Geriatrics Society*, 46, 517–524.

Suk, S. H., Sacco, R. L., Boden-Albala, B., Cheun, J. F., Pittman, J. G., Elkind, M. S., et al. (2003) Abdominal obesity and risk of ischemic stroke: The Northern Manhattan Stroke Study. *Stroke, 34,* 1586–1592.

Sullivan, K. (2004) Neuropsychological assessment of mental capacity. *Neuropsychology Review, 14,* 131–142.

Sullivan, K. A. and Katajamaki, A. (2009a) Stroke education: Promising effects on the health beliefs of those at risk. *Topics in Stroke Rehabilitation, 16,* 377–387.

Sullivan, K. A. and Katajamaki, A. (2009b) Stroke education: Retention effects in those at low- and high-risk of stroke. *Patient Education and Counseling, 74,* 205–212.

Sullivan, K. A., White, K. M., Young, R. M., Chang, A., Roos, C. and Scott, C. (2008a) Predictors of intention to reduce stroke risk among people at risk of stroke: An application of an extended health belief model. *Rehabilitation Psychology 53,* 505–512.

Sullivan, K. A., White, K. M., Young, R. M., Scott, C. and Mulgrew, K. (2008b) Developing a stroke intervention program: What do people at risk of stroke want? *Patient Education and Counseling, 70,* 126–134.

Sullivan, K. A., White, K. M., Young, R. M. and Scott, C. (2009) Predicting behaviour to reduce stroke risk in at-risk populations: The role of beliefs. *International Journal of Therapy and Rehabilitation, 16,* 499–496.

Sundell, L., Salomaa, V., Vartiainen, E., Poikolainen, K. and Laatikainen, T. (2008) Increased stroke risk is related to a binge drinking habit. *Stroke, 39,* 3179–3184.

Sunderland, A. (2000) Recovery of ipsilateral dexterity after stroke. *Stroke, 31,* 430–433.

Sunderland, A. (2007) Impaired imitation of meaningless gestures in ideomotor apraxia: A conceptual problem not a disorder of action control? A single case investigation. *Neuropsychologia, 45,* 1621–1631.

Sunderland, A., Bowers, M. P., Sluman, S. M., Wilcock, D. J. and Ardron, M. E. (1999) Impaired dexterity of the ipsilateral hand after stroke and the relationship to cognitive deficit. *Stroke, 30,* 949–955.

Sunderland, A., Harris, J. E. and Baddeley, A. D. (1983) Do laboratory tests predict everyday memory? A neuropsychological study. *Journal of Verbal Learning and Verbal Behaviour, 22,* 341–357.

Sunderland, A. and Shinner, C. (2007) Ideomotor apraxia and functional ability. *Cortex, 43,* 359–367.

Sunderland, A. and Sluman, S. M. (2000) Ideomotor apraxia, visuomotor control and the explicit representation of posture. *Neuropsychologia, 38,* 923–934.

Sunderland, A., Tinson, D. J., Bradley, E. L., Fletcher, D., Hewer, R. L. and Wade, D. T. (1992) Enhanced physical therapy improves recovery of arm function after stroke – a randomized controlled trial. *Journal of Neurology Neurosurgery and Psychiatry, 55,* 530–535.

Sundet, K., Finset, A. and Reinvang, I. (1988) Neuropsychological predictors in stroke rehabilitation. *Journal of Clinical and Experimental Neuropsychology, 10,* 363–379.

Surtees, P. G., Wainwright, N. W., Luben, R. N., Wareham, N. J., Bingham, S. A. and Khaw, K. T. (2008) Psychological distress, major depressive disorder, and risk of stroke. *Neurology, 70,* 788–794.

Sutcliffe, L. M. and Lincoln, N. B. (1998) The assessment of depression in aphasic stroke patients: The development of the Stroke Aphasic Depression Questionnaire. *Clinical Rehabilitation, 12,* 506–513.

Sutherland, G. R. and Auer, R. N. (2006) Primary intracerebral hemorrhage. *Journal of Clinical Neuroscience*, 13, 511–517.

Sutherland, H. J., Llewellyn-Thomas, H. A., Lockwood, G. A., Tritchler, D. L. and Till, J. E. (1989) Cancer patients their desire for information and participation in treatment decisions. *Journal of the Royal Society of Medicine*, 82, 260–263.

Swain, D., Ellins, J., Coulter, A., Heron, P., Howell, E., Magee, H., *et al.* (2007) *Accessing Information about Health and Social Care Services.* Oxford: Picker Institute Europe.

Swinburn, K., Porter, G. and Howard, D. (2004) *Comprehensive Aphasia Test.* Hampshire: Psychology Press.

Syder, D., Body, R., Parker, M. and Boddy, M. (1993) *Sheffield Screening Test for Acquired Language Disorders.* Windsor, UK: NFER-Nelson.

Tajfel, H. and Turner, J. C. (1979) An integrative theory of intergroup conflict. In W. G. Austin & S. Worchel (eds), *The Social Psychology of Intergroup Relations* (pp. 94–109). Monterey, CA: Brooks-Cole.

Takatori, K., Okada, Y., Shomoto, K. and Shimada, T. (2009) Does assessing error in perceiving postural limits by testing functional reach predict likelihood of falls in hospitalised stroke patients? *Clinical Rehabilitation*, 23, 568–575.

Tang, W., Chan, S., Chiu, H., Ungvari, G., Wong, K. and Kwok, T. (2004) Emotional incontinence in Chinese stroke patients. *Journal of Neurology*, 251, 865–869.

Tang, W. K., Chen, Y. K., Lam, W. W. M., Mok, V., Wong, A., Ungvari, G. S., *et al.* (2009a) Emotional incontinence and executive function in ischemic stroke: A case-controlled study. *Journal of the International Neuropsychological Society*, 15, 62–68.

Tang, W. K., Chen, Y. K., Lu, J. Y., Mok, V. C. T., Xiang, Y. T., Ungvari, G. S., *et al.* (2009b) Microbleeds and post-stroke emotional lability. *Journal of Neurology Neurosurgery and Psychiatry*, 80, 1082–1086.

Tang, W. K., Mok, V., Chan, S. S. M., Chiu, H. F. K., Wong, K. S., Kwok, T. C. Y., *et al.* (2005) Screening of dementia in stroke patients with Lacunar infarcts: Comparison of the Mattis Dementia Rating Scale and the Mini-Mental State Examination. *Journal of Geriatric Psychiatry and Neurology*, 18, 3–7.

Tant, M. L. M., Brouwer, W. H., Cornelissen, F. W. and Kooijman, A. C. (2002) Driving and visuospatial performance in people with hemianopia. *Neuropsychological Rehabilitation*, 12, 419–437.

Tapper, J. (2006) Working with stroke from the human gives approach. *Human Givens Journal*, 13, 35–39.

Tatemichi, T. K., Desmond, D. W., Stern, Y., Paik, M., Sano, M. and Bagiella, E. (1994) Cognitive impairment after stroke: Frequency, patterns and relationship to functional abilities. *Journal of Neurology, Neurosurgery and Psychiatry*, 57, 202–207.

Taylor, M. (1965) A measure of functional communication in aphasia. *Archives of Physical and Medical Rehabilitation*, 46, 101–107.

Taylor, M. J. and Heaton, R. K. (2001) Sensitivity and specificity of WAIS-III/WMS-III demographically corrected factor scores in neuropsychological assessment. *Journal of the International Neuropsychological Society*, 7, 867–874.

te Winkel-Witlox, A. C. M., Post, M. W. M., Visser-Meily, J. M. A. and Lindeman, E. (2008) Efficient screening of cognitive dysfunction in stroke patients: Comparison between the CAMCOG and the R-CAMCOG, Mini Mental State Examination and Functional Independence Measure-cognition score. *Disability & Rehabilitation*, 30, 1386–1391.

Teasell, R. W., McRae, M. P. and Finestone, H. M. (2000) Social issues in the rehabilitation of younger stroke patients. *Archives of Physical Medicine and Rehabilitation*, *81*, 205–209.

Tedeschi, R. G. and Calhoun, L. G. (1996) The posttraumatic growth inventory: Measuring the positive legacy of trauma. *Journal of Traumatic Stress*, *9*, 455–471.

Tennstedt, S., Howland, J., Lachman, M., Peterson, E., Kasten, L. and Jette, A. (1998b) A randomized, controlled trial of a group intervention to reduce fear of falling and associated activity restriction in older adults. *Journals of Gerontology Series B: Psychological Sciences and Social Sciences*, *53*, P384–P392.

Tennstedt, S., Peterson, E., Howland, J. and Lachman, M. (1998a) *A Matter of Balance: Facilitator Training Manual*. Boston: Boston University.

Teper, E. and O'Brien, J. (2008) Vascular factors and depression. *International Journal of Geriatric Psychiatry*, *23*, 993–1000.

Tham, K. and Tegner, R. (1996) The Baking Tray Task: A test of spatial neglect. *Neuropsychological Rehabilitation*, *6*, 19–25.

Thanvi, B. and Treadwell, S. (2009) Cannabis and stroke: Is there a link? *Postgraduate Medical Journal*, *85*, 80–83.

The AGREE Collaboration. (2003) Development and validation of an international appraisal instrument for assessing the quality of clinical practice guidelines: The AGREE project. *Quality and Safety in Health Care*, *12*, 18–23.

The Scottish Government. (2000) The Adults with Incapacity Act (Scotland) 2000. Edinburgh: TSO.

The Scottish Government. (2002) *Coronary Heart Disease and Stroke Strategy for Scotland*. Edinburgh: Scottish Executive Health Department.

The Scottish Government. (2003) Mental Health (Care and Treatment) (Scotland) Act 2003, Edinburgh: TSO.

Thickpenny-Davis, K. L. and Barker-Collo, S. L. (2007) Evaluation of a structured group format memory rehabilitation program for adults following brain injury. *Journal of Head Trauma Rehabilitation*, *22*, 303–313.

Thimm, M., Fink, G. R., Kust, J., Karbe, H. and Sturm, W. (2006) Impact of alertness training on spatial neglect: A behavioural and fMRI study. *Neuropsychologia*, *44*, 1230–1246.

Thimm, M., Fink, G. R., Kst, J., Karbe, H., Wilmes, K. and Sturm, W. (2009) Recovery from hemineglect: Differential neurobiological effects of optokinetic stimulation and alertness training. *Cortex*, *45*, 850–862.

Thoits, P. A. (1986) Social support as coping assistance. *Journal of Consulting and Clinical Psychology*, *54*, 416–423.

Thomas, C. and Parry, A. (1996) Research on users' views about stroke services: Towards an empowerment research paradigm or more of the same? *Physiotherapy*, *82*, 6–12.

Thomas, R. H. and Hughes, T. A. T. (2009) 'Can I drive, doctor?' LEAN thinking may help us answer the question. *Practical Neurology*, *9*, 71–79.

Thomas, S.A., Walker, M. F., J.A.B., Haworth, H. and Lincoln, N. B. (2010) *Communication and Low Mood: A Randomised Trial*. Submiited

Thomas, S. A. and Lincoln, N. B. (2006) Factors relating to depression after stroke. *British Journal of Clinical Psychology*, *45*, 49–61.

Thomas, S. A. and Lincoln, N. B. (2008a) Predictors of emotional distress after stroke. *Stroke*, *39*, 1240–1245.

Thomas, S. A. and Lincoln, N. B. (2008b) Depression and cognitions after stroke: Validation of the Stroke Cognitions Questionnaire Revised (SCQR) *Disability and Rehabilitation, 30,* 1779–1785.

Thommessen, B., Aarsland, D., Braekhus, A., Oksengaard, A. R., Engedal, K. and Laake, K. (2002) The psychosocial burden on spouses of the elderly with stroke, dementia and Parkinson's disease. *International Journal of Geriatric Psychiatry, 17,* 78–84.

Thommessen, B., Thoresen, G. E., Bautz-Holter, E. and Laake, K. (1999) Screening by nurses for aphasia in stroke – the Ullevaal Aphasia Screening (UAS) test. *Disability and Rehabilitation, 21,* 110–115.

Thompson, S. C., Sobolew-Shibin, A., Graham, M. A. and Janigan, A. S. (1989) Psychosocial adjustment following stroke. *Social Science and Medicine, 28,* 239–247.

Tiffin, J. (1968) *Purdue Pegboard Examiner's Manual.* Rosemont, IL: London House.

Tilling, K., Kunze, K. and Beech, R. (2002) League tables for outcome of chronic disease. In C. Wolfe, C. McKevitt and A. E. Rudd (eds), *Stroke Services: Policy and Practice across Europe.* Oxford: Radcliffe Medical Press.

Tinetti, M. E. and Powell, L. (1993) Fear of falling and low self-efficacy: A case of dependence in elderly persons. *Journal of Gerontology, 48,* 35–38.

Tinetti, M. E., Richman, D. and Powell, L. (1990) Falls efficacy as a measure of fear of falling. *Journals of Gerontology. Series B: Psychological Sciences and Social Sciences, 45,* P239–P242.

Tinson, D. J. and Lincoln, N. B. (1987) Subjective memory impairment after stroke. *International Disability Studies, 9,* 6–9.

Toedter, L. J., Schall, R., Reese, C. A., Hyland, D., Berk, S. and Dunn, D. S. (1995) Psychological measures: Reliability in the assessment of stroke patients. *Archives of Physical Medicine and Rehabilitation, 76,* 719–725.

Tombaugh, T. N. (1996) *Test of Memory Malingering.* New York: Multi-Health Systems.

Towle, D. and Lincoln, N. B. (1991) Development of a questionnaire for detecting everyday problems in stroke patients with unilateral visual neglect. *Clinical Rehabilitation, 5,* 135–140.

Towle, D. and Wilsher, C. (1989) The Rivermead Behavioural Memory Test: Remembering a short route. *The British Journal of Clinical Psychology, 28,* 287–288.

Townend, B. S., Sturm, J. W., Petsoglou, C., O'Leary, B., Whyte, S. and Crimmins, D. (2007a) Perimetric homonymous visual field loss post-stroke. *Journal of Clinical Neuroscience, 14,* 754–756.

Townend, B. S., Whyte, S., Desborough, T., Crimmins, D., Markus, R., Levi, C., *et al.* (2007b) Longitudinal prevalence and determinants of early mood disorder post-stroke. *Journal of Clinical Neuroscience, 14,* 429–434.

Townend, E. (2004) *Beliefs about 'Stroke' and 'Its Effects': A Study of Their Association with Emotional Distress.* Edinburgh: University of Edinburgh.

Townend, E., Brady, M. and McLaughlan, K. (2007c) A systematic evaluation of the adaptation of depression diagnostic methods for stroke survivors who have aphasia. *Stroke, 38,* 3076–3083.

Townend, E., Tinson, D., Kwan, J. and Sharpe, M. (2010) 'Feeling sad and useless': An investigation into personal acceptance of disability and its association with depression following stroke. *Clinical Rehabilitation, 24,* 555–564.

Townsend, S. (2003) *Regaining Confidence after Stroke: A Manual for Group Leaders.* Telford, Shropshire: Telford & Wrekin PCT.

Trahan, D. E. (1997) Relationship between facial discrimination and visual neglect in patients with unilateral vascular lesions. *Archives of Clinical Neuropsychology, 12,* 57–62.

Treadwell, S. D. and Robinson, T. G. (2007) Cocaine use and stroke. *Postgraduate Medical Journal, 83* (980), 389–394.

Treger, I., Shames, J., Giaquinto, S. and Ring, H. (2007) Return to work in stroke patients. *Disability and Rehabilitation, 29,* 1397–1403.

Treisman, A. and Gelade, G. (1980) A feature-integration theory of attention. *Cognitive Psychology, 12,* 97–136.

Truelsen, T., Nielsen, N., Boysen, G. and Grønbæk, M. (2003) Self-reported stress and risk of stroke: The Copenhagen City Heart Study. *Stroke, 34,* 856–862.

Tsouna-Hadjis, E., Vemmos, K. N., Zakopoulos, N. and Stamatelopoulos, S. (2000) First-stroke recovery process: The role of family social support. *Archives of Physical Medicine and Rehabilitation, 81,* 881–887.

Tsutsumi, A., Kayaba, K., Kario, K. and Ishikawa, S. (2009) Prospective study on occupational stress and risk of stroke. *Archives Internal Medicine, 169,* 56–61.

Tulving, E. (1972) Episodic and semantic memory. In E. a. D. Tulving (ed), *Organisation of Memory* (pp. 381–403) New York: Academic Press.

Turner, S. and Whitworth, A. (2006) Conversational partner training programmes in aphasia: A review of key themes and participants' roles. *Aphasiology, 20,* 483–510.

Turner-Stokes, L., Disler, R., Shaw, A. and Williams, H. (2008) Screening for pain in patients with cognitive and communication difficulties: Evaluation of the SPIN-screen. *Clinical Medicine, 8,* 393–398.

Turner-Stokes, L. and Hassan, N. (2002) Depression after stroke: A review of the evidence base to inform the development of an integrated care pathway: Part 2: Treatment alternatives. *Clinical Rehabilitation, 169,* 248–260.

Turner-Stokes, L., Hassan, N., Pierce, K. and Clegg, F. (2002) Managing depression in brain injury rehabilitation: The use of an integrated care pathway and preliminary report of response to sertraline. *Clinical Rehabilitation, 16,* 261–268.

Turner-Stokes, L., Kalmus, M., Hirani, D. and Clegg, F. (2005) The Depression Intensity Scale Circles (DISCS): A first evaluation of a simple assessment tool for depression in the context of brain injury. *Journal of Neurology Neurosurgery and Psychiatry, 76,* 1273–1278.

Turner-Stokes, L. and MacWalter, R. (2005) Use of antidepressant medication following acquired brain injury: Concise guidance. *Clinical Medicine, 5,* 268–274.

Turton, A. J., O'Leary, K., Gabb, J., Woodward, R. and Gilchrist, I. D. (2009) A single blinded randomised controlled pilot trial of prism adaptation for improving self-care in stroke patients with neglect. *Neuropsychological Rehabilitation, 20,* 180–196.

Tymchuk, A. J., Ouslander, J. G. and Rader, N. (1986) Informing the elderly – a comparion of 4 methods. *Journal of the American Geriatrics Society, 34,* 818–822.

Tymchuk, A. J., Ouslander, J. G., Rahbar, B. and Fitten, J. (1988) Medical decision-making among elderly people in long-term care. *Gerontologist, 28,* 59–63.

Tyson, S. F. and Turner, G. (1999) The process of stroke rehabilitation: What happens and why. *Clinical Rehabilitation, 13,* 322–332.

Tzeng, H. M., Ketefian, S. and Redman, R. W. (2002) Relationship of nurses' assessment of organisational culture, job satisfaction, and patient satisfaction with nursing care. *International Journal of Nursing Studies, 39,* 79–84.

Ubel, P. A. (2002) Is information always a good thing? Helping patients make 'good' decisions. *Medical Care, 40,* 39–44.

Uchino, B. N. (2006) Social support and health: A review of physiological processes potentially underlying links to disease outcomes. *Journal of Behavioral Medicine, 29,* 377–387.

UK Forum for Stroke Training. (2009) *Stroke-Specific Education Framework.* London: Department of Health.

Ulrich, L. P. (1999) *The Patient Self-Determination Act: Meeting the Challenges in Patient Care.* Washington, DC: Georgetown University Press.

Urban, P. P., Rolke, R., Wicht, S., Keilmann, A., Stoeter, P., Hopf, H. C., *et al.* (2006) Left-hemispheric dominance for articulation: A prospective study on acute ischaemic dysarthria at different localizations. *Brain, 129,* 767–777.

Valko, P. O., Bassetti, C. L., Bloch, K. E., Held, U. and Baumann, C. R. (2008) Validation of the Fatigue Severity Scale in a Swiss cohort. *Sleep, 31,* 1601–1607.

Vallar, G. and Ronchi, R. (2006) Anosognosia for motor and sensory deficits after unilateral brain damage: A review. *Restorative Neurology and Neuroscience, 24,* 247–257.

Vallar, G. and Ronchi, R. (2009) Somatoparaphrenia: A body delusion: A review of the neuropsychological literature. *Experimental Brain Research, 192,* 533–551.

van de Port, I. G. L., Visser-Meily, A. M. A., Post, M. W. M. and Lindeman, E. (2007) Long-term outcome in children of patients after stroke. *Journal of Rehabilitation Medicine, 39,* 703–707.

van de Weg, F. B., Kuik, D. J. and Lankhorst, G. J. (1999) Post-stroke depression and functional outcome: A cohort study investigating the influence of depression on functional recovery. *Clinical Rehabilitation, 13,* 268–272.

van den Berg, E., Nys, G. M. S., Brands, A. M. A., Ruis, C., van Zandvoort, M. J. E. and Kessels, R. P. C. (2009) The Brixton Spatial Anticipation Test as a test for executive function: Validity in patient groups and norms for older adults. *Journal of the International Neuropsychological Society, 15,* 695–703.

van den Broek, M. D. (2005) Why does neurorehabilitation fail? *Journal of Head Trauma Rehabilitation, 20,* 464–473.

Van den Broek, M. D., Downes, J., Johnson, Z., Dayus, B. and Hilton, N. (2000) Evaluation of an electronic memory aid in the neuropsychological rehabilitation of prospective memory deficits. *Brain Injury, 14,* 455–462.

van der Merwe, A. (2007) Self-correction in apraxia of speech: The effect of treatment. *Aphasiology, 21,* 658–669.

van der Smagt-Duijnstee, M. E., Hamers, J. P. H., Abu-Saad, H. H. and Zuidhof, A. (2001) Relatives of hospitalized stroke patients: Their needs for information, counselling and accessibility. *Journal of Advanced Nursing, 33,* 307–315.

Van der Werf, Y. D., Scheltens, P., Lindeboom, J., Witter, M. P., Uylings, H. B. and Jolles, J. (2003) Deficits of memory, executive functioning and attention following infarction in the thalamus: A study of 22 cases with localised lesions. *Neuropsychologia, 41,* 1330–1344.

Van der Werf, Y. D., Weerts, J. G. E., Jolles, J., Witter, M. P., Lindeboom, J. and Scheltens, P. H. (1999) Neuropsychological correlates of a right unilateral lacunar thalamic infarction. *Journal of Neurology, Neurosurgery and Psychiatry, 66,* 36–42.

Van der Wurff, F. B., Stek, M. L., Hoogendijk, W. L. and Beekman, A. T. (2003) Electroconvulsive therapy for the depressed elderly. *Cochrane Database Systematic Reviews* (2), CD003593.

Van Dulmen, S., Sluijs, E., Van Dijk, L., De Ridder, D., Heerdink, R. and Bensing, J. (2007) Patient adherence to medical treatment: a review of reviews. *Health Services Research, 7,* 55.

Van Dulmen, S., Sluijs, E., Van Dijk, L., De Ridder, D., Heerdink, R. and Bensing J and the International Expert Forum on Patient Adherence. (2008) Furthering patient adherence: A position paper of the international expert forum on patient adherence based on an internet forum discussion. *BMC Health Services Research 8*, 47.

van Herk, R., van Dijk, M., Baar, F. P. M., Tibboel, D. and de Wit, R. (2007) Observation scales for pain assessment in older adults with cognitive impairments or communication difficulties. *Nursing Research, 56*, 34–43.

van Heugten, C., Rasquin, S., Winkens, I., Beusmans, G. and Verhey, F. (2007) Checklist for cognitive and emotional consequences following stroke (CLCE-24): Development, usability and quality of the self-report version. *Clinical Neurology and Neurosurgery, 109*, 257–262.

van Heugten, C., Visser-Meily, A., Post, M. and Lindeman, E. (2006) Care for carers of stroke patients: Evidence-based clinical practice guidelines. *Journal of Rehabilitation Medicine, 38*, 153–158.

van Heugten, C. M., Dekker, J., Deelman, B. G., Stehmann-Saris, F. C. and Kinebanian, A. (1999) A diagnostic test for apraxia in stroke patients: Internal consistency and diagnostic value. *Clinical Neuropsychologist, 13*, 182–192.

van Zomeren, E. and Spikman, J. (2003) Assessment of attention. In P. W. Halligan, U. Kischka and J. C. Marshall (eds), *Handbook of Clinical Neuropsychology*. Oxford: Oxford University Press.

Vandrevala, T., Hampson, S. E., Daly, T., Arber, S. and Thomas, H. (2006) Dilemmas in decision-making about resuscitation: A focus group study of older people. *Social Science & Medicine, 62*, 1579–1593.

Vataja, R., Pohjasvaara, T., Mantyla, R., Ylikoski, R., Leppavuori, A., Leskela, M., *et al.* (2003) MRI correlates of executive dysfunction in patients with ischaemic stroke. *European Journal of Neurology, 10*, 625–631.

Vellas, B. J., Wayne, S. J., Romero, L. J., Baumgartner, R. N. and Garry, P. J. (1997) Fear of falling and restriction of mobility in elderly fallers. *Age and ageing, 26*, 189–193.

Vellinga, A., Smit, J. H., van Leeuwen, E., van Tilburg, W. and Jonker, C. (2004) Competence to consent to treatment of geriatric patients: Judgements of physicians, family members and the vignette method. *International Journal of Geriatric Psychiatry, 19*, 645–654.

Verdelho, A., Henon, H., Lebert, F., Pasquier, F. and Leys, D. (2004) Depressive symptoms after stroke and relationship with dementia: A three-year follow-up study. *Neurology, 62*, 905–911.

Vestling, M., Ramel, E. and Iwarsson, S. (2005) Quality of life after stroke: Well-being, life satisfaction, and subjective aspects of work. *Scandinavian Journal of Occupational Therapy, 12*, 89–95.

Vestling, M., Tufvesson, B. and Iwarsson, S. (2003) Indicators for return to work after stroke and the importance of work for subjective well-being and life satisfaction. *Journal of Rehabilitation Medicine, 35*, 127–131.

Vickery, C., Evans, C., Sepehri, A., Jabeen, L. and Gayden, M. (2009) Self-esteem stability and depressive symptoms in acute stroke rehabilitation: Methodological and conceptual expansion. *Rehabilitation Psychology, 54*, 332–342.

Vickery, C., Sepehri, A., Evans, C. and Lee, J. (2008) The association of level and stability of self-esteem and depressive symptoms in the acute inpatient stroke rehabilitation setting. *Rehabilitation Psychology, 53*, 171–179.

Vickery, C. D. (2006) Assessment and correlates of self-esteem following stroke using a pictorial measure. *Clinical Rehabilitation, 20*, 1075–1084.

Vig, E. K., Starks, H., Taylor, J. S., Hopley, E. K. and Fryer-Edwards, K. (2007) Surviving surrogate decision-making: What helps and hampers the experience of making medical decisions for others. *Journal of General Internal Medicine, 22,* 1274–1279.

Visser-Keizer, A. C., Meyboom-De Jong, B., Deelman, B. G., Berg, I. J. and Gerritsen, M. J. J. (2002) Subjective changes in emotion, cognition and behaviour after stroke: Factors affecting the perception of patients and partners. *Journal of Clinical and Experimental Neuropsychology, 24,* 1032–1045.

Visser-Meily, A. and Meijer, A. M. (2006) Stroke, consequences for the family and recommendations for rehabilitation. In D. M. Devore (ed), *Parent–Child Relations: New Research* (pp. 157–174) New York: Nova Science.

Visser-Meily, A., Post, M., Meijer, A. M., Maas, C., Ketelaar, M. and Lindeman, E. (2005a) Children's adjustment to a parent's stroke: Determinants of health status and psychological problems, and the role of support from the rehabilitation team. *Journal of Rehabilitation Medicine, 37,* 236–241.

Visser-Meily, A., Post, M., Meijer, A. M., van de Port, I., Maas, C. and Lindeman, E. (2005b) When a parent has a stroke: Clinical course and prediction of mood, behavior problems, and health status of their young children. *Stroke, 36,* 2436–2440.

Visser-Meily, A., Post, M., van de Port, I., Maas, C., Forstberg-Warleby, G. and Lindeman, E. (2009) Psychosocial functioning of spouses of patients with stroke from initial inpatient rehabilitation to 3 years poststroke course and relations with coping strategies. *Stroke, 40,* 1399–1404.

Visser-Meily, A., van Heugten, C., Post, M., Schepers, V. and Lindeman, E. (2005) Intervention studies for caregivers of stroke survivors: A critical review. *Patient Education and Counseling, 56,* 257–267.

Vohora, R. and Ogi, L. (2008) Addressing the emotional needs of stroke survivors. *Nursing Times, 104,* 32–36.

Vollmann, J., Kühl, K. P., Tilmann, A., Hartung, H. D. and Helmchen, H. (2004) Einwilligungsfähigkeit und neuropsychologische Einschränkungen bei dementen Patienten. *Nervenarzt, 75,* 29–35.

von Cramon, D. Y. and Cramon, G. M. (1992) Reflections on the treatment of brain-injured patients suffering from problem-solving disorders. *Neuropsychological Rehabilitation, 2,* 207–229.

von Cramon, D. Y., Matthes-von Cramon, G. and Mai, N. (1991) Problem solving deficits in brain-injured patients: A therapeutic approach. *Neuropsychological Rehabilitation, 1,* 45–64.

Wachters-Kaufmann, C. S. M. (2000) Personal accounts of stroke experiences. *Patient Education and Counseling, 41,* 295–303.

Waddell, G. and Burton, A. K. (2006) *Is Work Good for Health and Well Being?* London: HMSO.

Wade, D. T. (1999a) Goal planning in stroke rehabilitation: Evidence. *Topics in Stroke Rehabilitation, 6,* 37–42.

Wade, D. T. (1999b) Goal planning in stroke rehabilitation: Why? *Topics in Stroke Rehabilitation, 6,* 1–7.

Wade, D. T. (2009) Goal setting in rehabilitation: An overview of what, why and how. *Clinical Rehabilitation, 23,* 291–295.

Wade, D. T., Leghsmith, J. and Hewer, R. L. (1986) Effects of living with and looking after survivors of a stroke. *British Medical Journal, 293* (6544), 418–420.

Wade, D. T. and Troy, J. C. (2001) Mobile phones as a new memory aids: A preliminary investigation using case studies. *Brain Injury*, 15, 305–320.

Wagenaar, R. C., Van Wieringen, P. C. W., Netelenbos, J. B., Meijer, O. G. and Kuik, D. J. (1992) The transfer of scanning training effects in visual inattention after stroke: Five single-case studies. *Disability and Rehabilitation*, 14, 51–60.

Wahl, H. W., Martin, P., Minnemann, E., Martin, S. and Oster, P. (2001) Predictors of well-being and autonomy before and after geriatric rehabilitation. *Journal of Health Psychology*, 6, 339–354.

Walker, C. M., Sunderland, A., Sharma, J. and Walker, M. F. (2004a) The impact of cognitive impairments on upper body dressing difficulties after stroke: A video analysis of patterns of recovery. *Journal of Neurology, Neurosurgery and Psychiatry*, 75, 43–48.

Walker, M. F., Gladman, J. R. F., Lincoln, N. B., Siemonsma, P. and Whitely, T. (1999) Occupational therapy for stroke patients not admitted to hospital: A randomised controlled trial. *Lancet*, 354, 278–280.

Walker, M. F., Leonardi-Bee, J., Bath, P., Langhorne, P., Dewey, M., Corr, S., *et al.* (2004) Individual patient data meta-analysis of randomized controlled trials of community occupational therapy for stroke patients. *Stroke*, 35, 2226–2232.

Walker, M. F. and Lincoln, N. B. (1991) Factors influencing dressing performance after stroke. *Journal of Neurology, Neurosurgery & Psychiatry*, 54, 699–701.

Walker, M. F., Sunderland, A., Fletcher-Smith, J., Drummond, A., Logan, P., Edmans, J., *et al.* (In Press) Dressing Rehabilitation Stroke Study: A pilot randomised controlled trial (The DRESS study). Clinical Rehabilitation.

Walker, R., Findlay, J. M., Young, A. W. and Welch, J. (1991) Disentangling neglect and hemianopia. *Neuropsychologia*, 29, 1019–1027.

Wallston, B. and Wallston, K. (1978) Locus of control and health: A review of the literature. *Health Education Monographs*, 6, 107–117.

Walshe, M., Peach, R. K. and Miller, N. (2009) Dysarthria Impact Profile: Development of a scale to measure psychosocial effects. *International Journal of Language & Communication Disorders*, 44, 693–715.

Wambaugh, J. L., Duffy, J. R., McNeil, M. R., Robin, D. A. and Rogers, M. A. (2006) Treatment guidelines for acquired apraxia of speech: A synthesis and evaluation of the evidence. *Journal of Medical Speech-Language Pathology*, 14, 15–33.

Wambaugh, J. L., Kalinyak-Fliszar, M. M., West, J. E. and Doyle, P. J. (1998) Effects of treatment for sound errors in apraxia of speech and aphasia. *Journal of Speech Language and Hearing Research*, 41, 725–743.

Wang, X., Qin, X., Demirtas, H., Li, J., Mao, G., Huo, Y., *et al.* (2007) Efficacy of folic acid supplementation in stroke prevention: A meta-analysis. *Lancet*, 369, 1876–1882.

Wannamethee, S. G., Shaper, A. G., Whincup, P. H. and Walker, M. (1995) Smoking cessation and the risk of stroke in middle-aged men. *Journal of the American Medical Association*, 274, 155–160.

Warden, V., Hurley, A. C. and Volicer, L. (2003) Development and psychometric evaluation of the Pain Assessment in Advanced Dementia (PAINAD) scale. *Journal of the American Medical Directors Association*, 4, 9–15.

Wardlaw, J. M., del Zoppo, G. J., Yamaguchi, T. and Berge, E. (2003) Thrombolysis for acute ischaemic stroke. *Cochrane Database of Systematic Reviews* (3), CD000213.

Warrington, E. K. (1997) The graded naming test: A restandardisation. *Neuropsychological Rehabilitation*, 7, 143–146.

Warrington, E. K. and James, M. (1988) Visual apperceptive agnosia – a clinic-anatomical study of 3 cases. *Cortex, 24,* 13–32.

Warrington, E. K. and James, M. (1991) *The Visual Object and Space Perception Battery.* Bury St Edmunds, UK: Thames Valley Test Company.

Watanabe, Y. (2005) Fear of falling among stroke survivors after discharge from inpatient rehabilitation. *International Journal of Rehabilitation Research, 28,* 149–152.

Watkins, C., Daniels, L., Jack, C., Dickinson, H. and van den Broek, M. (2001a) Accuracy of a single question in screening for depression in a cohort of patients after stroke: A comparative study. *British Medical Journal, 323,* 1159.

Watkins, C., Leathley, M., Daniels, L., Dickinson, H., Lightbody, C. E., van den Broek, M., *et al.* (2001b) The signs of depression scale in stroke: How useful are nurses' observations? *Clinical Rehabilitation, 15,* 456.

Watkins, C. L., Auton, M. F., Deans, C. F., Dickinson, H. A., Jack, C. I. A., Lightbody, C. E., *et al.* (2007a) Motivational interviewing early after acute stroke: A randomized, controlled trial. *Stroke, 38,* 1004–1009.

Watkins, C. L., Lightbody, C. E., Sutton, C. J., Holcroft, L., Dickinson, H. A., van den Broek, M. D., *et al.* (2007b) Evaluation of a single-item screening tool for depression after stroke: A cohort study. *Clinical Rehabilitation, 21,* 846–852.

Watzlawick, P. and Coyne, J. C. (1980) Depression following stroke: Brief, problem-focused family treatment. *Family Process, 19,* 13–18.

Weathers, F.W., Litz, B.T., Herman, D.S., Huska, J.A. & Keane, T.M. (1993) The PTSD checklist: Reliability, validity, and diagnostic utility. Paper presented at the annual meeting of the International Society for Traumatic Stress Studies, San Antonio, TX.

Webster, J. S., McFarland, P. T., Rapport, L. J., Morrill, B., Roades, L. A. and Abadee, P. S. (2001) Computer-assissted training for improving wheelchair mobility in unilateral neglect patients. *Archives of Physical Medicine and Rehabilitation, 82,* 769–775.

Wechsler, D. (1997a) *Wechsler Memory Scale,* 3rd ed. San Antonio, TX: Psychological Corporation.

Wechsler, D. (1997b) *Wechsler Adult Intelligence Scale 3rd Edition Manual.* San Antonio, TX: Psychological Corporation.

Wechsler, D. (1999) *Wechsler Abbreviated Scale of Intelligence (WASI).* San Antonio, TX: Psychological Corporation.

Wechsler, D. (2001) *Wechsler Test of Adult Reading (WTAR).* San Antonio, TX: Psychological Corporation.

Wechsler, D. (2008) *Wechsler Adult Intelligence Scale,* 4th ed. San Antonio, TX: Pearson Assessment.

Wechsler, D. (2009) *Wechsler Memory Scale UK (WMS-IVUK),* 4th ed. London: Pearson Education.

Weinberg, J., Diller, L., Gordon, W. A., Gerstman, L. J., Lieberman, A., Lakin, P., *et al.* (1979) Training sensory awareness and spatial-organisation in people with right brain-damage. *Archives of Physical Medicine and Rehabilitation, 60,* 491–496.

Weinberg, J., Diller, L., Gordon, W. A., Gertman, L., Liebermann, A., Lakin, P., *et al.* (1977) Visual scanning training effect on reading related tasks in acquired right brain damage. *Archives of Physical Medicine and Rehabilitation, 58,* 479–486.

Weisman, C. and Nathanson, C. (1985) Professional satisfaction and client outcomes: A comparative organizational analysis. *Medical Care, 23,* 1179.

Wellwood, I., Dennis, M. and Warlow, C. (1995) Patients' and carers' satisfaction with acute stroke management. *Age and Ageing, 24,* 519–524.

Welsh Assembly Government. (2007) *Improving Stroke Services: A Programme of Work.* WHC (2007) 08. Cardiff: Welsh Assembly Government.

Wendel-Vos, G., Schuit, A., Feskens, E., Boshuizen, H., Verschuren, W., Saris, W., *et al.* (2004) Physical activity and stroke: A meta-analysis of observational data. *International Journal of Epidemiology, 33,* 787–798.

Wenke, R. J., Theodores, D. and Cornwell, P. (2008) The short- and long-term effectiveness of the LSVT for dysarthria following TBI and stroke. *Brain Injury, 22,* 339–352.

Wertz, R. T., LaPointe, L. L. and Rosenbek, J. C. (1984) *Apraxia of Speech in Adults: The Disorder and Its Management.* New York: Grune and Stratton.

Wertz, R. T., Weiss, D. G., Aten, J. L., Brookshire, R. H., Garcia-Bunel, L., Holland, A. L., *et al.* (1986) Comparison of clinic, home, and deferred language treatment for aphasia: A Veterans Administration Cooperative Study. *Archives of Neurology, 43,* 653–658.

West, C., Bowen, A., Hesketh, A. and Vail, A. (2008) Interventions for motor apraxia following stroke. *Cochrane Database of Systematic Reviews* (1), CD004132.

West, C., Hesketh, A., Vail, A. and Bowen, A. (2005) Interventions for apraxia of speech following stroke. *Cochrane Database of Systematic Reviews* (4), CD004298.

Westover, A. N., McBride, S., Robert, W. and Haley, R. W. (2007) Stroke in young adults who abuse amphetamines or cocaine: A population-based study of hospitalized patients. *Archives of General Psychiatry, 64,* 495–502.

Wetherell, J. L., Hopko, D. R., Diefenbach, G. J., Averill, P. M., Beck, J. G., Craske, M. G., *et al.* (2005) Cognitive-behavioral therapy for late-life generalized anxiety disorder: Who gets better? *Behavior Therapy, 36,* 147–156.

White, C. A. (2001) *Cognitive Behaviour Therapy for Chronic Medical Problems: A Guide to Assessment and Treatment in Practice.* Chicester: John Wiley.

White, C. L., Lauzon, S., Yaffe, M. J. and Wood-Dauphinee, S. (2004) Toward a model of quality of life for family caregivers of stroke survivors. *Quality of Life Research, 13,* 625–638.

White, C. S., Mason, A. C., Feehan, M. and Templeton, P. A. (1995) Informed consent for percutaneous lung-biopsy – comparison of 2 consent protocols based on patient recall after the procedure. *American Journal of Roentgenology, 165,* 1139–1142.

White-Bateman, S. R., Schumacher, H. C., Sacco, R. L. and Appelbaum, P. S. (2007) Consent for intravenous thrombolysis in acute stroke: Review and future directions. *Archives of Neurology, 64,* 785–792.

Whiting, S., Lincoln, N., Cockburn, J. and Bhavnani, G. (1984) *Rivermead Perceptual Assessment Battery.* Windsor, UK: NFER-Nelson.

Whurr, R. (1972) *Aphasia Screening Test.* London: Cole and Whurr.

Widar, M., Ahlstrom, G. and Ek, A. C. (2004) Health-related quality of life in persons with long-term pain after a stroke. *Journal of Clinical Nursing, 13,* 497–505.

Widar, M., Samuelsson, L., Karlsson-Tivenius, S. and Ahlstrom, G. (2002) Long-term pain conditions after a stroke. *Journal of Rehabilitation Medicine, 34,* 165–170.

Wilde, M. C. (2006) The validity of the repeatable battery of neuropsychological status in acute stroke. *Clinical Neuropsychologist, 20,* 702–715.

Wilkinson, P. R., Wolfe, C. D. A., Warburton, F. G., Rudd, A. G., Howard, R. S., RossRussell, R. W., *et al.* (1997) A long-term follow-up of stroke patients. *Stroke, 28,* 507–512.

Willey, J. Z., Moon, Y. P., Paik, M. C., Boden-Albala, B., Sacco, R. L. and Elkind, M. S. V. (2009) Physical activity and risk of ischemic stroke in the Northern Manhattan Study. *Neurology, 73,* 1774–1779.

Williams, B. (1994) Patient satisfaction – a valid concept. *Social Science & Medicine*, *38*, 509–516.

Williams, G. R., Jiang, J. G., Matchar, D. B. and Samsa, G. P. (1999) Incidence and occurrence of total (first-ever and recurrent) stroke. *Stroke*, *30*, 2523–2528.

Williams, L. S., Brizendine, E. J., Plue, L., Bakas, T., Tu, W. Z., Hendrie, H., *et al.* (2005) Performance of the PHQ-9 as a screening tool for depression after stroke. *Stroke*, *36*, 635–638.

Williams, L. S., Weinberger, M., Harris, L. E., Clark, D. O. and Biller, J. (1999) Development of a stroke-specific quality of life scale. *Stroke*, *30* (7), 1362–1369.

Williams, P. (2009) Reduction in incident stroke risk with vigorous physical activity: Evidence from 7.7-year follow-up of the National Runners' Health Study. *Stroke*, *40*, 1921–1923.

Williams, R., Davis, M. and Millsap, R. (2002) Development of the cognitive processing of trauma scale. *Clinical Psychology & Psychotherapy*, *9*, 349–360.

Williams, W. H. and Evans, J. J. (2003) Brain injury and emotion: An overview to a special edition on biopsychosocial approaches in neurorehabilitation. *Neuropsychological Rehabilitation*, *13*, 1–12.

Willis, S. L. (1996) Everyday cognitive competence in elderly persons: Conceptual issues and empirical findings. *Gerontologist*, *36*, 595–601.

Willoughby, D., Sanders, L. and Privette, A. (2001) The impact of a stroke screening program. *Public Health Nursing*, *18*, 418–423.

Wills, T. A. and Shinar, O. (2000) Measuring perceived and received social support. In L. G. U. S. Cohen & B. H. Gottlieb (eds), *Social Support Measurement and Intervention: A Guide for Health and Social Scientists* (pp. 86–135) New York: Oxford University Press.

Wilson, B. A. (1999) *Case Studies in Neuropsychological Rehabilitation*. New York: Oxford University Press.

Wilson, B. A. (2002) Towards a comprehensive model of neuropsychological rehabilitation. *Neuropsychological Rehabilitation*, *12*, 97–110.

Wilson, B. A. (2008) Neuropsychological rehabilitation. *Annual Review of Clinical Psychology*, *4*, 141–162.

Wilson, B. A., Alderman, N., Burgess, P., Emslie, H. and Evans, J. (1996) *Behavioural Assessment of the Dysexecutive Syndrome*. Bury St Edmunds: Thames Valley Test Company.

Wilson, B. A., Clare, L., Baddeley, A. D., Watson, P. and Tate, R. (1998) *Rivermead Behavioural Memory Test–Extended Version (RBMT-E)*. Bury St Edmunds: Thames Valley Test Company.

Wilson, B. A., Cockburn, J. M. and Baddeley, A. D. (2003) *The Rivermead Behavioural Memory Test–II*. Bury St Edmunds: Thames Valley Test Company.

Wilson, B. A., Cockburn, J. M. and Halligan, P. W. (1987) *Behavioural Inattention Test*. Bury St Edmunds: Thames Valley Test Company.

Wilson, B. A., Emslie, H. and Evans, J. (2001) Reducing everyday memory and planinng problems by means of a paging system: A randomised control crossover study. *Journal of Neurology, Neurosurgery and Psychiatry*, *70*, 477–482.

Wilson, B. A., Gracey, F., Evans, J. J. and Bateman, A. (eds) (2009) *Neuropsychological Rehabilitation: Theory, Models, Therapy and Outcome*. Cambridge: Cambridge University Press.

Wilson, P., Bozeman, S., Burton, T., Hoaglin, D., Ben-Joseph, R. and Pashos, C. (2008) Prediction of first events of coronary heart disease and stroke with consideration of adiposity. *Circulation*, *118* (2), 124.

Wing, J. K., Cooper, J. E. and Sartorious, N. (1974) *The Measurement and Classification of Psychiatric Symptoms.* Cambridge: Cambridge University Press.

Winkens, I., Van Heugten, C. M., Fasotti, L., Duits, A. A. and Wade, D. T. (2006) Manifestations of mental slowness in the daily life of patients with stroke: a qualitative study. *Clinical Rehabilitation, 20,* 827–834.

Winkler, R., James, R., Fatovich, B. and Underwood, P. (1982) *Migraine and Tension Headaches: A Multi-Modal Approach to the Prevention and Control of Headache Pain.* Perth: University of Western Australia.

Winward, C., Sackley, C., Metha, Z. and Rothwell, P. M. (2009) A population-based study of the prevalence of fatigue after transient ischemic attack and minor stroke. *Stroke, 40,* 757–761.

Wolf, P. A., D'Agostino, R. B., Kannel, W. B., Bonita, R. and Belanger, A. J. (1988) Cigarette smoking as a risk factor for stroke: The Framingham Study. *Journal of the American Medical Association, 259,* 1025–1029.

Wolfe, C., Rudd, A., McKevitt, C., Heuschmann, P. and Kalra, L. (2008) *Top Ten Priorities for Stroke Services Research: A Summary of an Analysis of Research for the National Stroke Strategy.* London: University of London.

Wolfe, P. L. and Scott, R. (2009) Effort indicators within the California Verbal Learning Test-II (CVLT-II). *The Clinical Neuropsychologist, 24,* 153–168.

Wolfenden, B. and Grace, M. (2009) Returning to work after stroke: A review. *International Journal of Rehabilitation Research, 32,* 93–97.

Wong, J. G., Clare, I. C. H., Gunn, M. J. and Holland, A. J. (1999) Capacity to make health care decisions: Its importance in clinical practice. *Psychological Medicine, 29,* 437–446.

Woolf, S. H., Grol, R., Hutchinson, A., Eccles, M. and Grimshaw, J. (1999) Clinical guidelines: Potential benefits, limitations, and harms of clinical guidelines. *British Medical Journal 318,* 527–530.

Woolsey, T. A., Hanaway, J. and Mokhtar, H. G. (2008) *The Brain Atlas,* 3rd ed. Hoboken, NJ: John Wiley & Sons.

World Health Organization. (1980) *The International Classification of Impairments, Disabilities and Handicaps: A Manual of Classification Relating to the Consequence of Disease.* Geneva: WHO.

World Health Organisation. (1992a) *International Classification of Diseases,* 10th ed. Geneva: WHO.

World Health Organisation. (1992b) *Schedules for Clinical Assessment in Neuropsychiatry.* Geneva: World Health Organisation.

World Health Organisation. (2001) *International Classification of Functioning, Disability and Health (ICF).* Geneva: World Health Organisation. http://www.who.int/classification/icf

World Health Organisation (WHO) (2003) *Adherence to Long Term Therapies: Evidence for Action.* Geneva: World Health Organisation.

World Health Organization. (2005) *International Classification of Functioning, Disability and Health.* Geneva, Switzerland: World Health Organization.

World Health Organisation. (2006) *WHO STEPS Stroke Manual: The WHO STEPwise Approach to Stroke Surveillance.* Geneva: World Health Organisation.

Worrall, L. and Yiu, E. (2000) Effectiveness of functional communication therapy by volunteers for people with aphasia following stroke. *Aphasiology, 14* (9), 911–924.

Worthington, A. (2005) Rehabilitation of executive deficits: Effective treatments of related disabilities. In P. W. Halligan and D. Wade (eds), *Effectiveness of Rehabilitation for Cognitive Deficits.* Oxford: Oxford University Press.

Worthington, A. D. (1996) Cueing strategies in neglect dyslexia. *Neuropsychological Rehabilitation*, 6, 1–17.

Wressle, E., Oberg, B. and Henriksson, C. (1999) The rehabilitation process for the geriatric stroke patient – an exploratory study of goal setting and interventions. *Disability and Rehabilitation*, 21, 80–87.

Yamashita, H. (2010) Right- and left-hand performance on the Rey-Osterrieth Complex Figure: A preliminary study in non-clinical sample of right handed people. *Archives of Clinical Neuropsychology*, 25, 314–317.

Yang, Z. H., Zhao, X. Q., Wang, C. X., Chen, H. Y. and Zhang, Y. M. (2008) Neuroanatomic correlation of the post-stroke aphasias studied with imaging. *Neurological Research*, 30, 356–360.

Yardley, L. (2004) Fear of falling: Links between imbalance and anxiety. *Reviews in Clinical Gerontology*, 13, 195–201.

Yardley, L., Beyer, N., Hauer, K., Kempen, G., Piot-Ziegler, C. and Todd, C. (2005) Development and initial validation of the Falls Efficacy Scale-International (FES-I). *Age and Ageing*, 34, 614–619.

Yardley, L. and Smith, H. (2002) A prospective study of the relationship between feared consequences of falling and avoidance of activity in community-living older people. *Gerontologist*, 42, 17–23.

Yeates, G. N., Gracey, F. and McGrath, J. C. (2008) A biopsychosocial deconstruction of 'personality change' following acquired brain injury. *Neuropsychological Rehabilitation*, 18, 566–589.

Yesavage, J. A., Brink, T. L., Rose, T. L., Lum, O., Huang, V., Adey, M., *et al.* (1983) Development and validation of a geriatric depression screening scale: A preliminary report. *Journal of Psychiatric Research*, 17, 37–49.

Young, G. C., Collins, D. and Hren, M. (1983) Effects of pairing scanning training with block design training in the remediation of perpetual problems in left hemiplegics. *Journal of Clinical Neuropsychology*, 5, 201–212.

Zarkowska, E. and Clements, J. (1994) *Severe Problem Behaviour: The STAR Approach*. London: Chapman and Hall.

Zeiss, A. and Lewinsohn, P. M. (1986) Adapting behavioral treatment for depression to meet the needs of the elderly. *The Clinical Psychologist*, 39, 98–100.

Zelinski, E. M., Gilewski, M. J. and Anthony-Bergstone, C. R. (1990) Memory Functioning Questionnaire: Concurrent validity with memory performance and self-reported memory failures. *Psychology and Aging*, 5, 388–399.

Zeloni, G., Farne, A. and Baccini, M. (2002) Viewing less to see better. *Journal of Neurology, Neurosurgery and Psychiatry*, 73, 195–198.

Zhang, S. Q., Liu, M. Y., Wan, B. and Zheng, H. M. (2008) Contralateral body half hypalgesia in a patient with lateral medullary infarction: Atypical Wallenberg syndrome. *European Neurology*, 59, 211–215.

Zigmond, A. S. and Snaith, R. P. (1983) The Hospital Anxiety and Depression Scale. *Acta Psychiatrica Scandinavia*, 67, 361–370.

Zihl, J. (1989) Cerebral disturbances of elementary visual function. In J. W. Brown (ed), *Neuropsychology of Visual Perception*. Hillsdale, NJ: Lawrence Erlbaum Associates.

Zihl, J. (1995) Visual scanning behavior in patients with homonymous hemianopia. *Neuropsychologia*, 33, 287–303.

Zihl, J. (2000) *Rehabilitation of Visual Disorders after Brain Injury*. Hove: Psychology Press.

Zijlstra, G. A. R., van Haastregt, J. C. M., van Rossum, E., van Eijk, J. T. M., Yardley, L. and Kempen, G. (2007) Interventions to reduce fear of falling in community-living older people: A systematic review. *Journal of the American Geriatrics Society, 55,* 603–615.

Zinn, S., Bosworth, H. B., Hoenig, H. M. and Swartzwelder, H. S. (2007) Executive function deficits in acute stroke. *Archives of Physical Medicine and Rehabilitation, 88,* 173–180.

Zoccolotti, P., Antonucci, G. and Judica, A. (1992) Psychometric characterisitcs of two semi-structured scales for the functional evaluation of hemi-inattention in extra-personal and personal space. *Neuropsychological Rehabilitation, 2,* 179–191.

Zoccolotti, P. and Judica, A. (1991) Functional evaluation of hemineglect by means of a semistructured scale: Personal extrapersonal differentiation. *Neuropsychological Rehabilitation, 1,* 33–44.

Zwakhalen, S. M. G., Hamers, J. P. H., Abu-Saad, H. H. and Berger, M. P. F. (2006a) Pain in elderly people with severe dementia: A systematic review of behavioural pain assessment tools. *Geriatrics, 6,* 3.

Zwakhalen, S. M. G., Hamers, J. P. H. and Berger, M. R. F. (2006b) The psychometric quality and clinical usefulness of three pain assessment tools for elderly people with dementia. *Pain, 126,* 210–220.

Zwinkels, A., Geusgens, C., van de Sande, P. and van Heugten, C. (2004) Assessment of apraxia: Inter-rater reliability of a new apraxia test, association between apraxia and other cognitive deficits and prevalence of apraxia in a rehabilitation setting. *Clinical Rehabilitation, 18,* 819–827.

Index

Printed and bound by CPI Group (UK) Ltd, Croydon, CR0 4YY
13/01/2022

03103716-0006